T0198287

THE NETTER COLLECTION OF MEDICAL ILLUSTRATIONS

3rd Edition

Integumentary System

A compilation of paintings prepared by **FRANK H. NETTER, MD**

VOLUME 4

Authored by

Bryan E. Anderson, MD
Professor of Dermatology
Pennsylvania State University
College of Medicine
Hershey, Pennsylvania

Additional illustrations by
Carlos A.G. Machado, MD

CONTRIBUTING ILLUSTRATORS
Tiffany S. DaVanzo, MA, CMI
Anita Impagliazzo, MA, CMI
Paul Kim, MS
James A. Perkins, MS, MFA
Kristen Wienandt Marzejon, MS, MFA

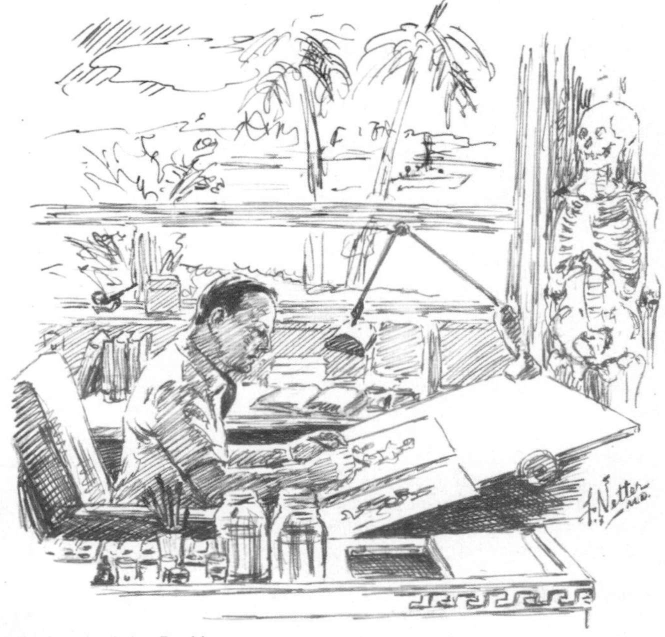

Self portrait by Dr. Netter

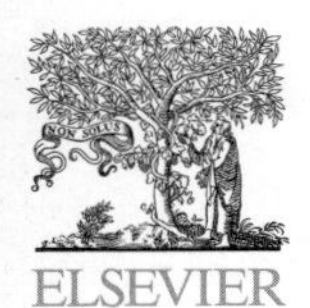

Elsevier
1600 John F. Kennedy Blvd.
Suite 1600
Philadelphia, Pennsylvania

THE NETTER COLLECTION OF MEDICAL ILLUSTRATIONS:
INTEGUMENTARY SYSTEM, VOLUME 4, THIRD EDITION ISBN: 978-0-323-88089-3

Publisher: Elyse O'Grady
Senior Content Strategist: Marybeth Thiel
Publishing Services Manager: Catherine Jackson
Senior Project Manager/Specialist: Carrie Stetz
Book Design: Patrick Ferguson

Printed in India

Last digit is the print number: 9 8 7 6 5 4 3 2 1

"Clarification is the goal. No matter how beautifully it is painted, a medical illustration has little value if it does not make clear a medical point."

-Frank H. Netter, MD

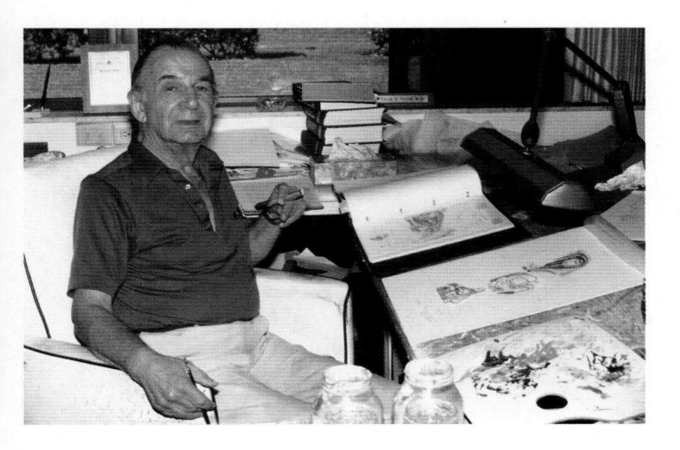

Dr. Frank Netter at work.

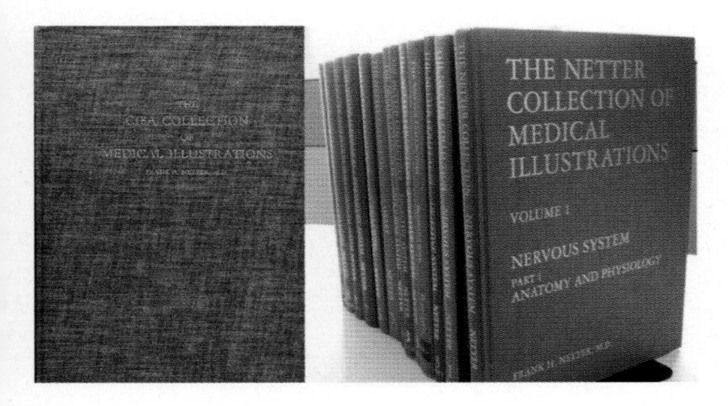

The single-volume "Blue Book" that preceded the multivolume *Netter Collection of Medical Illustrations* series, affectionately known as the "Green Books."

Dr. Frank Netter created an illustrated legacy unifying his perspectives as physician, artist, and teacher. Both his greatest challenge and greatest success was charting a middle course between artistic clarity and instructional complexity. That success is captured in *The Netter Collection,* beginning in 1948 when the first comprehensive book of Netter's work was published by CIBA Pharmaceuticals. It met with such success that over the following 40 years the collection was expanded into an 8-volume series—with each title devoted to a single body system. Between 2011 and 2016, these books were updated and rereleased. Now, after another decade of innovation in medical imaging, renewed focus on patient-centered care, conscious efforts to improve inequities in healthcare and medical education, and a growing understanding of many clinical conditions, including multisystem effects of COVID-19, we are happy to make available a third edition of Netter's timeless work enhanced and informed by modern medical knowledge and context.

Inside the classic green covers, students and practitioners will find hundreds of original works of art. This is a collection of the human body in pictures—Dr. Netter called them *pictures,* never paintings. The latest expert medical knowledge is anchored by the sublime style of Frank Netter that has guided physicians' hands and nurtured their imaginations for more than half a century.

Noted artist-physician Carlos Machado, MD, the primary successor responsible for continuing the Netter tradition, has particular appreciation for the Green Book series. "*The Reproductive System* is of special significance for those who, like me, deeply admire Dr. Netter's work. In this volume, he masters the representation of textures of different surfaces, which I like to call 'the rhythm of the brush,' since it is the dimension, the direction of the strokes, and the interval separating them that create the illusion of given textures: organs have their external surfaces, the surfaces of their cavities, and texture of their parenchymas realistically represented. It set the style for the subsequent volumes of *The Netter Collection*—each an amazing combination of painting masterpieces and precise scientific information."

This third edition could not exist without the dedication of all those who edited, authored, or in other ways contributed to the second edition or the original books, nor, of course, without the excellence of Dr. Netter. For this third edition, we also owe our gratitude to the authors, editors, and artists whose relentless efforts were instrumental in adapting these classic works into reliable references for today's clinicians in training and in practice. From all of us with the Netter Publishing Team at Elsevier, thank you.

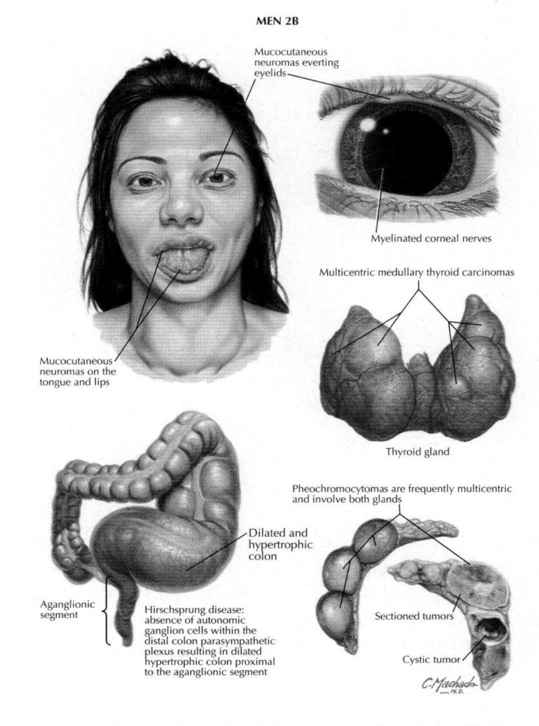

An illustrated plate painted by Carlos Machado, MD.

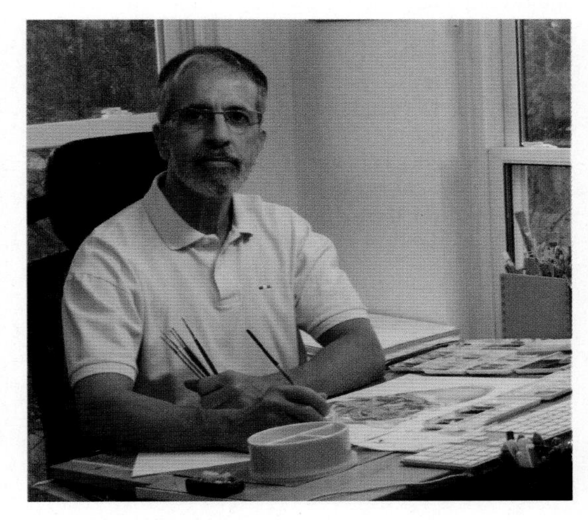

Dr. Carlos Machado at work.

The Netter Collection OF MEDICAL ILLUSTRATIONS

3rd Edition

- Volume 1: **Reproductive System**
- Volume 2: **Endocrine System**
- Volume 3: **Respiratory System**
- Volume 4: **Integumentary System**
- Volume 5: **Urinary System**
- Volume 6: **Musculoskeletal System**
- Volume 7: **Nervous System**
- Volume 8: **Cardiovascular System**
- Volume 9: **Digestive System**

ABOUT THE AUTHOR

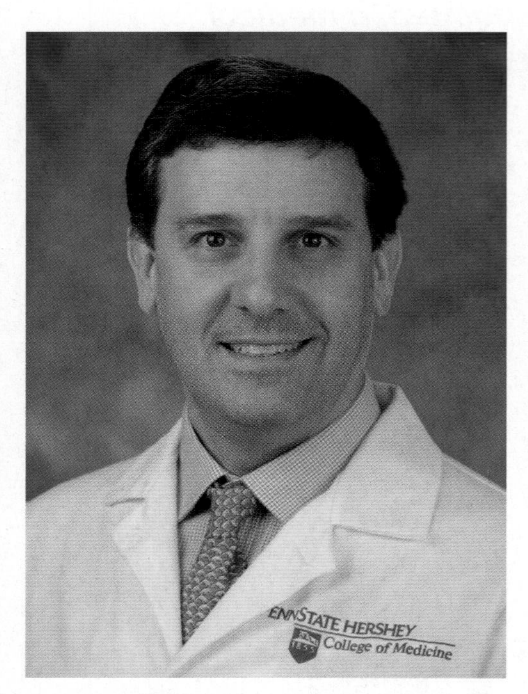

Bryan E. Anderson, MD, is Professor of Dermatology at the Pennsylvania State University College of Medicine. He is proud to have received both his undergraduate and medical degrees from The Ohio State University. He completed his internship and dermatology residency at the Pennsylvania State University College of Medicine in Hershey, Pennsylvania, where, upon completion thereof, he joined the faculty in the Department of Dermatology in 2002. There he works as a clinician, educator, and researcher. Dr. Anderson is currently the Vice Chair of Clinical Operations in the Department of Dermatology. He is also a part of the Milton S. Hershey Medical Center and Penn State Cancer Institute's Multidisciplinary Skin Oncology Clinic. His areas of interest and research include resident education and cutaneous malignancies, with an emphasis on melanoma. He is an active member of the American Academy of Dermatology and the American Contact Dermatitis Society. He has written numerous journal articles and book chapters. He currently lives in Hershey with his wife, Susan, and two daughters, Rachel and Sarah. In his leisure time he enjoys woodworking, cheering on his alma mater, and spending time with his family.

PREFACE

It has been an honor to continue my involvement with this newly updated edition of *The Netter Collection of Medical Illustrations: Integumentary System*. I am grateful for the opportunity to contribute to the legacy that *The Netter Collection* deserves with its timeless quality and continued contribution to medical education. My hope is that this volume is appreciated by those with vast experience as well as individuals just beginning their journey of lifelong learning, which I feel so accurately describes the medical world.

My sincerest gratitude is extended to the people behind the scenes at Elsevier, as well as the artists who were able to bring the slightest nuance to life for the benefit of clinicians and patients alike.

I would like to thank all those who have positively influenced, taught, and mentored me, whose impact on my career has been immeasurable. I have had the pleasure of crossing paths with so many fine people—too many to list. Additionally, I would like to thank my colleagues at the Milton S. Hershey Medical Center, whose encouragement and support have always been a part of our culture.

Finally, I would like to recognize and express appreciation for my family and friends. Their presence in my life is my greatest joy!

Bryan E. Anderson, MD

ABOUT THE ARTIST

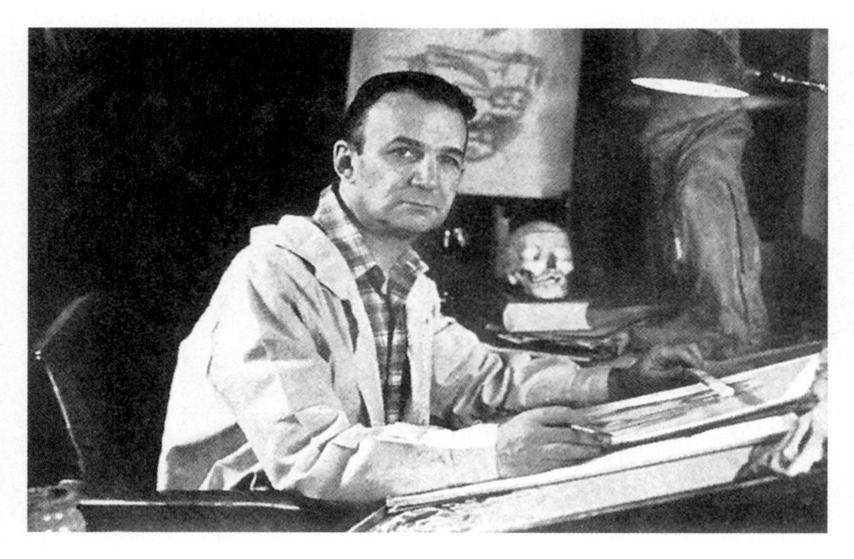

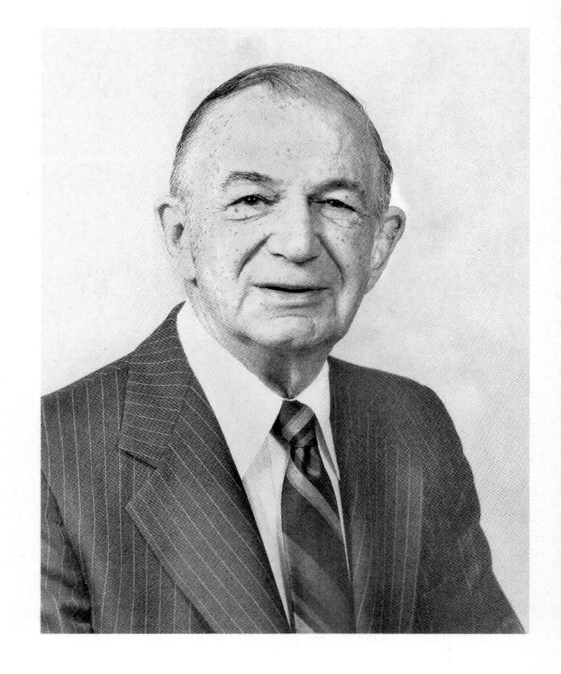

Celebrated as the foremost medical illustrator of the human body and how it works, Dr. Frank H. Netter began his career as a medical illustrator in the 1930s when the CIBA Pharmaceutical Company commissioned him to prepare illustrations of the major organs and their pathology. Dr. Netter's incredibly detailed, lifelike renderings were so well received by the medical community that CIBA published them in a book. This first successful publication in 1948 was followed by the series of volumes that now carry the Netter name, *The Netter Collection of Medical Illustrations*. Even years after his death, Dr. Netter is still acknowledged as the foremost master of medical illustration. His anatomic drawings are the benchmark by which all other medical art is measured and judged. "As far back as I can remember, ever since I was little tot, I studied art," said Dr. Netter during an interview in 1986. At the time he was hailed by *The New York Times* as "The Medical Michelangelo." "All I wanted to do was to make pictures," he reflected. Born in New York in 1906, Dr. Netter had already established himself as a successful commercial artist in the 1920s when, at the advice of his parents, he changed careers. "I gave up art at the urging of my family," he said. "They felt that artists led a very dissolute life, which, of course, was really not true."

To find a more "dependable" career, Dr. Netter entered New York University Medical School. But even as he pursued his training as a surgeon, Dr. Netter found that it was easier for him to take notes in pictures than in words. "Mine was a graphic viewpoint. My notebooks were crammed with illustrations. It was the only way I could remember things." Soon faculty members recognized his artistic talents, and Dr. Netter began to pay for part of his medical education by illustrating lectures and textbooks.

Starting out as a young physician during the Great Depression, Dr. Netter found that there was more interest in his medical artwork than his surgical capabilities. "I thought I could do drawings until I had my practice on its feet," he recalled, "but the demand for my pictures grew much faster than the demand for my surgery. As a result, I gave up my practice entirely."

In 1938, Dr. Netter was hired by the CIBA Pharmaceutical Company to work on a promotional flyer for a heart medication. He designed a folder cut in the shape of and elaborately depicting a heart, which was sent to physicians. Surprisingly, many of the doctors wrote back asking for more heart flyers—without the advertising copy. Dr. Netter went on to design similar product advertisements depicting other organs, and all were extremely well received. After that project was concluded, Dr. Netter was commissioned to prepare small folders of pathology plates that were later collected into the first *CIBA Collection of Medical Illustrations*. Following the success of these endeavors, Dr. Netter was asked to illustrate a series of atlases that became his life's work. They are a group of volumes individually devoted to each organ system and cover human anatomy, embryology, physiology, pathology, and pertinent clinical features of the diseases arising in each system. Dr. Netter has completed volumes on the nervous system, reproductive system, lower and upper digestive tracts, liver, biliary tract and pancreas, endocrine system, kidney, ureters, urinary bladder, respiratory system, and musculoskeletal system.

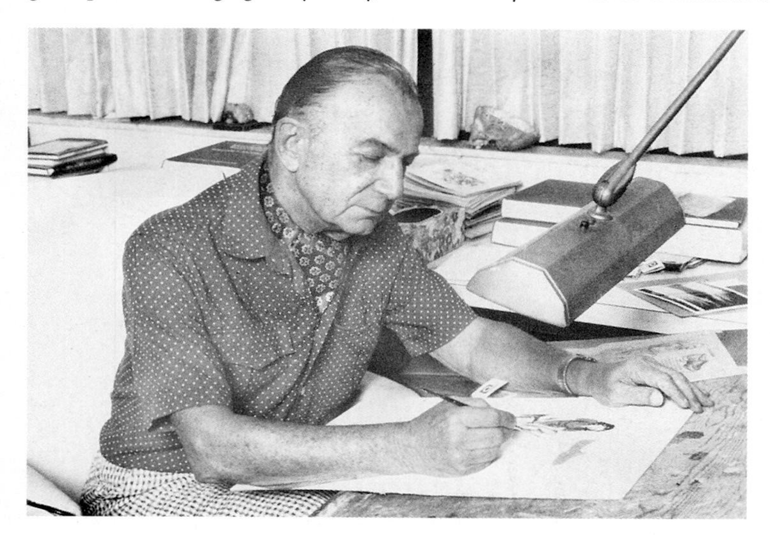

Dr. Netter's beautifully rendered volumes are now found in every medical school library in the country, as well as in many doctors' offices around the world, and his work has helped to educate and enlighten generations of physicians. In 1988 *The New York Times* called Netter "an artist who has probably contributed more to medical education than most of the world's anatomy professors taken together."

Dr. Netter's career has spanned the most revolutionary half-century in medicine's history. He chronicled the emergence of open heart surgery, organ transplants, and joint replacements. To learn firsthand about a variety of diseases and their effects on the body, Dr. Netter traveled widely. In the early 1980s, Dr. William Devries asked Netter to be present at the first artificial heart transplant, a procedure that Netter illustrated in full detail. Dr. Netter also developed a variety of unusual medical art projects, including building the 7-foot "Transparent Woman" for the San Francisco Golden Gate Exposition, which depicted the menstrual process, the development and birth of a baby, and the physical and sexual development of a woman. When asked whether he regretted giving up his surgical practice, Dr. Netter replied that he thought of himself as a clinician with a specialty that encompasses the whole of medicine. "My field covers everything. I must be a specialist in every specialty; I must be able to talk with all physicians on their own terms. I probably do more studying than anyone else in the world," he said.

In his work, Dr. Netter made pencil sketches, which he then copied, transferred, and painted to portray gross anatomy, microscopic anatomy, radiographic images, and drawings of patients. "I try to depict living patients whenever possible," Dr. Netter said. "After all, physicians do see patients, and we must remember we are treating whole human beings." Into his eighth decade, Dr. Netter continued to create his medical illustrations and added to the portfolio of thousands of drawings that encompass his long and illustrious career. Dr. Netter died in 1991, but his work lives on in books and electronic products that continue to educate millions of healthcare professionals worldwide.

CONTENTS

SECTION 1 ANATOMY, EMBRYOLOGY, AND PHYSIOLOGY

SECTION 2 BENIGN GROWTHS

SECTION 3 MALIGNANT GROWTHS

SECTION 4 RASHES

SECTION 5 AUTOIMMUNE BLISTERING DISEASES

SECTION 6 INFECTIOUS DISEASES

SECTION 7 HAIR AND NAIL DISEASES

SECTION 8 NUTRITIONAL AND METABOLIC DISEASES

SECTION 9 GENODERMATOSES AND SYNDROMES

SECTION 1

ANATOMY, EMBRYOLOGY, AND PHYSIOLOGY

EMBRYOLOGY OF THE SKIN

The human skin develops from two special embryonic tissues, the ectoderm and the mesoderm. Epidermal tissue is derived from the embryonic ectoderm. The dermis and subcutaneous tissue are derived from the embryonic mesoderm. The developmental interactions between mesoderm and ectoderm ultimately determine the nature of human skin. Neural tissue and epidermal tissue are both derived from the ectoderm. It is believed that calcium signaling pathways are critical in determining the fate of the ectoderm and its ultimate differentiation into epidermal or neural tissue.

At approximately 4 weeks after conception, a single layer of ectoderm (cuboidal undifferentiated cells) is present surrounding a thicker layer of mesoderm. Two weeks later, this ectodermal layer has separated into two different components: an outer periderm (flattened simple squamous cells) and an inner basal layer, which is connected to the underlying mesoderm and separated by a basement membrane. At 8 weeks after conception, the epidermis has developed into three separate layers: the periderm, an intermediate layer, and the basal cell layer. The dermal subcutaneous tissue is now beginning to develop, and a distinct basement membrane (dermal subcutaneous boundary) can be seen by the end of the eighth week. One function of the periderm is to produce fluid. This fluid, along with desquamated periderm cells, becomes a source of amniotic fluid. There is active fluid and electrolyte transfer between the amniotic fluid and the fetus across the ectodermal layers. This transfer will end when the basement membrane is fully matured at 12 weeks after conception. Once the basement membrane is fully matured, it is called the *basement membrane zone*.

Between weeks 10 and 15 after conception, the beginning of the skin appendages can be seen. The formation of hair follicles is initiated by a complex genetic mechanism that causes the dermis to direct certain basal epidermal cells to congregate and form the rudimentary hair follicle. This process occurs in a highly organized fashion beginning from the scalp and working caudally to the lower extremity. At the same time the hair follicles are forming, the epidermis invaginates into the dermis, forming the beginning of the dermal papillae. The hair follicles continue to differentiate throughout the second trimester, and the hair of the fetus can be seen at approximately 20 weeks after conception. This first hair is known as *lanugo hair* and is almost always shed before delivery.

The fingernails and toenails develop from ectoderm that invaginates into the underlying mesoderm by the fourteenth week after conception. By the fifth month, the fetus has fully developed fingernails and toenails. The fingernails fully develop slightly before the toenails.

Melanocytes are specialized cells derived from neural crest tissue. These cells form along the neural tube. Melanocytes migrate in a specific pattern laterally and then outward along the trunk. Melanocytes can be seen in the epidermis by the middle of the first trimester, but they do not begin to function until the end of the second trimester. The density of melanocytes is highest during the fetal period and decreases thereafter until young adulthood. Melanocytes are beginning to make their first melanosomes and are capable of transferring melanin pigment to adjacent keratinocytes by approximately 5 months after conception. Melanocytes are not fully functional until birth. Langerhans cells are specialized immune surveillance cells that appear within the epidermis at approximately 40 days after conception. In contrast to melanocytes, the density of Langerhans cells increases with time.

By late in the second trimester, the periderm begins to shed. This shedding results in the vernix caseosa, a whitish, cheese-like material that covers the fetus. It is believed to have a protective function. At the beginning of the third trimester, the individual epidermal layers can be seen, including the stratum basale, stratum granulosum, stratum spinosum, and stratum corneum. Keratinization begins to occur during the second trimester, first in the appendageal structures and then in the epidermis. The thickness of the epidermis in a newborn closely approaches that in an adult. The significant difference is that the skin barrier function in a newborn is not as fully developed as in an adult and therefore is more vulnerable to water loss, infection, thermal regulatory dysfunction, and external insults.

Midsagittal section of folding gastrula

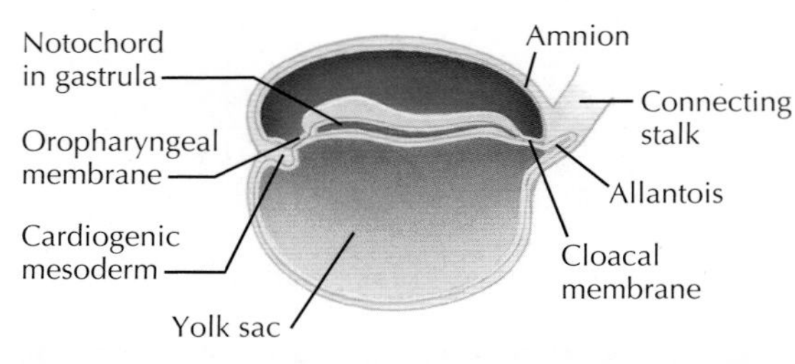

Cross section of folding gastrula

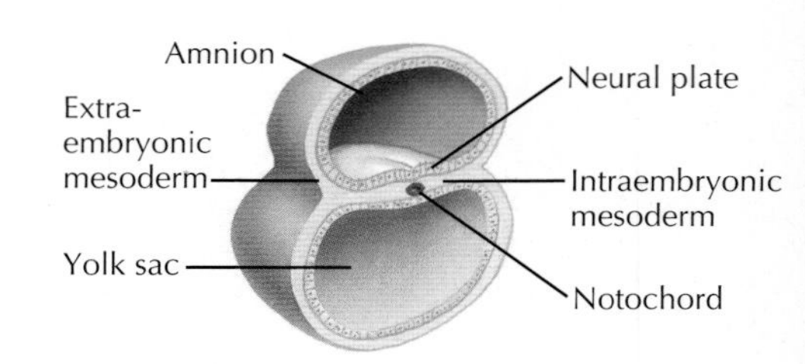

Vertebrate body plan after 4 weeks

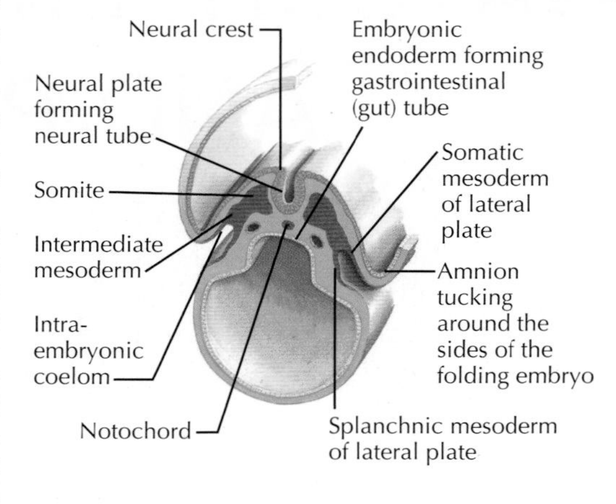

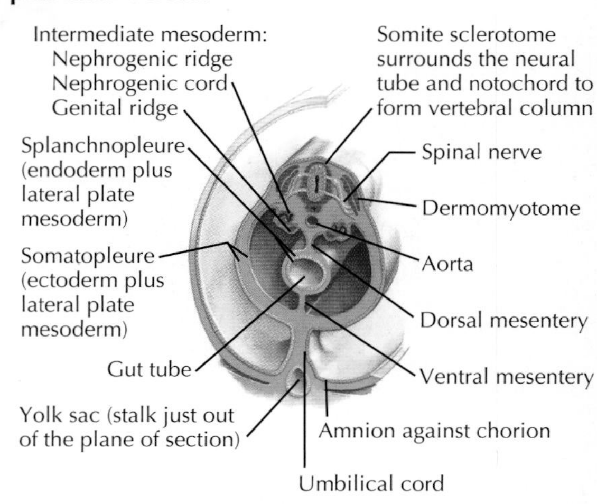

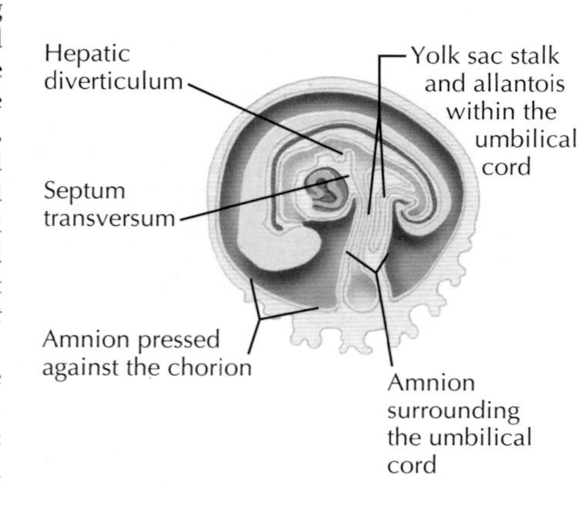

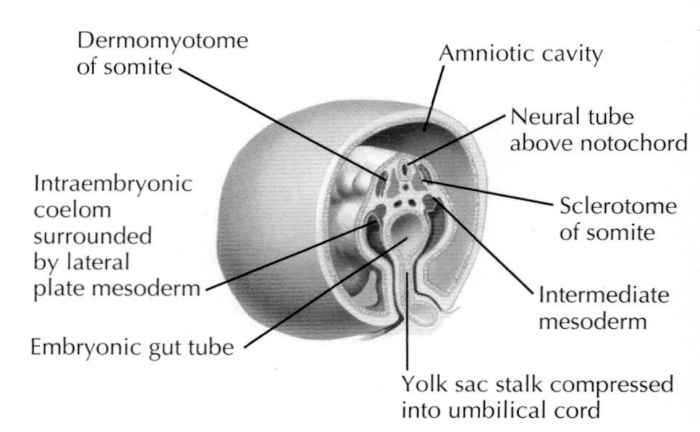

Dorsal views

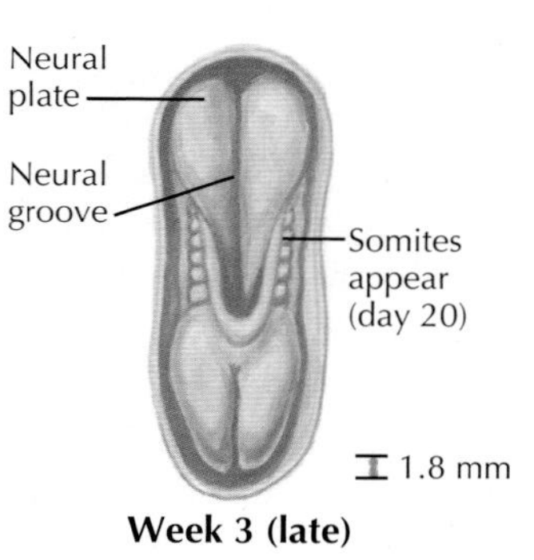

Week 3 (late)

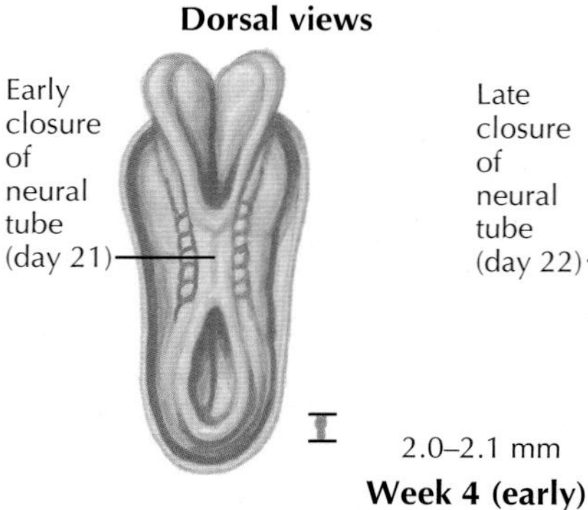

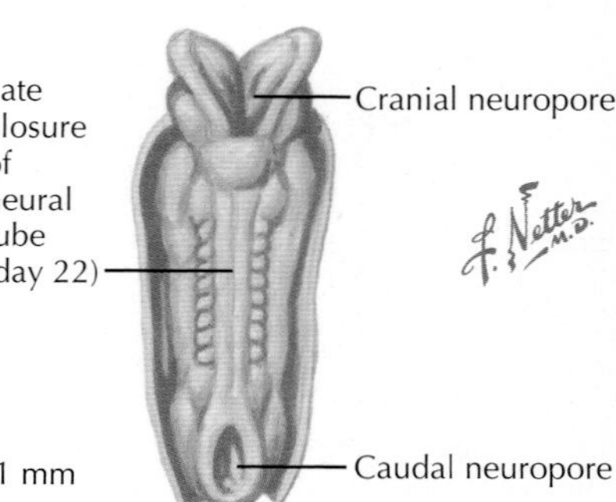

Week 4 (early)

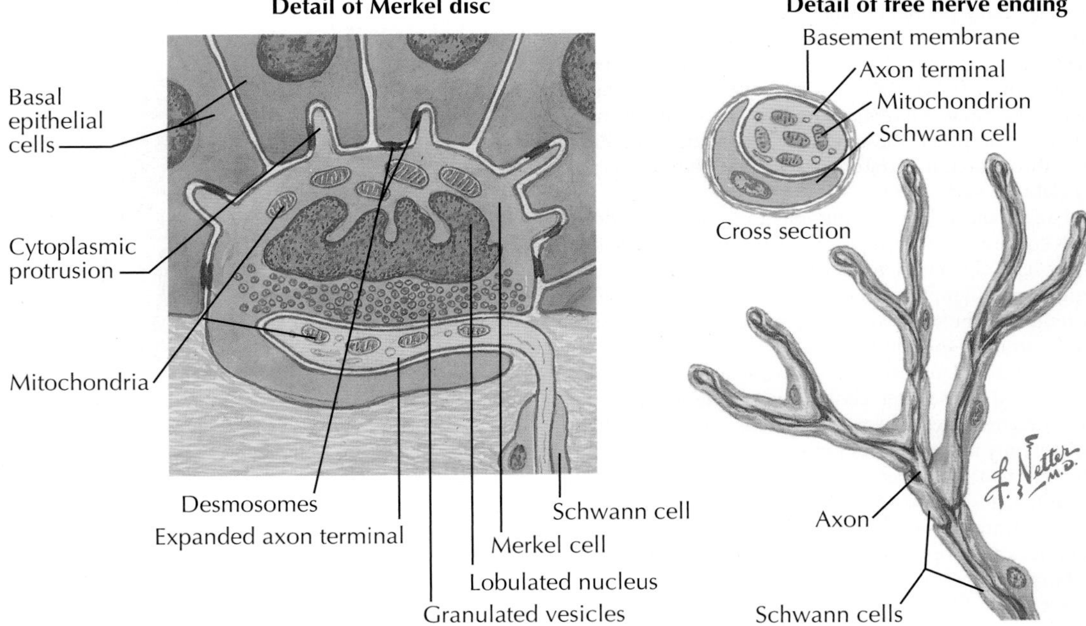

Normal Skin Anatomy

The human skin, taken collectively, is the largest organ in the human body. On average, it weighs between 4 and 5 kg. It is vitally important to life. The skin is made up of three distinct layers: the epidermis, dermis, and subcutaneous tissue. Each of these layers plays a pivotal role in the execution of the day-to-day functions of the skin. The skin's primary function is to protect the interior of the body from the exterior environment. It performs this role in many fashions: It acts as a semipermeable barrier to both hydrophilic and hydrophobic substances, it is the first line of immunologic defense against invading microbes, it blocks harmful ultraviolet radiation, and it contains many components of the adaptive and innate immune system. The skin is not just a barrier; it plays a critical role in physiologic vitamin D metabolism.

The majority of the epidermis is made up of keratinocytes. It also contains melanocytes, Langerhans cells, and Merkel cells. The epidermis is avascular and receives its nutrition from the superficial vascular plexus of the papillary dermis.

Melanocytes are derived from the neural crest and are responsible for producing the melanin family of pigments, which are packaged in melanosomes. Melanocytes are found in equal density in all humans, but darker-skinned individuals have a higher density of melanosomes than those with lighter skin. This is the reason for color variation among humans. Eumelanin, the predominant type of melanin protein, is responsible for brown and black pigmentation. Pheomelanin is a unique variant of melanin that is found in humans with red hair.

The skin is found in continuity with the epithelial lining of the digestive tract, including the oral mucosa and the anal mucosa. Distinct transition zones are seen at these interfaces. The skin also abuts the conjunctival mucosa of the globe and the mucosa of the nasal passages. The skin and its neighboring epithelial components supply the human body with a continuous barrier to protect it from the external world.

Many appendageal structures are present throughout the skin. The major ones are the hair follicles, their associated sebaceous glands, and the eccrine glands. Most of the skin is hair-bearing. Fine vellus hairs make up the preponderance of the skin's hair production. Terminal hairs are much thicker and are found on the scalp, eyebrows, and eyelashes; in the axilla and groin areas; and in the beard region in men. Glabrous skin, which is devoid of hair follicles, includes the vermilion border of the lips, palms, soles, glans penis, and labia minora.

Human skin varies in thickness. It is thickest on the back, and the thinnest areas are found on the eyelids and the scrotum. Regardless of thickness, all skin possesses the same immunologic function and barrier activity.

Appendageal structures are found in varying concentrations based on location. Sebaceous glands are located predominantly on the face, upper chest, and back. Sebaceous glands are attached to hair follicles and are found only on hair-bearing skin. Eccrine sweat glands, on the other hand, are found ubiquitously. Eccrine glands are found in the highest density on the palms and soles. The other main sweat glands of the skin, the apocrine glands, are found almost exclusively in the axillae and the groin. Apocrine glands can be found in the external ear canal (ceruminous glands), the eyelid (Moll's glands), and the areola. The apocrine glands, like sebaceous glands, are found only in conjunction with hair follicles.

Nails are composed of specialized keratin proteins. These keratins make a hard nail plate that is important for protection, grasp, and defense. Fingernails and toenails are made of the same keratin structure and in the same manner. Fingernails grow slightly faster than toenails. The average thumbnail takes 6 months to replace itself, whereas the average great toenail takes 8 to 12 months.

Touch is mediated through specialized nerve receptors within the skin. Meissner's corpuscles, lamellar (pacinian) corpuscles, Merkel cell receptors, and Ruffini receptors are specialized nerve endings that help mediate light touch, vibration, sustained touch, deep touch, and stretch sensations. There are also free nerve endings and type C fibers in the skin, which are important for pain and temperature detection and itching, respectively.

NORMAL SKIN HISTOLOGY

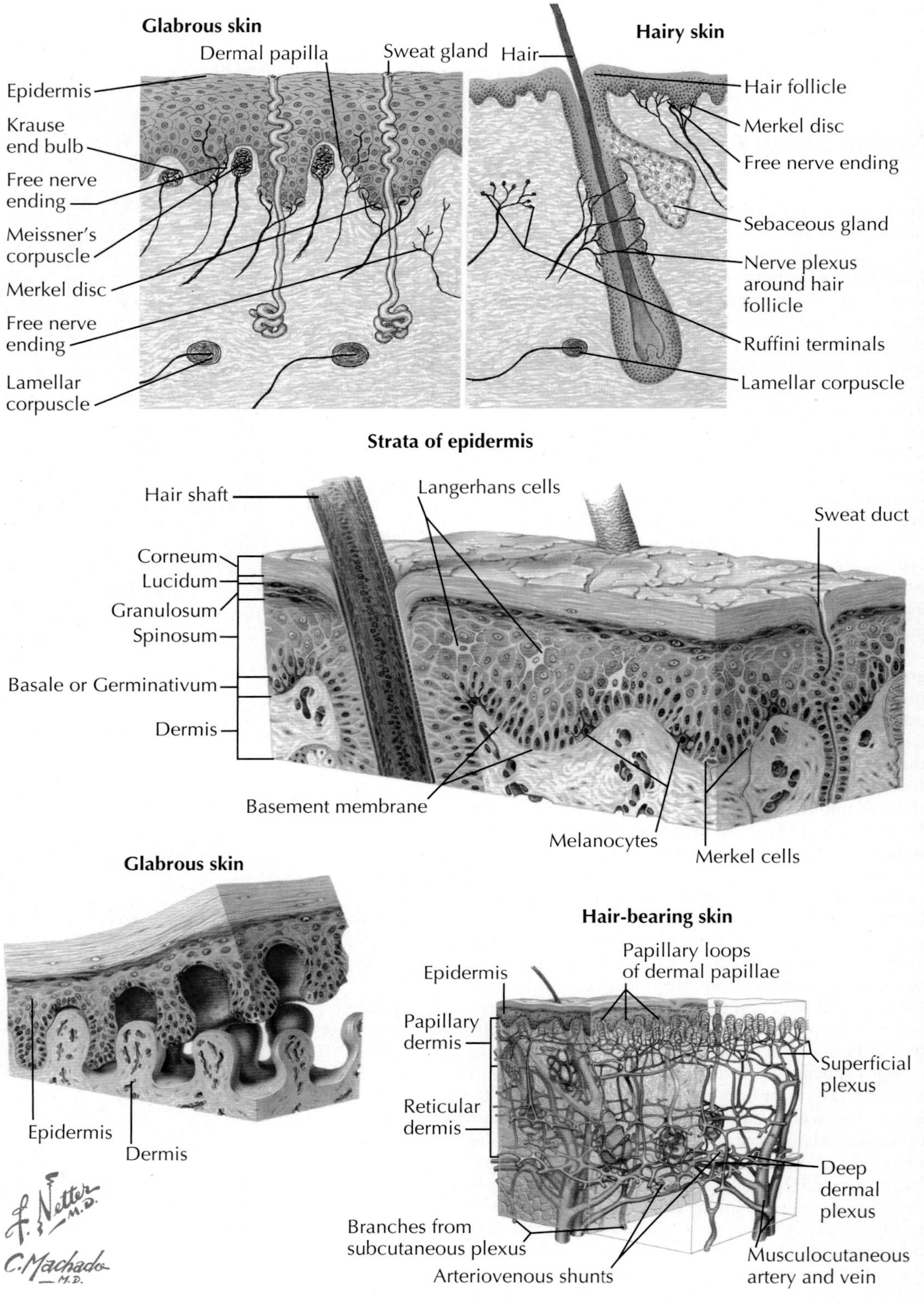

The integumentary system is composed of multiple interconnected subunits that work in unison. The skin and its appendageal structures make up the integumentary system. The three main layers of the skin are the epidermis, dermis, and subcutaneous tissue. Within the epidermis, the principal skin cell is the keratinocyte. Other cells found in the epidermis include melanocytes, Merkel cells, and Langerhans cells. The main cell type found within the dermis is the fibroblast. Fibroblasts make collagen, which forms the foundation and mechanical support for the overlying epidermis. The dermis is a region of high vascularity. Subcutaneous fat tissue is found directly beneath the dermis and is composed primarily of adipocytes.

The normal human epidermis varies extensively in thickness over the body. It is thickest on the back and thinnest on the eyelids. The epidermis can be subdivided into five components: stratum basale, stratum spinosum, stratum granulosum, stratum lucidum, and stratum corneum. The stratum lucidum is found only on the skin of the palms and soles. Each layer of the epidermis has important anatomic and physiologic functions.

The stratum basale is the deepest layer. It consists of cuboidal epithelium sitting atop a basement membrane zone. The stratum basale contains proliferating keratinocytes, which are constantly undergoing replication to replace the overlying epidermis. It takes approximately 28 days for a basal keratinocyte to mature and progress to the outermost layer of the stratum corneum. Melanocytes and Merkel cells can also be found within the stratum basale. Melanocytes are pigment-forming cells; they transfer their pigment, which is packaged in melanosomes, to neighboring keratinocytes. Melanocytes have arm-like extensions that reach out and touch approximately 10 to 15 keratinocytes. Merkel cells are modified nerve endings and have been found to be as important as mechanoreceptors. These cells are present in small numbers throughout the stratum basale, with higher densities in glabrous skin.

Langerhans cells are immunologically active dendritic cells and are critically important in immune surveillance. They have the ability to move from the epidermis and migrate to lymph nodes. These cells can be found throughout the epidermis but are most frequently seen in the stratum spinosum.

The stratum spinosum is many cell layers thick and is recognized by the intercellular connections among adjacent keratinocytes. These connections are seen on light microscopy as tiny spines between adjacent cells. From the lower to the upper layers of the stratum spinosum, keratinocytes progressively become flatter in appearance.

The stratum granulosum is recognized by the large number of basophilic keratohyalin granules within its keratinocytes. This stratum is typically two to four cell layers thick. The keratohyalin granules are composed primarily of the protein profilaggrin; they vary from 1 to 4 μm in diameter. Profilaggrin is the precursor to filaggrin, an essential protein that is required for the integrity of the epidermis.

The stratum lucidum occurs only in the skin of the palms and soles. It is composed of tightly packed squamous keratinocytes and appears as a translucent eosinophilic layer.

The stratum corneum, the outermost layer of skin, is made up of anucleate, cornified keratinocytes. Keratinization (cornification) is a complex process that results in the appearance of the stratum corneum. As cells progress up the stratum corneum, they are shed in the process known as desquamation.

The dermis is primarily composed of fibroblast-manufactured collagen. The dermis contains a highly vascular network that is responsible for thermoregulation and nutrition of the skin. This network includes a deep dermal plexus and a superficial plexus. The superficial plexus is responsible for thermoregulation. It undergoes vasoconstriction during exposure to cold temperatures and vasodilation in times of warm temperature. The dermis can be split into two regions, the papillary and the reticular portions. The papillary dermis is juxtaposed to the overlying epidermis and interdigitates with it. The papillary dermis and the epidermis are connected by the basement membrane zone. The reticular dermis makes up the largest portion of the dermis.

The subcutaneous tissue is composed of adipocytes. This tissue's main functions are storage of energy, insulation, and cushioning. The adipocytes are closely packed in a connective tissue septum with associated blood vessels and nerve endings.

There are many types of skin appendages, including hair follicles, sebaceous glands, eccrine glands, apocrine glands, and various nerve endings.

Skin Physiology: The Process of Keratinization

Keratinization, also known as *cornification*, is unique to the epithelium of the skin. Keratinization allows humans to live on dry land. The process of keratinization begins in the basal layer of the epidermis and continues upward until full keratinization occurs within the stratum corneum.

The keratinized skin of the stratum corneum is highly organized and is relatively strong and resistant to physical and chemical insults. This layer is critically important in keeping out microorganisms, is the first line of defense against ultraviolet radiation, and contains many enzymes that can degrade and detoxify external chemicals. The stratum corneum is also a semipermeable structure that selectively allows passage of hydrophilic and lipophilic agents. However, the most studied aspect of the stratum corneum is its ability to protect against excessive water and electrolyte loss. It acts as a barrier to keep chemicals out, but, more importantly, it keeps water and electrolytes within the human body. Transepidermal water loss increases as the stratum corneum is damaged, thinned, or disrupted. The main lipids responsible for protection against water loss are the ceramides and the sphingolipids. These molecules are capable of binding many water molecules, thus protecting the body from excessive water loss.

As keratinocytes migrate from the stratum basale and journey through the layers of the epidermis, they undergo characteristic morphologic and biochemical changes. The keratinocytes flatten and become more compacted and polyhedral. The resulting corneocytes become stacked, like bricks in a wall. These corneocytes are still bonded together by desmosomes, which are now called *corneodesmosomes*.

The stratum granulosum gets its name from the appearance of multiple basophilic keratohyalin granules present within the keratinocytes. These granules are largely composed of the protein profilaggrin. Profilaggrin is converted into filaggrin by various proteases and other biochemical modifications. Filaggrin is so named because it is a filament-aggregating protein. Filaggrin interacts with keratin intermediate filaments. This interaction allows for the cells to become compacted and makes it possible for the development of an insoluble keratin matrix. Over time, filaggrin is broken down into natural moisturizing factor (NMF), urocanic acid, and, ultimately, its precursor amino acids. NMF is a metabolite of filaggrin that slows water evaporation from the corneocytes.

The intercellular space is composed of lipids and water. The lipids are derived from the release of the lamellar bodies (Odland bodies). Lamellar bodies begin to form in the uppermost basal layer and are secreted into the extracellular space in the outer layers of the stratum granulosum. Ceramides make up the overwhelming majority of the contents of the lamellar bodies. Other components include free fatty acids, cholesterol esters, and proteases. The lamellar bodies fuse with the cell surface and release their contents into the intercellular space. The fusion of the lamellar body with the cell surface is dependent on the enzyme transglutaminase I.

Concurrently, the cornified cell envelope (CCE) develops. The CCE proteins envoplakin, loricrin, periplakin, small proline-rich proteins, and involucrin are cross-linked in various arrangements by transglutaminase I and transglutaminase III, forming a sturdy scaffolding along the inner surface of the keratinocyte cell membrane. As the keratinocyte migrates upward, the cell membrane is lost, and the ceramides that are released begin cross-linking with the CCE proteins. The cells continue to move toward the surface of the skin and begin to lose their nucleus and cellular organelles. The loss of these organelles is mediated by the activation of certain proteases that can quickly degrade protein, DNA, RNA, and the nuclear membrane.

Once the cells reach the outer layers of the stratum corneum, they begin to be shed. On average, a keratinocyte spends 2 weeks in the stratum corneum before being shed from the skin surface in a process called desquamation. Shedding is achieved by the final degradation of the corneodesmosomes by proteases that destroy the desmoglein-1 protein.

Keratinization is especially important in the diseases of cornification. Many skin diseases have been found to involve defects in one or more proteins that are critical in the process of cornification. Examples are lamellar ichthyosis, which is caused by a defect in the transglutaminase I enzyme, and Vohwinkel syndrome (keratoma hereditarium mutilans), which results from a genetic mutation in the loricrin protein and a resultant defective CCE.

Cornified layer
Granular layer
Spinous layer
Basal layer
Dermis
Bricks (keratinocytes)
Mortar (intercellular space of the stratum corneum)
Corneodesmosomes
Cornified cell envelope cross linked with ceramides replaces plasma membrane
Corneodesmosome
Filaments of keratin
LM
Corneocyte
SG cell
LB
Keratohyalin granules
Golgi apparatus
Lamellar bodies (LB) that are seen today as part of a branched tubular structure like the trans-Golgi network migrate to the surface of the cell of the stratum granulosum (SG) and release their content into the intercellular space. The released lipids are rearranged into lamellar membrane (LM).
C. Machado M.D.

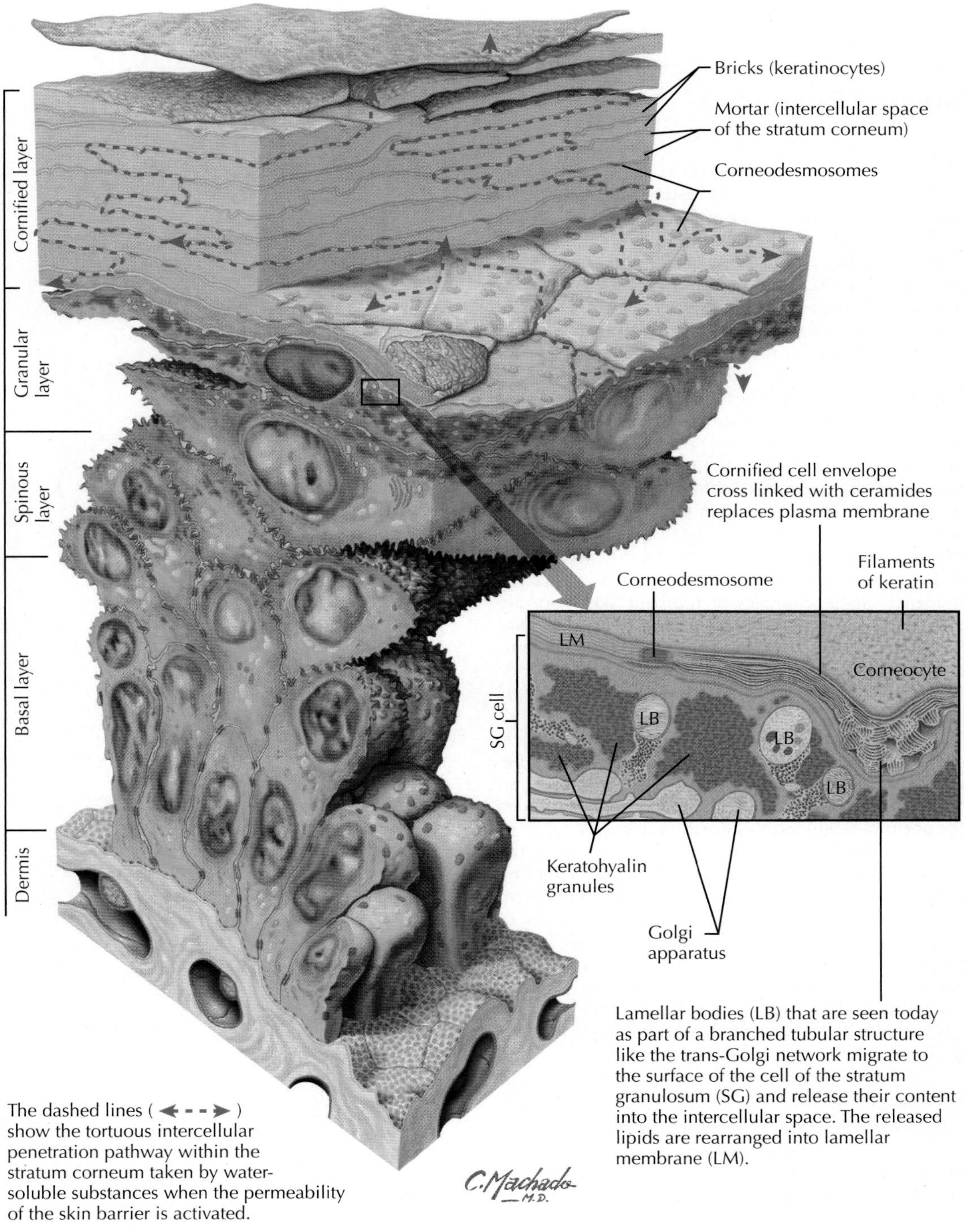

The dashed lines (◄- - -►) show the tortuous intercellular penetration pathway within the stratum corneum taken by water-soluble substances when the permeability of the skin barrier is activated.

Normal Skin Flora

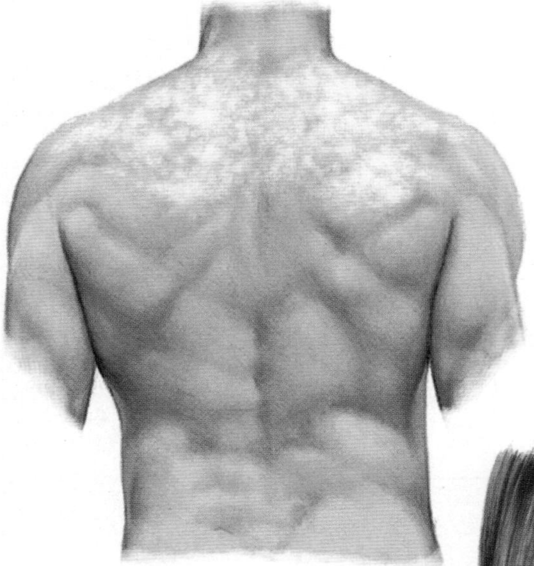

The skin contains normal microflora that are universally found on all humans. It has been estimated that the number of bacteria on the surface of the human skin is greater than the number of cells in the human body. The normal skin flora includes the bacteria *Staphylococcus epidermidis*, *Corynebacterium* species, *Propionibacterium acnes*, *Micrococcus* species, and *Acetobacter* species. *Demodex brevis* and *Demodex folliculorum*, collectively referred to as *demodex mites*, are the only parasites that are part of the normal flora. *Pityrosporum* species are the only fungi considered to be normal skin flora.

The microbes that make up the normal skin flora under most circumstances do not cause any type of disease. They are able to reproduce and maintain viable populations, living in harmony with the host. In stark contrast, transient skin flora can sustain growth only in certain skin environments. Transient microbes are not able to produce long-lasting, viable reproductive populations and therefore are unable to maintain a permanent residence. Some examples of transient skin flora are *Staphylococcus aureus*, including methicillin-resistant *S. aureus* (MRSA), *Enterobacter coli*, *Pseudomonas aeruginosa*, *Streptococcus pyogenes*, and some *Bacillus* species. Normal and transient flora can become pathogenic under the correct environmental conditions.

Normal bacterial colonization begins immediately after birth. Once newborns are exposed to the external environment, they are quickly colonized with bacteria. *S. epidermidis* is often the first colonizing species and is the one most commonly cultured in neonates.

The innate ability of certain bacteria to colonize the human skin is dependent on a host of contributing factors, thus allowing them to evolve a competitive advantage over the transient skin flora. Availability of nutrients, pH, hydration, temperature, and ultraviolet radiation exposure all play a role in allowing certain bacteria to develop in a synergistic balance. The normal skin flora use these factors to their survival advantage, which allows them to thrive in a symbiotic relationship with the human skin.

Under certain circumstances, normal skin flora can become pathogenic and cause overt skin disease. Overgrowth of *Malassezia furfur* (previously known as *Pityrosporum ovale*) causes tinea versicolor, an exceedingly common superficial fungal infection. Warm and humid environments are believed to be factors in the pathogenesis. Tinea versicolor manifests as fine, scaly patches with hyperpigmentation and hypopigmentation. Other *Malassezia* species have been implicated in causing neonatal cephalic pustulosis, *Pityrosporum* folliculitis, and seborrheic dermatitis.

The common skin bacterium *S. epidermidis* is a gram-positive coccus that can become a pathogenic microbe under certain circumstances. Conditions that increase the chance that this bacterium will cause pathogenic skin disease include use of immunosuppressive medications, an immunocompromised state (e.g., human immunodeficiency virus infection), and presence of a chronic indwelling intravenous catheter. *S. epidermidis* creates a biofilm on indwelling catheters, which can lead to transient bacteremia and sepsis in immunocompromised patients and occasionally in the immunocompetent.

P. acnes is a gram-positive organism that is found within the pilosebaceous unit. These bacteria occur in high densities in the sebum-rich regions of the face, back, and chest. It is the major species implicated in the pathogenesis of acne vulgaris. In immunocompromised individuals, it has been reported to cause abscesses.

Corynebacterium species, when in an environment of moisture and warmth, can produce an overgrowth on the terminal hairs of the axilla and groin regions, resulting in the condition known as *trichomycosis axillaris*. Different colonies of this bacterium can produce superficial red, yellow, or black nodules along the terminal hair shafts. Corynebacteria can also cause pitted keratolysis, a superficial infection of the outer layers of the epidermis on the soles.

The only parasites that can be found normally on human skin are the *Demodex* mites, which live in various regions of the pilosebaceous unit. *Demodex brevis* live within the sebaceous gland ducts, whereas *Demodex folliculorum* live in the hair follicle infundibulum. *Demodex* mites can cause *Demodex* folliculitis, an infection of the hair follicles that manifests as superficial, follicle-based pustules.

The most important skin microbes, based on their ability to cause pathology, are the transient microbes. The best-known species is *S. aureus*. The ability of *S. aureus* to cause folliculitis, boils, abscesses, and bacterial sepsis is well documented and presents a major cause of morbidity and mortality.

The normal skin flora includes *Malassezia furfur*, which under pathologic conditions may cause tinea versicolor.

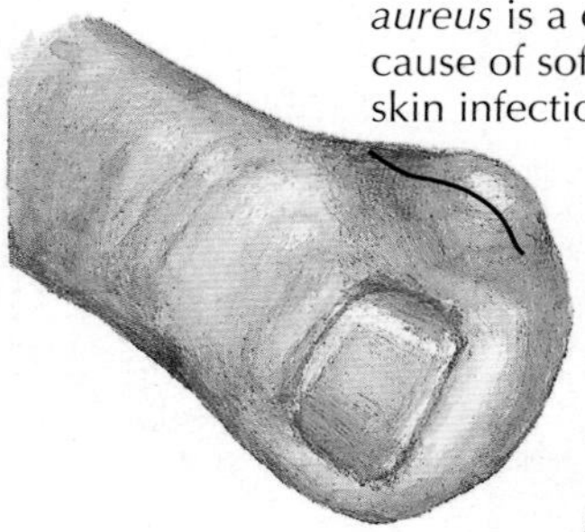

Staphylococcus aureus is a common cause of soft tissue skin infections.

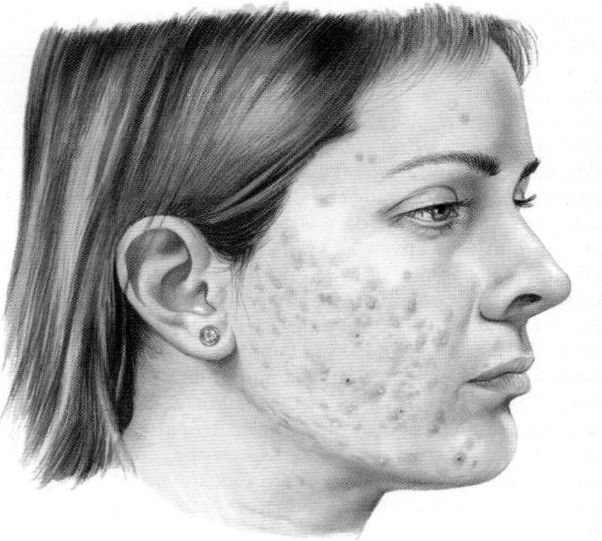

The normal skin flora *Propionibacterium acnes* is partially responsible for the pathomechanism of acne vulgaris.

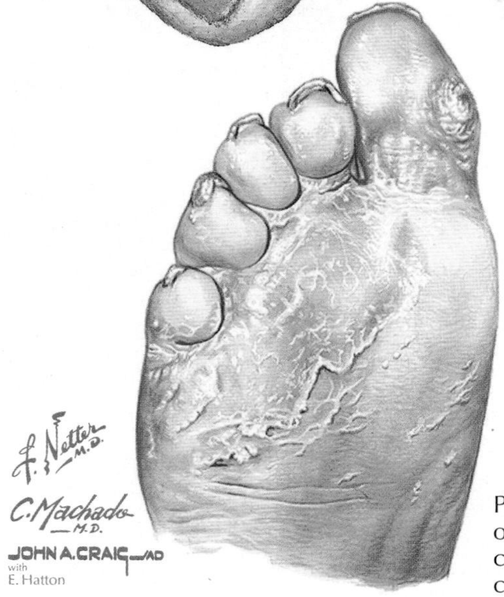

Pitted keratolysis may be caused by overgrowth of *Corynebacterium* species. Under normal circumstances, *Corynebacterium* species are considered normal skin flora.

VITAMIN D METABOLISM

The skin plays a critical role in the production of vitamin D and thus in calcium and phosphate hemostasis. When skin is exposed to sunlight, it immediately begins production of vitamin D_3. The epidermis turns provitamin D_3 (7-dehydrocholesterol) into vitamin D_3 (cholecalciferol) through interaction with ultraviolet B (UVB) radiation. Previtamin D_3 is converted into vitamin D_3 via a spontaneous endothermic reaction. Vitamin D is then transported to the liver and kidneys, leading to the production of 1,25-dihydroxyvitamin D_3. This biologically active metabolite is critical in calcium metabolism, bone metabolism, and endocrine and neuromuscular transmission and is important in immune system regulation.

Vitamin D_3 produced in the skin can act locally or be absorbed into the systemic circulation and added to the concentration of vitamin D_3 absorbed by the gastrointestinal tract. Vitamin D is transferred in the blood bound to the vitamin D–binding protein. Within the liver, it is hydroxylated to 25-hydroxyvitamin D_3. This then travels to the kidney and is again hydroxylated into 1,25-dihydroxyvitamin D_3, known as *calcitriol*. 1,25-Dihydroxyvitamin D_3 is the main biologically active form of vitamin D in the human body. An elevated level of vitamin D_3 in the general circulation causes increased absorption of calcium and phosphate through the gastrointestinal tract, increased mobilization of calcium stores from bone tissue, and increased release of parathyroid hormone (PTH), which results in a lowering of the serum phosphate concentration.

The earliest sign of vitamin D deficiency is an often subtle and transient decrease in the serum calcium level. This decrease causes the pituitary gland to secrete PTH, which acts on the kidneys to increase calcium reabsorption, decrease phosphate retention, and increase osteoclast activity. This increase in osteoclast activity also increases the serum calcium level. Vitamin D deficiency is manifested by normal serum calcium levels, increased PTH levels, and decreased phosphorous levels.

Vitamin D_3 synthesis in the skin is dependent on contact with UVB radiation. Sunscreens, clothing, and glass all block UVB radiation and diminish the local production of vitamin D_3 in the skin. The keratinocytes within the epidermis contain enzymes that can convert vitamin D_3 into 25-hydroxyvitamin D_3 and 1,25-dihydroxyvitamin D_3. These are believed to act locally within the skin, directing keratinocyte proliferation and differentiation, and are not thought to contribute to the body's hydroxyvitamin D_3 stores.

Immunologically, 1,25-dihydroxyvitamin D_3 has been found to regulate the maturation of dendritic cells, monocytes, and T-lymphocytes. Vitamin D and its analogs are believed to inhibit tumor cell proliferation and to cause apoptosis of tumor cells. Because the vitamin D receptor (VDR) forms heterodimers with the retinoid X receptor (RXR) and other retinoid receptors, the combination of vitamin D and vitamin A analogs may ultimately be found to be responsible for the immunologic effects of both of these vitamins.

Rickets is a disease of childhood that is caused by severe vitamin D deficiency. It is rarely seen in the United States, but it is not uncommon in developing countries. Vitamin D deficiency in adults more commonly manifests as osteomalacia, which occurs throughout the world. This deficiency leads to decreased bone mineralization and can cause osteopenia and osteoporosis. The normal concentration of vitamin D in serum is believed to be between 35 and 200 nmol/L.

1,25-Vitamin D_3 exerts its effect by binding with the VDR and then interacting with DNA to directly modulate the transcription of specific genes. The VDR is a member of the nuclear receptor family. 1,25-Vitamin D_3 enters a cell, binds with VDR in the cytoplasm, and then enters the nucleus of the cell. There, the complex interacts with cellular DNA by binding to various regulatory sites. In this way, vitamin D_3 and the VDR are able to modulate gene transcription. The VDR also forms heterodimers with other members of the nuclear receptor family, mainly the RXR. Most VDR signaling involves this heterodimer form.

Vitamin D is one of the fat-soluble vitamins. It is found in many foods, such as cod liver oil, many fish, egg yolks, and liver. Vitamin D is commonly present as a supplement in many foods, such as milk, breads, and cereals. Oral vitamin D supplements are easily obtained and well tolerated.

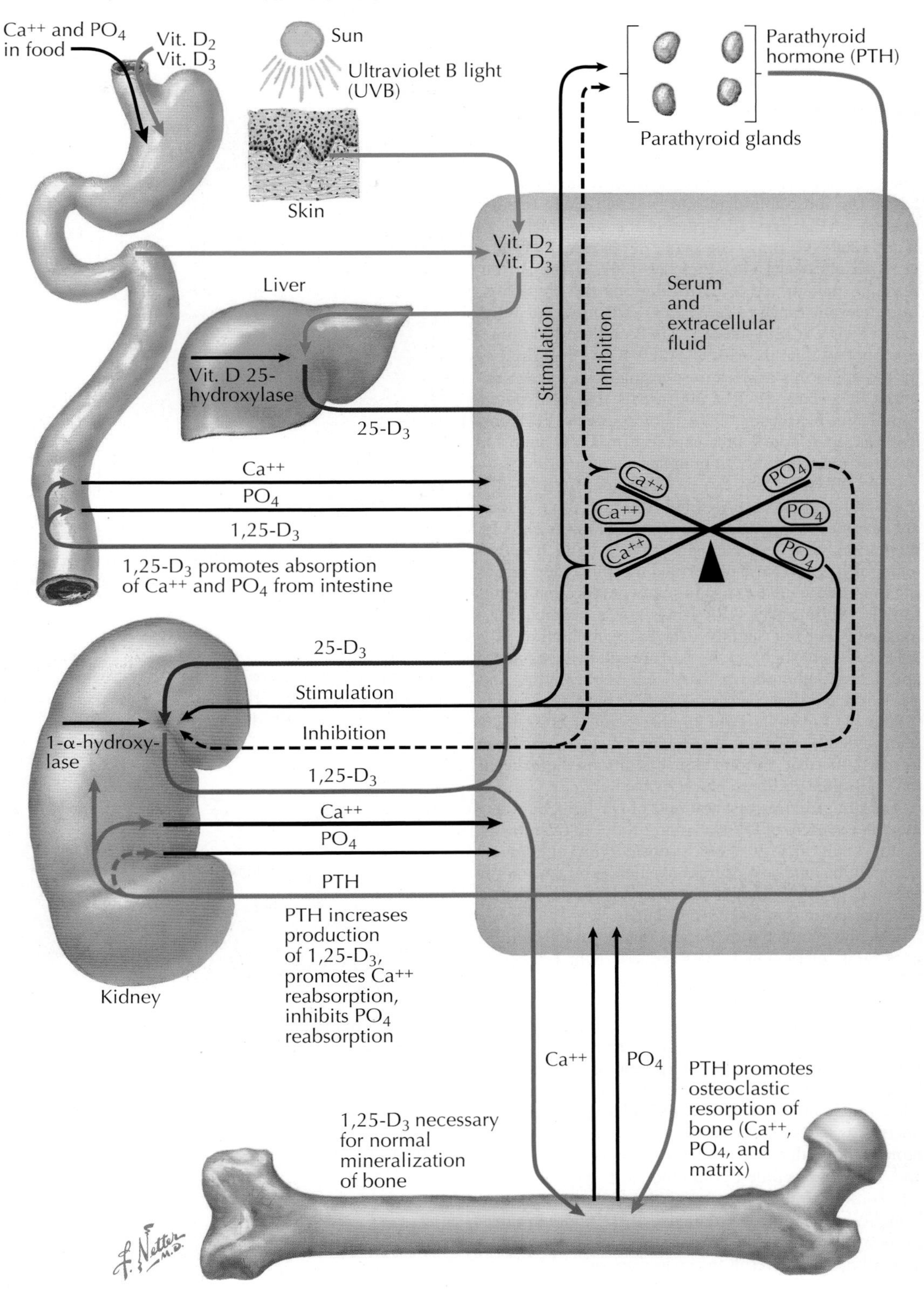

PHOTOBIOLOGY

The skin interacts with some form of light on a daily basis. The most abundant and physiologically relevant portion of the light spectrum is the ultraviolet (UV) range (200–400 nm). The ozone layer essentially prevents all ultraviolet C (UVC) rays (200–280 nm) from reaching the surface of Earth, limiting the physiologically relevant range to UVB (280–320 nm) and ultraviolet A (UVA; 320–400 nm). UVB rays are 1000 times more potent than those of UVA. UVB rays are absorbed by the epidermis and are responsible for causing sunburns. It is believed that 300 nm is the most potent wavelength for causing DNA photoproducts. Erythema begins 2 to 6 hours after exposure to UVB light and peaks at approximately 10 hours postexposure.

The UVA spectrum can be subdivided into UVA II (320–340 nm) and UVA I (340–400 nm). UVA II rays are responsible for the immediate but transient pigmentation seen after exposure to UV light. It causes melanocytes to release preformed melanosomes, resulting in a mild increase in skin pigmentation that begins to fade within a day. UVA I rays are responsible for a longer-lasting but slightly delayed pigmentation. The effects of visible light on the skin are still being explored and defined. Photodermatoses such as porphyria cutanea tarda and solar urticaria can flare with exposure to visible light. Visible light in the form of laser light, photodynamic therapy, or low-level light therapy can be used to treat various skin conditions. Sunscreens have a limited ability to block visible light.

The sun produces vast amounts of UV light, but there are other sources of UV radiation produced by humans. A thorough history should consider an individual's occupations and exposures. Welders are commonly exposed to UVC and, if not properly protected, can develop severe skin and corneal burns.

UV rays interact with skin in many ways. The most important interaction is between UV light (especially UVB) and the DNA of keratinocytes. Because UVB is limited in its depth of penetration into the epidermis, it affects only keratinocytes, melanocytes, and Langerhans cells. The photons of UV light interact with cellular DNA, inducing a number of specific and nonspecific effects. These interactions can result in DNA photoproducts, which are formed between adjacent pyrimidine nucleoside bases on one strand of DNA. The most common photoproducts are cyclobutane pyrimidine dimers and the pyrimidine-pyrimidone 6,4 photoproduct. The common cyclobutane pyrimidine dimer mutation is highly specific for UV damage. These photoproducts cause a decrease in DNA replication and mutagenesis and ultimately can result in carcinogenesis.

The cell nucleus is well equipped to handle DNA damage caused by photoproducts. A series of DNA repair proteins are in constant surveillance. Once a photoproduct is found, the DNA repair mechanism is called into service. There are at least seven well-described proteins that help in recognition, removal of the damage, and repair of the DNA strand. These seven proteins were named XPA through XPG after studies of numerous patients with the photosensitivity disorder xeroderma pigmentosum. Each protein is uniquely responsible for some part of the DNA repair mechanism. Defects in any of these XP proteins result in a differing phenotype of xeroderma pigmentosum. Patients with xeroderma pigmentosum are prone to develop multiple skin cancers at a young age.

Proteins within the cells are also susceptible to damage from UV light exposure. The amino acids histidine and cysteine are susceptible to oxidation reactions after interaction with UV light. Melanin pigment absorbs UV light, and this is one of the mechanisms by which the skin defends itself against UV assault. Absorption of UV light by cell membranes, organelles, RNA, and other components of the living cell can cause oxidative stress and cellular damage.

When exposed to UV radiation, the skin increases production of melanin, which in turn helps in photoprotection. Melanin can be considered a naturally produced sunscreen. Many organic and inorganic compounds have been used as sunscreens to help neutralize the effects of UV radiation on skin. The main protective mechanisms are absorption, reflection, and physical blockade.

Comparison of penetration of radiation with different wavelengths into human skin

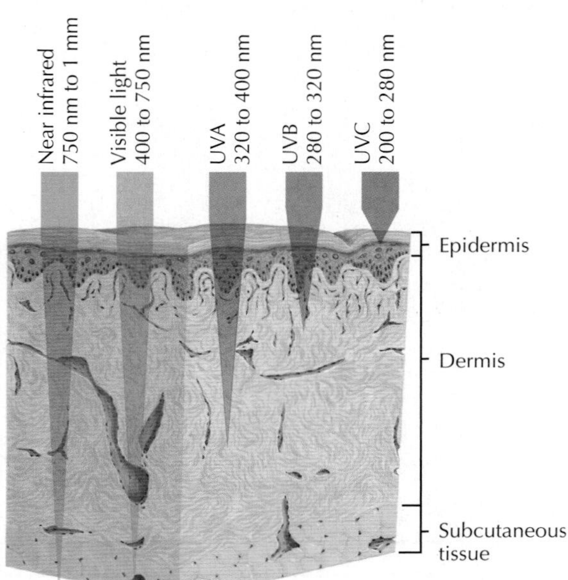

Erythema and tanning onset and duration are ultraviolet (UV) wavelength dependent. By comparison, UVA radiation induces transient erythema. The erythema from UVB takes 6–24 hours to induce and is much longer lasting.

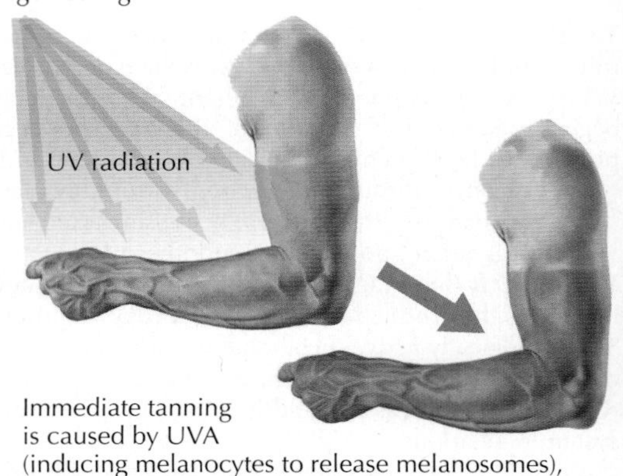

Nucleotide excision repair (NER) is a major DNA repair mechanism in eukaryotic cells for removing several DNA lesions caused by different agents, including UV-induced damage such as thymine-thymine dimer, the most common cyclobutane pyrimidine dimer mutation. NER comprises the following steps:

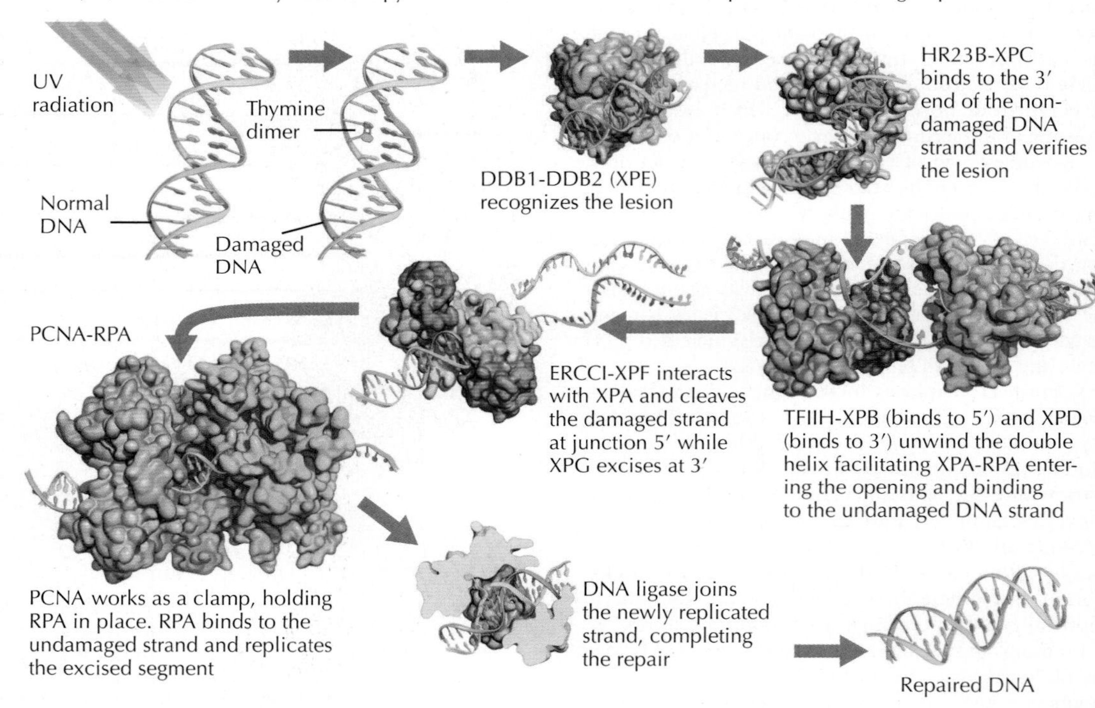

XP (XPA XPB, XPC...) = Xeroderma pigmentosum (A, B, C...), **HR23B** or **hHRD23B** = Human Homologue of Yeast Rad23, **DDB** = Damaged DNA-binding protein, **TFIIH** = Transcription factor IIh, **PCNA** = Proliferating cell nuclear antigen, **RPA** = Replication protein A, **ERCC** = Excision repair cross-complementing

WOUND HEALING

Wound healing is a complex process that involves an orderly and sequential series of interactions among multiple cell types and tissue structures. Classically, wound healing has been divided into phases: hemostasis, inflammation, new tissue formation, and matrix formation/remodeling. Each of these phases is unique, and particular cell types play key roles in the different phases.

Once a disruption of the skin barrier occurs, a cascade of inflammatory mediators is released and wound healing begins. The disruption of dermal blood vessels allows extravasation of blood into the tissues. The ruptured vessels undergo immediate vasoconstriction. Platelets begin the process of coagulation and initiate the earliest phase of inflammation. The formation of the earliest blood clot provides the foundation for future cell migration into the wound. Many inflammatory mediators are released during this initial phase. Once initial hemostasis is achieved, the platelets discharge the contents of their alpha granules into the extravascular space. Alpha granules contain fibrinogen, fibronectin, von Willebrand factor, factor VIII, and many other proteins. The fibrinogen is converted into fibrin, which aids in formation of the fibrin clot. Platelets also play a critical role in releasing growth factors and proteases. The best known of these is platelet-derived growth factor (PDGF), which helps mediate the formation of the initial granulation tissue.

During the late portion of the inflammatory phase, leukocytes are seen for the first time. Neutrophils make up the largest component of the initial leukocyte response. Neutrophils are drawn into the area by various cytokines and adhere to the activated vascular endothelium. They enter the extravascular space by a process of diapedesis. These early-arriving neutrophils are responsible for the recruitment of more neutrophils, and they also begin the process of killing bacteria by use of their internal myeloperoxidase system. Through the production of free radicals, neutrophils are efficient at killing large numbers of bacteria. Neutrophil activity continues for a few days unless the wound is contaminated with bacteria. Once the neutrophil activity has cleared the wound of bacteria and other foreign particles, monocytes are recruited into the wound and activated into macrophages. Macrophages are critical in clearing the wound of neutrophils and any remaining cellular and bacterial debris. Macrophages are capable of producing nitrous oxide, which can kill bacteria and has also been shown to decrease viral replication. Macrophages release various cytokines, including PDGF, interleukin-6, and granulocyte colony-stimulating factor, which in turn recruit more monocytes and fibroblasts into the wound.

At this point, new tissue formation, the proliferative phase of wound healing, has begun. This phase typically begins on the third day and ends about 14 days after the initial insult. It is marked by reepithelialization and formation of granulation tissue. Reepithelialization occurs by the movement of epithelial cells (keratinocytes) from the free edge of the wound slowly across the wound defect. The migrating cells have the distinct phenotype of basal keratinocytes. It is believed that a low calcium concentration in the wound causes the keratinocytes to take on the characteristics of basal keratinocytes. PDGF is an important stimulant for keratinocytes and is partially responsible for this migration across the wound. The migrating keratinocytes contain the keratin pairs 5,14 and 6,16. They secrete vascular endothelial growth factor, which promotes the production of dermal blood vessels. At the same time the keratinocytes are migrating, the underlying fibroblasts are synthesizing a backbone matrix, made up predominantly of type III collagen and some proteoglycans. Some of the fibroblasts are converted into myofibroblasts by PDGF and tumor growth factor-β1. These myofibroblasts are important in that they cause the overlying wound to contract, decreasing its surface.

The final phase of wound healing involves scar maturation and tissue remodeling. This phase overlaps in time with the first two phases; it is said to begin with the production of the first granulation tissue. This phase extends for months and is complete when most of the collagen III and fibronectin have been replaced by mature type I collagen. In the final mature scar, the collagen fibers are oriented in large bundles running perpendicular to the basement membrane zone. The resulting scar has only 80% of the tensile strength of the uninjured skin.

HEALING OF INCISED, SUTURED SKIN WOUND

Immediately after incision
Blood clot with fine fibrin network forms in wound. Epithelium thickens at wound edges.

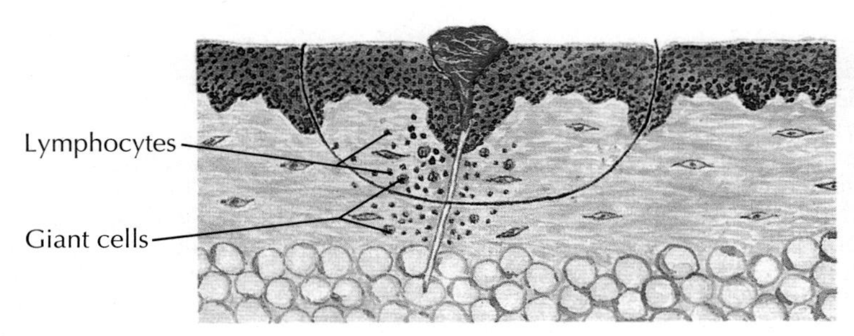

24–48 hours
Epithelium begins to grow down along cut edges and along suture tract. Leukocyte infiltration, chiefly round cells (lymphocytes) with few giant cells, occurs and removes bacteria and necrotic tissue.

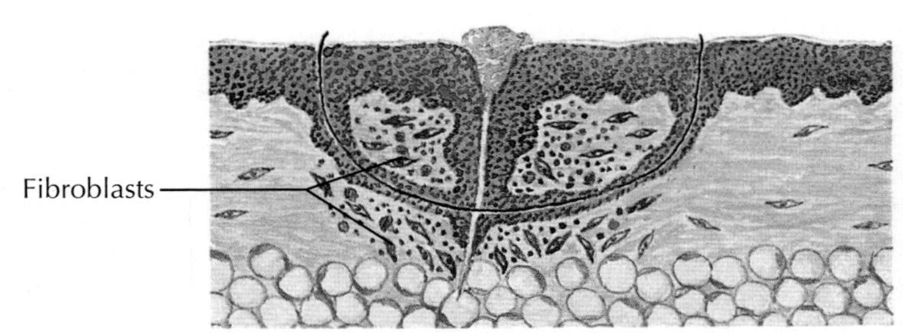

5–8 days
Epithelial downgrowth advances. Fibroblasts grow in from deeper tissues and add collagen precursors and glycoproteins to matrix. Cellular infiltration progresses.

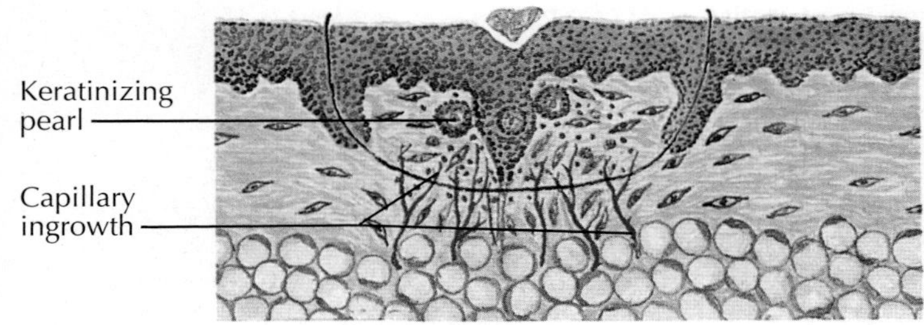

10–15 days
Capillaries grow in from subcutaneous tissue, forming granulation tissue. Epithelium bridges incision; epithelial downgrowths regress, leaving keratinizing pearls behind. Fibrosed clot (scab) is being pushed out. Collagen formation progresses and cellular infiltration abates.

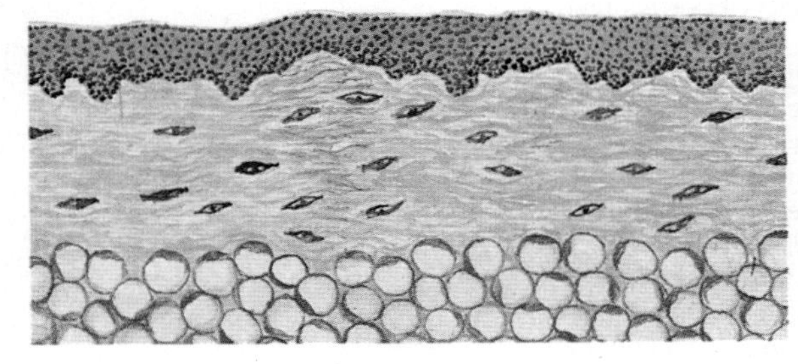

3 weeks–9 months
Epithelium is thinned to near normal. Tensile strength of tissue is increased owing to production and cross-linking of collagen fibers; elastic fibers reappear later.

MORPHOLOGY: LICHENIFICATION, PLAQUES, AND FISSURES

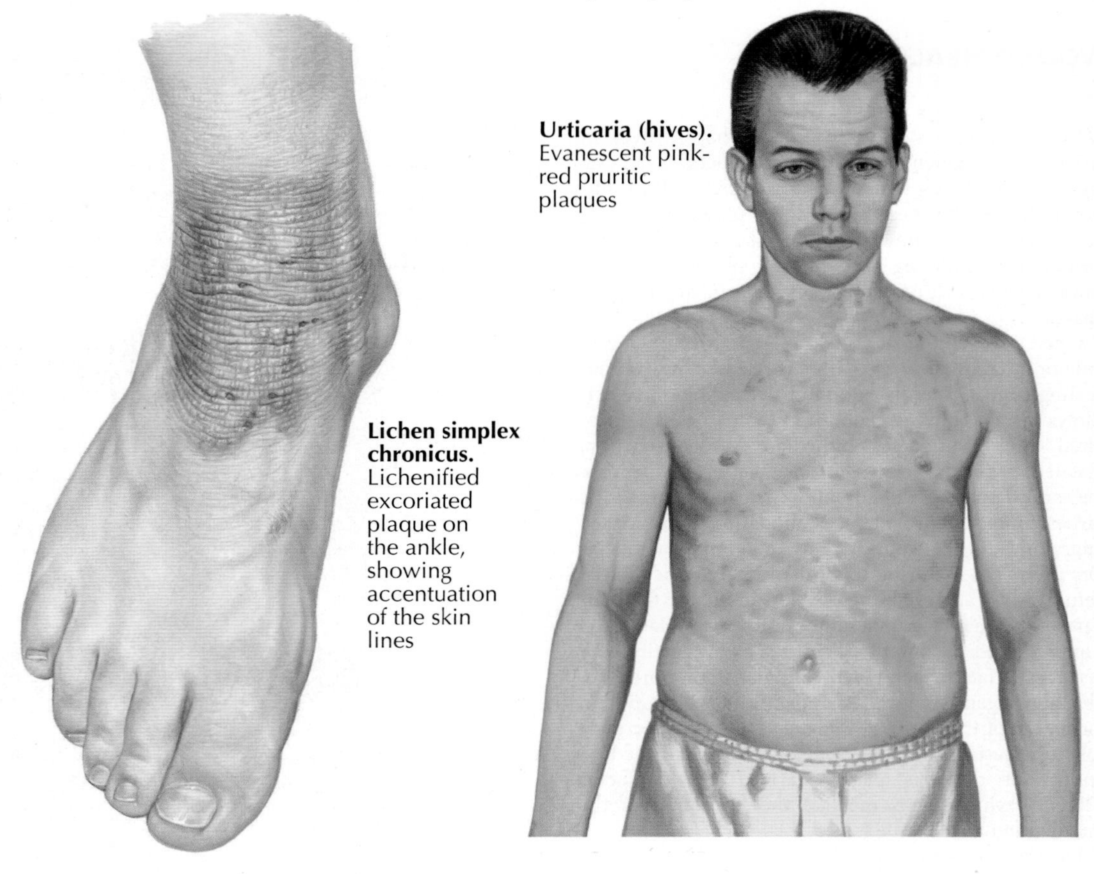

Lichen simplex chronicus. Lichenified excoriated plaque on the ankle, showing accentuation of the skin lines

Urticaria (hives). Evanescent pink-red pruritic plaques

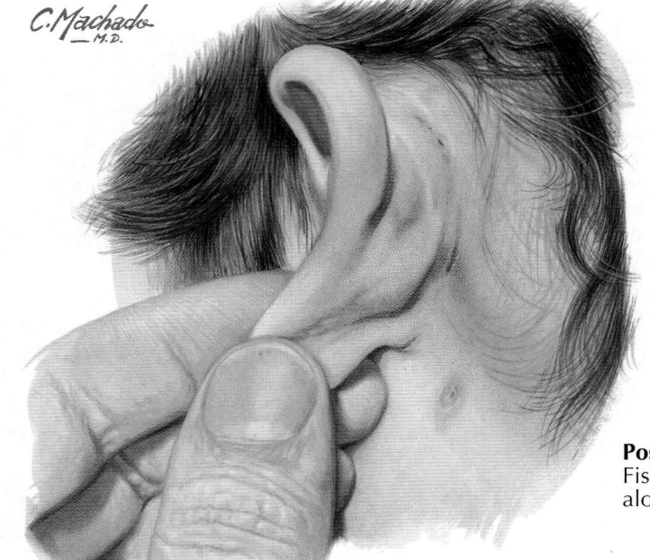

Postauricular fissures. Fissures are linear thin erosions or ulcers along skin lines.

MORPHOLOGY

The first lesson a student of dermatology must learn is how to properly describe skin diseases. Skin morphology has been well defined over the years and is the basis for all discussions about skin disorders. One must be adept at describing skin lesions before it is possible to develop a differential diagnosis. For example, once it has been determined that a rash is in the morphologic category of macule, all rashes in the blistering and nodular categories can easily be excluded from the differential diagnosis. To get a firm grasp of dermatology and to effectively communicate with other medical professionals, one must have an excellent foundation in description and morphology. The most common descriptors used in the dermatology lexicon are discussed here.

Skin lesions and rashes can be described as primary or secondary lesions. The primary category includes bullae, comedones, hives, macules, nodules, papules, patches, plaques, pustules, tumors, and vesicles. The secondary lesions are best described as burrows, crusts, erosions, excoriations, fissures, lichenification, scars, scales, and ulcerations.

Many adjectives are used in conjunction with primary and secondary descriptive terms to better characterize the lesion and to help determine a differential diagnosis and, ultimately, a diagnosis for the patient. Color is of utmost importance and is universally used in the description of skin lesions. For example, a good description of melanoma would include color, size, regularity, and the primary morphology, such as "a dark black, 2 cm, irregularly shaped macule with a central nodule."

Other descriptive terms often used in dermatology deal with the configuration of the lesion, such as a linear or annular configuration. Words such as *arcuate*, *polycyclical*, *nummular*, and *agminated* are commonly used. Some skin rashes tend to follow specific types of skin lines, most commonly Langer lines (skin tension lines) and Blaschko's lines (embryologic cleavage lines).

The distribution of skin lesions is also important because some skin diseases have a propensity to occur in specific areas of the body. A classic example is acne, which typically affects the face, upper back, and chest. It would be inappropriate to consider acne in the differential diagnosis of a rash on the hands and feet.

Starting with the primary skin lesions, a macule is most often thought of as a well-circumscribed, flat area on the skin with a distinct color change. The macule may have an irregular or a regular border. Macules are not raised or scaly and are essentially nonpalpable. An example of a macule is vitiligo.

A papule is a well-circumscribed, small (<5 mm in diameter) elevation in the skin of variable color. A papule is solid and should not be confused with a vesicle. Papules may be described as flat-topped or umbilicated, and their consistency may be characterized as soft or firm. An example of an umbilicated papule is molluscum contagiosum.

Comedones are seen in acne and in a few less-common conditions. They come in two forms: open and closed. Open comedones are also known as *blackheads*, which are easily recognized. Each comedo represents a dilated follicular infundibulum with a buildup of an oxidized keratin plug. Closed comedones are seen as tiny white papules, which are produced when the follicular epithelium sticks together and seals the follicular orifice. These tiny plugs of keratin can be easily expressed from the skin with lateral pressure.

The word *patch* is sometimes used to describe a large macule. A more precise definition of a patch is an area of the skin that is not elevated but has surface change such as scale or crust. The classic example of a patch is seen in tinea corporis. Depending on the source or reference review, the term patch can include either of these two definitions.

A plaque is a well-defined lesion that has a plateau-like elevation and is typically larger than 5 mm in diameter. The term plaque can also be used to describe a confluence of papules. An example of a plaque is a lesion of psoriasis.

A nodule is defined as a space-occupying lesion in the dermis or subcutaneous tissue. Its breadth is

MORPHOLOGY (Continued)

MORPHOLOGY: MACULES, PATCHES, AND VESICULOPUSTULES

Vitiligo. Depigmented macules

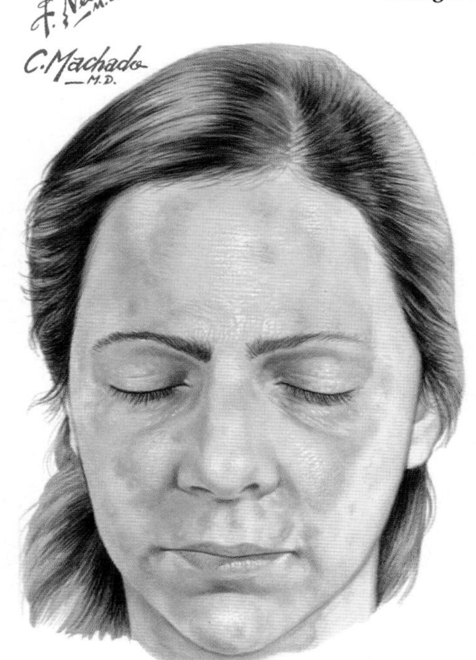

Tinea faciei. Annular scaly patches with a leading edge of scale

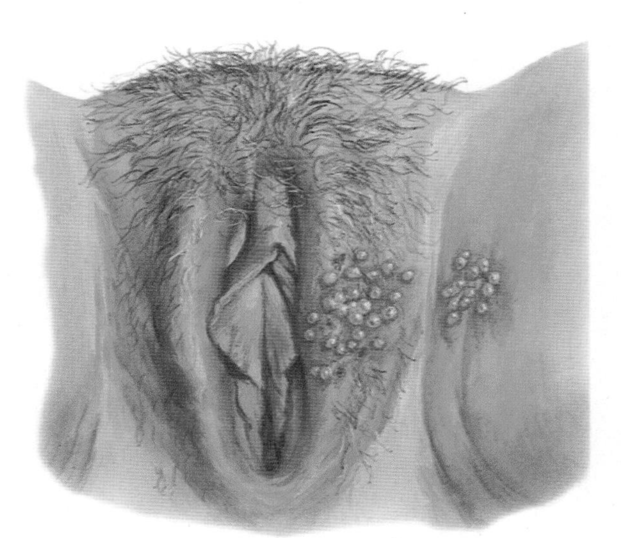

Herpes simplex virus. Tender vesiculopustule on a red base

typically larger than its height. Surface changes may or may not be present. Most authors agree that nodules are typically larger than 1 cm in diameter, and they can be much larger.

A tumor is generally considered to be larger than 2 cm in diameter, and the term should be reserved exclusively for the description of malignant neoplasms. The words *tumor* and *nodule* are sometimes used interchangeably, which can cause confusion. Tumors can be elevated from the skin and located entirely in the epidermis, or they can be space-occupying lesions in the dermis or subcutaneous tissue. Tumors often develop necrosis over time because of their neoplastic nature. A classic example is a fungating skin tumor, as seen with mycosis fungoides.

Hives or wheals are also known as *urticaria*; this is a very specific term used to describe evanescent, pink-red, pruritic plaques that spontaneously develop and remit within 24 hours. Dermatographism is commonly seen in association with hives.

Blistering disorders are common pathologic conditions, and their lesions may be described as vesicles or bullae. A vesicle is defined as a fluid-filled elevation less than 1 cm in diameter. A bulla is a fluid-filled epidermal cavity larger than 1 cm in diameter. Blisters are most often filled with serous fluid, but they can be filled with a purulent exudate or a hemorrhagic infiltrate. Bullae are often described as flaccid and fragile or as firm and intact. Intact firm bullae are seen in bullous pemphigoid, whereas flaccid fragile bullae are seen in pemphigus vulgaris.

Pustules are small elevations in the epidermis that are filled with neutrophilic debris. The infiltrate within a pustule may be sterile or infectious in nature. An example of a sterile pustule is pustular psoriasis. An example of an infectious pustule is folliculitis.

Secondary lesions are often encountered in the dermatology clinic and are of utmost importance when describing skin lesions and rashes. The word *scale* is used to describe exfoliating keratinocytes that have typically built up in such a mass that there is obvious surface change to the skin. Normal shedding of keratinocytes occurs on a daily basis, so a small amount of scale is found on every human's skin. It is the collection in large quantities that allows one to use scale as a descriptive term. Scale must be differentiated from crust. Crust is produced by the drying of blood, serum, or purulent drainage. Most commonly, a crust is described as a scab. Lesions of psoriasis will often form a characteristic silvery scale.

Excoriations are secondary lesions that develop as a result of repetitive scratching. They are typically linear but can be seen in many bizarre configurations.

Erosions are seen in many skin disorders, most commonly superficial blistering diseases, in which the upper layers of the epidermis have been removed, leaving a shallow, denuded erosion. Erosions are defined as breaks in the epidermis. This is in contrast to ulceration, which is defined as a break in the skin that extends into the dermis or subcutaneous tissue or, in severe cases, muscular tissue. A fissure is often seen on the palms or soles; it is a full-thickness epidermal break that follows the skin lines. Fissures have very sharply defined borders and are typically only a few centimeters long.

Scar is another secondary descriptive term used to describe the healing of the epidermis and dermis, usually in a linear or a geographic pattern, caused by some form of trauma or end-stage inflammatory process. Fresh scars are typically pink to red; over time, they mature, becoming flattened and dyspigmented. Lichenification is seen as an end process in chronically rubbed skin. The skin lines become accentuated, and the entire skin becomes thickened from chronic rubbing. A classic example of lichenification is lichen simplex chronicus.

The last of the secondary descriptive lesions discussed here are burrows. Burrows are seen as tiny, irregularly shaped, serpiginous or linear scale, often with a tiny black dot at one end. They are pathognomonic for the diagnosis of scabies, and the tiny black dot represents the scabies mite.

BENIGN GROWTHS

ACROCHORDON

Acrochordons are better known by their common name of skin tag or fibroepithelial polyp. They are found universally in adulthood, and it is possible that every adult has at least one skin tag located somewhere across the surface of his or her skin. Except for a few loose associations with certain syndromes, skin tags are benign growths and have no medical importance and are most often clinically ignored.

Clinical Findings: Skin tags can be found throughout the adult population. They have no sex or race predilection. They are completely benign skin growths that have no malignant potential. They are most commonly located in the axillae, on the neck, in the groin area, and on the eyelids but can be found in other locations. Skin tags are almost never seen in children. The finding of a skin tag in a child should lead one to perform a biopsy to rule out a basal cell carcinoma. Basal cell carcinoma syndrome has been well documented to manifest in children and has been shown to mimic the appearance of skin tags in this population. If a skin tag in a child is discovered to be basal cell carcinoma, the patient should immediately be evaluated for basal cell carcinoma syndrome.

Most skin tags are minute, 1 to 5 mm in length, with a skin-colored to slightly hyperpigmented appearance. They are pedunculated papules that appear as outpouchings of the skin with a stalk-like base. They are soft and nontender. Occasionally, larger skin tags are found with a thickened or a more sessile stalk. These larger skin tags may approach 1 to 1.5 cm in length with a 5-mm base. Most individuals have more than one skin tag, and some individuals are afflicted with hundreds of them.

On occasion a patient will present with a painful, necrotic skin tag. This is most commonly caused by trauma to the skin tag or twisting of the base that results in strangulation of the blood supply and subsequent necrosis. In these cases, removal is advised. If the appearance or clinical history is not classic, the specimen should be sent for pathologic evaluation.

Many investigations have looked at the association of skin tags and underlying medical disorders with conflicting and confusing results. Patients with multiple skin tags may be at a higher risk for glucose intolerance. Some studies have even suggested that patients with multiple skin tags are at a higher risk for colonic polyps, but this is subject to debate.

Pathogenesis: The pathogenesis of skin tags is believed to be a localized overgrowth of fibroblasts within the dermis. The incidence increases with age. They may be more common during pregnancy, and they have been shown to be increased in patients with increased weight. This has led some to implicate insulin-like growth factor-1 as a possible driver of skin tag formation. The initiating factor, however, is not completely understood.

Histology: The overlying epidermis is essentially normal. The skin tag appears as an outgrowth of the skin. The dermis appears normal, and there is minimal, if any, inflammatory infiltrate. Thrombosed or strangulated skin tags show necrosis of the dermis and epidermis and thrombosis of the superficial supplying blood vessels. There is no atypia present.

Treatment: No therapy is necessary for these extraordinarily common skin growths. They are mostly overlooked and not even mentioned on routine skin examination. The rare strangulated or thrombosed skin tag can be removed easily with a forceps and skin tag removal scissors after injection of a local anesthetic. If cosmetic removal is desired, it can easily be done by cleaning the skin with alcohol or chlorhexidine and removing individual skin tags with a forceps and skin tag removal scissors. Application of aluminum chloride after removal causes the superficial bleeding to stop.

Screening of individuals with skin tags for errors in glucose metabolism or for colonic polyps is controversial but should be performed if other findings in the review of systems or the clinical history and physical examination suggest one of these underlying disorders.

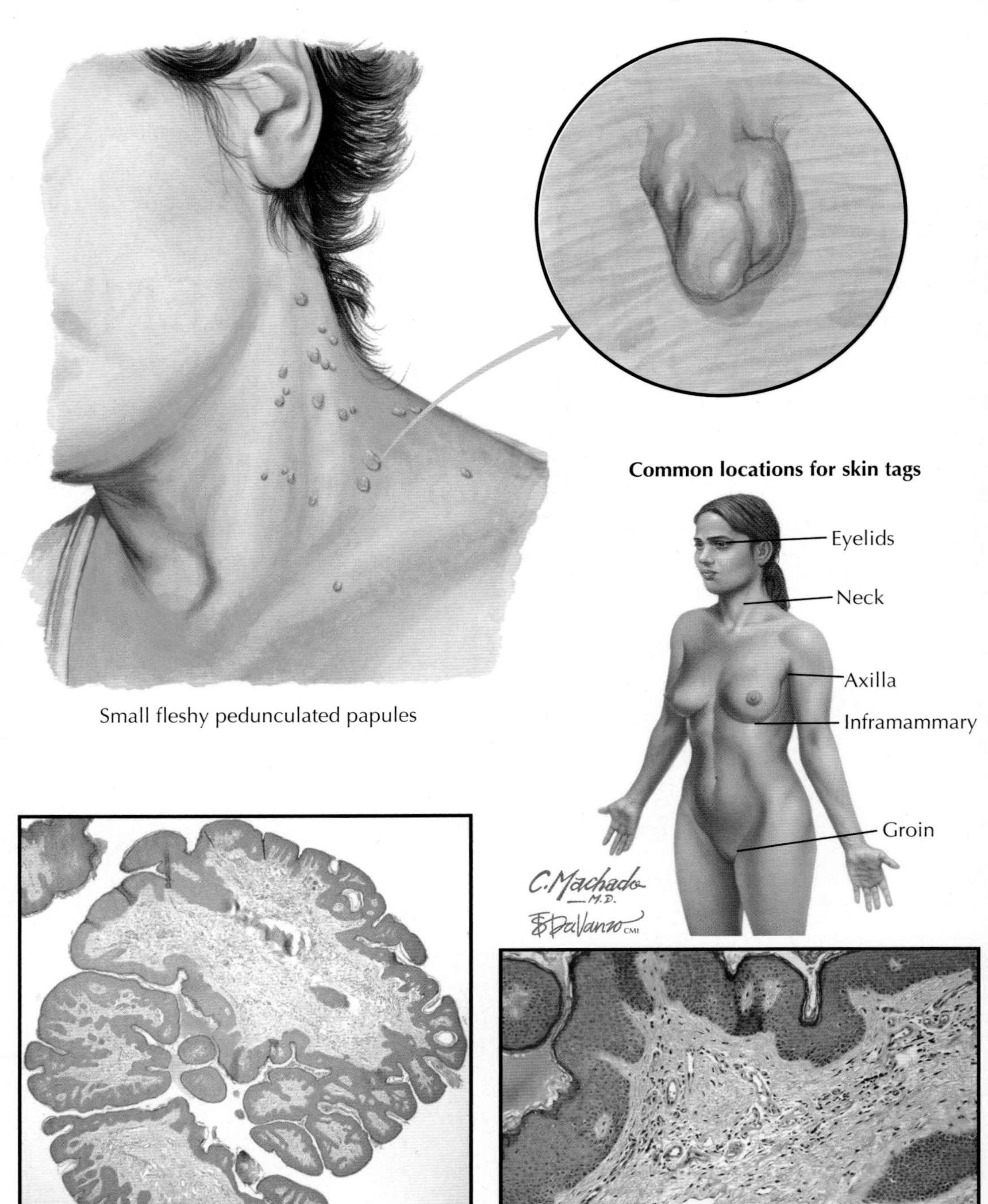

Small fleshy pedunculated papules

Low power. The pedunculated skin tag is bisected horizontally. It has a symmetrical appearance, with many small dermal capillaries present within a background of collagen bundles.

High power. A slightly acanthotic epidermis is seen overlying a vascular dermis with plentiful collagen.

Becker's Nevus (Smooth Muscle Hamartoma)

Becker's nevi most commonly appear on the shoulder or upper limb girdle of prepubescent boys. It is a rather common benign condition that is seen in up to 0.5% of the male population. It is less commonly seen in females. Becker's nevi are acquired nevi that can develop at birth or any time before puberty but are most often recognized around puberty. The average age of onset has been estimated at 10 years. Becker's nevus is classified as a smooth muscle hamartoma. It does not contain melanocytic nevus cells and is not considered to be a melanocytic nevus. It was named for the dermatologist Samuel Becker, who first described this condition.

Clinical Findings: Becker's nevi begin as ill-defined, slightly hyperpigmented macules, most frequently on the upper limb girdle, from a few centimeters in size to over 20 cm. Within a year of puberty, the hyperpigmented region often develops hypertrichosis, resulting in its characteristic appearance. Becker's nevi may occur anywhere on the body, but by far the most common locations are on the shoulder, upper chest, and back. The area of hypertrichosis is limited to the underlying hyperpigmented area. The clinical significance of Becker's nevi is its differentiation from large congenital nevi and café-au-lait macules. Becker's nevi confer no increased risk for development of melanoma, and they are rarely associated with any underlying abnormalities. The most common underlying abnormality is unilateral hypoplasia of the breast. Hypoplasia of the breast may require reconstructive surgery. Rarely, a patient with a Becker's nevus has underlying hypoplasia of bone and soft tissue, the cause of which is unknown. The differential diagnosis includes a giant congenital nevus and a café-au-lait macule. These two conditions should be easily differentiated from Becker's nevi because they both are typically apparent at birth or soon thereafter, whereas Becker's nevi are typically acquired at about the age of 10 years.

The diagnosis is typically made on clinical findings, but a skin biopsy is sometimes needed to confirm the diagnosis if the nevus is in an unusual anatomic location. The punch biopsy is the best method for obtaining tissue.

Pathogenesis: The pathogenesis of Becker's nevus is unclear. It is believed to be caused by the dermal presence of hamartomatous smooth muscle tissue. Research has shown that the tissue in Becker's nevi has an increased number of androgen receptors. It is thought that increased androgen levels at puberty interact with the excessive androgen receptors and cause the clinical findings.

Histology: The biopsy specimen shows a smooth muscle hamartoma. Multiple smooth muscle fascicles are seen within the dermis. There is an increased ratio of terminal to vellus hairs and a lack of melanocytic nevus cells. The hyperpigmentation results from an increased formation of pigmentation within the melanocytes of the stratum basalis. Melanosomes are increased in number and are enlarged. There is no increase in the number of melanocytes. Varying amounts of acanthosis and hyperkeratosis are seen.

Becker's nevus is the most common type of smooth muscle hamartoma in the skin. Smooth muscle hamartomas by themselves are rarely found within the skin. Non-Becker's smooth muscle hamartomas are usually present at birth or soon thereafter and manifest as small, flesh-colored plaques located anywhere on the body. All smooth muscle hamartomas may at some point exhibit the pseudo-Darier's sign. To clinically elicit this sign, gently rub the smooth muscle hamartoma; the lesion may fasciculate because of smooth muscle activity, or the region may develop an urticarial appearance. This sign has nothing to do with histamine release; rather, it is caused by a neurally mediated contraction of the underlying hamartomatous smooth muscle tissue.

Treatment: No therapy is required. Surgical excision is likely to produce a mutilating scar unless the nevus is extraordinarily small. The hypertrichosis can be treated for cosmetic purposes with any of a multitude of therapies, including laser removal, shaving, and electrolysis. Most patients prefer to not treat the area. With improvements in laser therapy, the hyperpigmentation can been treated with varying results. The best results have been with the use of a combination of various laser wavelengths.

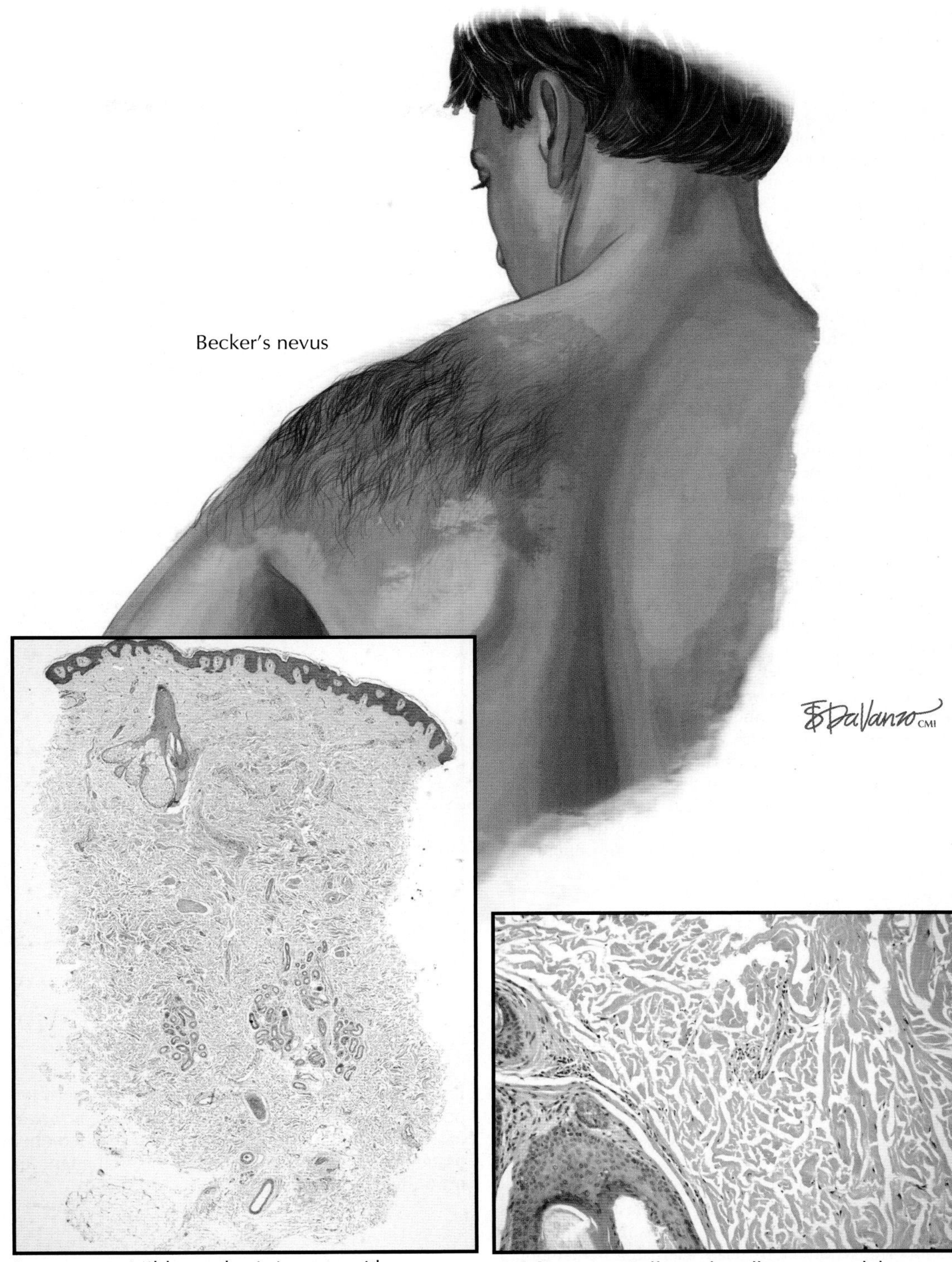

Low power. Mild acanthosis is seen, with hyperpigmentation present within the basal cell layer. Prominent sebaceous glands are present.

High power. Collagen bundles surround the prominent adnexal structures.

DERMATOFIBROMA (SCLEROSING HEMANGIOMA)

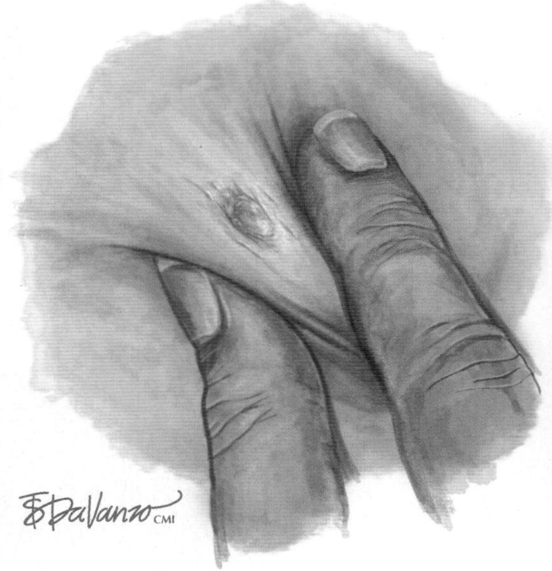

Dermatofibroma. Demonstrating the "dimple sign"

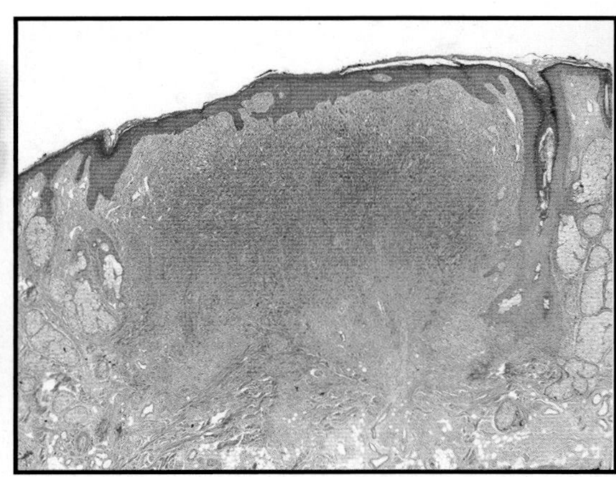

Low power. There is a dermal proliferation of spindle-shaped fibroblasts. The epidermis centrally shows acanthosis and basilar hyperpigmentation. The tumor cells do not reach to the subcutaneous tissue.

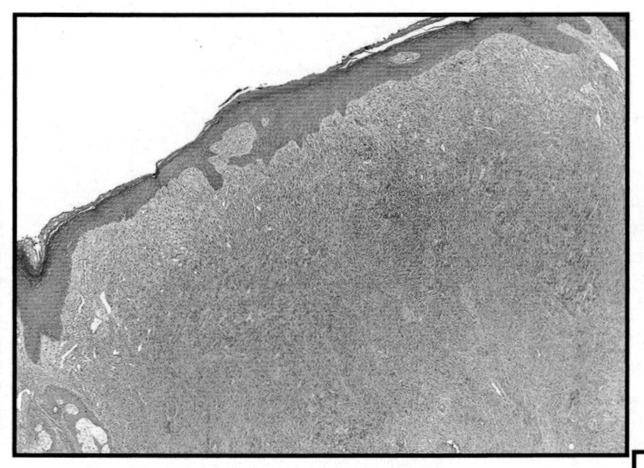

High power. Multiple spindle-shaped fibroblasts are arranged in a whorled pattern.

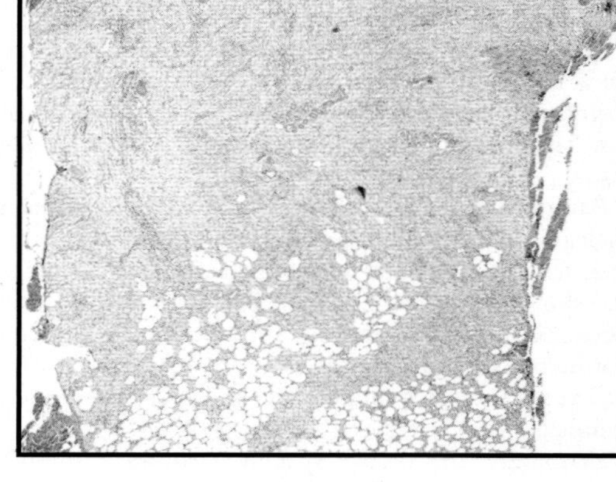

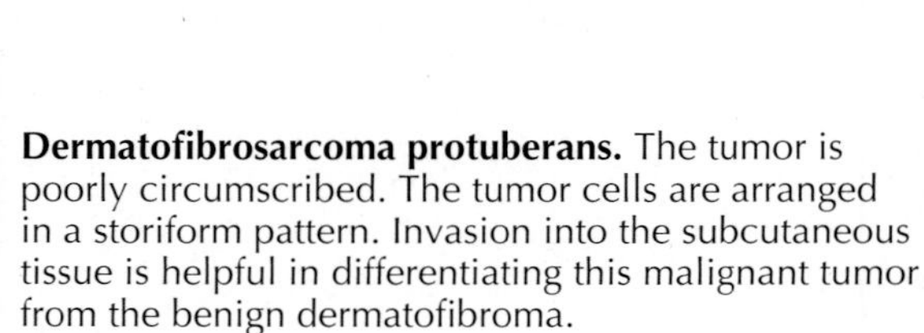

Dermatofibrosarcoma protuberans. The tumor is poorly circumscribed. The tumor cells are arranged in a storiform pattern. Invasion into the subcutaneous tissue is helpful in differentiating this malignant tumor from the benign dermatofibroma.

Dermatofibromas are among the most common types of benign skin growths. They usually occur on the extremities, with a predilection for the legs. There is some debate as to whether this is a true neoplasm or an inflammatory reaction.

Clinical Findings: Dermatofibromas are seen almost exclusively in adults, and females tend to be afflicted slightly more often than males. There is no race predilection. Dermatofibromas can range in diameter from 2 mm to 2 cm. They are round or oval. Most often they are solitary, but numerous dermatofibromas may be present in an individual. Dermatofibromas are usually small (4–5 mm), firm, red to slightly purple papules that dimple with lateral pressure. This "dimple sign" is often used clinically to differentiate dermatofibromas from other growths. There are many variations of dermatofibromas clinically. Elevated dome-shaped papules or plaques may be seen. The surface may have a slight amount of scale, and occasionally there is hyperpigmentation. Dermoscopic evaluation of dermatofibromas may show a central white scar-like area. On the lower legs of females, they are often excoriated as a result of shaving, which is often the reason the patient presents for evaluation. Dermatofibromas are most frequently asymptomatic, but they can be slightly pruritic. They are rarely tender.

Individuals often develop more than one dermatofibroma but rarely more than four or five. If dermatofibromas are numerous and located in different regions of the body, the clinician should consider a possible association with an underlying immunodeficiency state. There have been reports of multiple eruptive dermatofibromas, with more than 10 in patients with systemic lupus erythematosus, human immunodeficiency virus infection, and other immunosuppressive states. Dermatofibromas in these patients have been shown to contain more mast cells.

The differential diagnosis of a dermatofibroma can be broad. If the dermatofibroma does not exhibit the dimple sign or presents a diagnostic challenge, the lesion can be biopsied to help differentiate it from a melanocytic nevus, melanoma, basal cell carcinoma, dermatofibrosarcoma protuberans (DFSP), prurigo papules, and other epidermal and dermal tumors.

Pathogenesis: The precipitating factor that initiates the formation of a dermatofibroma is thought to be superficial trauma, such as from a bug bite, which causes the fibrous tissue proliferation. The exact etiology is unknown.

Histology: Dermatofibromas are made up of a collection of dermal spindle-shaped fibroblasts. Histiocytes and myofibroblasts are also found throughout the lesion. The synonymous term sclerosing hemangioma arises when numerous extravasated red blood cells are seen within the dermatofibroma. Characteristically, the overlying epidermis is acanthotic with broadening of the rete ridges. The rete ridges are slightly hyperpigmented, which is sometimes referred to as "dirty feet" or "dirty fingers." This finding explains the hyperpigmentation seen clinically.

Dermatofibromas stain positively for factor XIIIa and negatively for CD34. This is the opposite of the staining pattern seen in DFSP. Immunohistochemical staining also provides a marker that can be used to help distinguish the benign dermatofibroma (which stains with stromelysin-3) from the malignant DFSP (which does not). In contrast to DFSP, dermatofibromas do not infiltrate the underlying adipose tissue. Dermatofibromas can push down or displace the adipose tissue, but they never truly demonstrate an infiltrative pattern as does a DFSP. There are numerous histologic variants of dermatofibromas, including fibrous, cellular, hemosiderotic, epitheloid, and atrophic, to name a few.

Treatment: Most dermatofibromas are not treated in any manner. Complete elliptical excision with a minimal 1- to 2-mm margin is curative. The resulting scar may be more noticeable than the initial dermatofibroma. For dermatofibromas that are 5 mm or less in size, a punch biopsy can be used with good cosmetic results. The specimen can be sent for pathologic evaluation, and the resulting punch biopsy can be sutured with one or two fine sutures. There is no evidence to support the routine removal of these common tumors to prevent malignant degeneration into a DFSP. One must remember that dermatofibromas are extraordinarily common, whereas DFSP is exceedingly rare. Malignant degeneration of dermatofibromas into DFSP has been reported, but this is likely the exception and not the rule.

ECCRINE POROMA

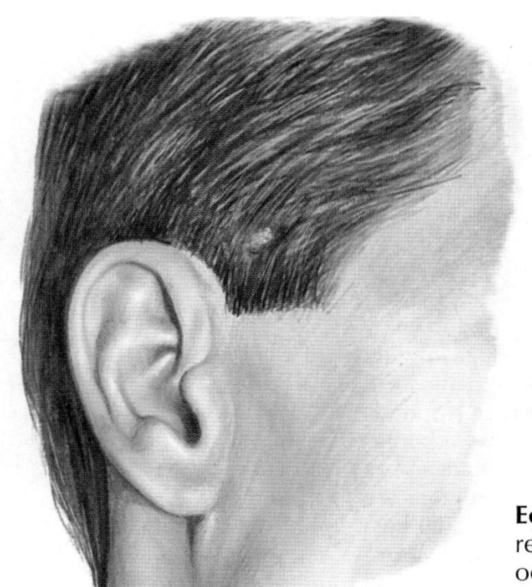

Eccrine poroma on the scalp. Glistening red papule or nodule that can be located at any location.

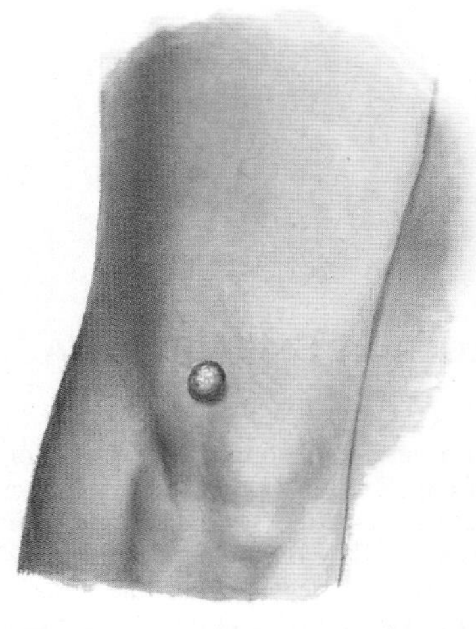

Eccrine porocarcinoma. Nondescript red papule or nodule. Ulceration may occur. A biopsy is required to diagnose this rare form of skin cancer.

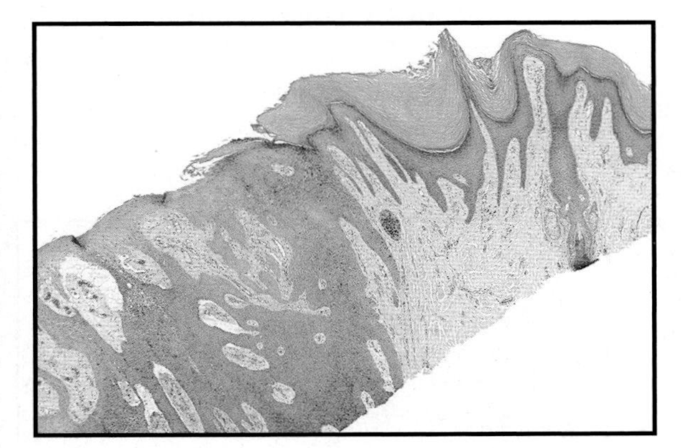

Low power. The tumor appears as an extension of the epidermis. The finger-like projections of tumor cells extend into the dermis. There is a clear difference between keratinocytes and the smaller tumor cells. Many blood vessels are present within the tumor stroma.

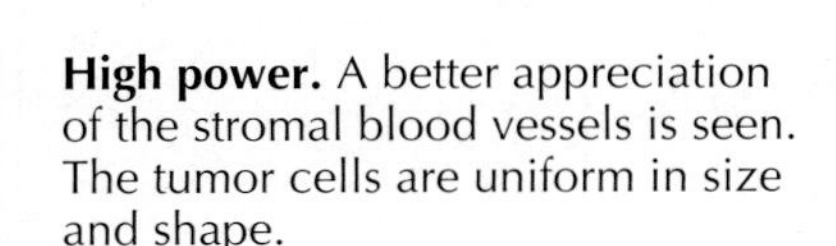

High power. A better appreciation of the stromal blood vessels is seen. The tumor cells are uniform in size and shape.

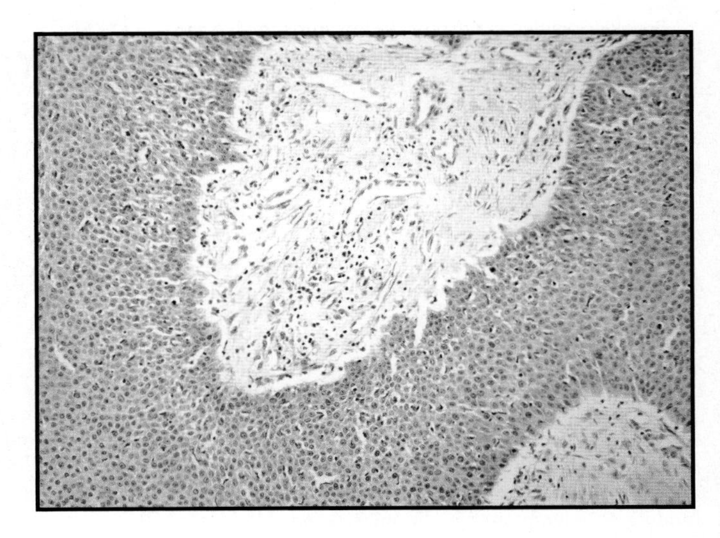

Eccrine poromas are the most common tumors in the poroma family of skin tumors. Other tumors in this family include the dermal ductal tumor, the poroid hidradenoma, and the hidroacanthoma. In general, these are rare tumors with a low incidence. Eccrine porocarcinoma is the rare malignant counterpart to the eccrine poroma. Eccrine poromas develop from the appendageal structures of the skin. These are benign adnexal tumors of the skin. The all-encompassing term *poroma* is more accurate in that it appears that not all of these tumors are derived from eccrine structures. There is evidence that the cell of origin is actually apocrine. Other possibilities for the cell of origin include the sebaceous gland and the follicular epithelium.

Clinical Findings: Eccrine poromas are uncommon tumors of the skin. They occur equally in men and women and almost exclusively in the adult population. These tumors are most often seen in the sixth to eighth decades of life. They are typically small tumors, ranging from 5 to 20 mm. They are most frequently found on the soles and palms. As many as 50% to 60% of these tumors have been found on the sole, but they have can occur in any skin location. Pain and bleeding are the two most common symptoms encountered. A poroma may be found secondarily in a nevus sebaceus or after radiation treatment. Eccrine poromas tend to have a vascular appearance and often manifest as a friable red or purplish papule or nodule. They are almost always solitary in nature, and they easily bleed when traumatized. On inspection, the eccrine poroma often has a slight, dell-like depression surrounding the tumor. This is more commonly seen on acral skin. This dell, when seen by the perceptive clinician, often leads to a differential diagnosis that includes an eccrine poroma. There are no specific clinical criteria used to make the diagnosis. The differential diagnosis includes vascular tumors, metastatic lesions (particularly the vascular renal cell carcinoma metastasis), pyogenic granuloma, and melanoma because some eccrine poromas exhibit pigmentation. The diagnosis is made by histologic examination after biopsy.

Histology: Eccrine poromas show varying degrees of ductal differentiation. The tumor is well circumscribed and has characteristic features. The keratinocytes have been described as cuboidal. They tend to be small and have an increased nuclear to cytoplasmic volume. Necrosis is often seen in parts of the tumor. The ductal portions of the tumor are lined by an eosinophilic layer or cuticle. The stromal portions of the tumor are rich in vascular components. This vascular element imparts the red appearance to the tumor. Eccrine poromas can be histologically classified as other members of the poroma family of tumors based on their location in the skin. The necrosis and vascular components of the tumors can explain the pain and bleeding that these tumors often exhibit. As an example, the hidroacanthoma, a member of this family, is defined as an eccrine poroma that is entirely located in the epidermis.

The eccrine porocarcinoma is very uncommon; histologically, it is a tumor that is poorly circumscribed and often found in conjunction with an eccrine poroma. Cells with multiple large nuclei and multiple mitoses help make the diagnosis. Eccrine porocarcinomas can mimic metastatic adenocarcinomas, and immunohistochemical staining is required to confirm the diagnosis.

Treatment: Although they are benign tumors, eccrine poromas often are located on the sole or palm and require removal from a functional standpoint. Surgical excision with a small (1–2 mm), conservative margin is curative. Because porocarcinomas have been shown to develop from a preexisting poroma, complete surgical excision is often recommended for most poromas. The recurrence rate is very low after surgical excision. Electrodesiccation and curettage have been used successfully. Eccrine porocarcinomas require surgical excision and close clinical follow-up for recurrence. Chemotherapy is reserved for cases of metastatic disease. The role of sentinel lymph node sampling in these tumors has yet to be defined.

ECCRINE SPIRADENOMA

Eccrine spiradenomas are uncommon benign tumors of the skin. Most often they are solitary in nature. On occasion a patient will be afflicted with multiple spiradenomas. They occur in conjunction with cylindromas in Brooke-Spiegler syndrome. Eccrine spiradenomas can arise in any location on the human body but are most frequently found on the head and neck. The next most common region is the ventral trunk; they are rarely seen on the extremities. Spiradenomas tend to appear between the ages of 15 and 40 years, although they have been reported to occur at any age. Malignant degeneration is extremely rare, and when it does occur, it is often fatal.

Clinical Findings: A spiradenoma usually manifests as a solitary dermal nodule or papule ranging from 5 to 20 mm in diameter, with an average size of approximately 10 mm. They are typically seated deep in the dermis and can be very painful to light touch. Most will be tender to palpation to some extent. The tumors grow very slowly and, except for the pain, can go unnoticed for some time. The pain tends to have a waxing and waning course, and it is typically the reason the patient seeks medical advice. The overlying epidermis is almost always normal. The dermal nodule sometimes takes on a purple or bluish coloration. Although they are most commonly solitary, multiple spiradenomas may be seen in association with multiple cylindromas in Brooke-Spiegler syndrome.

Brooke-Spiegler syndrome is an autosomal dominant inherited skin condition caused by a genetic defect in the *CYLD* gene. This syndrome is characterized by multiple cylindromas, spiradenomas, and trichoepitheliomas. The tumors usually begin in the third decade of life and increase in number and size throughout the patient's life. *CYLD* encodes a tumor suppressor protein that is an important downregulator of the nuclear factor-κB pathway. The clinical phenotype varies depending on the type of mutation in this gene. Patients with familial cylindromatosis also have defects in this gene. The gene has been localized to the long arm of chromosome 16.

The eccrine spiradenoma is considered one of the group of unique tumors that can cause painful dermal nodules. This group also includes angiolipomas, neuromas, glomus tumors, and leiomyomas. This collection of tumors makes up the clinical differential diagnosis when evaluating these painful dermal nodules. If the nodule is asymptomatic, lipomas, cysts, and other adnexal tumors would also be considered in the differential diagnosis. A skin biopsy is required for diagnosis.

The exact cell type from which the spiradenomas are derived is still undetermined. They were originally believed to arise from eccrine tissue, but increasing evidence points to a derivation from apocrine tissue.

Histology: The histologic hallmark of an eccrine spiradenoma is the appearance of large nests of basophilic cells in the dermis. There are no epidermal changes, and the multilobulated tumors do not connect with the epidermis. This gives rise to the description "blue balls in the dermis." The tumor is composed of two unique cell types. Large, pale cells predominate, with surrounding aggregates of smaller basophilic cells that contain hyperchromatic nuclei. The tumor is well circumscribed and is surrounded by a fibrous capsule.

Treatment: Surgical excision is curative. Surgical removal with carbon dioxide laser ablation has also been found to be highly successful. Because of the number and size of the tumors in patients with Brooke-Spiegler syndrome, a multidisciplinary approach is often taken. Malignant degeneration is believed to be a rare occurrence. If malignant transformation occurs, it is typically in a long-standing lesion that has changed in some manner. Rapid growth, ulceration, and drastic change in tenderness may be clues to malignant transformation and warrant evaluation and biopsy. There is currently no consensus on appropriate surgical margins for removal of these tumors. Dermatologic and plastic surgeons are often the primary physicians removing these tumors.

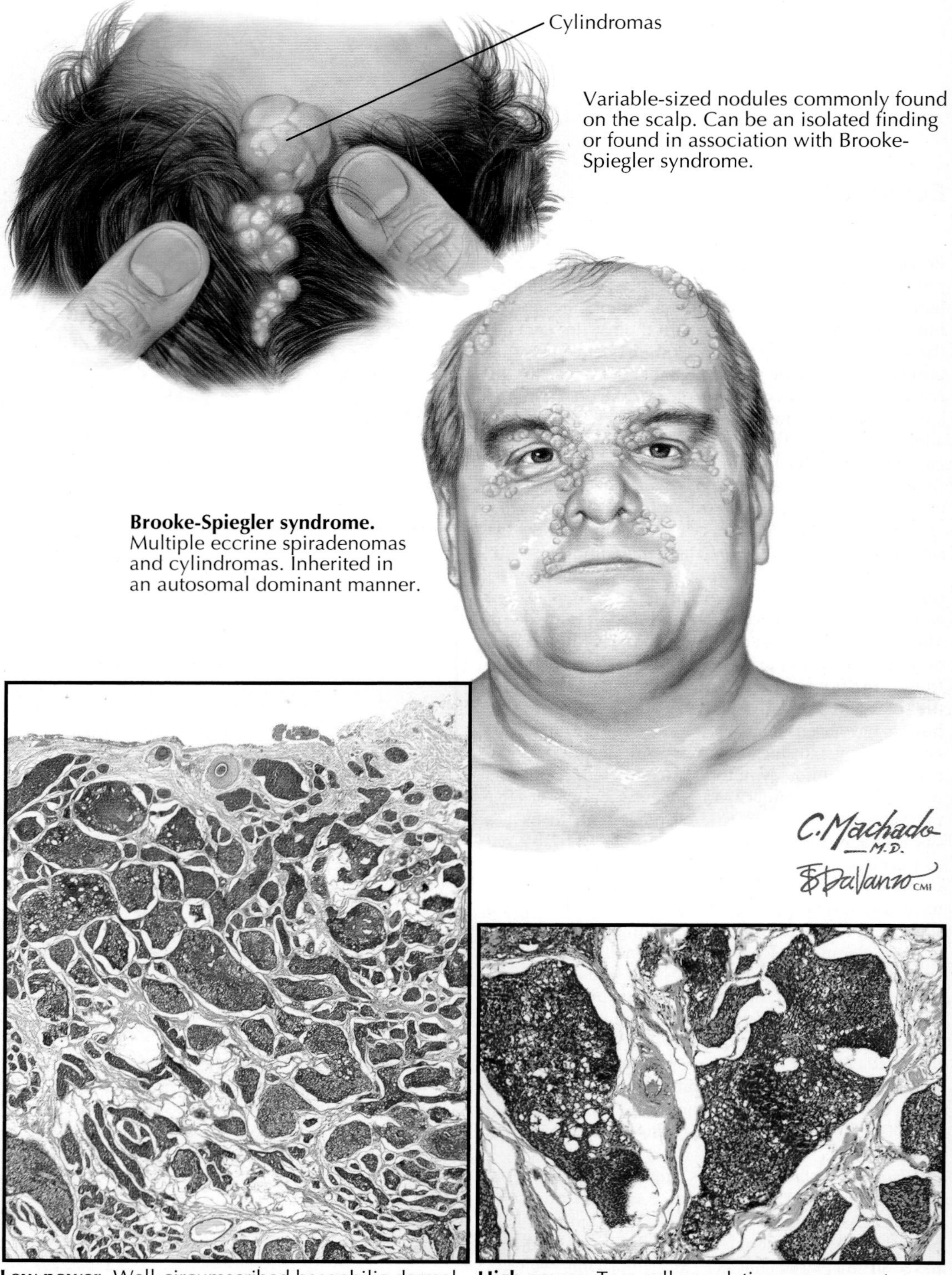

Low power. Well-circumscribed basophilic dermal nodule within the dermis

High power. Two cell populations are present, a larger pale cell type and a peripheral smaller basophilic cell type.

ECCRINE SYRINGOMA

Eccrine syringomas are extremely common benign skin growths. They are most often found on the lower eyelids and malar cheek regions of adults. These small tumors are of no clinical significance and are routinely ignored in clinical practice.

Clinical Findings: Eccrine syringomas are one of the most common benign skin tumors. They are believed to be more common in women than in men. They typically manifest in adulthood as small (2–4 mm), firm, flesh-colored papules on the lower eyelids or upper cheek regions. They are usually multiple and symmetric. Some have a slight yellow or tan hue. Syringomas are also seen on the upper eyelids, neck, and chest. They have been reported to occur on any region of the body. When located on the eyelids and cheeks, they have a characteristic clinic appearance and are diagnosed on clinical appearance alone. On locations other than the face, syringomas are not often in the clinical diagnosis, and the ultimate diagnosis of a syringoma in one of these locations will require a biopsy.

Plaque-like syringomas have been reported to occur on the forehead, and they have the appearance of a flesh-colored to slightly yellow, broad, flat plaque with minimal to no surface change. They can be quite large, up to 4 to 5 cm in diameter. They are essentially asymptomatic, but occasionally a patient complains of slight intermittent itching or of an increase in size with strenuous physical activity. This is possibly explained by the eccrine nature of the tumors: under conditions of activity, an increase in sweating causes the tumors to transiently appear to enlarge. There are specific variants seen in patients with diabetes mellitus (clear cell). Individuals with Down syndrome have a much higher incidence of syringomas, and eruptive syringomas are also more common in this population. Eruptive syringomas have been described and typically afflict the anterior trunk and the penile shaft. Linear syringomas have been reported to occur on a unilateral limb; these have been termed unilateral linear nevoidal syringomas.

The clinical differential diagnosis of eccrine syringomas is relatively limited when the clinician encounters symmetric small papules on the lower eyelids. The differential diagnosis for a solitary syringoma is broad and includes other adnexal tumors as well as basal cell carcinoma. The greatest difficulty arises when reviewing the histologic features of a syringoma that has been biopsied in a superficial manner. If the pathologist is not given a deep enough specimen, the eccrine syringoma can mimic a microcystic adnexal carcinoma. These two tumors, one benign and the other malignant, can have very similar histologic features in the superficial dermis. In some cases, only a full-thickness biopsy can confidently differentiate the two tumors.

Pathogenesis: Eccrine syringomas are believed to be an overgrowth of the eccrine sweat ductal apparatus. Researchers have proposed that this proliferation is caused by an inflammatory response to an as-yet undetermined antigen. The precise pathogenesis of eccrine syringomas is unclear. Familial patterns suggest a genetic predisposition, but most patients do not have a family history to support genetic transmission.

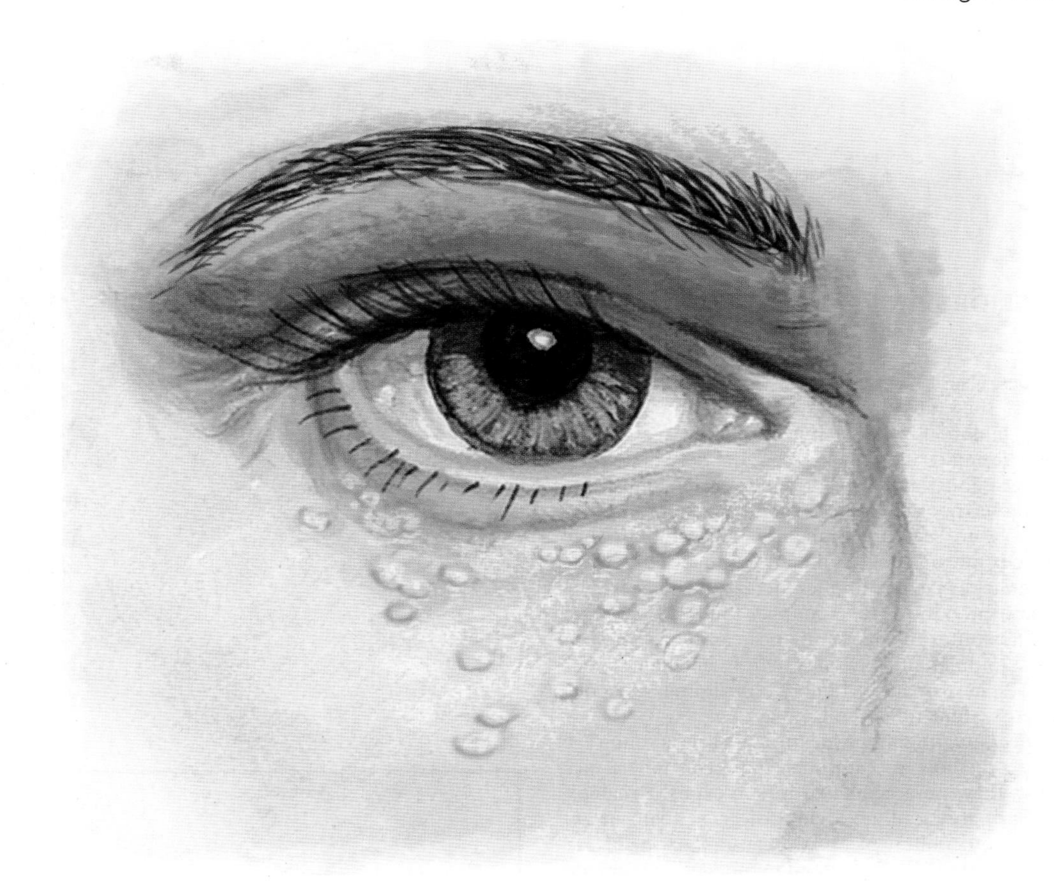

Syringoma. The most common location for syringomas is on the lower eyelid.

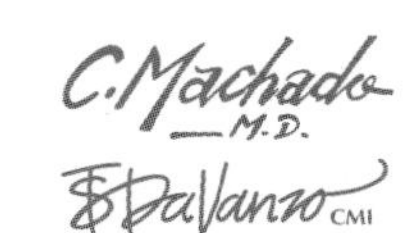

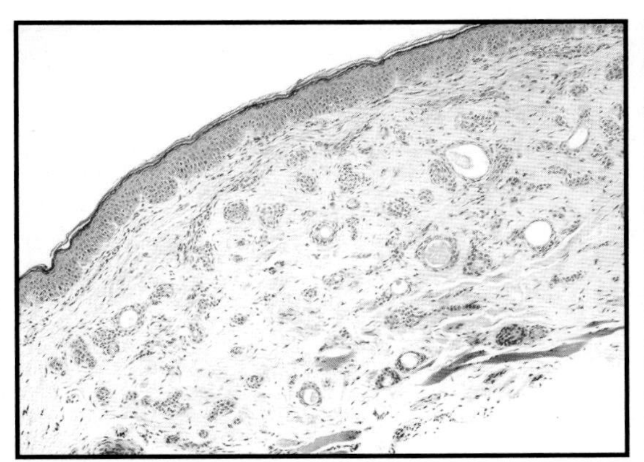

Low power. The overlying epidermis is normal. The tumor is located in the superficial dermis and is made up of comma-shaped dilated ductal eccrine glands.

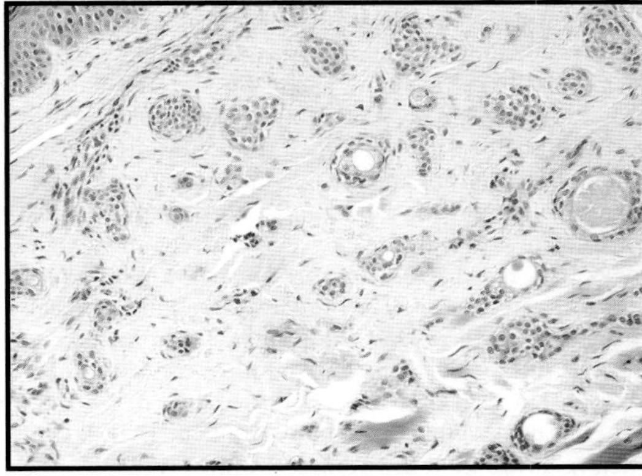

High power. Clusters of cells with a pale cytoplasm are found throughout the tumor. There is a background of sclerotic stromal tissue. The comma-shaped dilated ductal eccrine gland apparatus is apparent.

Histology: The overlying epidermis is normal. The tumor is based within the dermis and is sharply circumscribed. The syringoma typically does not penetrate deeper than the upper third of the dermis. Clusters of cells with a pale cytoplasm are found throughout the tumor. A background of sclerotic stromal tissue is always appreciated. A characteristic finding is the "tadpole" sign. The tadpole- or comma-shaped, dilated ductal eccrine gland apparatus is pathognomonic for eccrine syringoma. Clear cell variants are associated with diabetes mellitus. A microcystic adnexal carcinoma is poorly circumscribed, is asymmetric, and infiltrates into the underlying subcutis.

Treatment: No treatment is necessary. If therapy is desired, it should be done with caution because treatment experiences are anecdotal, and scarring may have a worse appearance than the syringoma itself. Variable results have been reported with electrocautery, light cryotherapy, chemical peels, laser resurfacing, dermabrasion, and excision.

Ephelides and Lentigines

Ephelides, also known as freckles, are common benign findings. They typically manifest in sun-exposed areas during childhood in fair-skinned individuals, especially those with red or blond hair color. The development of ephelides is inherited in an autosomal dominant pattern.

Lentigines are sun-induced proliferations of melanocytes. They are seen predominantly in adulthood. They also occur more frequently in fair-skinned individuals, and the incidence of lentigines increases with age. They may be seen in individuals younger than 20 years after repetitive sun exposure. Lentigines can be almost impossible to differentiate clinically from ephelides. Solar lentigines have many synonyms, including sunspots, liver spots, and lentigo senilis.

Clinical Findings: Ephelides occur at a very young age and tend to show an autosomal dominant inheritance pattern. They are accentuated in sun-exposed regions, particularly the head, neck, and forearms. Exposure to the sun or other ultraviolet source causes the ephelides to become darker and clinically more noticeable. They do not occur within the oral mucosa. They are usually uniform in coloration but can have many different sizes and shapes. Some are round or oval; others are angulated or have a bizarre shape. Their color is usually a uniform light to dark brown; they are never black. They have no malignant potential. Patients with multiple ephelides may have a higher risk for skin cancer because their presence may be an indication of increased exposure to ultraviolet radiation. The differential diagnosis is usually very narrow and includes lentigines and common acquired nevi. The clinical location, age at onset, family history, and skin type usually make the diagnosis straightforward. Difficulty can occur when trying to differentiate a solitary lentigo from an ephelide in an adult patient.

Solar lentigines most often arise in the adult population and are distributed evenly among males and females. They can occur in anyone but are much more common in light-skinned persons. The number of lentigines typically increases with the age of the patient. Lentigines are induced by ultraviolet radiation, the most common source being chronic sun exposure. Lentigines tend to get darker with ultraviolet light exposure and lighten over time when removed from the exposure. Unlike ephelides, they never completely fade away. They are clinically highly uniform in color and size within an individual patient. They can be small (1–5 mm), but some are much larger (2–3 cm in diameter). They are most commonly located in sun-exposed areas but in some syndromes can be located anywhere on the body, including mucosal regions. Over time, some lentigines merge together to form rather large lentigines, which can mimic lentigo maligna.

There are some important variants of lentigines. Lentigo simplex and the ink spot lentigo are two very common versions. Lentigo simplex is believed to occur at any age and to have no or minimal relationship to sun exposure. The lesions are found anywhere on the body. Ink spot lentigines are variants of lentigo simplex that are differentiated by their characteristic dark brown to almost black coloration. Under dermatoscopic evaluation, they have a characteristic uniform pigment network, with accentuation of pigment in the rete ridge regions. They are so named because they have the appearance of a tiny drop of dark ink dropped onto the skin. Neither of these two forms of lentigines has malignant potential.

One of the more important and unique variants of lentigines are the psoralen plus ultraviolet A light (PUVA) lentigines. PUVA lentigines are iatrogenic in nature and occur after medical therapy with PUVA phototherapy treatment. Patients who have undergone long-term therapy with PUVA have a high risk of developing PUVA lentigines. These lentigines are darkly pigmented macules that occur across the entire body except in the areas that were not exposed to the PUVA therapy. More than half of patients who have undergone prolonged PUVA treatment will develop PUVA lentigines. They are more common in patients with fair skin types and rarely occur in darker-skinned individuals. The lentigines induced by PUVA therapy are permanent and can have disastrous cosmetic consequences. Like all patients undergoing ultraviolet phototherapy, these patients must be routinely monitored for their entire

Ephelides

Ephelides, also known as freckles, are most frequently encountered in fair-skinned individuals on sun-exposed skin. Sun exposure causes accentuation.

C. Machado M.D.
DalIanzo CMI

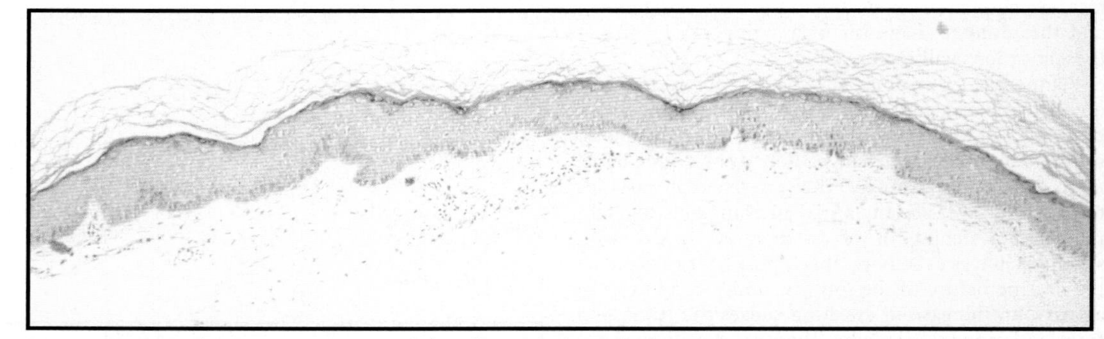

Low power. Basilar pigmentation is uniformly seen along the biopsy specimen. There is no increase in the density of melanocytes present.

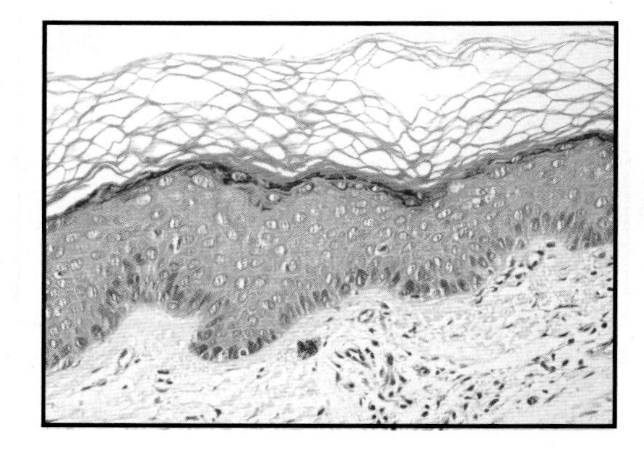

High power. Pigmentation is isolated to the basal layer. A basketweave stratum corneum is seen with a well-formed granular layer.

EPHELIDES AND LENTIGINES (Continued)

lives because they are at increased risk for melanoma and nonmelanoma skin cancer.

Patients with Peutz-Jeghers syndrome have clinical findings of multiple lentigines of the oral mucosa, lips, and hands. These patients are at increased risk for gastrointestinal carcinomas, particularly colon cancer. Peutz-Jeghers syndrome is inherited in an autosomal dominant fashion and is caused by a defect in the *STK11 (LKB1)* tumor suppressor gene.

LEOPARD syndrome is another well-described genetic syndrome associated with lentigines. This syndrome is composed of **l**entigines, **e**lectrocardiographic abnormalities, **o**cular hypertelorism, **p**ulmonary stenosis, **a**bnormal genitalia, **r**etardation of growth, and **d**eafness. It is caused by a genetic mutation in *PTPN11*, which encodes a tyrosine phosphatase protein.

Pathogenesis: Ephelides are thought to be genetically inherited in an autosomal dominant pattern. They become more prominent with sun exposure and fade with less exposure to ultraviolet radiation. The increase in pigment is caused by an increase in the production of melanin and an increase in the transfer of melanosomes from melanocytes to keratinocytes. There is no increase in the number of melanocytes in ephelides. The exact reason for this has not been determined.

Histology: Histopathologic evaluation is one method to differentiate a lentigo from an ephelide. This is rarely done. The most common use of histology is to differentiate the benign lentigo from its malignant counterpart, lentigo maligna (melanoma in situ).

On histopathologic evaluation, ephelides show no change in the epidermis. There is no increase in the number of melanocytes. The only finding is an increase in the amount of melanin and an increased rate of transfer of melanosomes from melanocytes to keratinocytes.

Lentigines, on the other hand, show an increased number of melanocytes within the area of involvement. The hyperpigmentation is obvious along the club-like configuration of the rete ridges. The increase in the number of melanocytes is not associated with any nesting of those melanocytes, as is seen in melanocytic nevi. In solar lentigines, the dermis often shows signs of chronic sun damage, with a thinning of the dermis and solar elastosis. The epidermis is also thinned in some cases.

A biopsy of a lentigo maligna will show a higher density of melanocytes, with some melanocytes being large and bizarre appearing. There is pagetoid spread of the melanocytes and an asymmetry to the lesion. Differentiating lentigines and lentigo maligna may be difficult. Lentigo simplex has also been shown to lack defects in the *BRAF* gene, in contrast to melanoma, which may be one way to differentiate the two. Genetic markers are sure to be used more in the future to distinguish malignant from benign melanocytic lesions.

Lentigines are caused by an increased proliferation of melanocytes locally within the skin. The cause of this proliferation is most likely ultraviolet light in the case of solar lentigines. The cause of lentigo simplex is unknown. The increased number of melanocytes ultimately leads to an increase in the amount of melanin produced, resulting in the overlying hyperpigmentation.

The cause of lentigines in some genetic disorders is probably the underlying genetic defect. The exact mechanism of how the various gene defects lead to an increase in lentigines is being researched. A better understanding of how lentigines form in certain genetic syndromes may lead to discovery of the entire pathogenesis of solar lentigines and lentigo simplex.

Treatment: No therapy is needed other than to recommend sun protection, sunscreen use, and routine skin examinations. For cosmetic reasons, lentigines can be removed in a myriad of ways. Light cryotherapy is effective, easy to perform, and easily available in most dermatology clinics. This treatment can leave hypopigmented areas and should be used with caution in darker-skinned individuals. Many different chemical peels and dermabrasion techniques have been used to help decrease the appearance of lentigines. With the proliferation of medical laser devices in dermatology, lasers with unique wavelengths have been developed to target the melanin in lentigines. These laser devices have shown promise in lightening and removing solar lentigines.

LENTIGINES

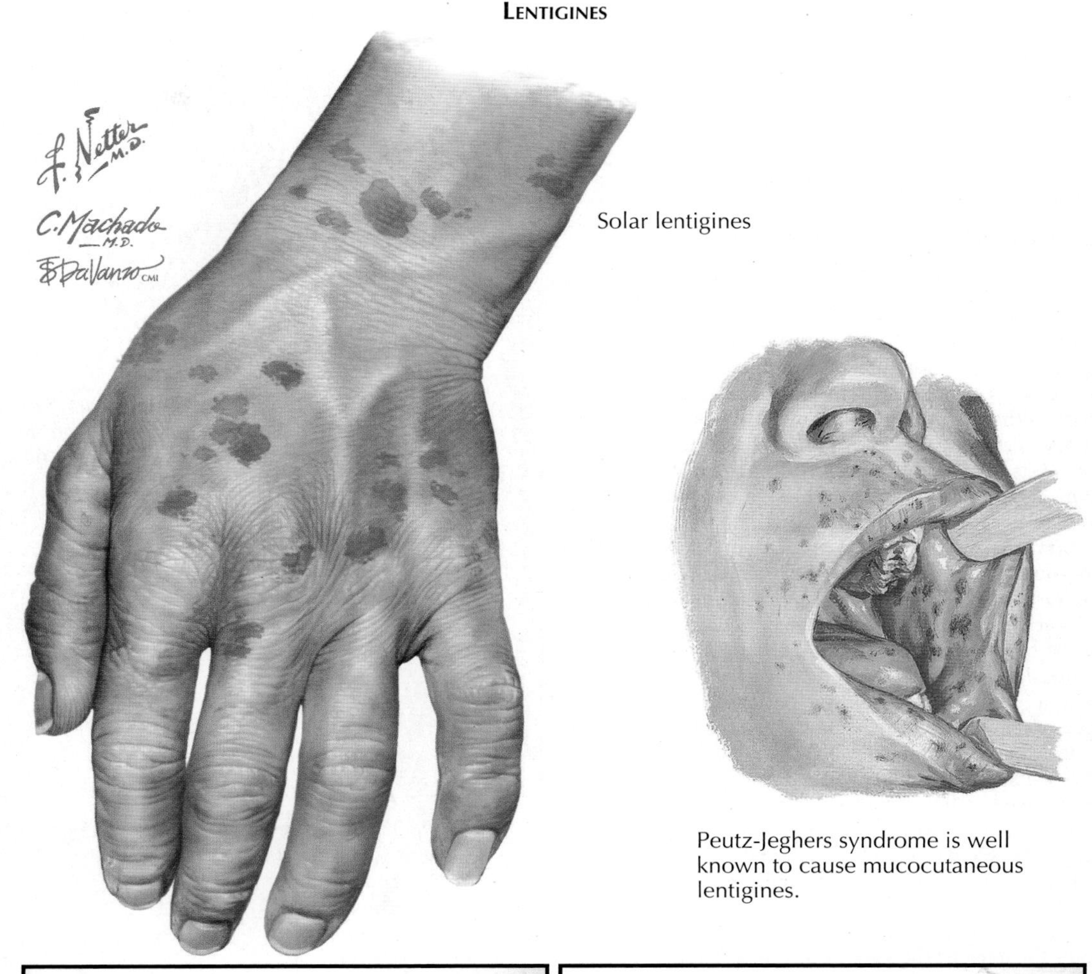

Peutz-Jeghers syndrome is well known to cause mucocutaneous lentigines.

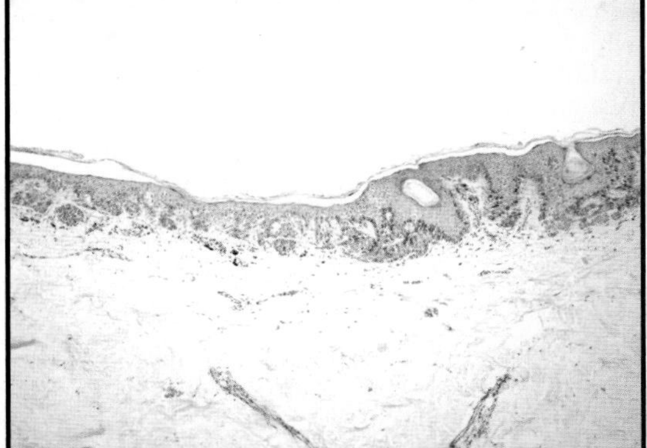

Low power. Basilar hyperpigmentation is prominent. There is an increase in the production of melanin and an increase in the number of melanocytes. The rete ridge pattern is altered and appears club shaped. Solar elastosis is prominent in the dermis.

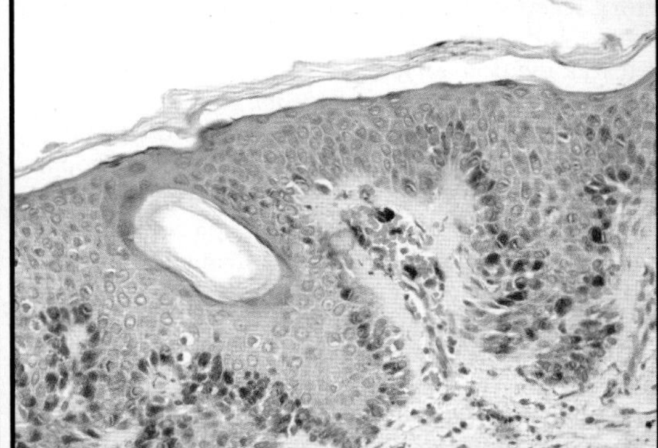

High power. An increase in the number of melanocytes is appreciated. No pagetoid spread is seen. A few melanophages are seen in the dermis.

Epidermal Inclusion Cyst

Epidermal inclusion cysts are the most common benign cysts derived from the skin. They are also known as epidermoid cysts or follicular infundibular cysts. The name "sebaceous cyst" has been used to describe these cysts, although it is a misnomer because epidermal inclusion cysts are not derived from sebaceous epithelium. The cysts, which are derived from hair follicle epithelium, can occur anywhere on the skin except the palms, soles, glans, labia minora, and vermilion border.

Clinical Findings: Most epidermal inclusion cysts are subcutaneous nodules that vary in size from 5 mm to more than 5 cm. They have no race predilection but are seen more commonly in males than in females. Onset most commonly occurs during the third decade of life. The nodules characteristically have an overlying central punctum. The central punctum may show a plug of oxidized keratin, similar to an open comedone. From this punctum, drainage of odiferous white, cheese-like material, which represents a buildup of macerated keratin debris, can occur. Most small epidermal inclusion cysts are asymptomatic, and they rarely cause a problem.

Larger epidermal inclusion cysts can become irritated and inflamed. If the inflammation is severe enough, the cyst wall ruptures. When the cyst contents enter the dermis, the keratin sets off a massive inflammatory reaction, which manifests clinically as edema, redness, and pain. Once this has occurred, patients often seek medical advice.

The main differential diagnosis for a ruptured epidermal inclusion cyst is a boil or furuncle. Ruptured epidermal inclusion cysts are almost never infected, although infection can occur within a long-standing ruptured cyst that has not been treated. The main differential diagnosis of an unruptured, noninflamed epidermal inclusion cyst is a pilar cyst. Pilar cysts do not have an overlying central punctum; this is the easiest means of differentiating the two cyst types. Pilar cysts are also more common on the scalp. Milia are considered to be tiny epidermal inclusion cysts.

Pathogenesis: The epidermal inclusion cyst is derived from the infundibulum of the hair follicle. Epidermal inclusion cysts occur as the result of direct implantation of epidermis into the underlying dermis; from there, the epidermal component continues to grow into the cyst lining. As the lining grows, it sheds keratin into the center of the cyst, causing the cyst to enlarge. Many researchers have looked at the roles of ultraviolet light and human papillomavirus infection in the etiology, but no definitive conclusions on either have been drawn.

Histology: The epidermal inclusion cyst is a true cyst with an epithelial lining of stratified squamous epithelium and an associated granular cell layer. The central cavity is filled with keratin debris. The cyst is derived from follicular epithelium.

Treatment: Small cysts that are asymptomatic do not need to be treated. Patients should be advised not to manipulate or squeeze the cysts. Such trauma could cause rupture of the cyst wall and set off an inflammatory reaction. Small cysts can be cured by a complete elliptical excision, making sure to remove the entire cyst wall. If a small portion of the cyst wall is left behind, the cyst is likely to recur. Excising a previously inflamed cyst or a recurrent cyst is often more challenging because of the associated scar tissue that can inhibit confident identification of the cyst wall.

Inflamed cysts should be treated initially with an incision and drainage technique. The region is anesthetized and then incised with a No. 11 blade. The resulting cheesy, white, macerated keratin debris is removed with lateral pressure, and a curette is used to break apart internal loculations. The drainage material has a pungent odor. The resulting cyst cavity can be packed or left open until the patient returns in 2 to 3 weeks for definitive removal of the cyst lining by excision. Intralesional triamcinolone is very effective in decreasing the inflammation and pain in these inflamed cysts. Long-standing cysts should be cultured and the patient should be given the appropriate antibiotic therapy based on the culture results.

Origin of pilosebaceous unit cysts

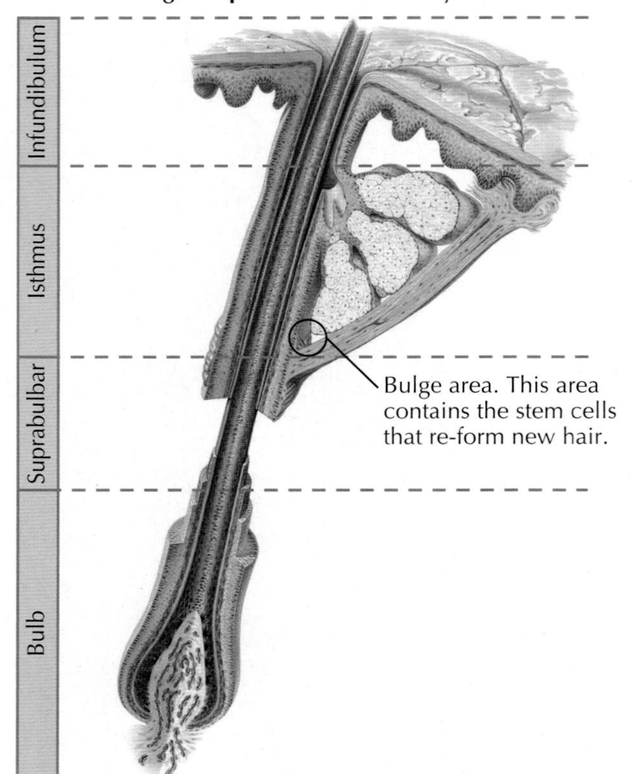

Epidermal inclusion cyst, sometimes referred to as a sebaceous cyst. The upper cyst is red and inflamed. The lower noninflamed cyst has a central punctum.

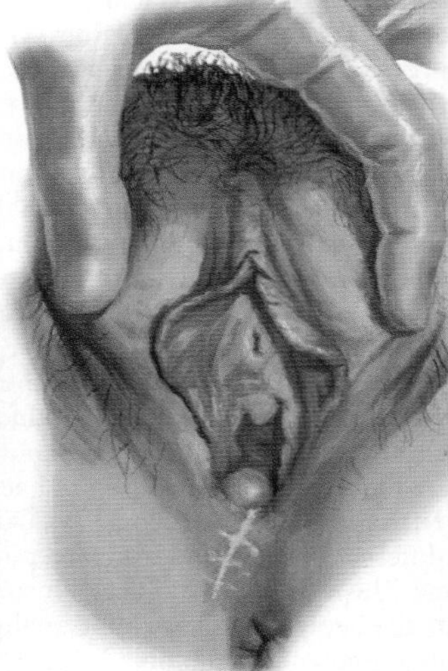

Epidermal inclusion cyst arising at the site of scar

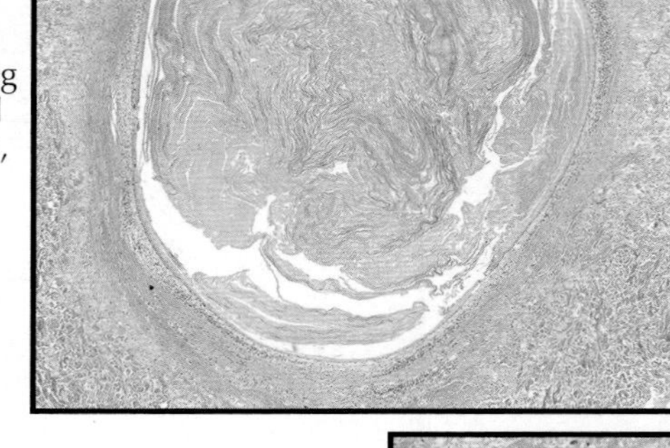

Low power. A well-circumscribed cyst is seen within the dermis. The cyst lining is formed by stratified squamous epithelium, which contains a granular cell layer. A slight amount of dermal inflammation is seen surrounding the cyst.

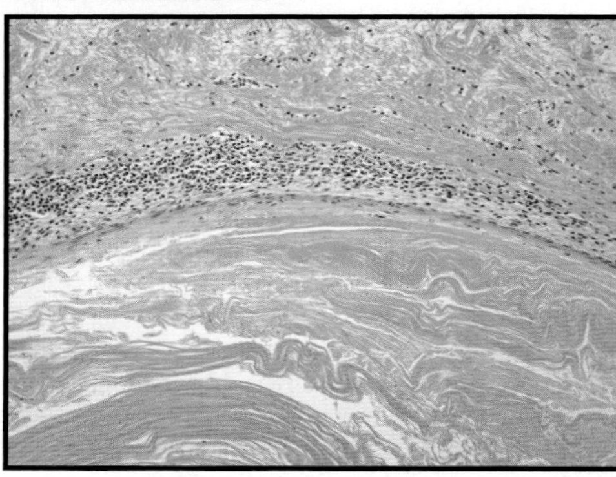

High power. The stratified squamous lining is better appreciated in this high-power image. An intact granular layer is seen. The cyst contents appear as wavy eosinophilic material.

F. Netter M.D.
K. Marzejon
C. Machado M.D.

EPIDERMAL NEVUS

Epidermal nevi are benign epidermal hamartomatous growths that most commonly occur as small plaques but can be widespread and can have associated systemic findings. Epidermal nevi tend to follow the embryologic lines of Blaschko. The lines of Blaschko are well defined and follow a whorl-like pattern. Why these lesions follow Blaschko's lines is not fully understood, but it is somehow caused by an interruption of normal epidermal migration during embryogenesis.

Clinical Findings: Epidermal nevi typically manifest in childhood as a solitary linear plaque. Epidermal nevi do not have a race predilection, and they can be found equally in males and females. This type of nevus is not melanocytic in nature; rather, it is composed of a proliferation of keratinocytes. The nevus initially has a smooth surface and often develops a mamillated or verrucal surface over time. Epidermal nevi appear to occur most commonly on the head and neck region but can occur anywhere. After puberty, the lesions do not change dramatically. Most are flesh colored to slightly hyperpigmented. If found on the scalp, an epidermal nevus can mimic a nevus sebaceus and can be associated with hair loss, but more commonly it does not cause alopecia.

The epidermal nevus is usually small and slightly linear. Some are large, encompassing the entire length of an extremity, and still others cover a large percentage of the body surface area. Intraoral mucosal involvement has rarely been reported. Larger epidermal nevi are more likely to be associated with systemic findings, such as underlying bone abnormalities. The most common bony abnormality is shortening of the unilateral underlying limb. The epidermal nevus syndrome is a rare disorder associated with a large or widespread epidermal nevus and many systemic findings.

Epidermal nevus syndrome is composed of a constellation of findings. Children with this syndrome often present with neurologic deficits, including seizures and developmental delay. They can have a multitude of bony abnormalities, cataracts, and glaucoma. The finding of a widespread epidermal nevus in an infant should alert the clinician to the possibility of this syndrome and the need for a multidisciplinary approach to patient care.

Pathogenesis: The epidermal nevus is a hamartomatous proliferation of the epidermal components. The exact cause is unknown. These lesions are believed to be caused by a developmental abnormality of the ectoderm. Epidermal nevus syndrome has not been shown to have any appreciable inheritance pattern and is believed to be sporadic in nature. The exact genetic defect is unknown; it is most likely a result of genetic mosaicism. The involvement of fibroblast growth factor has been studied, but no firm conclusions have been made. These lesions do not show any abnormalities of melanocytes. There is no increased malignant transformation potential.

Histology: The findings in this condition are all located within the epidermis. Significant acanthosis and hyperkeratosis with papillomatosis predominate. A variable degree of pigmentation is seen in the involved keratinocytes; however, this is not a disorder of melanocytes, and the number of melanocytes is normal. The granular cell layer is expanded. Many unique histologic variants of epidermal nevi have been described.

Treatment: Small, isolated epidermal nevi can be removed with the shave removal technique. They have a high rate of recurrence with this technique, but recurrence may take many years. The advantages of this technique are that it is relatively easy, noninvasive, and quick, and it provides an opportunity for histopathologic evaluation of the tissue for evidence of epidermolytic hyperkeratosis. The disadvantage of shave removal is that it is appropriate only for small epidermal nevi. Cryotherapy with liquid nitrogen has been used successfully, but it may leave unsightly hypopigmentation in darker-skinned individuals and should be used with caution.

Complete surgical excision is curative for small epidermal nevi. However, it leaves a scar that may be more noticeable than the nevus. Laser resurfacing, dermabrasion, and chemical peels have been used to help smooth out the appearance of epidermal nevi.

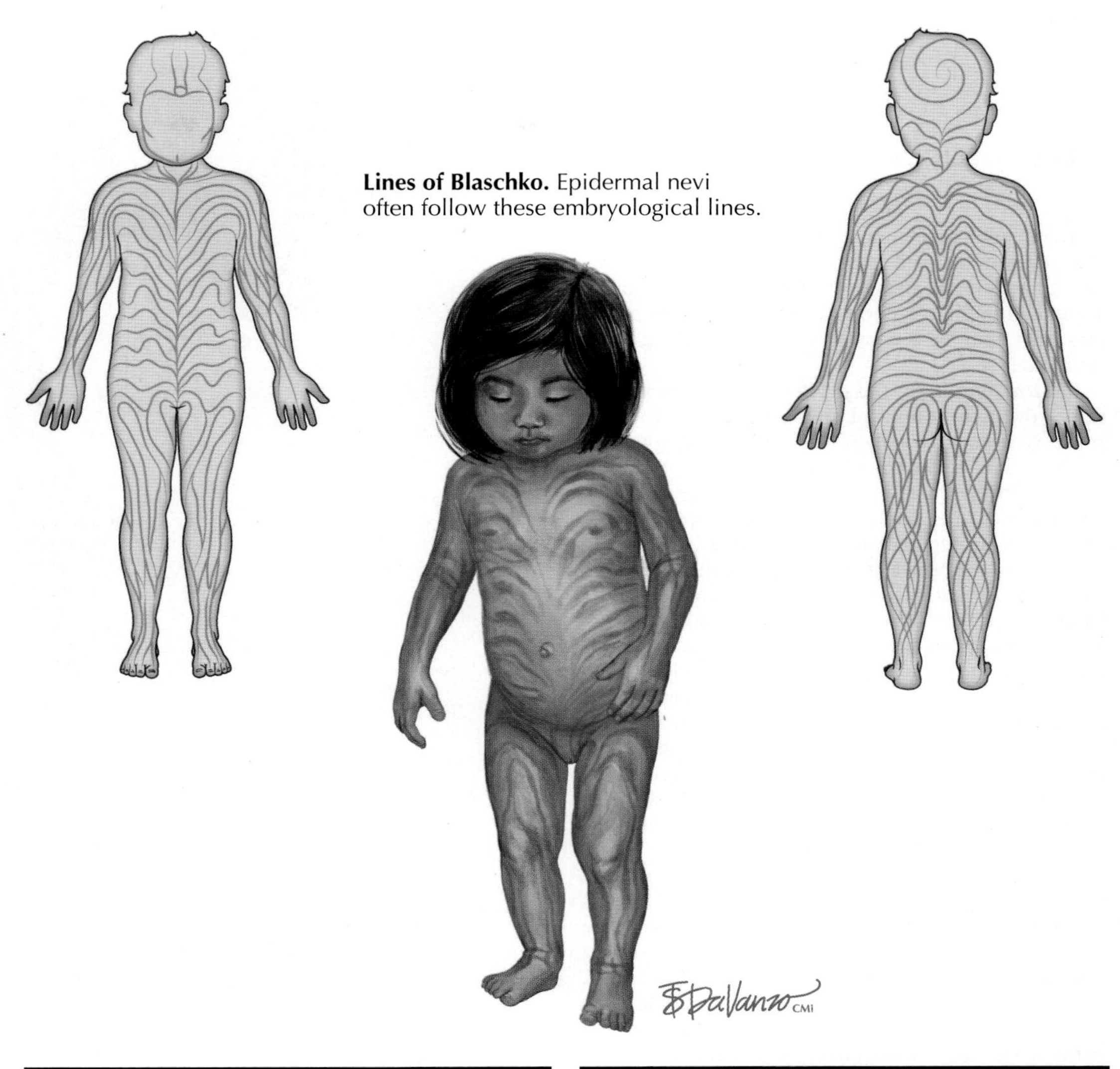

Lines of Blaschko. Epidermal nevi often follow these embryological lines.

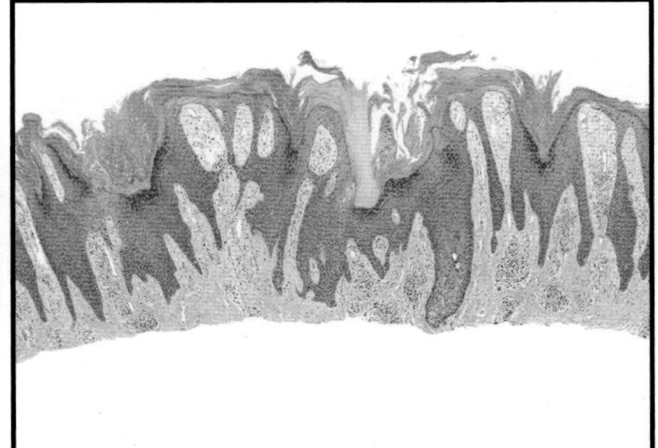

Epidermal nevus, low power. Hyperkeratosis, acanthosis, papillomatosis, and basilar hyperpigmentation are prominent.

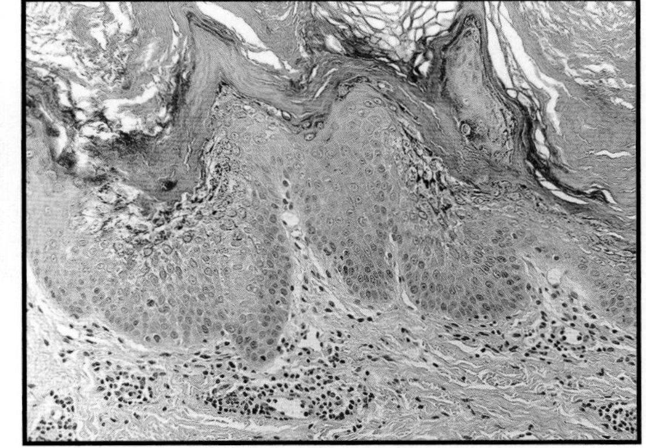

Epidermolytic hyperkeratosis, low power. The same architecture as an epidermal nevus is seen; however, prominent vacuolar changes are seen within the epidermis.

FIBROFOLLICULOMA

Fibrofolliculomas are uncommon benign tumors of the skin. They are derived from the hair follicle epithelium and show a unique mantle differentiation. These tumors are uncommonly seen, but if they are seen in multiples, they may be a constellation of Birt-Hogg-Dubé syndrome.

Clinical Findings: These tumors are often solitary skin growths on the head and neck region. They are small (2–5 mm), firm, flesh-colored to tan-yellow nontender papules. Fibrofolliculomas most commonly manifest in the third or fourth decade of life. They are asymptomatic and rarely, if ever, get inflamed or bleed spontaneously. On occasion, a small hair is seen emanating from the center of the lesion. The main differential diagnosis clinically includes compound nevus, basal cell carcinoma, fibrous papule, and other types of adnexal tumor. No characteristic clinical findings allow for an accurate clinical diagnosis, and definitive diagnosis is impossible without histologic examination. Solitary fibrofolliculomas are usually found incidentally on routine skin examination. Some patients present with an enlarging new papule, often expressing concern for or fear of skin cancer. A biopsy is performed to rule out skin cancer, and a fibrofolliculoma is determined to be the cause on histologic evaluation.

Multiple fibrofolliculomas are seen in association with Birt-Hogg-Dubé syndrome. The fibrofolliculomas in this syndrome can often be found on the neck in a postauricular location. This syndrome is caused by a genetic defect in the tumor suppressor gene *FLCN,* which has been localized to the short arm of chromosome 17. It is inherited in an autosomal dominant fashion. Other cutaneous constellations include trichodiscomas and skin tags. The most important aspect of diagnosing this syndrome early is to screen patients for the possibility of renal tumors, both benign and malignant. Renal oncocytomas are the most common malignant renal tumor seen in this syndrome. Another rare renal cancer, chromophobe renal cell carcinoma, also may be seen. This very rare tumor is seen in a higher percentage of patients with Birt-Hogg-Dubé syndrome than in the general population. It has a less aggressive behavior than other forms of renal cell carcinoma. Patients with this syndrome are also at higher risk for spontaneous pneumothorax; the reason for this is unclear. Some pathologists believe that trichodiscomas are the same type of tumor as the fibrofolliculoma and that the difference in histologic appearance is caused by sampling and processing artifact (i.e., the identical tumor processed at different tissue surface levels).

Pathogenesis: Fibrofolliculomas are believed to be derived from the upper part of the follicular epithelium. The tumors are thought to be hamartomatous processes that develop within the dermis. Mantle-like structures, as seen in sebaceous glands, are often present and may be the derivation of these tumors. Some consider the mantleoma (an extremely rare benign skin tumor) to be in the same spectrum of tumors as the fibrofolliculoma and the trichodiscoma.

Histology: The tumor surrounds a well-formed terminal hair shaft. The upper portion of the hair shaft is slightly dilated. Emanating from the central hair shaft epithelium are cords or epithelial strands that project into the surrounding dermis. These cords interconnect at various positions and form a weave-like pattern. Clinically, trichodiscomas do not contain a hair shaft; a proliferation along a hair follicle of a fibrovascular stroma is seen, akin to an angiofibroma. It is postulated that these two tumors are indeed the same but appear to be two distinct tumors because of routine processing and sampling at various tissue plane levels.

Treatment: Solitary fibrofolliculomas can be removed completely with the shave removal technique. This gives excellent cosmetic results, and the tumors are unlikely to recur. Multiple tumors are more difficult to remove; laser resurfacing, cryotherapy, dermabrasion, and chemical peeling have all been used with varying results. The recognition of multiple fibrofolliculomas or trichodiscomas necessitates screening for Birt-Hogg-Dubé syndrome. If diagnosed, patients with Birt-Hogg-Dubé syndrome should be evaluated regularly by a urologist because of their risk for developing renal carcinoma.

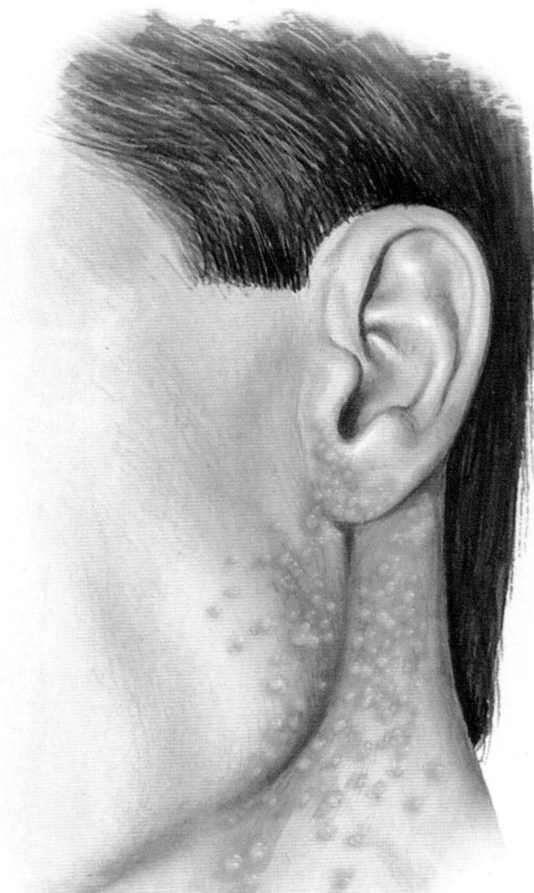

Fibrofolliculomas. Note the periauricular and retroauricular location of monomorphous papules. They are most commonly seen in association with Birt-Hogg-Dubé syndrome.

Skin Findings in Birt-Hogg-Dubé
1. Fibrofolliculomas
2. Skin tags
3. Trichodiscomas
4. Lipomas
5. Angiolipomas
6. Angiofibromas

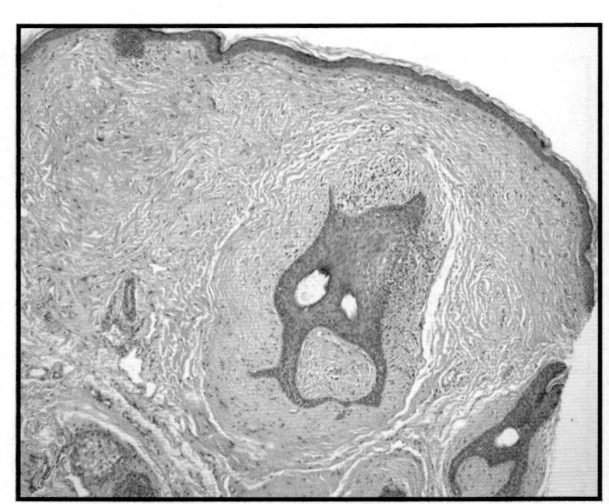

Low power. The tumor is made up of a centrally located basophilic tumor lobule with what appears to be a hair shaft forming within the lobule.

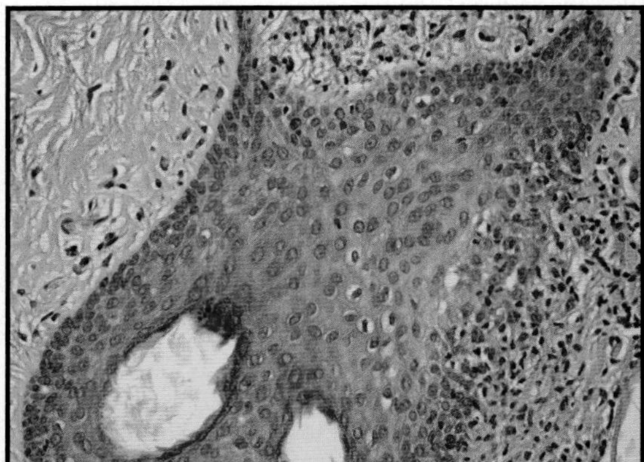

High power. Close-up view shows the basophilic tumor lobule and the fine hair shaft with keratin debris.

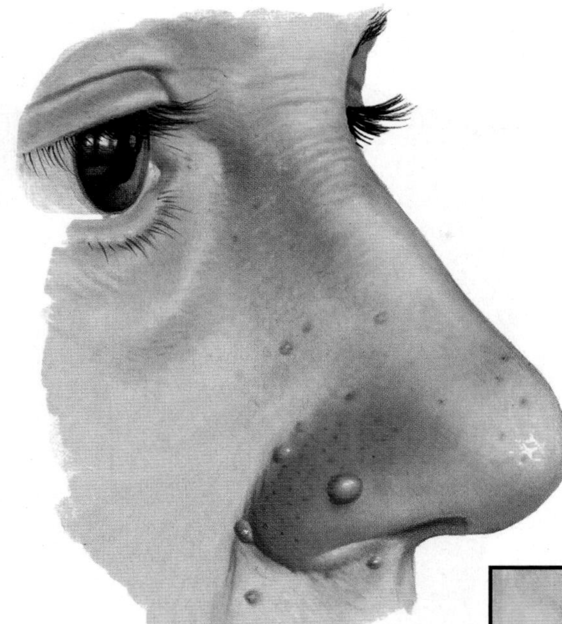

Angiofibromas. Also termed *fibrous papules*. Can be seen in isolation. Multiple angiofibromas associated with tuberous sclerosis are termed adenoma sebaceum.

FIBROUS PAPULE

Fibrous papules are common benign skin growths encountered in clinical practice. Individuals often present with a concern for skin cancer due to a small growth on or near the nose. They are often overlooked or ignored during routine skin examinations. The exact incidence is unknown, but they are believed to be extraordinarily common. These skin growths are most frequently found on the nose, but they can occur anywhere, especially on the face.

Clinical Findings: Fibrous papules are typically small, 0.5 to 5 mm in diameter. They are slightly oval and dome shaped with an overlying smooth surface. Most commonly, they are flesh colored to slightly hyperpigmented. Fibrous papules can also have a hypopigmented appearance. These benign tumors are almost entirely asymptomatic. Most patients do not even know they are present. On occasion, a patient notices a slight itching sensation; less frequently, a patient may describe spontaneous bleeding or bleeding after minor trauma. These growths are most often solitary in nature, but multiple fibrous papules have been reported. Fibrous papules most commonly occur in young adults, especially in the third to fifth decades of life. The most common location is the face, with the nose and chin most commonly involved.

Fibrous papules are considered angiofibromas. Multiple angiofibromas can be part of a constellation known as the tuberous sclerosis complex. The differential diagnosis in a teenager with multiple angiofibromas should always include tuberous sclerosis complex. However, solitary fibrous papules are extraordinarily common and should not trigger investigation for an underlying syndrome such as tuberous sclerosis. Pearly penile papules are small, dome-shaped, 1- to 2-mm papules found along the corona of the glans. These pearly penile papules are histologically indistinguishable from fibrous papules and are also considered angiofibromas.

The differential diagnosis of a fibrous papule can be quite broad, and a biopsy is often required to differentiate the potential mimickers. The entities most commonly included in the differential diagnosis are common acquired melanocytic nevus and basal cell carcinoma. In these cases, a shave biopsy is required to make a firm diagnosis.

Pathogenesis: Fibrous papules are believed to be a benign proliferation of fibroblasts and blood vessels in a collagen-filled stroma. Immunohistochemical staining has shown that the dermal dendrocyte is the most likely precursor cell to the abnormal fibroblasts seen in fibrous papules. The underlying cause has yet to be determined. The multiple angiofibromas of tuberous sclerosis complex are directly related to an underlying defect in the tumor suppressor gene *tuberin (TSC2)*. Patients with tuberous sclerosis complex also have angiofibromas in a periungual location as well as hundreds to thousands of angiofibromas located symmetrically on the face and nose.

Adenoma sebaceum (multiple angiofibromas) over both cheeks and nasal bridge. This is a sign of tuberous sclerosis.

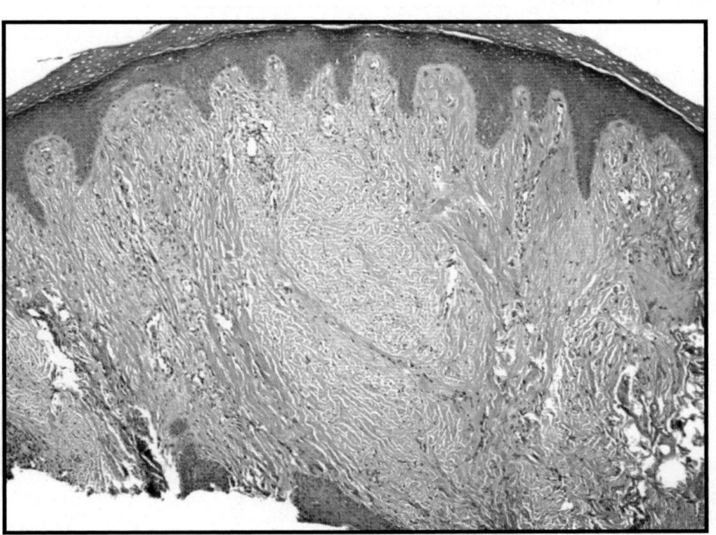

High power. Fibroblasts are the main cell type along with the blood vessels.

Histology: There are multiple histologic variants of fibrous papules. The most commonly encountered fibrous papules are typically dome shaped and small (up to 5 mm in diameter), and they show a proliferation of fibroblasts with a stroma of fibrotic collagenized material. Dilated blood vessels are often found within the papules. An inflammatory infiltrate is frequently seen, but it is typically sparse. The combination of clinical findings with the typical histopathologic findings solidifies the diagnosis.

Multiple histologic variants have been described, including pleomorphic, pigmented, granular cell, hypercellular, and clear cell variants. These variants are believed to be much less common than the classic type of fibrous papule. They have been described in detail and are well-accepted and recognized histopathologic variations.

Treatment: No treatment is necessary, although a small shave biopsy is often all that is required to remove the fibrous papule, with an excellent cosmetic result. Most fibrous papules are removed because they are mistaken for basal cell carcinomas or for relief of some underlying irritation, such as itching or bleeding.

GANGLION CYST

Ganglion cysts are commonly encountered in the general population. They are fluid-filled cavities that occur most commonly on the dorsal aspect of the hands and wrists. They are believed to be derived from the synovial lining of various tendons. They typically manifest as asymptomatic, soft, rubbery nodules below the skin.

Clinical Findings: Ganglion cysts are common benign growths that occur on the distal upper extremity, and in most cases are located on the dorsal aspect of the hand or wrist. Ganglion cysts are almost always solitary, but some patients present with more than one, and occasionally the individual ganglion cysts coalesce into one large area that can overlie the entire wrist. Most are relatively small, 1 cm in diameter, but some can get very large (2–3 cm). The overlying epidermis is normal, and the cyst is located in the subcutaneous space below the adipose tissue. They are smooth, dome-shaped, fluid-filled cysts that are slightly compressible. The cyst is a direct extension of the synovial lining of the tendon. The cysts form by various mechanisms and fill with synovial fluid. This fluid is critical in the normal lubrication of the tendon space to decrease friction and allow the tendon to easily slide back and forth within its synovial covering. These cysts can occur at any age, but they are much more common in the younger population and often manifest in the third or fourth decade of life. Women are much more likely than men to develop these cysts.

Most cysts are asymptomatic, but they can cause discomfort and pain if they become large enough to press on underlying structures. Patients are concerned by the appearance of the cysts, which is often the main reason for seeking medical attention. Rarely, the cyst compresses an underlying nerve, resulting in symptoms of pain, numbness, or muscle weakness. The differential diagnosis is limited, and most often the diagnosis is made clinically. Occasionally, a biopsy is required to differentiate ganglion cysts from giant cell tumors of the tendon sheath. Giant cell tumors of the tendon sheath are much more likely to be firm in nature. Ganglion cysts have no malignant degeneration potential. In difficult cases, an ultrasound examination can be performed; it is highly sensitive in detecting these fluid-filled cysts.

Pathogenesis: Ganglion cysts are believed to be caused by an outgrowth of the underlying synovial lining of the tendon sheath. Trauma is likely the leading culprit in initiating the formation of these cysts. Patients with osteoarthritis are also at increased risk for development of ganglion cysts, most likely because of the mechanical trauma that the synovial lining repetitively undergoes when it rubs against osteoarthritic bone.

Histology: Ganglion cysts are not true cysts in that they do not have a well-formed epithelial lining that surrounds the entire cystic cavity. The lining is a loose collection of fibrous connective tissue composed mostly of collagen. The cyst lining is multilobulated in most cases and typically has no connection to the underlying joint capsule or tendon sheath. The contents of the cyst are made of mucopolysaccharides.

Treatment: No therapy is required for small, asymptomatic ganglion cysts. Some smaller ganglion cysts will spontaneously resolve without therapy. If a patient desires removal or if the cyst is causing symptoms, especially weakness and numbness, therapy is needed. Needle aspiration is often used as a first-line treatment option; a pressure bandage is applied to try to keep the cyst from reexpanding. After the aspiration, intralesional injection of triamcinolone is used to try to scar down the lining of the cyst to prevent it from re-forming. This has shown excellent results. If aspiration and injection are not successful, surgical excision is necessary. It is important to have a hand surgeon evaluate and treat these cysts because of their proximity to multiple vital nerve and tendon structures.

Firm, rubbery, sometimes lobulated swelling over carpus, most prominent on flexion of wrist. *Broken line* indicates line of skin incision.

Extensor tendon retracted

Carpal ligaments and capsule

Excision of ganglion via transverse incision. Excision is one of the therapies with the lowest recurrence rate. The surgeon must expose the entire cyst and remove the entire lining to limit recurrence.

Intralesional steroid injections have been used with success.

Loss of strength can be diagnosed on physical exam. Muscle weakness may occur from pressure on an underlying nerve by the cyst.

F. Netter M.D.

K. Marzen

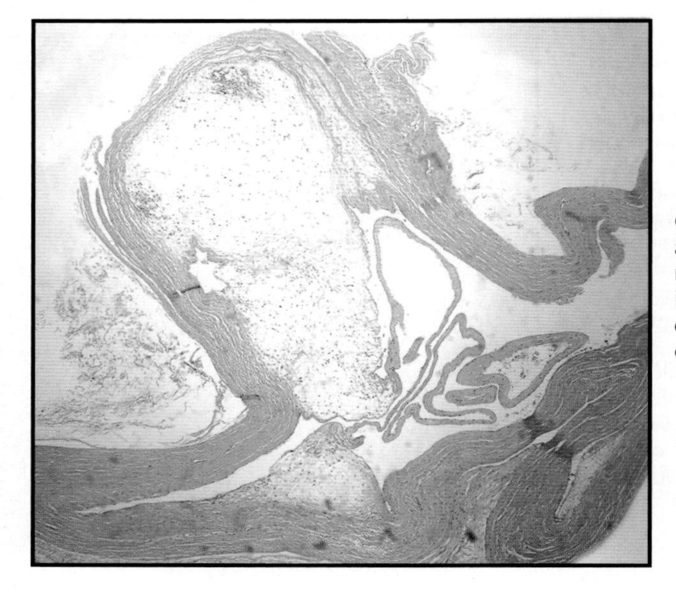

Ganglion cyst. No epidermis is appreciated. The ganglion cyst does not have a true epithelial lining; rather, it is surrounded by a loose collection of collagen and fibrous material. The cyst contains mucopolysaccharides.

GLOMUS TUMOR AND GLOMANGIOMA

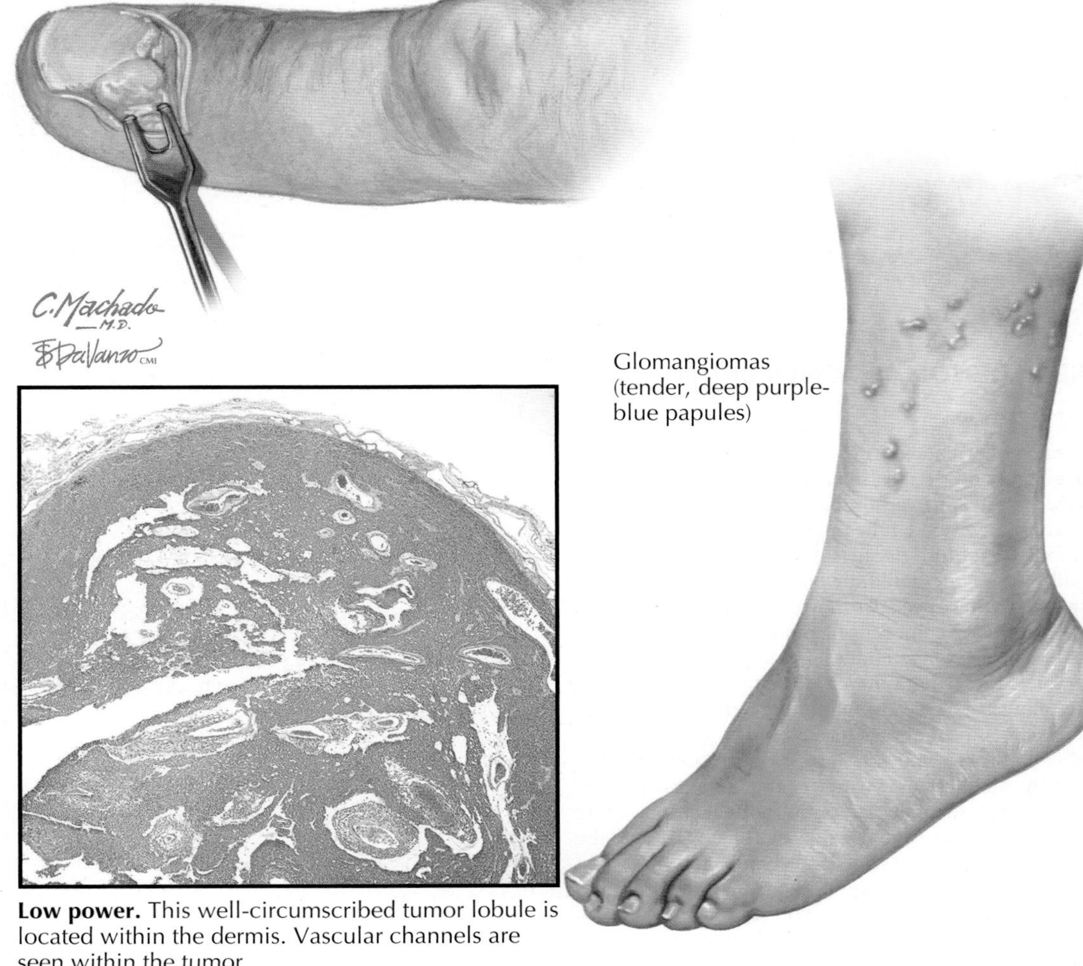

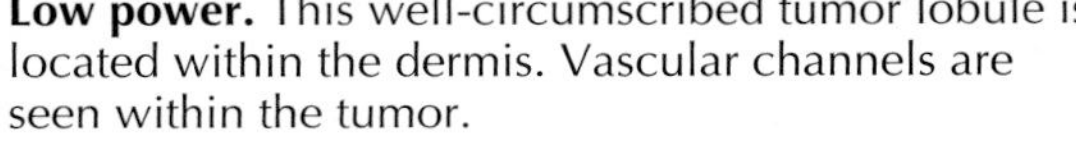

Low power. This well-circumscribed tumor lobule is located within the dermis. Vascular channels are seen within the tumor.

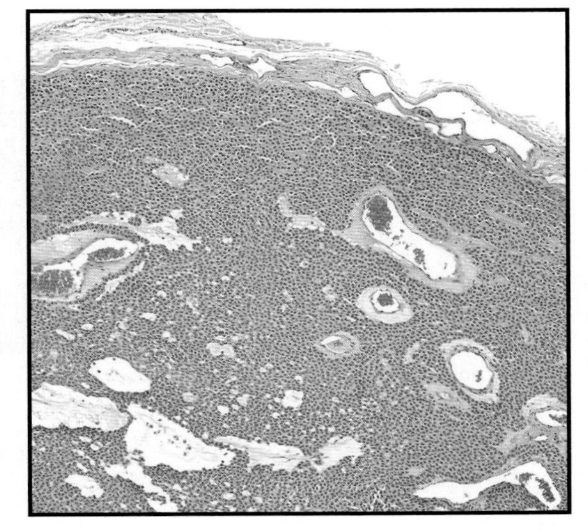

High power. The uniform-appearing glomus cells are seen surrounding the vascular structure. The glomus cells are eosinophilic in nature with uniformly basophilic nuclei.

Glomus tumors are benign tumors derived from the glomus body. The glomus body is a component of the vascular thermoregulatory unit. These tumors are most frequently encountered in early adulthood and are most commonly found on the digits, with the fingers more frequently involved than the toes. Glomus tumors are solitary in nature, and the term glomangioma is used when describing the glomuvenous malformation. This usually manifests as a congenital defect in infants and young children and appears to be a multifocal grouping or mass of coalescent glomus tumors.

Clinical Findings: The solitary glomus tumor is often found on the digit in a subungual location. The tumors occur equally in men and in women. Lesions have been described in all regions of the skin and also in extracutaneous locations. These tumors are small, well localized, and almost always tender or painful. The glomus tumor is in the differential diagnosis of any painful dermal nodule. Examination often reveals a 1- to 2-cm, well-circumscribed, blue to purple dermal nodule. It is tender to palpation and can be extremely painful with changes in the ambient temperature.

Glomangiomas are frequently congenital and manifest as a multifocal cluster of coalescing blue-purple nodules and papules. There is occasionally some surface change over the top of the tumors. The Hildreth sign is a diagnostic maneuver that can be used to help make the diagnosis. The sign is positive if the pain from the glomus tumor decreases or disappears when a blood pressure cuff is placed proximal to the tumor and inflated to a pressure greater than the patient's systolic blood pressure. Glomangiomas can be confused with hemangiomas or other vascular malformations. The differential diagnosis of a solitary glomus tumor includes angiolipoma, neuroma, eccrine spiradenoma, leiomyoma, and other vascular tumors. The differential diagnosis of a glomangioma includes hemangiomas and other vascular malformations.

Pathogenesis: Glomus tumors arise from the Sucquet-Hoyer canal. This canal, which is part of the glomus body, is an arteriovenous shunt found in the small vasculature of the skin. The glomus body is made up of a small arteriole, the Sucquet-Hoyer canal, a venule, and the sympathetic nerve ending supplying the vessels. These canals have been found in a higher density within the blood vessels of the digits. They are responsible for thermoregulation and cause shunting of blood in response to neurologic and temperature changes. The exact initiating factor is unknown. Anecdotal reports of glomus tumors occurring after trauma have led some to believe that trauma is causative. This may explain the preponderance of the tumors on the digits, where they are prone to trauma. Trauma is unlikely to be the true initiating factor because these tumors are quite rare and trauma to the digits occurs frequently.

Some glomangiomas have been described to be inherited in an autosomal dominant fashion. These cases are caused by a deletion defect in the *glomulin (GLMN)* gene, which is located on the short arm of chromosome 1. This gene encodes a protein that has been found to be important in the normal development of vascular tissue.

Histology: The tumor manifests as a well-circumscribed nodule of even glomus cells surrounding a number of small capillaries. The glomus cells are distinctive and uniform. They appear round and have round nuclei, with a near identical appearance to the adjacent cells of the tumor. The cytoplasm is scarce and eosinophilic. The background stroma is myxoid, and there is often a fibrous capsule surrounding the entire tumor.

Treatment: Glomus tumors are successfully treated with complete surgical excision. Glomangiomas, because of their size, can be excised in a staged approach or with the help of tissue expanders. Reports of treatment with laser ablation, electrocauterization, and sclerotherapy, with some success, have been documented in the literature.

Hidradenoma papilliferum is most frequently located on the external genitalia of women.

HIDRADENOMA PAPILLIFERUM

Hidradenoma papilliferum is a rare benign tumor of the genital and perianal regions. It is most commonly located on the vulva, although extragenital locations have been described. It has a predilection for women in the fourth and fifth decades of life. Typically, these are small tumors a few millimeters in diameter, but some large tumors have been described. There is no connection to the overlying epidermis or mucosa.

Clinical Findings: Hidradenoma papilliferum is an extremely rare benign tumor located in the dermis. It is seen almost exclusively in middle-aged women. The lesions are almost always located in the genital region. Individuals are often unaware they are present. They typically manifest as asymptomatic nodules that are discovered incidentally on routine annual exams. There are usually no overlying epidermal changes, and the tumor is well circumscribed, freely movable, and firm in consistency. They range in size from a few millimeters to a centimeter in diameter. They do not have a connection with the overlying epithelium. In rare instances, they can be tender or pruritic and can bleed or ulcerate. Most of these tumors are found on routine gynecologic examination. The most common location is the labia majora. The differential diagnosis of a solitary, firm dermal nodule in the genital region is very broad, and a biopsy for histopathologic examination is required in all cases to make the diagnosis. It is essential for dermatologists and gynecologists to be aware of this tumor and its common locations. These tumors have also been rarely found in extragenital locations, such as the axilla and areola of the breast. These are areas rich in apocrine glands.

Pathogenesis: Hidradenoma papilliferum is a tumor that is believed to be derived from apocrine glands. For this reason, it is considered to be a type of apocrine adenoma. Apocrine glands are found in higher density in the anogenital region, which may be one reason for the unequal cutaneous distribution of this tumor. Apocrine glands are also found in higher densities in the axilla and breast regions. The tumor is benign and is closely related to another benign adnexal tumor, the syringocystadenoma papilliferum. The latter tumor is more common on the head and neck, with a predilection for the scalp. Histologically, these two tumors are almost identical, with the major differentiating factor being that the syringocystadenoma papilliferum has a connection to the overlying epidermis. Clinically, the syringocystadenoma papilliferum usually manifests as an ulcerated papule or plaque. Both of these tumors can develop within a nevus sebaceus.

Histology: Hidradenoma papilliferum is a well-circumscribed dermal tumor. It almost never has any overlying epithelial abnormalities. Syringocystadenoma papilliferum, on other hand, has a connection with the overlying epidermis. They both can commonly arise in conjunction with a nevus sebaceus. On closer inspection, the hidradenoma papilliferum is composed of vascular papillary projections into the center of the tumor lobule. These projections are lined by cells with an apocrine origin that have a columnar configuration. Apocrine secretion (decapitation secretion) is often noted in various sections of the tumor. There is also a thin layer of myoepithelial cells. Within the papillary projections is a background stroma composed of many vascular spaces and lymphocytes.

Syringocystadenoma papilliferum has almost identical central characteristics. Compared with hidradenoma papilliferum, it has a denser plasma cell infiltrate and has an attachment to the overlying epidermis, which usually manifests as an invagination of the epidermis into the tumor lobule.

Treatment: A complete excision is diagnostic and curative at the same time. Often, a biopsy is performed to ascertain the diagnosis, followed by the curative complete excision. These are rare and benign tumors. There have been reports of malignant degeneration, but this is exceedingly rare.

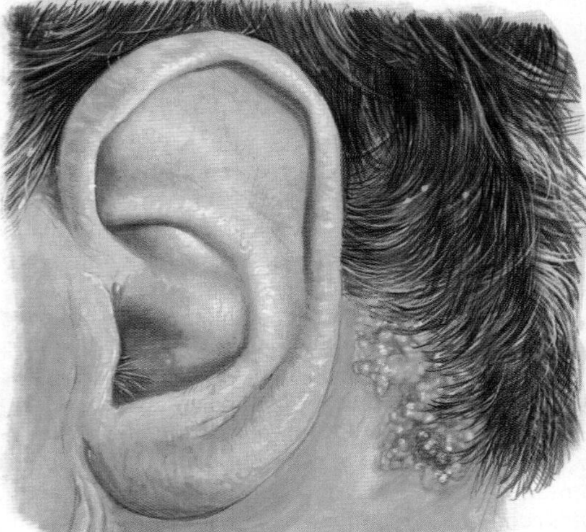

Syringocystadenoma papilliferum arising within a nevus sebaceus. Transformation of a nevus sebaceus into various tumors, including syringocystadenoma papilliferum and basal cell carcinoma, occurs most frequently after puberty.

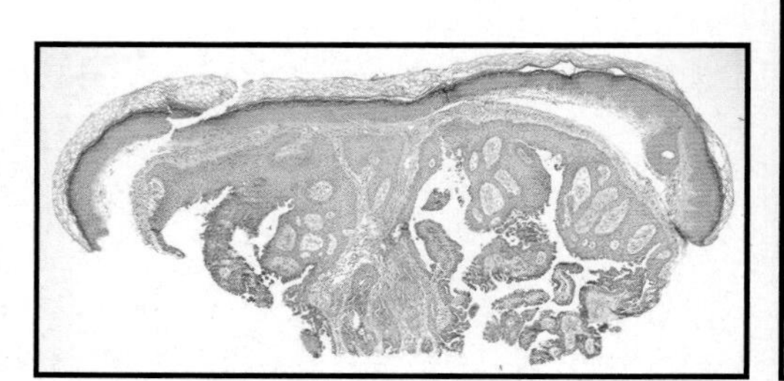

Low power. Symmetrically arranged dermal tumor with multiple papillary projections.

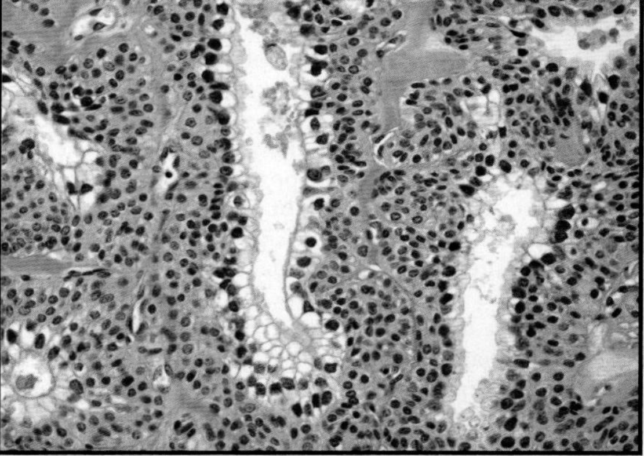

High power. Close-up of the papillary projections. The projections are lined by cells with an apocrine origin. Apocrine secretion (decapitation secretion) is often noted in various sections of the tumor.

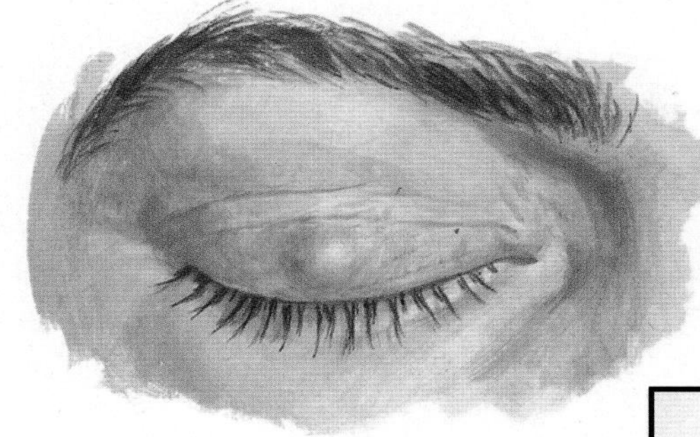

Hidrocystomas of the eyelid may appear similar to a chalazion or a basal cell carcinoma. They may appear translucent and easily rupture. They are almost always asymptomatic.

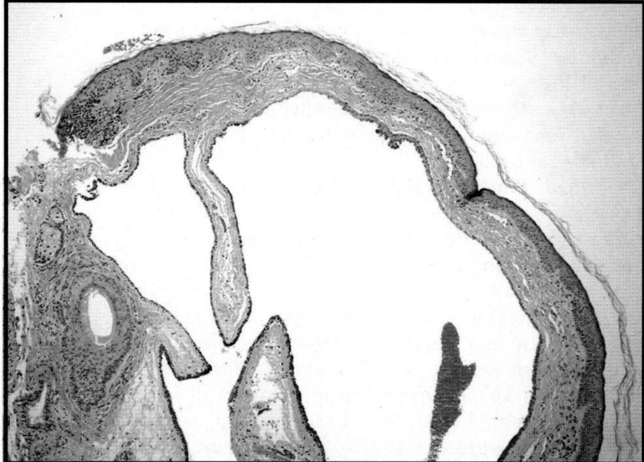

Low power. A well-circumscribed cystic lining is seen in the dermis. Minimal surrounding inflammation is present.

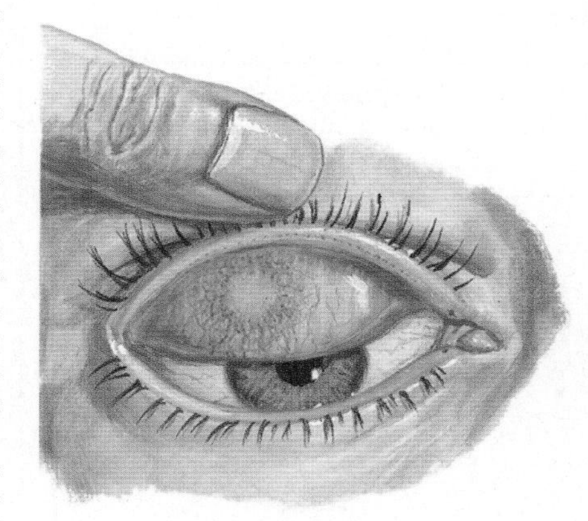

Chalazion; lid everted. Tender nodule of the eyelid.

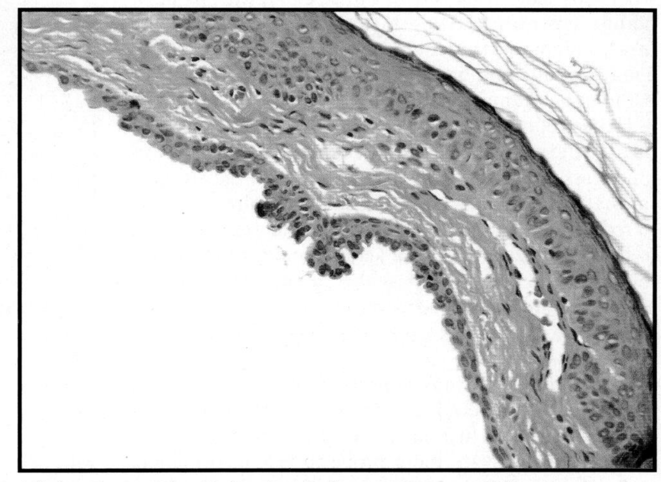

High power. The lining is made up of two cell layers of cuboidal epithelium. There is a small amount of dermis between the cyst and the overlying epidermis.

HIDROCYSTOMA

Hidrocystomas, also known as eccrine hidrocystomas, are common benign skin tumors most frequently found along the eyelid margin. These benign tumors have a typical appearance and no malignant potential. Most often they manifest as solitary, asymptomatic, translucent papules. These are frequently encountered and often overlooked by the individual who has them because of their asymptomatic and subtle nature.

Clinical Findings: Eccrine hidrocystomas manifest as solitary, translucent, pale, clear to blue or light purple papules. They have a smooth surface and a dome shape. Eccrine hidrocystomas are soft; they feel as if pressure could easily rupture their cystic wall. Puncturing of the cyst wall with a 30-gauge needle causes drainage of a thin, watery fluid. These tumors are almost always asymptomatic. Large hidrocystomas may drape over the eyelid margin and potentially interfere with peripheral vision. They can occur at any age but are far more common after the fourth decade of life. No difference in incidence has been observed based on race or sex. Lesions are typically small, 5 mm to 1 cm in diameter, and can fluctuate in size. It is not uncommon for a patient to relate that the tumor enlarges during physical exercise, only to shrink after a few days. If ruptured, these tumors drain a thin, watery liquid, and the cystic cavity deflates. Although they are almost always solitary, there are reports of hundreds of these tumors developing in some patients. Large eccrine hidrocystomas occurring in atypical locations have also been described.

The main differential diagnosis is between eccrine hidrocystoma and basal cell carcinoma. Cystic basal cell carcinomas can have an identical appearance; however, the patient history will be quite different. Basal cell carcinomas typically enlarge over time and ulcerate, causing bleeding of the ulcerated papule. Hidrocystomas rarely, if ever, ulcerate or bleed. If left alone, they only transiently increase in size and never get much larger than 1 cm in diameter, and they are usually much smaller. A biopsy for pathologic evaluation is diagnostic but is only done when there is concern for the diagnosis of skin cancer. Typically, the diagnosis of hidrocystoma is clinical and no tissue is required.

Pathogenesis: Hidrocystomas develop from the eccrine apparatus. It is believed that a portion of the eccrine duct within the dermis becomes occluded. This occlusion causes a buildup of eccrine secretions proximal to the blockage. Once enough fluid collects, a translucent papule becomes evident on the surface of the skin. No genetic abnormalities of the involved eccrine duct have been discovered, and this cystic formation is most likely caused by damage from superficial trauma to the skin and the underlying eccrine ducts. Sun damage to the eccrine ducts has been theorized to play a role, although this theory has yet to be vigorously tested.

Histology: A lone cystic space is seen within the dermis. The cyst is well circumscribed, and the lining of the cyst contains two layers of cells. The cells are cuboidal and have an eosinophilic cytoplasm. The cell wall has no myoepithelial cell component. The cysts are found near eccrine gland structures. There is minimal to no inflammatory infiltrate surrounding the cyst. The central cavity of the cyst contains a small amount of lightly eosinophilic material that is consistent with eccrine gland secretions. There is no evidence for sebaceous gland or apocrine gland secretion or derivation.

Treatment: No therapy is necessary in most cases. Most eccrine hidrocystomas are biopsied to ensure they are not basal cell carcinomas. They rarely recur after biopsy. If they do recur, no treatment is required. Surgical excision is the definitive treatment and is curative. Hidrocystomas almost never recur after excision.

Hypertrophic scars

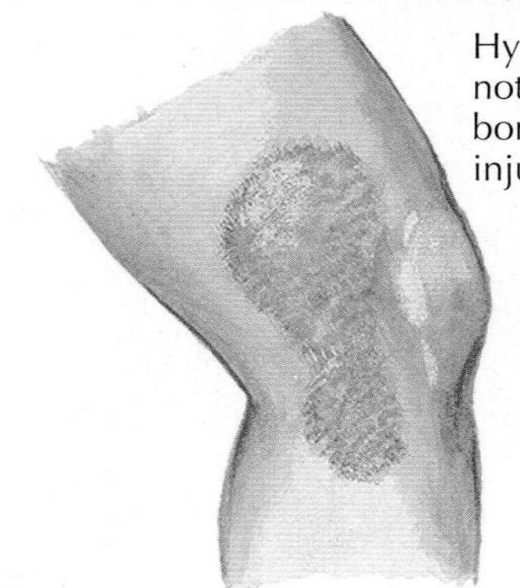

Hypertrophic scars do not extend beyond the border of the original injury.

Keloids

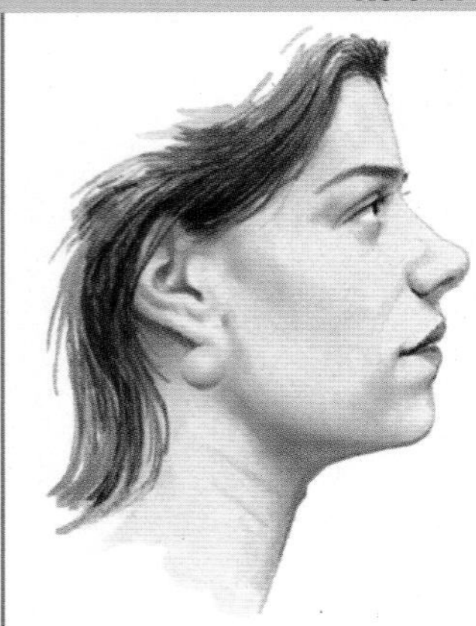

One of the most common locations for a keloid is the earlobe, and it can occur after ear piercing.

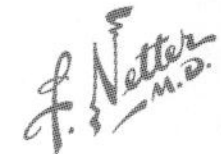

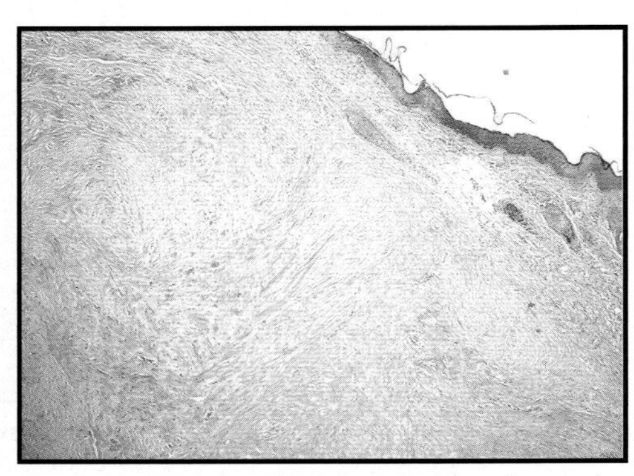

Hypertrophic scar, low power. Nonelevated scar made of numerous collagen bundles, fibroblasts, and blood vessels.

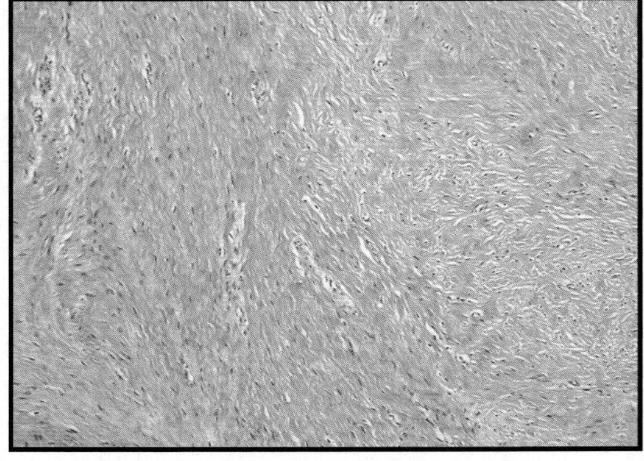

Hypertrophic scar, high power. Numerous fibroblasts with an increased number of vascular channels. The collagen bundles are arranged in the same direction.

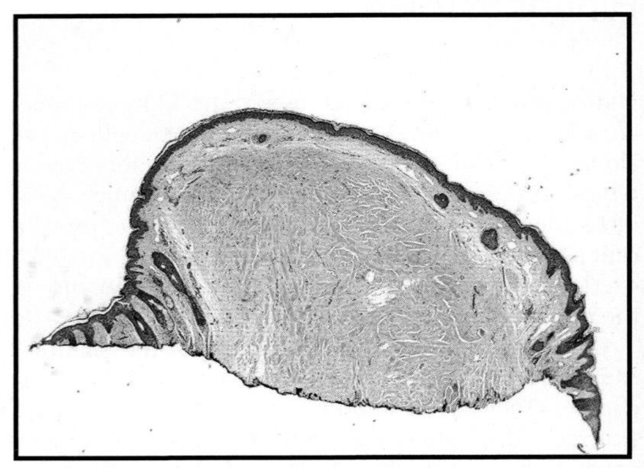

Keloid, low power. Haphazardly arranged collagen bundles. Thick eosinophilic bundles of collagen with surrounding fibroblasts.

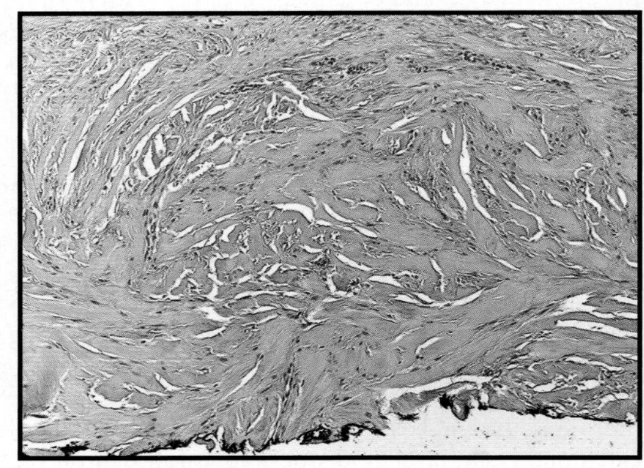

Keloid, high power. Thickened eosinophilic collagen bundles.

KELOID AND HYPERTROPHIC SCAR

Keloids are common benign skin tumors that consist of excessive scar tissue that forms after trauma or inflammatory skin conditions such as acne vulgaris. The keloid proliferates uncontrolled and expands beyond the borders of the underlying scar produced by the traumatic event. Hypertrophic scars, on the other hand, are exuberant scar formation that stays within the confines of the original scar border.

Clinical Findings: Keloids are often large overgrowths of scar tissue that expand over the original border of the underlying scar and affect previously normal-appearing skin. They may occur anywhere on the body but are more common on the earlobe, chest, and deltoid region of the upper arms. They can affect any age group and occur in males and females equally. Individuals of African or Asian descent have a higher incidence of keloid-type scarring. Almost all keloids manifest after a traumatic event such as a cut, ear piercing, burn, or surgical excision. Many other causes have been found to initiate the formation of keloids, including acne lesions and bug bites. Keloids often start as small, red, itchy papules that quickly enlarge into plaques and nodules. They usually have a smooth surface with a firm, hard consistency. Itching is a frequent complaint and often precedes the growth stage. Keloids are diagnosed clinically in a patient with the appropriate history. The differential diagnosis of early keloids includes hypertrophic scars. Difficulty sometimes arises when a patient presents with a firm, enlarging plaque or nodule but no preceding history of trauma. In these cases, a biopsy is prudent to rule out a dermatofibrosarcoma protuberans or other dermal tumor. The histopathologic findings easily differentiate the two lesions.

Hypertrophic scars occur after trauma and are confined to the area of the original trauma or scar. Hypertrophic scars, unlike keloids, do not grow into the adjacent normal skin. They can be quite large and often are pink to red in color and pruritic. Hypertrophic scars tend not to reach the size or extent of keloids, and for that reason they are a bit easier to manage therapeutically. Hypertrophic scars are diagnosed clinically in a patient with a typical history of preceding trauma and the characteristic clinical findings.

Pathogenesis: Keloids appear to be more common during the first 3 decades of life. Keloids may have a genetic pathogenesis that has yet to be discovered. Certain areas of the body are more prone to keloid formation, including the chest and earlobes, and there may be some local skin cytokine profile that allows for their formation. The keratinocytes within the keloid have been shown to express higher levels of various cytokines, which may play a role in keloid development. The majority of research has focused on the dermal fibroblasts and their role in the development of keloids. Biologic studies have looked at several cytokines, and elevated levels of transforming growth factor-β (TGF-β) have been found in keloids. TGF-β causes recruitment of fibroblasts into the region and induces them to produce more collagen. Sorafenib is a kinase inhibitor used to treat various cancers. It has been shown experimentally to antagonize the TGF-β pathway and decrease keloids. Local blockade of this cytokine may be developed as a therapy in the future with the goal of avoiding many of the systemic side effects.

Histology: Keloids show an increase in collagen production, which is arranged in a disorganized fashion. The overlying epidermis is typically thin due to the mass effect of the keloid tumor pressing on the undersurface of the epidermis, which causes attenuation of the surface epithelium. Mucopolysaccharides are found between the collagen fibers.

Hypertrophic scars are smaller and not exophytic in nature, and the collagen bundles are arranged parallel to the epidermis. There may be an increase in mast cells in both hypertrophic scars and keloids.

Treatment: Hypertrophic scars do not need to be treated because most will mature over time and eventually flatten and blend with the surrounding skin. Intralesional triamcinolone may be used to help speed the process, but care should be taken not to inject too much and thereby cause atrophy. Daily massage by the patient has also been shown to be effective in decreasing the outward appearance of the scar. The redness of both hypertrophic and keloid scars can be treated successfully with pulsed dye laser.

Keloids are more challenging to treat. They have a high rate of recurrence after excisional removal; for this reason, adjunctive therapy should always be used after excision. Serial injections with intralesional triamcinolone monthly for 4 to 6 months may help avoid a recurrence after surgery. Postoperative radiation therapy has also been very successful in decreasing the recurrence rate. There are anecdotal reports of treatment with imiquimod and cryotherapy, but they are of questionable value.

LEIOMYOMA

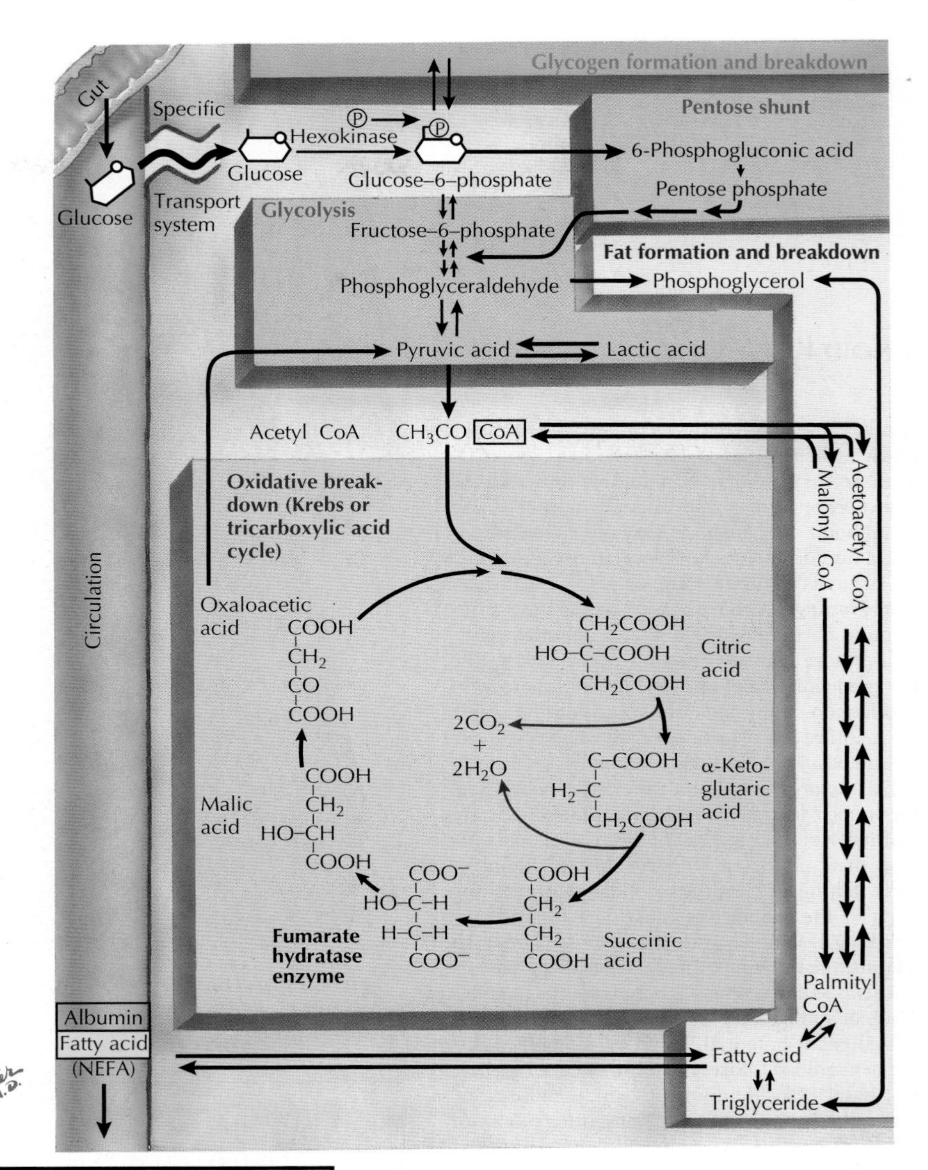

Cutaneous leiomyomas are uncommon benign tumors of the arrector pili muscle of the skin. They can occur as a solitary tumor or as multiple lesions. Both types can be associated with underlying genetic defects. Genetic defects occur more commonly in multiple cutaneous leiomyomatosis, and one needs to look for systemic findings in affected patients. Other muscle sources of cutaneous leiomyoma formation include the smooth muscle of blood vessel walls and the dartos muscle. These rare forms of cutaneous leiomyomas are named angioleiomyomas and solitary genital leiomyomas, respectively.

Clinical Findings: Leiomyomas manifest as dermal papules or nodules with a slight hyperpigmentation of the overlying epidermis. They can also have a reddish or brownish hue. The tumors are typically 1 to 2 cm in diameter. They occur equally in males and females and affect all races. They may occur anywhere on the skin, but the anterior chest and the genital region are more common areas of involvement. They are typically tender and can be painful. Most leiomyomas will become more painful and more sensitive to touch and temperature over time. Cold temperatures have been shown to exacerbate the pain. Leiomyomas exhibit the pseudo-Darier's sign. This sign is elicited by gently rubbing the leiomyoma; on manipulation, the lesion begins to twitch or fasciculate. It does not form an urticarial plaque as would be seen with a true Darier's sign (e.g., in cutaneous mastocytosis). Malignant transformation is exceedingly rare.

Multiple cutaneous leiomyomas occur most commonly on the trunk and proximal extremities. They are the same size as their solitary counterparts, but they can become so numerous that they appear to coalesce into large plaques. In most patients, onset occurs in the third to fifth decades of life. There is an autosomal dominant inheritance pattern to multiple cutaneous leiomyomas. These patients have a genetic defect in the *FH* gene (also called *MCUL1*), which encodes the Krebs cycle protein fumarate hydratase. The fumarate hydratase protein has been found to have tumor suppressor functions. Many different types of mutations have been described, ranging from frameshift mutations to deletion of the entire gene. This explains the variety of phenotypes seen. The most concerning and life-threatening aspect of this mutation is the possibility of developing an aggressive and deadly form of papillary renal cell carcinoma. This tumor in patients with multiple cutaneous leiomyomas tends to be highly aggressive and metastasizes early. Early screening of the patient and genetic screening of family members may help decrease the risk of metastatic renal carcinoma. Patients should be seen by a urologist familiar with this condition and should be evaluated routinely for kidney disease.

The term Reed syndrome is used for women with cutaneous leiomyomas and uterine leiomyomas.

Pathogenesis: Solitary leiomyomas not associated with the fumarate hydratase protein defect are believed to be caused by an abnormal proliferation of myocytes. The cause for this proliferation is unknown. Fumarate hydratase mutations result in a lack of tumor suppressor function. The role of this tumor suppressor protein in the production of multiple leiomyomas has yet to be fully determined, but defects in this enzyme lead to changes in cell cycle energy production and an upregulation of hypoxic pathway genes.

Histology: The tumor is located within the dermis and is composed of interconnected fascicles of spindle-shaped cells. The cells are arranged in a whorl-like pattern. The cells are uniform and bland appearing. Mitosis should be absent. The cells have been described as cigar shaped, meaning that they have a long, plump central region with blunt tip ends. The cell of origin is the myocyte. Immunohistochemical staining can be used to help differentiate difficult tumors. Leiomyomas stain with muscle markers such as smooth muscle actin. The overlying epidermis is usually normal.

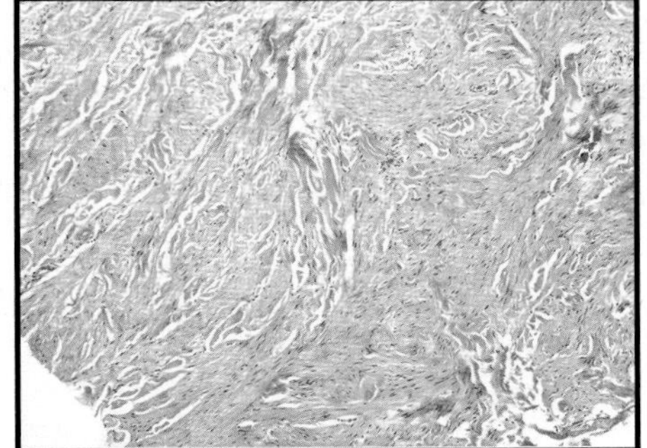
Low power. Tumor is located within the dermis and is composed of interlacing fascicles of spindle-shaped muscle cells.

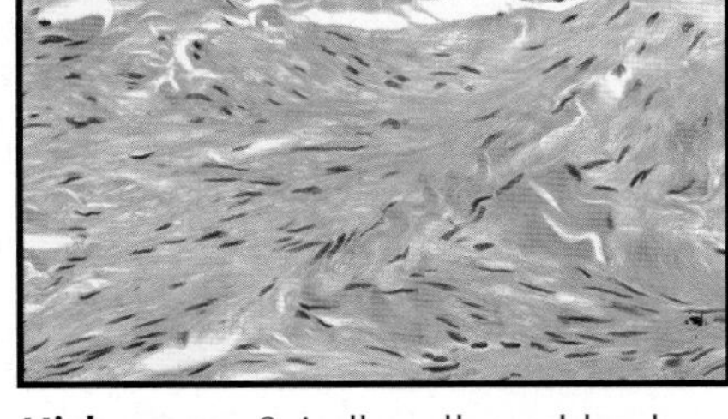
High power. Spindle cells are bland appearing with blunt-tipped ends.

Treatment: Surgical excision of the solitary form of leiomyoma is curative. Multiple cutaneous leiomyomatosis can be treated with a number of medications to help control the discomfort and pain. Use of α_1-adrenergic receptor blockers has been reported most frequently. Doxazosin and phenoxybenzamine have been efficacious. Calcium channel blockers such as nifedipine have been anecdotally successful. Gabapentin and botulinum toxin have also been described as therapeutic. Surgical excision is warranted for any lesion that is painful and not responding to therapy. Patients with multiple cutaneous leiomyomas should be evaluated for the genetic defect in the fumarate hydratase protein and should have appropriate lifelong screening for kidney disease.

Lichenoid Keratosis

Lichenoid keratoses are common benign skin growths also known as lichen planus–like keratoses. These are most often solitary, benign skin tumors and may be found anywhere on human skin. They are more common during adulthood. The keratosis may be clinically confused with a nonmelanoma skin cancer, most commonly a superficial basal cell carcinoma.

Clinical Findings: Lichenoid keratoses are most frequently found on the upper trunk and upper extremities and are more common in sun-exposed skin. The incidence is equal in males and females, and there is no race predilection. They are rare in childhood. They typically manifest as pruritic, red to slightly purple patches and thin plaques. Occasionally, a patient notices that the area arises in a preexisting seborrheic keratosis or solar lentigo. Most lichenoid keratoses are 1 cm or smaller in their largest diameter. Most patients present to their physician with a chief complaint of tenderness, itching, or bleeding secondary to scratching or rubbing of the lesion. The individual lesions may have a striking resemblance to the lesions of the rash lichen planus; the differentiating factor is that a lichenoid keratosis is solitary, whereas lichen planus includes a multitude of similar skin lesions. These skin growths have no malignant potential. It can be difficult to differentiate lichenoid keratoses from inflamed seborrheic keratoses, basal cell carcinomas, actinic keratoses, or squamous cell carcinoma in situ. Therefore a biopsy of the lesion is prudent to discern a pathologic diagnosis.

There are a few unusual clinical variants, including an atrophic form and a bullous type of lichenoid keratosis. The differential diagnosis of these two variants includes conditions such as lichen sclerosis for the former and autoimmune blistering diseases for the latter. The dermatoscope has become an indispensable tool and can be helpful in diagnosing lichenoid keratosis. Lichenoid keratoses have been shown to have a localized or diffuse granular-type pattern under dermatoscopic viewing. This finding should help differentiate these tumors from melanocytic tumors.

Pathogenesis: The exact etiology of lichenoid keratosis is unknown. It is believed to be caused by an inflammatory response to a lentigo or a thin seborrheic keratosis. The specific precipitating factor may be trauma. Chronic rubbing has been implicated in inducing lichenoid keratoses from lentigines. The role of human papillomavirus in causing lichenoid keratoses has been studied, but no firm conclusions have been made.

Histology: On histologic examination, a lichenoid keratosis has a symmetric, well-circumscribed area of intense lichenoid inflammation along the basement membrane region. There is disruption of the basilar keratinocytes. This leads to the appearance of a number of necrotic keratinocytes, also called Civatte bodies. Civatte bodies are seen in almost all cases of lichenoid keratosis and also in lichen planus. There is pronounced sawtooth hypergranulosis and pronounced acanthosis. There is no atypia of the involved keratinocytes, thus ruling out an inflamed actinic keratosis. The underlying inflammatory infiltrate is made up almost entirely of lymphocytes. However, it is not uncommon to find a rare eosinophil or plasma cell in the infiltrate. The pathologic differential diagnosis includes lichen planus. The clinical history is very important: whereas a lichenoid keratosis is a solitary lesion, the same findings in a biopsy specimen taken from a widespread rash of purple, flat-topped papules would be more consistent with the diagnosis of lichen planus. This example illustrates the importance of including the clinical history on a pathology report.

Treatment: Most biopsies of a lichenoid keratosis result in complete resolution of the lesion. Even if the entire lesion was not removed with the biopsy specimen, no treatment is necessary. Use of a topical corticosteroid cream or ointment twice daily for 1 to 2 weeks after healing of the biopsy site is likely to lead to complete resolution of the lichenoid keratosis. Other treatment options include light cryotherapy or a light curettage after anesthesia. Benign lichenoid keratoses rarely recur.

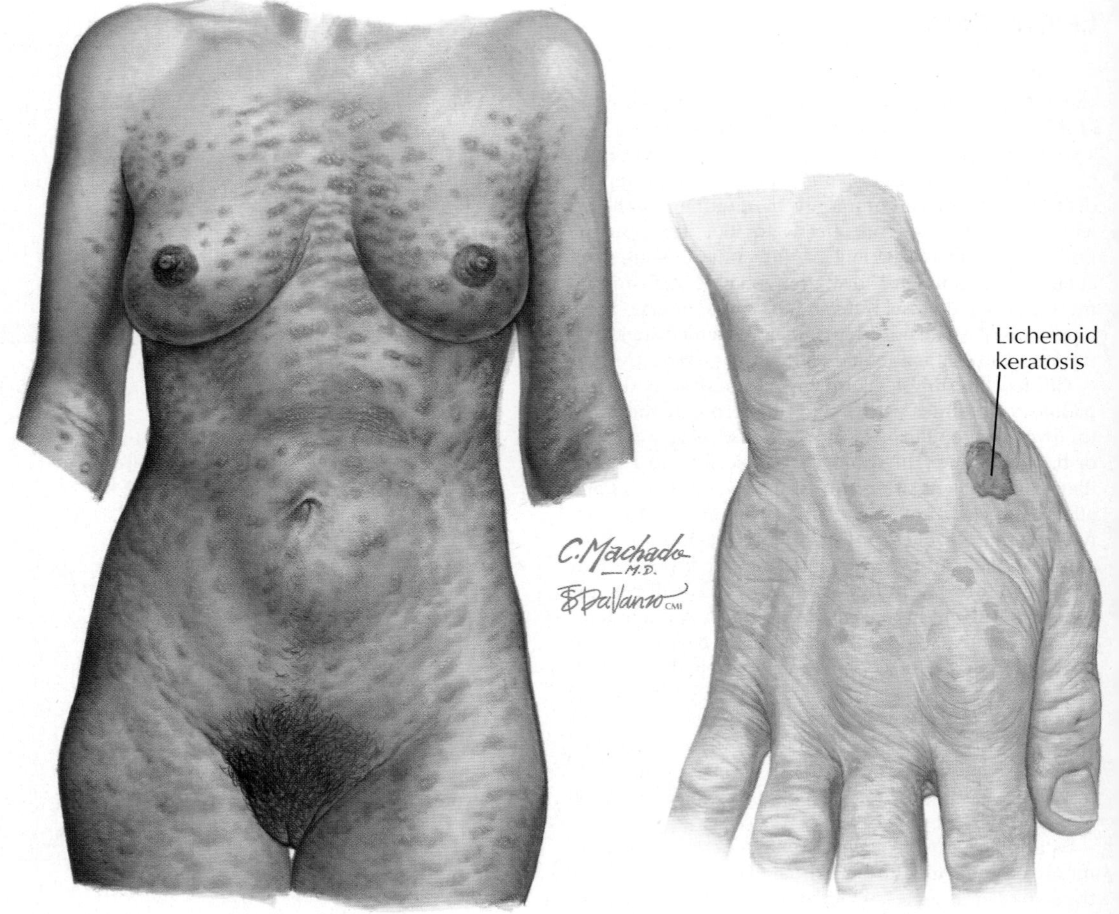

Lichen planus. Widespread pruritic purplish papules and plaques, some with Wickham striae.

Lichenoid keratosis. A solitary growth in comparison to the widespread nature of lichen planus. Histology can be identical.

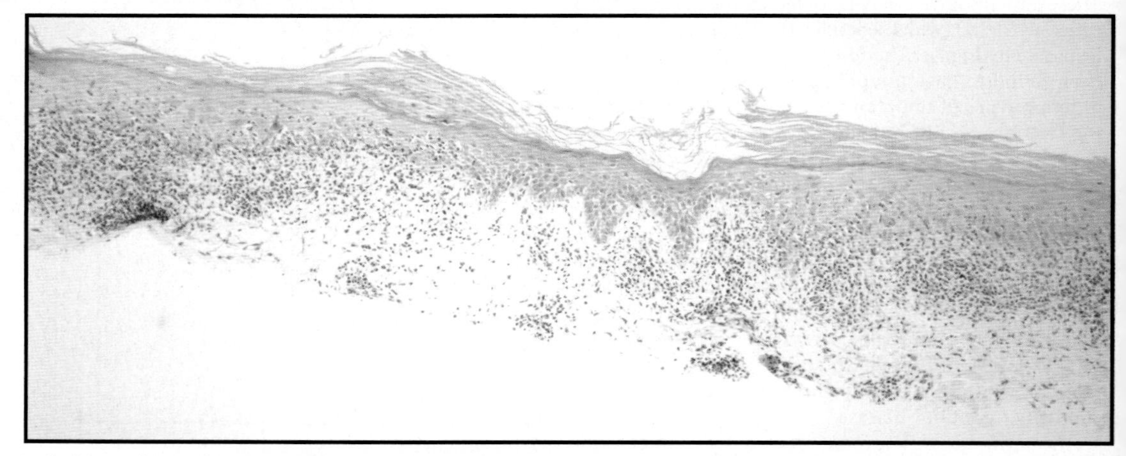

A lichenoid lymphocytic infiltrate is seen along the dermal-epidermal junction. Disruption of the dermal-epidermal junction is prominent. Necrotic keratinocytes are seen in the epidermis.

LIPOMA

Lipomas are common benign skin growths that can be seen as solitary lesions and frequently as multiple dermal nodules scattered about the skin. The lipoma is an overgrowth of the fibrofatty adipose tissue in the subcutaneous tissue plane. Patients with multiple lipomas often describe a familial inheritance pattern.

Clinical Findings: Lipomas are often small (1–2 cm), soft, subcutaneous nodules that are slow growing and freely movable underneath the skin. Some lipomas become quite large (>5 cm in diameter) and can be a cause for concern due to interference with movement and the possibility of malignant degeneration into a liposarcoma. There are no overlying epidermal changes, and there is no connection to the epidermis. Most often they are asymptomatic, but they can become painful if traumatized.

In stark contrast, a rare variant called the angiolipoma is almost always tender and multiple in nature. Angiolipomas contain a much higher percentage of blood vessels throughout the lobule of adipose tissue, and the diagnosis is made based on this histopathologic finding. These tumors are benign and have no familial inheritance pattern.

The differential diagnosis of a lipoma is broad and can include other dermal tumors; however, the clinical examination findings are often diagnostic. Occasionally, a small lipoma can be confused with an epidermal inclusion cyst, pilar cyst, lymph node, or adnexal tumor. Large, freely movable, soft, rubbery nodules that are slow growing are easily diagnosed clinically as lipomas. When palpating larger lipomas, the clinician may be able to palpate various fat lobules, thus further solidifying the clinical diagnosis.

Lipomas occur most commonly on the trunk and extremities. They most often affect women in their third through fifth decades of life but can affect people of any age and sex. There is no race predilection. They rarely affect the face, except for the subfrontalis lipoma, which occurs underneath the frontalis muscle on the forehead.

Rare syndromes of adipose tissue have been described, including benign symmetric lipomatosis, adiposis dolorosa (Dercum disease), and familial multiple lipomatosis. The best described of these syndromes is benign symmetric lipomatosis, also known as Madelung disease. In this condition, there is massive proliferation of adipose tissue on the neck and upper arms of men. The patients take on the appearance of a body builder. Numerous forms of lipoatrophy and lipodystrophy have been described in the literature.

Pathogenesis: The exact cause of lipomas is unknown. They are believed to be an overgrowth of normal tissue in a normal location. The tumor lobules are indistinguishable from normal adipose tissue. A genetic pattern of inheritance has been described, but no specific gene defect has been located. Angiolipomas contain a higher percentage of normal blood vessels within the tumor's fibrous septa compared with the typical lipoma.

Histology: Lipomas are composed of mature adipose tissue. The lobules are separated by fibrous septa that contain the blood supply for the adipose cells. Lipomas have a fibrous capsule enclosing the adipose lobules. Angiolipomas are described as fatty tumors in which 10% to 50% of the mass is composed of blood vessels. The various rare lipomatosis variants are identical in appearance histologically to a common lipoma.

Treatment: No therapy is required for these benign skin tumors. Solitary lipomas can be treated with a simple excision or with liposuction. Subfrontalis lipomas are more difficult to remove because the surgeon must dissect below the frontalis muscle to locate the lipoma. Small lipomas have been treated with intralesional steroid injection to take advantage of the steroid's atrophogenic effects. Injections with deoxycholate have also been effective. Large, fast-growing lipomas should be removed or biopsied to rule out malignant transformation into a liposarcoma. Compared with lipomas, liposarcomas are typically faster growing, firmer, and tender in nature.

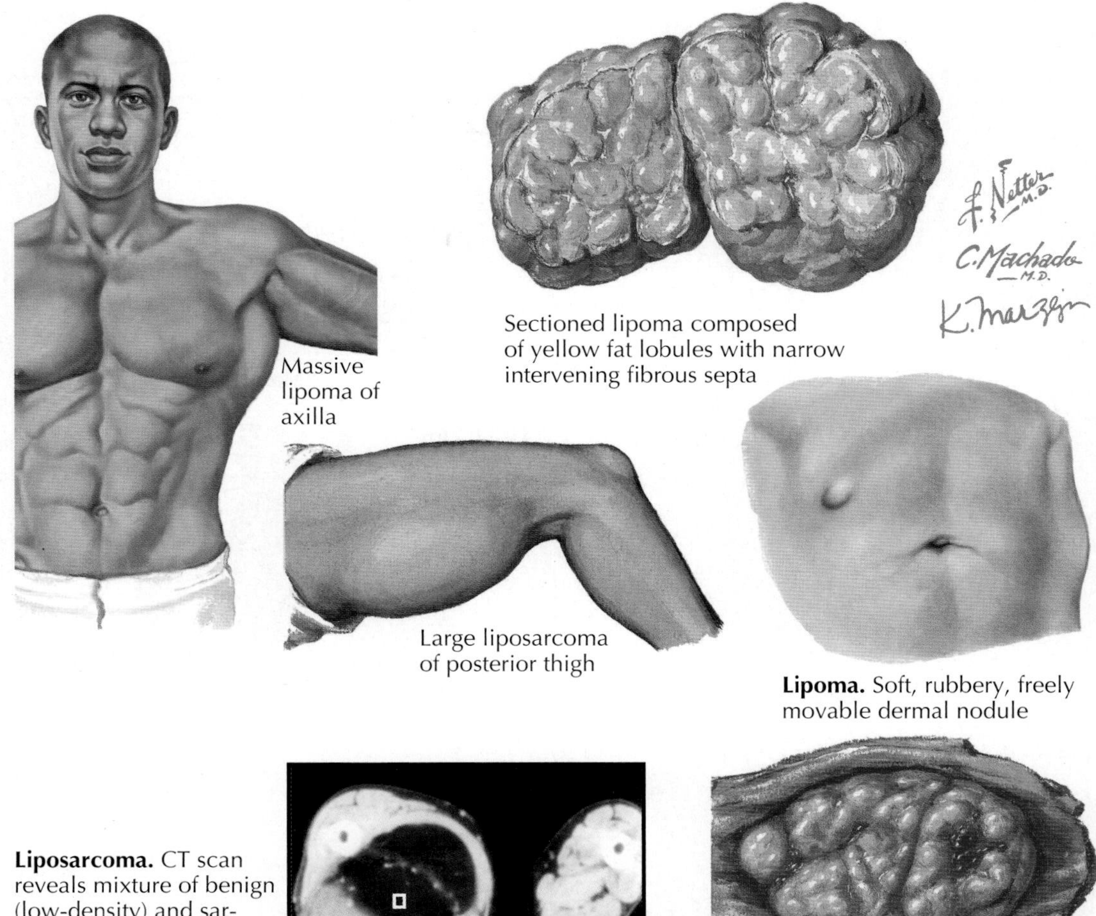

Massive lipoma of axilla

Sectioned lipoma composed of yellow fat lobules with narrow intervening fibrous septa

Large liposarcoma of posterior thigh

Lipoma. Soft, rubbery, freely movable dermal nodule

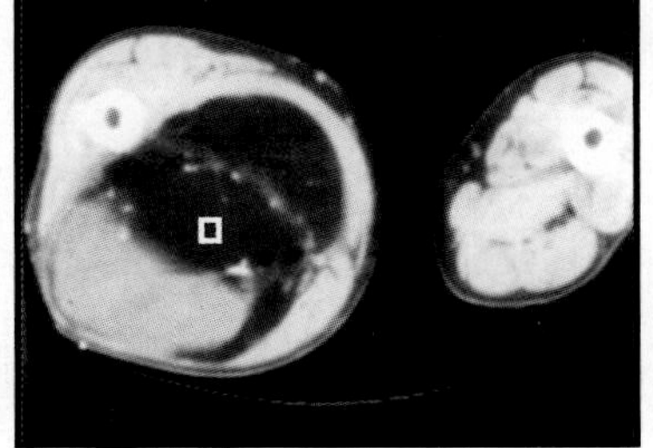

Liposarcoma. CT scan reveals mixture of benign (low-density) and sarcomatous (high-density) areas of tumor.

Liposarcoma. Excised tumor with muscle at margin; tumor darker and firmer than benign lipoma

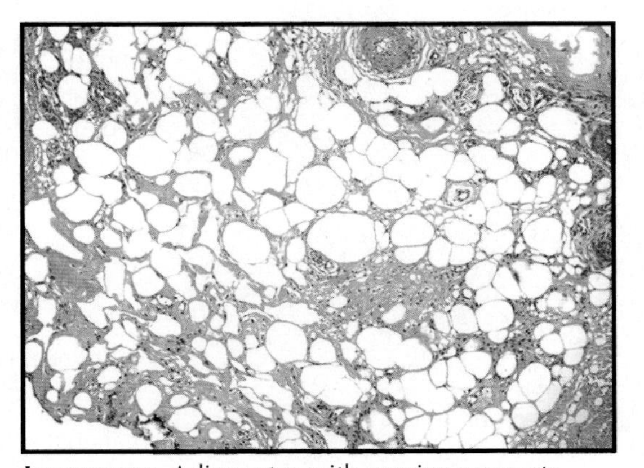

Low power. Adipocytes with varying amounts of fibrous tissue and blood vessels.

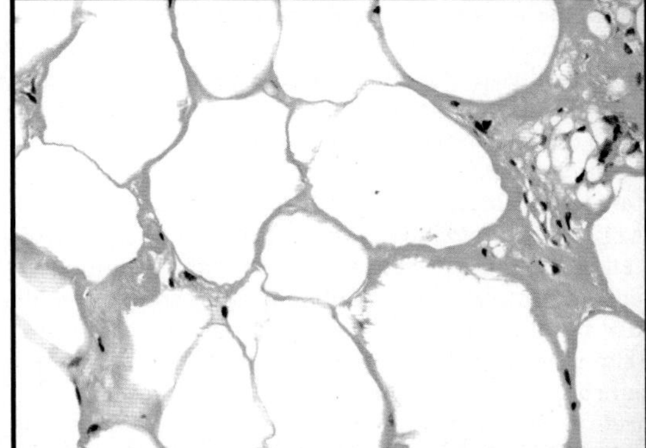

High power. Mature adipocytes are the main component of the tumor.

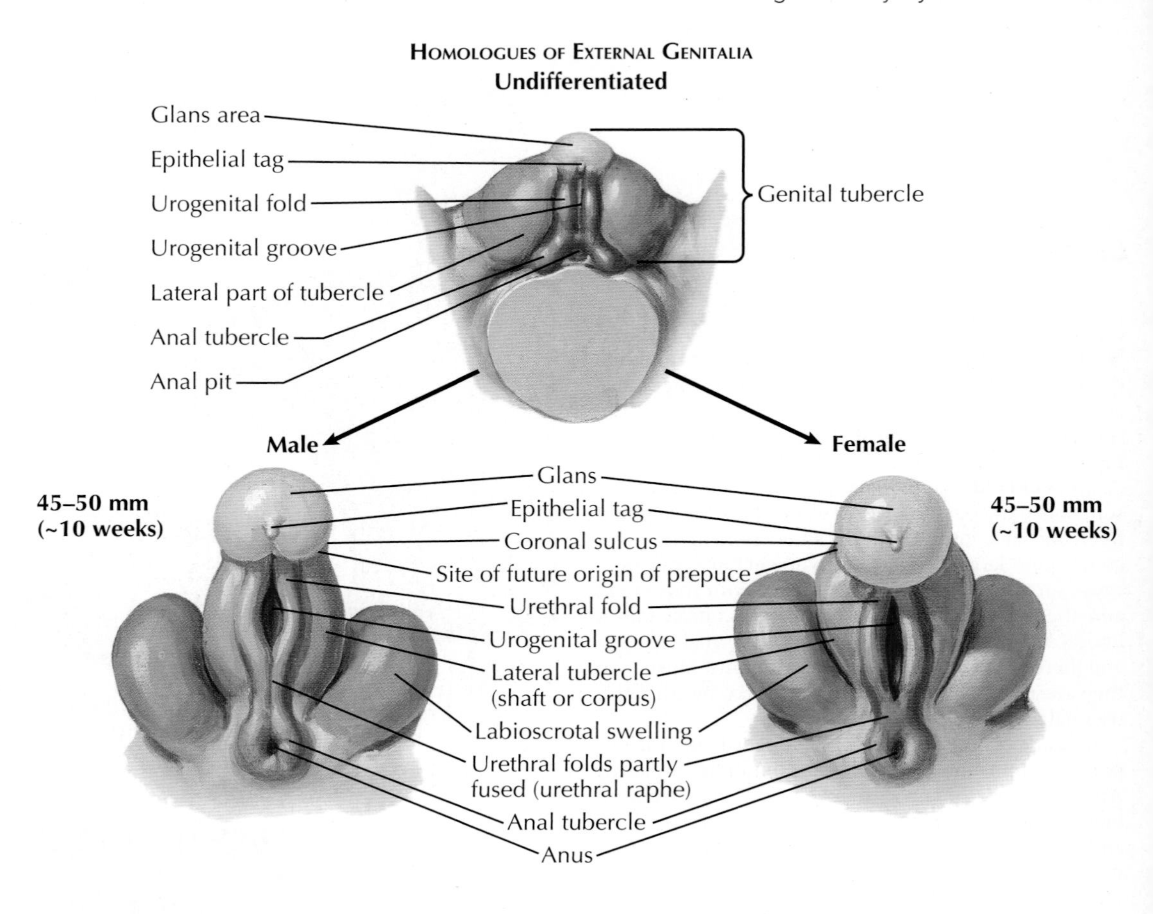

MEDIAN RAPHE CYST

Median raphe cysts are uncommon benign cysts that form in the midline region of the perineum. In males, they most commonly occur on the ventral shaft of the penis but can occur anywhere from the urethral opening along the ventral surface of the penis, in the midline across the scrotum, and to the anus. In females, they are most commonly found between the inferior aspect of the introitus to the anus. Abnormal urethral folding during embryologic development is believed to be the cause of these developmental cysts.

Clinical Findings: Most median raphe cysts are diagnosed in infants and young boys on the ventral surface of the penis and midline scrotum. They have no race predilection. They are present at birth but may go unnoticed for some time, even into adulthood. They appear as small (0.5–1 cm), solitary, soft, translucent cystic nodules. They are almost always asymptomatic. On occasion, they can rupture and drain serous fluid. The cyst rarely connects to the underlying urethra or other structures. The clinical differential diagnosis can be very broad, and the only way to make a definitive diagnosis is to perform a biopsy or complete excision.

Pathogenesis: These cysts are believed to be caused by an abnormal folding or fusing of the paired urogenital/urethral folds during embryologic development. These folds normally combine and fuse to form the external genitalia at the eighth to tenth week of gestation. In the male the folds form the shaft of the penis, and in females they form the labia minora. Hypospadias is another congenital abnormality caused by improper folding of these embryologic tissues. The cause of the abnormal folding has yet to be determined. Median raphe cysts have been reported to occur in conjunction with hypospadias.

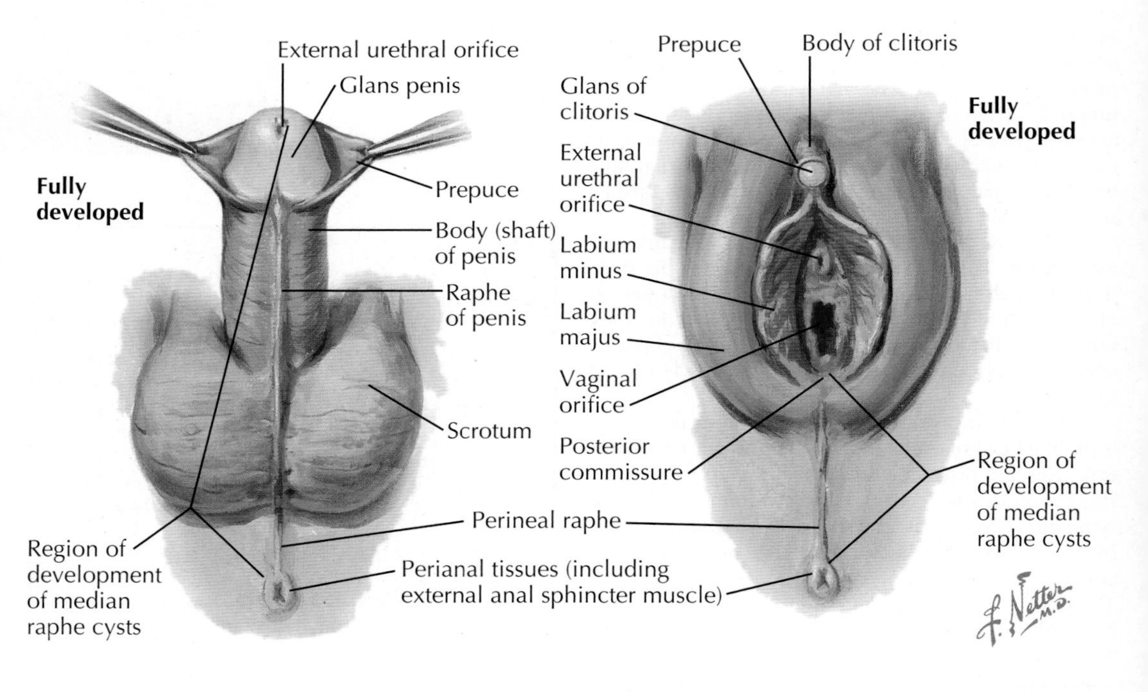

Histology: The cysts are lined with a pseudostratified or stratified columnar epithelium. The epithelium can closely approximate the appearance of transitional urethral cell epithelium. The lining surrounds a central cavity filled with serous fluid. Large mucinous cells are scattered throughout the columnar epithelium. The luminal cells have been shown to stain with cytokeratin 7, cytokeratin 13, epithelial membrane antigen, and carcinoembryonic antigen. Histologically, these cysts have a very characteristic appearance. The main pathologic differential diagnosis is between the median raphe cyst and an apocrine cystadenoma. Immunohistochemical staining can be used to differentiate the two.

Treatment: Individuals are often seen by pediatric urology for evaluation, diagnosis, and treatment. Simple surgical excision is the cure. They will not recur because they are developmental cysts. Care should be taken not to damage underlying structures, so a urologic surgeon typically performs the procedure.

Melanocytic Nevi

There are numerous types of melanocytic nevi, including the benign congenital melanocytic nevi, the blue nevi, and the common acquired melanocytic nevi. Atypical and dysplastic nevi are discussed with melanoma in the section on malignant growths. Evaluation of melanocytic nevi is one of the dermatologist's most common and important tasks. Every patient who enters a dermatologist's office should be offered the opportunity to have a full-body skin examination, specifically to evaluate melanocytic nevi for any signs of malignant transformation or de novo melanoma production. The importance of evaluating melanocytic nevi is to screen for melanoma. Melanoma is a life-threatening skin cancer that, if discovered early, can be cured. Different types of melanocytic nevi have varying rates of malignant transformation, and it is critical for the clinician to be aware of nevi that are likely to be encountered on a daily basis.

Clinical Findings: Melanocytic nevi can be classified both clinically and histopathologically. The common acquired melanocytic nevus is a clinical diagnosis; if the lesion is biopsied, it may show some evidence of atypia or dysplasia of melanocytes. Because of this, a universally accepted classification of melanocytic nevi has yet to be adopted.

Benign melanocytic nevi are extremely common. Virtually all humans have some form of these growths on their body. Common acquired melanocytic nevi are universally found and can have varying morphologies. They affect males and females equally. They are uncommon at birth but increase in number over the first 4 decades of life, after which the number typically stabilizes. As one ages, the nevi tend to slowly involute. They can be macular or papular in appearance. Most are uniform and symmetric in size and color. They can be flesh colored or varying shades of brown. They tend to grow proportionally as a child grows or as an adult gains weight. They also can become slightly larger and darker during pregnancy.

There is a risk for malignant degeneration into melanoma, and changes in color, size, symmetry, or border should be assessed. Nevi that become symptomatic, especially pruritic, and nevi that spontaneously bleed should be evaluated and biopsied appropriately.

Blue nevi are unique benign melanocytic tumors that have a characteristic clinical and histologic pattern. These nevi tend to be small, are located on the dorsal aspect of the hands or feet, and have a bluish to blue-gray coloration because of their location within the dermis. The blue color is believed to result from the Tyndall effect. This is a process by which various wavelengths of light are absorbed preferentially, and the reflected light or color that is seen depends on the material and depth of the substance being illuminated. Blue nevi share similar histologic characteristics with the nevus of Ota, nevus of Ito, and congenital dermal melanocytosis. However, the clinical appearance is so different that these lesions are not considered in the differential diagnosis of a blue nevus.

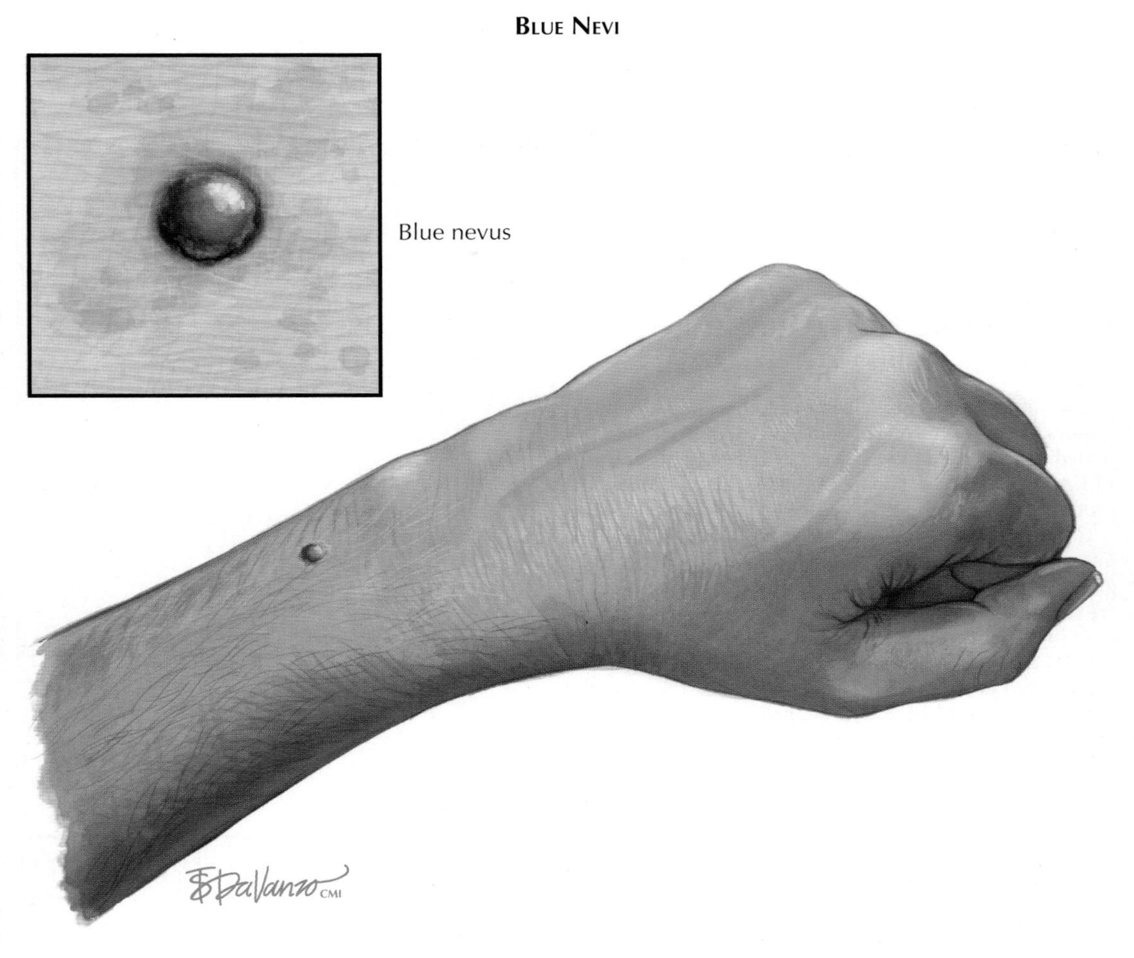

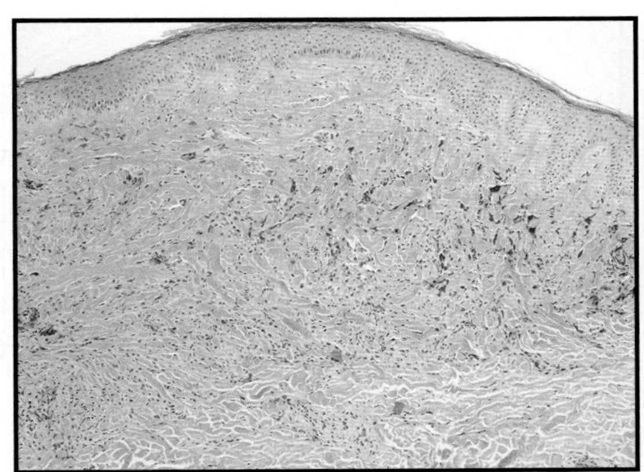

Low power. The epidermis appears normal. The dermis is filled with spindle-shaped melanocytes and many melanophages.

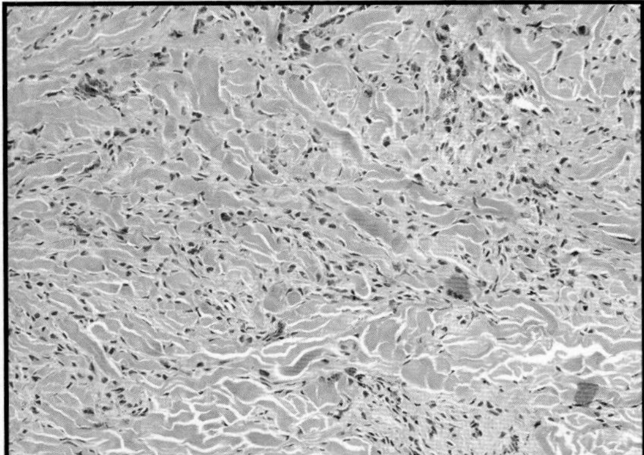

High power. Elongated pigmented melanocytes are appreciated with multiple dermal melanophages. The melanocytes are interspersed between the collagen bundles.

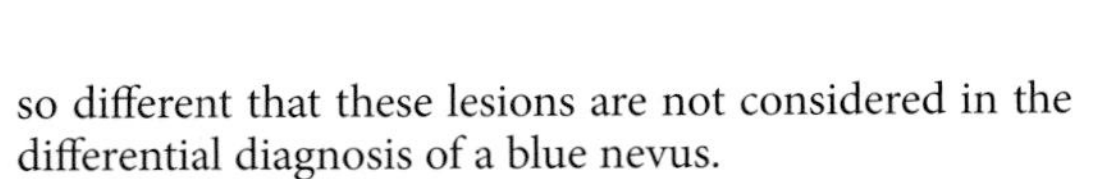

Blue nevi can occur at any age, and they appear equally often in men and in women. They typically manifest as small (2–5 mm), oval or round macules or papules. They are well circumscribed with distinct borders. They are commonly located on the dorsal aspect of the hands and feet but have been reported to occur anywhere, including the mucous membranes. They are frequently biopsied because of their unusual coloration. They are small and usually can be removed easily with a punch biopsy that is 1 mm larger than the lesion. Patients often state they were pierced with a pencil during childhood and believe that the lesion is a graphite tattoo. This occasionally is the case, but most of these lesions are actually blue nevi. Malignant transformation of blue nevi is extremely rare.

Multiple blue nevi can be seen in the Carney complex, also known by the mnemonics NAME or LAMB syndrome. This complex of clinical findings includes multiple blue nevi, lentigines, ephelides, myxomas, atrial myxomas, testicular tumors, pituitary tumors,

Melanocytic Nevi (Continued)

psammomatous melanotic schwannomas, and adrenal tumors. This is a rare syndrome that has been determined to be caused by a genetic defect in the gene *PRKAR1A,* a tumor suppressor gene that encodes a protein kinase A subunit.

Congenital melanocytic nevi can be divided clinically into distinct subtypes based on size (small, medium, and giant). Small congenital nevi are the most common; they are defined as nevi smaller than 2 cm in greatest diameter. These nevi occur with equal frequency in males and females and have no race predilection. Their prevalence is estimated at about 1% of the population. These nevi are typically described as well-defined macules, papules, or plaques. They are hyperpigmented compared with the normal surrounding skin. They are almost always uniform in color and symmetric. Over time, 50% develop terminal hair growth within the nevi. The risk of malignant transformation in these small congenital nevi is low and approaches that of the common acquired melanocytic nevi. Melanoma can arise in these nevi at any point in the patient's life but usually after puberty.

Medium-sized congenital melanocytic nevi are defined as having a diameter between 2 and 20 cm. They have the same risk of malignant transformation as small congenital nevi. They occur equally in males and females and can be seen in about 1% of the population. They can occur anywhere on the body.

Giant or large congenital melanocytic nevi, sometimes known as "bathing trunk" nevi, are important clinically in many ways. First, they have an increased risk of malignant transformation. This transformation can be difficult to discern clinically until the lesions are quite large. Most melanomas develop in a dermal or subcutaneous location, which makes them difficult to assess clinically. Melanomas typically occur before puberty and have been reported to occur in as many as 15% of giant congenital nevi. The risk of malignant transformation is higher in axial nevi than in acral nevi. For this reason, these lesions are treated more aggressively, and patients with large congenital melanocytic nevi need lifelong, frequent routine follow-up. These nevi occur equally in men and women and in any racial group. They affect the truncal region more often than any other region of the body.

The significant finding of neurocutaneous melanosis occurs at a higher rate in patients with large congenital nevi of the trunk. These nevi almost always occur over the majority of the trunk, and they can have any number of satellite melanocytic nevi. Individuals with a higher number of satellites (>50) have a higher risk of neurocutaneous melanosis. Patients with large truncal congenital melanocytic nevi should undergo magnetic resonance imaging of the nervous system to evaluate for neurocutaneous melanosis. Patients with neurocutaneous melanosis are at a high risk (almost 50%) for development of leptomeningeal melanoma, which is almost always fatal. A multidisciplinary approach to care for these patients is required, including the patient's pediatrician, dermatologist, neurologist, and neurosurgeon.

Common Acquired Nevi and Giant Congenital Melanocytic Nevi

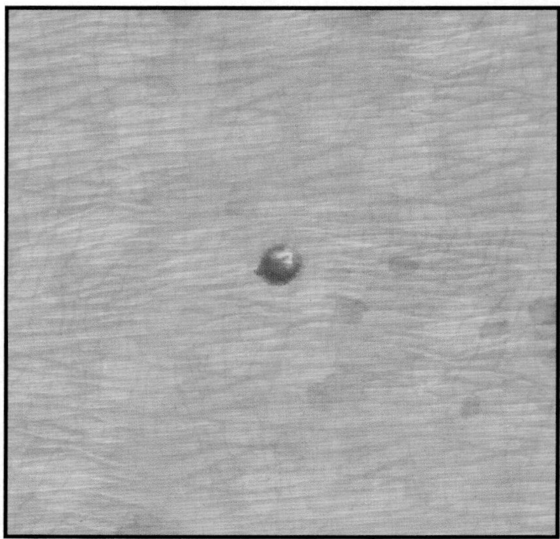

Common acquired nevus

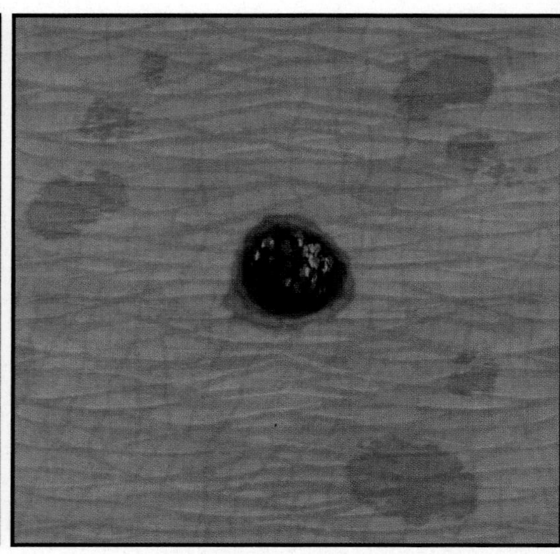

Atypical/dysplastic nevus with surrounding solar lentigines

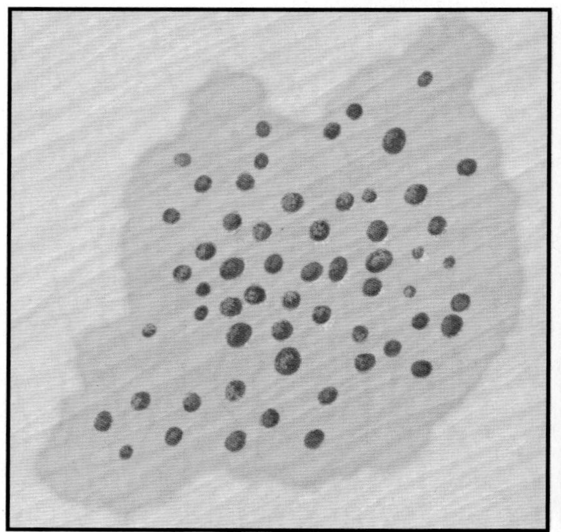

Nevus spilus

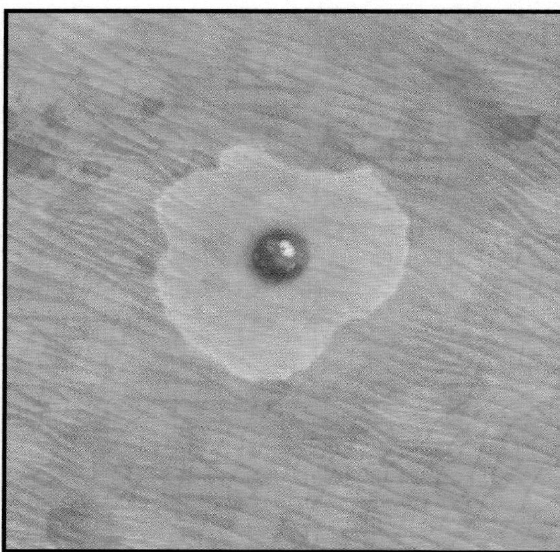

Halo nevus

Histology: In common acquired melanocytic nevi, the melanocytes are arranged symmetrically in a lateral fashion and in nests. The nested melanocytes do not have the typical dendritic appearance of normal melanocytes found within the stratum basalis. They are round and uniform in shape and show increasing maturation with depth in the dermis. Maturation of nevi cells implies a decrease in the ratio of nuclear to cytoplasmic volume and an overall decrease in the size of the melanocytes. The melanocytes are still uniform in size and shape at various depths within the dermis; they are not symmetric vertically. Many forms are seen histologically. Based on the location of the melanocyte nests, they can be classified as junctional, intraepidermal, dermal, or compound nevi. A junctional nevus has nests arranged along the basement membrane zone, whereas a compound nevus has epidermal and dermal nests.

Blue nevi are located entirely within the dermis. These nevi are made of melanocytes that resemble dendrites.

Melanocytic Nevi (Continued)

The dendritic processes contain melanin pigment, which is responsible for the coloration of the lesion. Collagen is interwoven between the dermally located melanocytes. Melanophages are almost always seen in and around the lesion. A grenz zone is sometimes appreciated above the melanocytic lesion. Numerous histologic subtypes of blue nevi have been described, including the dendritic blue nevus (common blue nevus), amelanotic blue nevus, cellular blue nevus, and epithelioid blue nevus.

Small, medium, and large congenital nevi all show the same histologic characteristics, and they cannot be distinguished on pathologic evaluation. The major criteria used to separate congenital nevi from other types of nevi are size and location. The nests are found deep within the dermis and can also be found within the subcutaneous tissue, fascia, and underlying muscle. Infiltration of muscle is unusual and is more likely to be seen in large congenital nevi. The nests of nevus cells accumulate around adnexal structures and are frequently seen juxtaposed to hair follicles, sebaceous glands, and eccrine glands. The melanocytes can penetrate the arrector pili muscles. The nevus cells show proper maturation and are uniform in appearance.

Pathogenesis: There are many conflicting theories as to the pathogenesis of common acquired melanocytic nevi and blue nevi. Some think there is an abnormal migration of melanocytes embryologically, whereas others believe that stem cells are located within the dermis or epidermis and melanocytes migrate upward or downward to form the nevi. Perhaps a combination of these processes occurs, but no definitive pathogenic mechanism has been universally accepted.

Congenital melanocytic nevi are thought to be caused by an embryologic malfunction of melanocyte migration. The precise mechanism that causes the disrupted or abnormal migration of melanocytes into the involved areas has not been determined. Migration in these cases is believed to be controlled by a complex but abnormal growth and regulatory signaling pathway.

Treatment: Common acquired melanocytic nevi do not need to be treated. They can be removed by various means for cosmetic purposes. Shave removal and punch biopsy removal are two highly successful techniques. Elliptical excision should be reserved for larger lesions in areas where the scar can be camouflaged. Only highly skilled physicians should consider removing pigmented lesions with laser therapy because there is no tissue left for histologic evaluation.

Blue nevi are easily removed by punch biopsy or elliptical excision. They are often removed for cosmetic reasons, and a small excision gives an excellent cosmetic result.

Removal of small and medium congenital nevi should be done with surgical excision. This removes the entire lesion and allows for pathologic evaluation. Most of these small and medium congenital melanocytic nevi can be observed over time and removed if there are changes. Serial photographs are invaluable in monitoring these nevi for changes. Some of these lesions occur in cosmetically sensitive areas, such as the face, and patients should be referred to a cosmetic surgeon for evaluation. The social and psychological well-being of the child can be enhanced by removing a disfiguring congenital nevus.

Large congenital nevi present the biggest treatment difficulty because of the high rate of malignant transformation. If possible, serial excisions to remove large nevi are the best option. Tissue expanders are often used to help decrease the need for skin grafting. The goal should be 100% removal, although in some cases this is not feasible. If the nevi cover 10% to 30% or more of body surface area, they become almost impossible to remove. In these cases, as in all the others, the importance of lifelong surveillance must be taught to the parents, the affected individuals, and the clinical team. The goal in these cases is to biopsy and remove any changing areas of the nevi in an effort to prevent metastasis if a melanoma were to develop.

Congenital Nevi

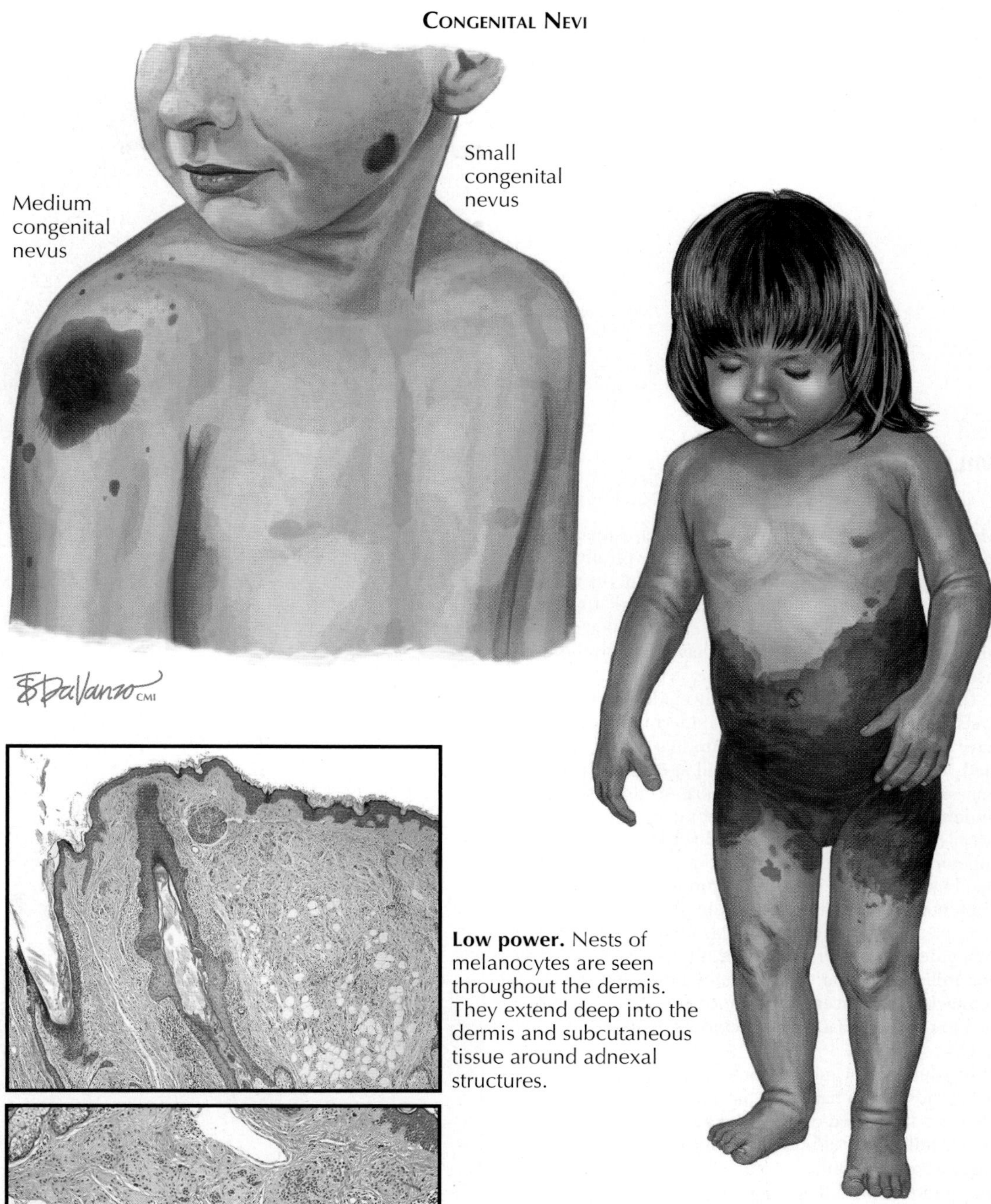

Low power. Nests of melanocytes are seen throughout the dermis. They extend deep into the dermis and subcutaneous tissue around adnexal structures.

Giant congenital bathing trunk nevus

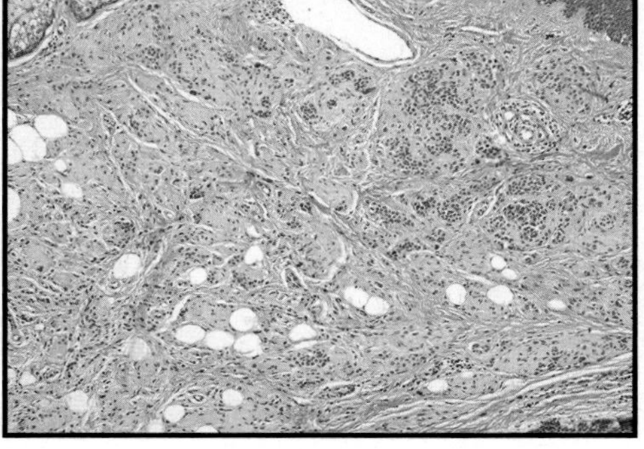

High power. Melanocytes are seen adjacent to adnexal structures. This is one characteristic finding in congenital nevi.

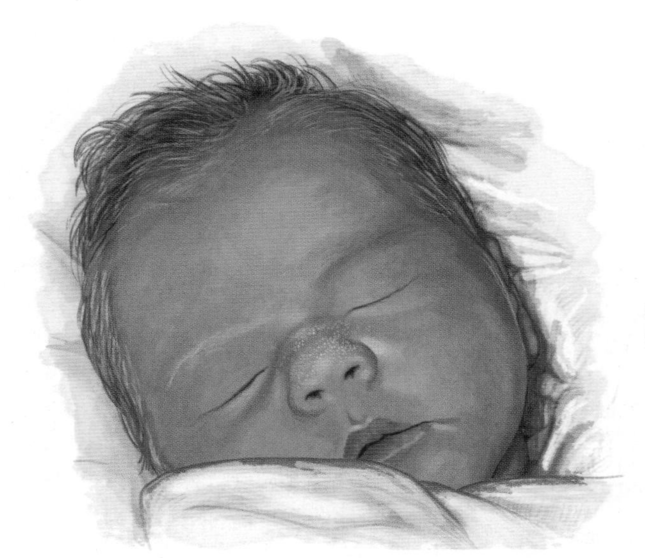

Congenital milia in a newborn. This is a common incidental finding.

MILIA

Milia are tiny (1–3 mm or smaller), superficially located epidermal inclusion cysts. They typically have a characteristic porcelain-white color. Patients can have a solitary milium or multiple milia. These tiny skin growths are entirely benign and cause no harm. It is highly probable that all humans have had a milium or two at some point in their lifetime.

Clinical Findings: Milia are tiny epidermal inclusion cysts located superficially in the epidermis. They do not have an overlying central punctum that can be appreciated. They occur in all races, at all ages, and equally in males and females. Primary milia occur without an underlying skin disorder. Secondary milia occur because of an underlying skin disorder, most often a subepidermal blistering condition. As the subepidermal blister heals, it is not uncommon to see the development of milia in the area of the previous blister. For example, patients with porphyria cutanea tarda develop subepidermal blisters and typically heal with scarring and milia formation. Occasionally, a milium can have a somewhat translucent appearance and should be biopsied to rule out a basal cell carcinoma or an intradermal nevus.

In adults, milia most commonly occur on or around the eyelids. Up to half of all newborns have milia. These are typically located on the head and are known as congenital milia. They almost always resolve without therapy. Unique forms of milia eruptions have been described in the literature, including eruptive multiple milia, grouped milia, and generalized milia. Eruptive milia manifest over a period of weeks, with the appearance of 10 to 100 milia. This has been described in teenagers and adults. Grouped milia and milia en plaque are rare; these terms describe a nodular grouping and a plaque-like grouping of milia, respectively.

Certain genetic syndromes show an association with milia, the best recognized one being Bazex syndrome. This syndrome is defined as a constellation of milia, basal cell carcinomas, hypotrichosis, and follicular atrophoderma. A few other genetic syndromes that have milia are Rombo syndrome, familial milia syndrome, and atrichia with papular lesions. Many other syndromes with milia have been reported.

Pathogenesis: The etiology is unknown, but the cysts are believed to be caused by the disruption of the hair follicle, sebaceous gland, or eccrine gland epithelium. Secondary milia occur after subepidermal blistering or trauma that interrupts the epidermal-dermal junction. The pathogenesis of milia associated with an underling genetic syndrome is unknown.

Milia in an adult. Small white papules just underneath the epidermis. They represent small cysts and are very commonly located on the eyelids.

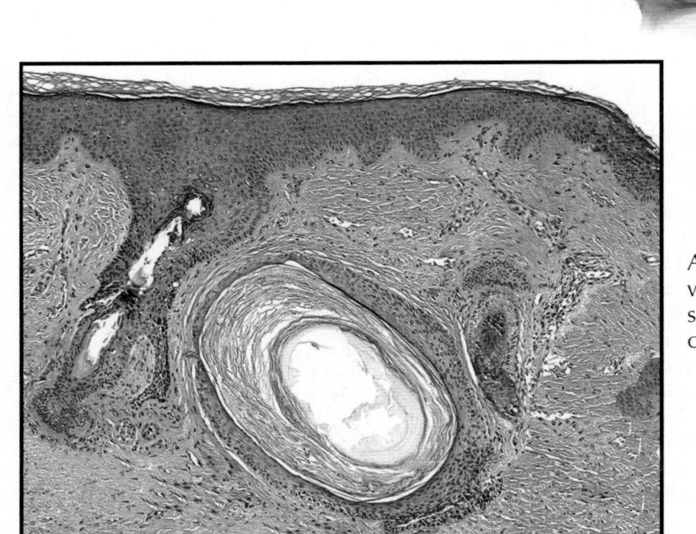

A small well-circumscribed cyst is seen within the dermis. The lining is stratified squamous epithelium with a granular cell layer.

Histology: Milia are tiny cysts in the superficial epidermis. The cyst has a true lining of stratified squamous epithelium. A granular cell layer is present in the cyst wall lining. The center of the cyst is filled with a small amount of keratin debris. There is typically no surrounding inflammation in a primary milium. The overlying epidermis is normal.

Treatment: No therapy is required. Most milia are found during routine skin examinations and are brought to the attention of the patient for education. Patients are often unaware of the milia. If a patient is bothered by the appearance of the cyst, extraction can be performed with a comedone extractor after creating a tiny (1-mm) incision with a No. 11 blade. Once the cyst is removed, it almost never recurs, although other milia may develop after extraction. Treatment of congenital milia in infants is not required because they almost all resolve spontaneously. Plaque-like milia can be removed in the same fashion as a solitary milium.

NEUROFIBROMA

Neurofibromas are uncommon benign skin tumors that can be solitary but are more commonly found in multiples in patients with neurofibromatosis. Neurofibromatosis is one of the more common genodermatoses, afflicting 1 in every 3000 to 4000 individuals. It is caused by a defective tumor suppressor gene.

Clinical Findings: Neurofibromas are small (up to 1 cm on average) papules or nodules that have a soft, rubbery feel. They are flesh colored to slightly hyperpigmented. When pressed, they show a characteristic "buttonholing" phenomenon, in which the neurofibroma invaginates into the underlying dermis and subcutaneous fat. The neurofibroma returns to its natural location once it is unconfined. Most solitary neurofibromas are asymptomatic. The clinical differential diagnosis is between a neurofibroma and a common acquired melanocytic nevus (compound or intradermal nevus). When multiple neurofibromas are seen in an individual patient, the clinician should look for other signs of neurofibromatosis.

Neurofibromatosis type 1 (previously known as von Recklinghausen disease) is a common genetic systemic disease with cutaneous findings. It is inherited in an autosomal dominant pattern but can also result from a spontaneous mutation. The gene that has been implicated, known as *NF1*, is located on the long arm of chromosome 17 and encodes the tumor suppressor protein, neurofibromin. This guanosine triphosphatase protein is critical in the regulation of the Ras cell signaling pathway. Other forms of neurofibromatosis have been described and show variations of the clinical phenotype. Neurofibromatosis type 2 is caused by a defect in *NF2*, a gene on the long arm of chromosome 22.

Patients with neurofibromatosis type 1 begin developing neurofibromas at puberty, and the lesions increase in number dramatically over their life span. They are often larger than solitary neurofibromas and can range from a handful to thousands. The sheer number of neurofibromas can cause significant disfigurement and can affect social and psychological well-being. In this genetic disease, neurofibromas can occur not only in the skin but along any nerve in the body. Neurofibromas that occur in areas where there is minimal room for expansion (e.g., in the intervertebral foramen) can cause significant morbidity and need for surgical intervention.

Patients with neurofibromatosis type 1 have many other skin findings, including multiple café-au-lait macules, axillary freckling, and plexiform neurofibromas. Plexiform neurofibromas are a unique variant of the neurofibroma and are considered pathognomonic for this disease. They are composed of multiple individual neurofibromas grouped into a large plaque. Systemic findings seen in neurofibromatosis include optic gliomas, Lisch nodules on the iris, multiple bony findings, various impairments of the central nervous system, and a number of endocrine disorders. The varying phenotypes of this disease may result from different mutations in the involved gene. These patients are also at much higher risk for malignancy than unaffected controls.

Pathogenesis: Solitary neurofibromas have not been found to contain defects in the neurofibromin protein. They arise as a result of unknown factors that cause proliferation within the dermis of all the components of a nerve filament. The neurofibromas found in neurofibromatosis are believed to be caused by the genetic defect in the tumor suppressor gene. How this defect ultimately regulates the formation of neurofibromas is not fully understood.

CUTANEOUS LESIONS IN NEUROFIBROMATOSIS (NF)

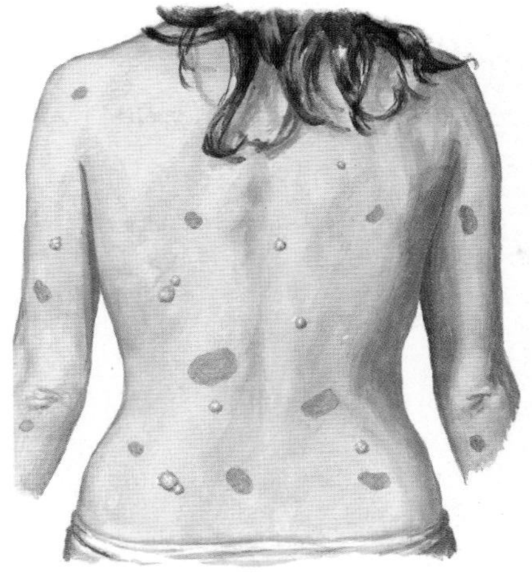
Multiple café-au-lait spots and neurofibromas are the most common manifestations of NF.

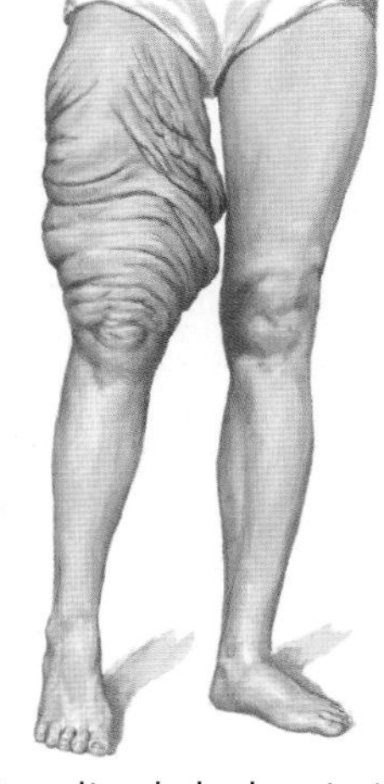
Localized elephantiasis of thigh with redundant skin folds

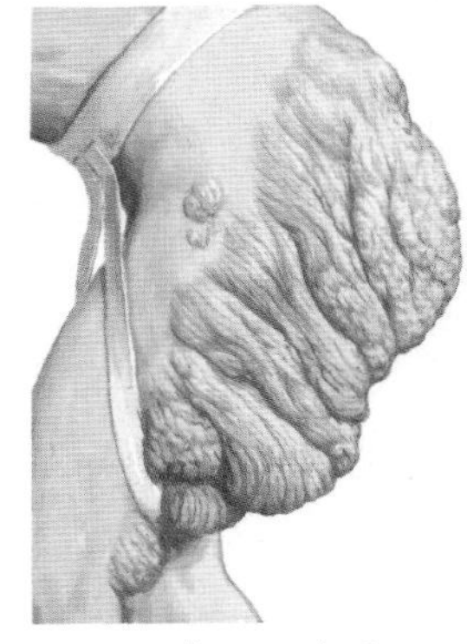
Verrucous hyperplasia. Maceration of velvety-soft skin may cause weeping and infection in crevices.

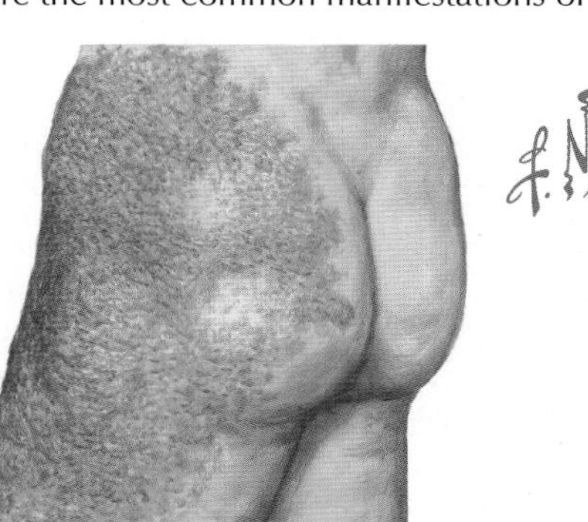
Plexiform neurofibroma. Characteristically localized to one side of trunk and thigh.

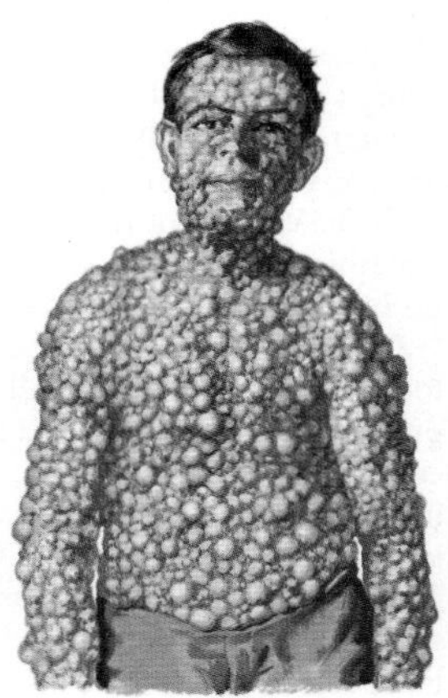
von Recklinghausen disease. One of von Recklinghausen's original patients had extensive neurofibromas but no neurologic symptoms. Fortunately, such widespread skin involvement is uncommon.

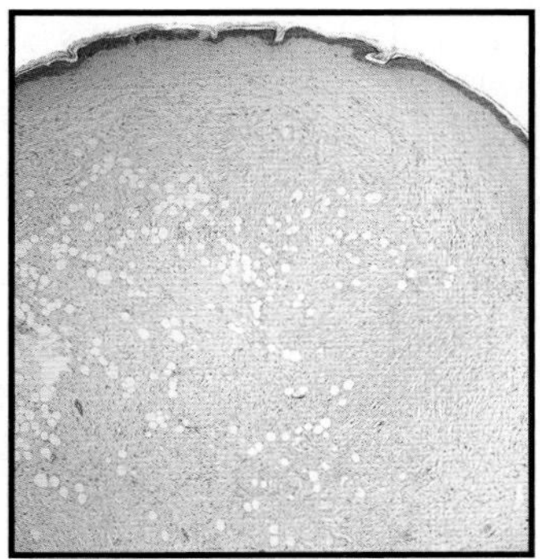
Low power. A nonencapsulated dermal tumor of cells with spindle-shaped nuclei. A small grenz zone is appreciated.

High power. Wavy-appearing nuclei seen within the center of the tumor. Mast cells are often found in the tumor.

Histology: Individual neurofibromas have a well-circumscribed, spindle-shaped proliferation within the dermis. No capsule is present. Schwann cell proliferation and proliferation of the axonal components of the nerve are seen. Many mast cells are present in these tumors. The epidermis is uninvolved, and a small grenz zone is often appreciated.

Treatment: Definitive treatment of a solitary neurofibroma is complete excision. This is curative and results in a very low recurrence rate. No other treatment is necessary because the transformation into malignancy is extremely low.

Any neurofibroma that starts growing or becomes hard or tender should be removed to look for degeneration into neurofibrosarcoma.

Patients with neurofibromatosis require a multidisciplinary approach and require an internist to manage all the potential systemic complications. The neurofibromas may be removed surgically. This approach is not ideal because the number of lesions typically precludes removal of only the bothersome ones. Plexiform neurofibromas should be removed by a plastic surgeon because they can have large subcutaneous extensions that are not visible clinically. There is no cure for this disease; lifelong screening and follow-up are required, and the patient should be referred for genetic counseling before reaching child-bearing age.

NEVUS LIPOMATOSUS SUPERFICIALIS

Nevus lipomatosus superficialis is a not-uncommon benign skin growth considered to be a hamartomatous proliferation of adipose tissue located in the dermis. It was originally named nevus lipomatosus cutaneous superficialis of Hoffman-Zurhelle. There are no known systemic associations with this benign skin growth, and no inheritance pattern has been described.

Clinical Findings: These nevi are most commonly found along the pelvic girdle. They have no sex or race predilection. They may occur at any age but are most common before the third decade of life. The lesions usually have a soft, bag-like appearance, often mimicking a large skin tag, and are flesh colored to yellow-tan. They are soft, nontender, easily movable papules with a sessile base or pedunculated plaques with a thick stalk-like projection. The main differential diagnosis includes a skin tag, a compound nevus, and a connective tissue nevus. However, these lesions are typically much larger than the common skin tag.

Although the diagnosis can be considered clinically, definitive diagnosis can be ascertained only after pathologic evaluation. These lesions are often solitary, but reports of multiple lesions have been described in the literature. In the case of multiple tumors, the lesions are typically described as flesh-colored to slightly red dermal nodules that tend to coalesce into larger plaques. Some of the tumors have a cerebriform appearance to their surface. They can become very large (>10 cm in diameter) if left untreated. However, most never grow larger than 1 to 2 cm in diameter. A generalized variety of this condition has been described, but it is exceedingly uncommon.

Children present after their parents notice the growth, and a skin biopsy is often used to determine the diagnosis. Adults often present because of a slowly enlarging plaque that has an unsightly appearance or has become eroded or ulcerated due to trauma from its size.

Pathogenesis: This condition is believed to be a hamartomatous process of adipose tissue located in the dermis. For an unknown reason, this normal-appearing adipose tissue proliferates within the dermis, often causing an outward herniation of the overlying epidermis, which ultimately leads to the distinctive clinical findings. The exact mechanism has not been elucidated. No genetic abnormalities of the adipose tissue have been established, and there is no known malignant potential.

Histology: Nevus lipomatosus superficialis has a characteristic pathology. It shows mature normal adipose tissue within the dermis. The key finding is lack of connection of the abnormally located dermal adipose tissue with the normally located subcutaneous adipose tissue. Variable amounts of fat tissue make up the individual lesions. No definitive percentage has been established to make the diagnosis, but as little as 10% to more than 50% of each lesion is made up of adipose tissue. The overlying epidermis can be normal or can exhibit acanthosis and papillomatosis. The more cerebriform appearing the lesion is clinically, the more likely it is that epidermal changes will be seen on pathologic examination. Skin tags do not have adipose tissue present, which is a key discriminating factor.

Treatment: These solitary lesions are best excised surgically. A shave excision or elliptical excision give the best cosmetic result and the best cure rate. Multiple lesions can be left alone after a diagnosis is made. If the group of lesions is amenable to surgical excision without the potential for disfiguring scarring, or if the scarring would result in a better cosmetic outcome, surgical excision can be undertaken.

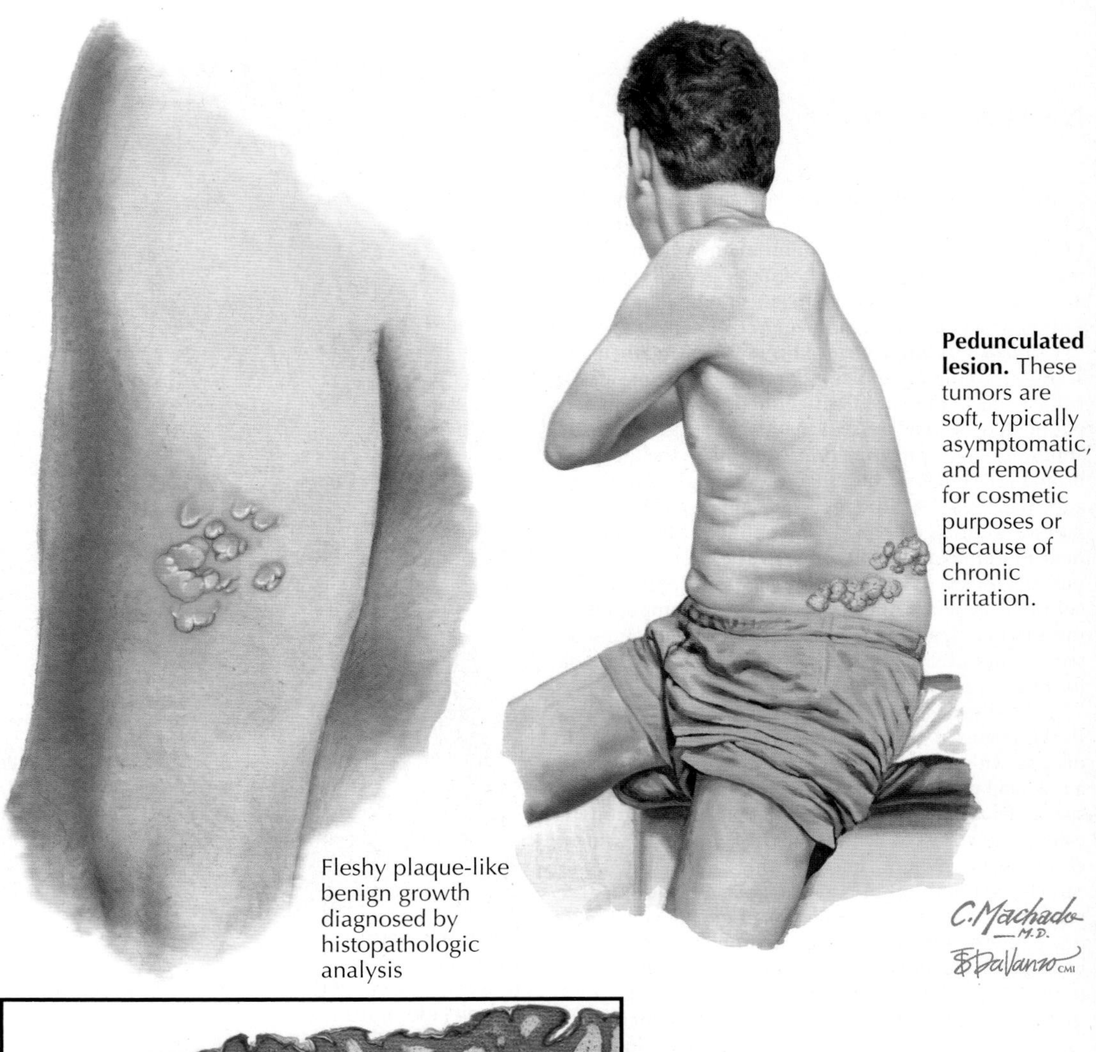

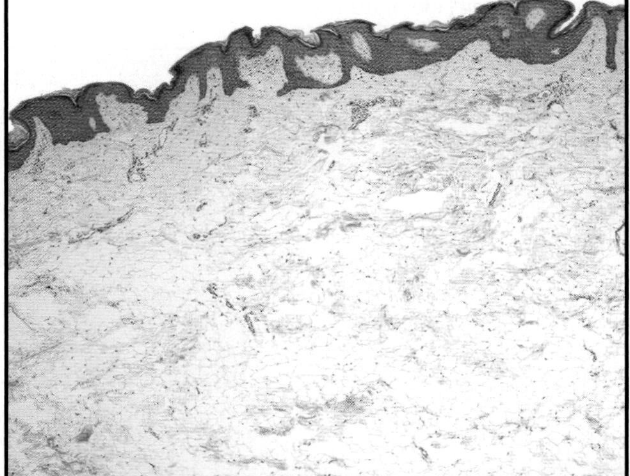

Low power. The dermis is almost entirely replaced with adipose tissue.

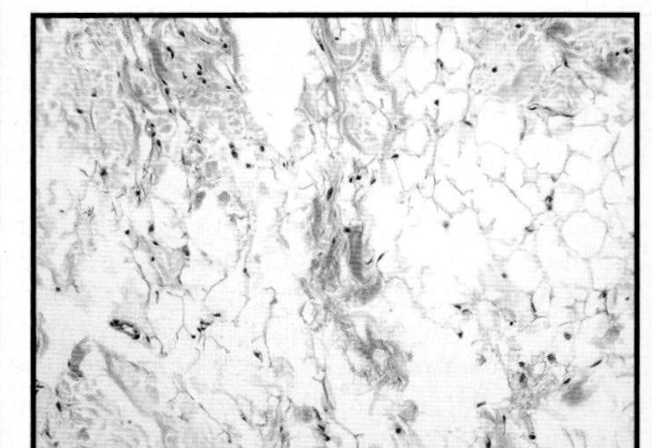

High power. The adipose tissue is normal in appearance.

Nevus of Ota and Nevus of Ito

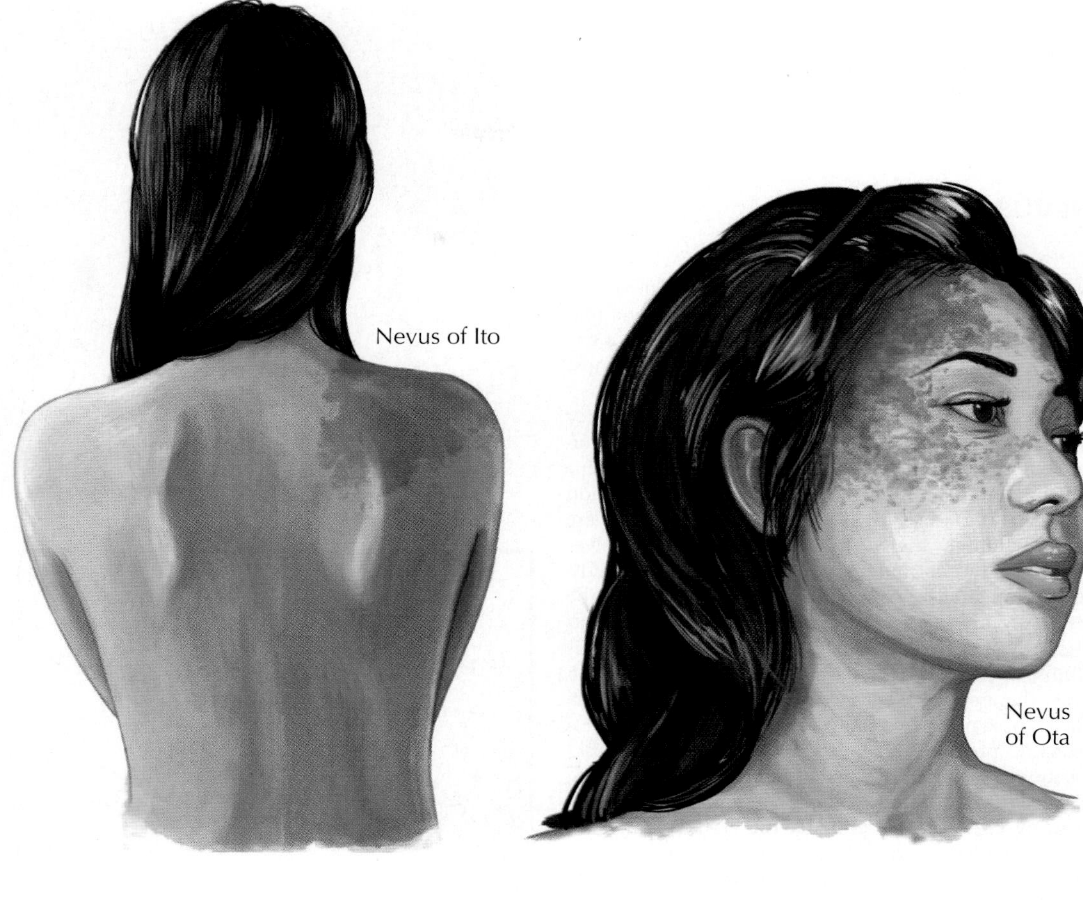

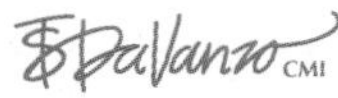

Both nevus of Ota (oculodermal melanocytosis, nevus fuscoceruleus ophthalmomaxillaris) and nevus of Ito (nevus fuscoceruleus acromiodeltoideus) are considered benign hamartomatous overgrowths of melanocytes. These two processes are located on the face and upper shoulder, respectively. They share a common pathogenesis and histology with congenital dermal melanocytosis and are most likely caused by abnormal embryologic migration of melanocytes.

Clinical Findings: The diagnosis of these conditions is most often made on clinical grounds, and a skin biopsy is rarely, if ever, needed to make the diagnosis. Nevus of Ota and nevus of Ito have characteristic locations, which helps the clinician make the ultimate diagnosis. The closely related congenital dermal melanocytosis is located on the lower back of infants and manifests as a deep blue, asymptomatic macule that almost always fades slowly until it disappears by adulthood. It has a higher prevalence in children of Asian or Mayan Indian descent.

Nevus of Ota occurs in a periocular location and can affect the bulbar conjunctiva. It is almost always unilateral in nature. Nevus of Ota manifests as a bluish to blue-gray macule with indistinct borders that fade into the surrounding normal-colored skin. It is usually located over the distribution of the first two branches of the trigeminal nerve. If the bulbar conjunctiva is involved, the color may vary from bluish gray to dark brown. This condition occurs much more commonly in women and individuals of Asian descent. Nevus of Ota is most often seen in isolation, but on occasion it can be seen with a coexisting nevus of Ito.

Nevus of Ito has a similar clinical appearance; however, the location is on the shoulder girdle and neck. Unilateral lesions are the rule. The blue to blue-gray macules can be large and can cause the patient considerable dismay. These lesions are asymptomatic but can be a cosmetic concern for patients and can cause considerable psychological and social difficulties.

Both nevus of Ota and nevus of Ito are more prevalent in the Asian population. Nevus of Ota appears to have a very small malignant potential. It is believed that White females with a nevus of Ota are at higher risk for transformation into malignant melanoma. Nevus of Ito does not appear to have a malignant potential.

Pathogenesis: Under normal circumstances, melanocytes migrate during embryogenesis from the neural crest outward to their final locations (e.g., skin, retina). Nevus of Ota and nevus of Ito are believed to be caused by abnormal migration of these melanocytes. During their migration, an unknown signal causes the melanocytes to collect on the face or on the shoulder, respectively. There does not appear to be a genetic inheritance pattern.

Histology: The histologic findings in nevus of Ota, nevus of Ito, and congenital dermal melanocytosis are identical and resemble those of common blue nevi. Within the lesion, nodular collections of melanocytes are found in the dermis, with noticeable elongation of the melanocytes in the superficial dermis. There is surrounding fibrosis in the dermis with a number of melanophages present.

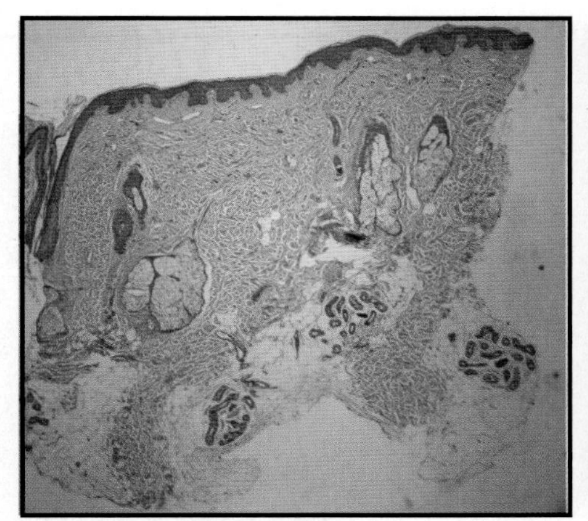

Nevus of Ota, low power. Pigmented melanocytes are spread out within the dermis.

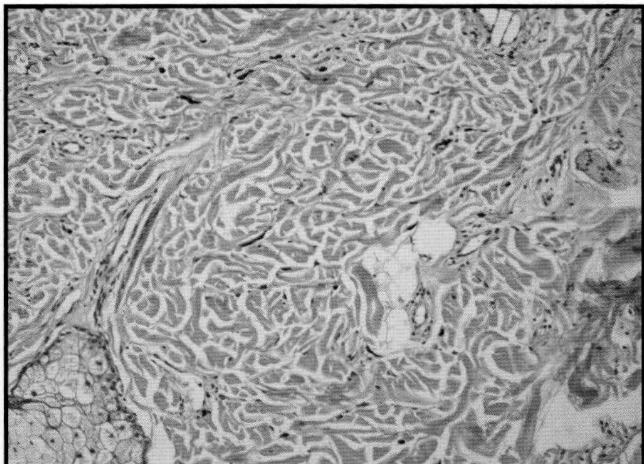

Nevus of Ota, high power. Pigmented melanocytes with elongated dendritic processes are seen among the dermal collagen bundles.

Treatment: These are benign lesions that require no therapy. It is not unreasonable to monitor them clinically for the rare development of malignant transformation. Most patients present for therapy because they are bothered by the appearance of the lesions. If only small areas are involved, cosmetic makeup may be used to camouflage the region. Topical therapies with hydroquinone and tretinoin have shown minimal to no effect on the pigmentation.

Use of the 1064-nm neodymium:yttrium-aluminum-garnet (Nd:YAG) laser has resulted in the most success in treating these lesions, and it can be used in patients of almost any skin type. Q-switching of the laser is a method that has been shown to increase its efficacy. Q-switched ruby, alexandrite, and 1064-nm Nd:YAG lasers have all been used successfully.

Nevus Sebaceus

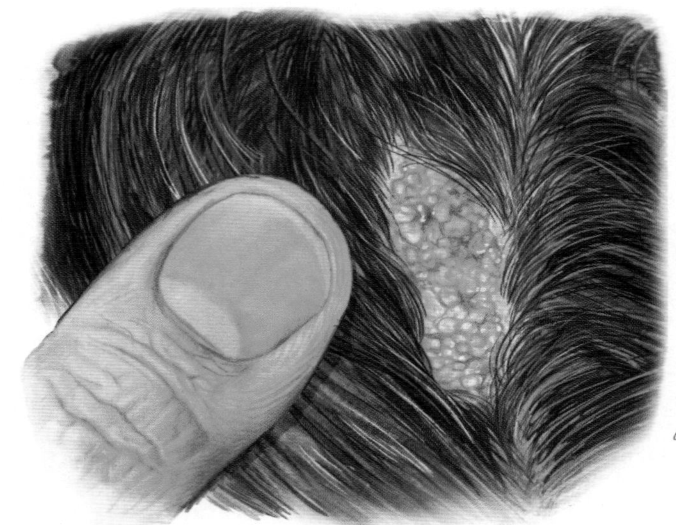

Nevus sebaceus. Flesh- to yellow-colored plaque, typically on the scalp with associated overlying alopecia.

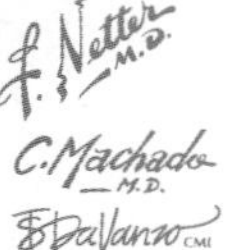

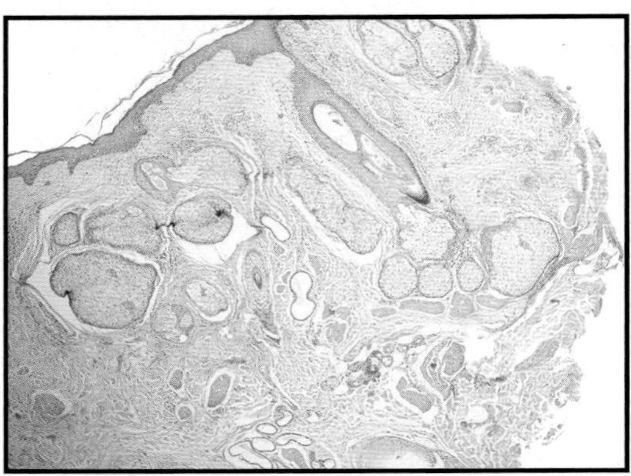

Low power. Acanthosis seen with an increased number of sebaceous glands and hair follicles.

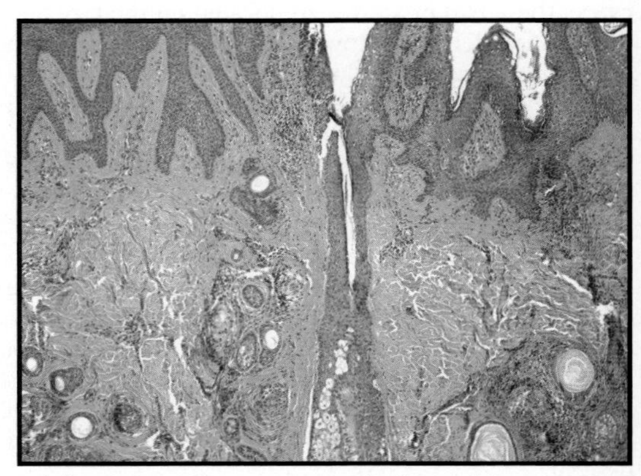

High power. Characteristic finding of the emptying of a sebaceous gland directly onto the surface of the epidermis.

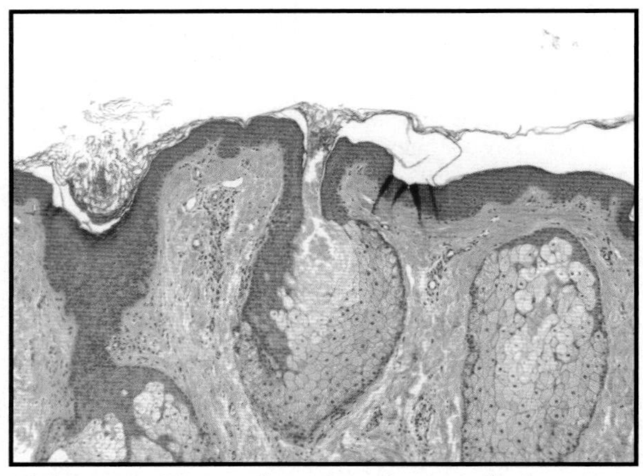

High power. Increased number of enlarged sebaceous glands, with the central sebaceous gland emptying onto the surface of the skin.

Nevus sebaceus, also known as organoid nevus or nevus sebaceus of Jadassohn, is a benign tumor that manifests in infancy or early childhood. This tumor has a risk of malignant transformation after puberty, most frequently basal cell carcinoma.

Clinical Findings: Most of these growths are very small, and some escape detection for years. Others can be obvious at birth. They show a large range in dimensions, and most are solitary. The most common location is within the scalp. Together, the scalp and face are overwhelmingly the most common areas of involvement; it is rare to find a lesion elsewhere on the body. At or soon after birth, an area of the scalp is seen to be obviously affected. Nevus sebaceus typically start off as a thin, yellowish-brown patch or plaque. The area is almost universally devoid of terminal hair shafts. With time, the area becomes more cobblestoned in appearance. These nevi are usually asymptomatic but can be a cosmetic problem depending on their size and exact location. They occur in males and females with equal frequency. The lesions enlarge in proportion to the growing child. Before puberty, the risk of malignant transformation is very low. After puberty, approximately one-third of these lesions develop a secondary growth, which usually manifests as a new nodule within the nevus sebaceus. The nodule can vary in color, but a light, translucent purple color is not infrequently seen. It is also common for a bleeding nodule or papule to develop within the underlying nevus sebaceus.

Most commonly, the growths that occur within the nevus sebaceus are benign in nature. The syringocystadenoma papilliferum is the most common benign tumor to develop within a nevus sebaceus. Because of the connection to the epidermis, these growths usually manifest as a draining or bleeding nodule that is slowly enlarging. The most common malignant growth to develop in a nevus sebaceus is a basal cell carcinoma. These usually manifest as a pearly colored papule with a central ulceration and varying amounts of bleeding or crusting. The transformation to malignancy has been shown to increase with the age of the patient. It is estimated that about 1% of nevus sebaceus lesions will develop a malignant growth over the patient's lifetime. There have been multiple reports of various tumors arising within a nevus sebaceus as well as multiple tumors arising within the same nevus sebaceus.

Nevus sebaceus syndrome is a very rare finding. It is similar in nature to the epidermal nevus syndrome. This syndrome can have a varying phenotype. The neurologic system, including the eye, and the musculoskeletal, cardiovascular, and genitourinary systems can all be involved to varying degrees. Patients with this syndrome usually have abnormally large areas of cutaneous involvement. The lesions can be found anywhere on the body and are often multiple.

Pathogenesis: Nevus sebaceus is considered a hamartomatous process of the epidermis and adnexal structures of the skin. The exact mechanism and cause have not been determined.

Histology: The histologic picture depends on the age of the patient. Before puberty, the findings are more subtle. Prepubertal lesions most commonly show undeveloped adnexal structures. After puberty, the lack of terminal hair follicles is a universal finding. Fine vellus hair follicles are often present but in reduced numbers. Prominent sebaceous glands are seen. Many of the sebaceous glands empty directly onto the surface of the epidermis. The overlying epidermis shows acanthosis and papillomatosis. The presence of apocrine glands is often appreciated.

Treatment: If treatment is undertaken, complete surgical excision is the treatment of choice. This not only removes the lesion but also removes the risk of malignant potential. Another approach is to watch and wait, with routine observation. If the nevus sebaceus develops any areas of change, a prompt biopsy is warranted. The timing of the surgical removal is controversial, and because the risk of malignancy is low, it is acceptable to wait until the patient is old enough to make the decision. The size and location of the nevus sebaceus dictate the type of surgical excision and repair required. Treatment of the rare nevus sebaceus syndrome requires a multidisciplinary team approach.

OSTEOMA CUTIS

Osteoma cutis is a rare benign tumor in which bone formation occurs within the skin. There are two types of osteoma cutis, primary and secondary. Primary osteoma cutis is idiopathic in nature, whereas secondary osteoma cutis is caused by bone formation in an area of trauma or another form of cutaneous inflammation. It can also be seen secondary to abnormalities of parathyroid hormone metabolism; this form of osteoma cutis is called metastatic ossification. Secondary osteoma cutis is much more common than the primary idiopathic form.

Clinical Findings: Primary osteoma cutis is not associated with any defined underlying disorder and can manifest as a solitary nodule, plaque, or plate-like hardening of the skin. Some are quite small, whereas others are large and cause discomfort. Males and females are equally affected, and there is no race predilection. The age at onset is variable. Plate-like or plaque-like osteoma cutis is a form of primary osteoma cutis that occurs during the first few months of life and can even be present at birth. The acral regions are most commonly affected. Over time, these osteomas tend to develop ulcerations or erosions of the overlying epidermis. With this ulceration, small parts of the osteoma are extruded from the underlying dermis and expelled from the skin. This may be the cause for presentation to the clinician. Most patients present with a thickened or hardened area of skin with no preceding trauma or inflammatory condition. There is no malignant potential.

Primary osteomas of the skin may be seen in Albright hereditary osteodystrophy. This condition is characterized by a constellation of findings, including short stature, osteoma cutis, mental and physical delay, and brachydactyly. Varying degrees of obesity and a round appearance to the face are also seen. This condition is caused by an underlying defect in the *GNAS* gene. This gene encodes a stimulatory G protein responsible for cell signaling through the eventual production of cyclic adenosine monophosphate. Albright hereditary osteodystrophy has been reported to manifest with resistance to parathyroid hormone, but other patients with this disorder have not shown this resistance. These differences are likely because of the complex inheritance pattern and depend on whether the defective gene was inherited from the maternal or paternal side, or both. Most patients have associated hypocalcemia and hyperphosphatemia.

Secondary osteoma cutis is far more common, by a ratio of about 9:1. Bone formation may occur in any area of previous skin trauma, acne cysts, or epidermal inclusion cysts and is commonly seen in pilomatricomas. Pilomatricomas are benign tumors that most often manifest in childhood. Inflammatory conditions associated with osteoma cutis include dermatomyositis and scleroderma.

Fibrodysplasia ossificans progressiva is a rare genetic condition in which connective tissue is turned into bone after minor trauma, causing secondary osteomas. The skin can be involved, as can the muscle and other underlying tissue. This disease is progressive and can result in premature death. This condition is unique in that it is caused by endochondral bone formation.

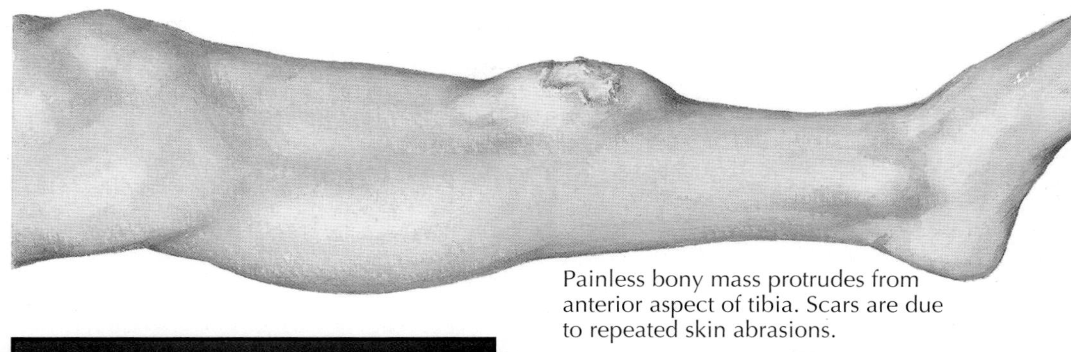

Painless bony mass protrudes from anterior aspect of tibia. Scars are due to repeated skin abrasions.

Radiograph reveals globular outgrowth on tibial cortex with sloping extensions (Codman's triangles).

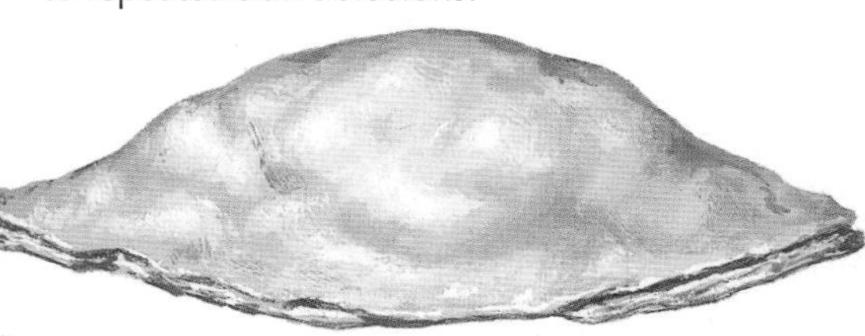

Specimen demonstrates continuity of tumor with overlying periosteum.

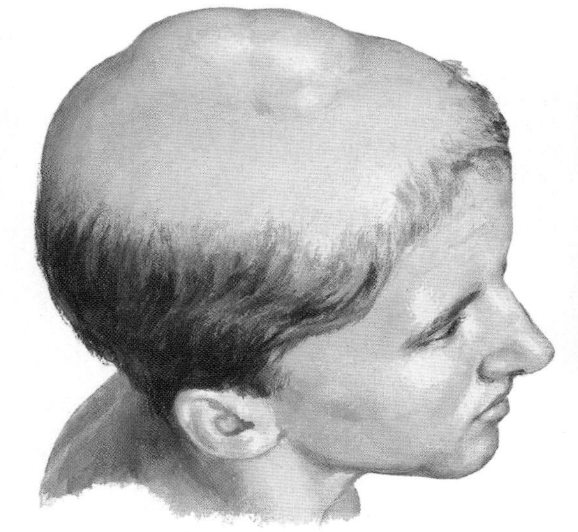

Slowly enlarging, asymptomatic bony mass on dome of head

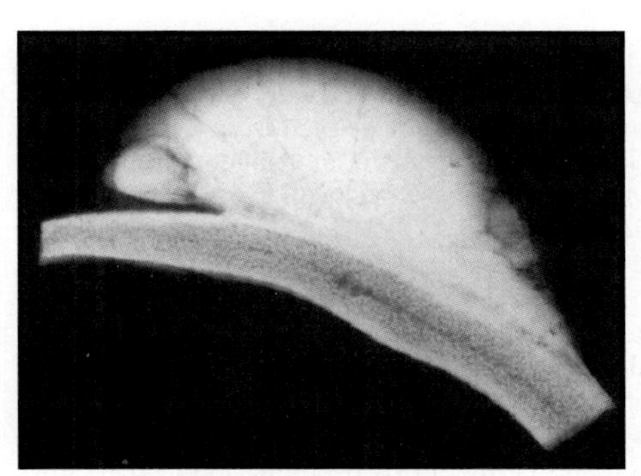

Radiograph of excised tumor reveals densely ossified cortical mass protruding from outer table of skull.

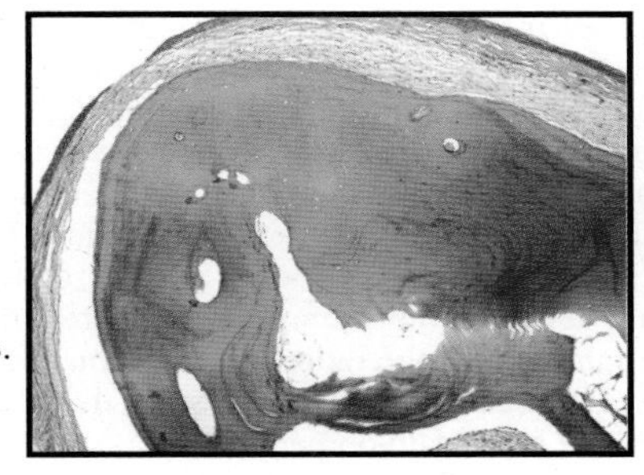

High power. A well-circumscribed nodule of bone formation just underneath the epidermis. A few haversian canals are present.

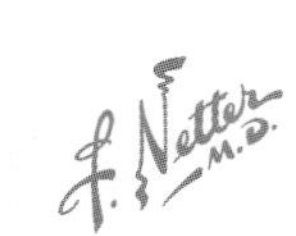

Pathogenesis: Primary forms of osteoma cutis show intramembranous ossification that is centered within the dermis. There is no preceding cartilage formation to act as a scaffolding for the bone to form. The exact cause is unknown. The G protein that is defective in Albright hereditary osteodystrophy has been found to be important in bone regulation. The precise reason why some areas of skin are involved while others are left intact is not well understood.

Histology: Areas of bone formation are seen ectopically in the dermis or subcutaneous tissue. The bone is formed by an intramembranous mechanism without the assistance of a preceding cartilage scaffolding.

Treatment: Secondary osteoma cutis can be removed with a number of surgical techniques. Creation of a small, nick-like incision over the area of osteoma formation and removal with a small curette or laser resurfacing has produced the best results. This treatment can be very time-consuming and labor intensive in cases of multiple secondary osteoma cutis (e.g., in some cases of acne-associated osteoma cutis).

The treatment of primary plaque-like osteoma cutis is surgical removal. Albright hereditary osteodystrophy and fibrodysplasia ossificans progressiva are rare diseases that require a multidisciplinary approach at centers with experience treating these conditions.

Palisaded Encapsulated Neuroma

The palisaded encapsulated neuroma (PEN) is an uncommon benign tumor derived from nerve tissue. It is also known as solitary circumscribed neuroma of the skin. Most of the tumors occur on the head and neck.

Clinical Findings: The lesions of PEN most often manifest on the head and neck region of patients in the fourth and fifth decades of life. They afflict men and women equally and have no race predilection. They are firm, dome-shaped papules or dermal nodules. They are almost always solitary in nature. The overlying epidermis is unaffected and is flesh colored. These benign tumors tend to grow slowly over a period of years until they reach a size (often <1 cm in diameter) that makes them worrisome to the patient. They are commonly misdiagnosed as compound nevi or basal cell carcinomas, and it is not until they are biopsied that the true diagnosis is made. These tumors have a propensity to develop on the eyelid margin and at the interface between keratinized skin and the mucous membranes. Many are seen and removed by ophthalmologists. Most of these tumors are completely asymptomatic. On occasion, they are tender. This tumor is not associated with any underlying neural or systemic symptoms. In contrast, traumatic neuromas occur at sites of trauma, especially at amputation stump sites, and are caused by hypertrophy and proliferation of the damaged nerve ending. Traumatic neuromas are solid, hard dermal nodules that cause pain on palpation.

Pathogenesis: PEN is derived from neural tissue. The Schwann cell is believed to be the cell type of origin for this growth. The proliferation of Schwann cells forms the tumor lobule. The exact mechanism or signal that causes this proliferation has not been discovered. Schwann cell origin is important to recognize and helps differentiate this tumor from other neurally derived tumors. The capsule is derived from perineural cells and collagen bundles. The capsule is believed to occur as a reaction to the underlying Schwann cell proliferation.

Histology: PEN has a clear and well-demarcated capsule lining derived from collagen and perineural cells. The tumor is located entirely within the dermis, and the overlying epidermis is normal in appearance. There is no inflammatory infiltrate. The tumor is composed of spindle-shaped cells that form a tight, interweaving pattern. Immunohistochemical staining is often used to help differentiate these tumors from other neurally derived tumors such as schwannomas, neurofibromas, and traumatic neuromas. Neurofibromas do not have a true capsule circumventing the tumor. The capsule stains with epithelial membrane antigen. This stain helps indicate the location of the perineural capsular cell components. The tumor proper stains with S100, vimentin, and type IV collagen. This staining pattern has been described for Schwann cells, so a positive result helps determine the derivation of this tumor. Schwannomas are differentiated by their characteristic Antoni A and B regions and their subcutaneous location. Traumatic neuromas are not encapsulated and are composed of all the individual components that make up the previously normal traumatized nerve tissue.

Treatment: Complete excision is diagnostic and curative. The tumors rarely recur after elliptical excision. They have no malignant potential, and patients can be reassured that they do not have an underlying neural syndrome. Traumatic neuromas can be cured by surgical removal. There is a small risk of recurrence. Pain control is also critical in the management of traumatic neuromas.

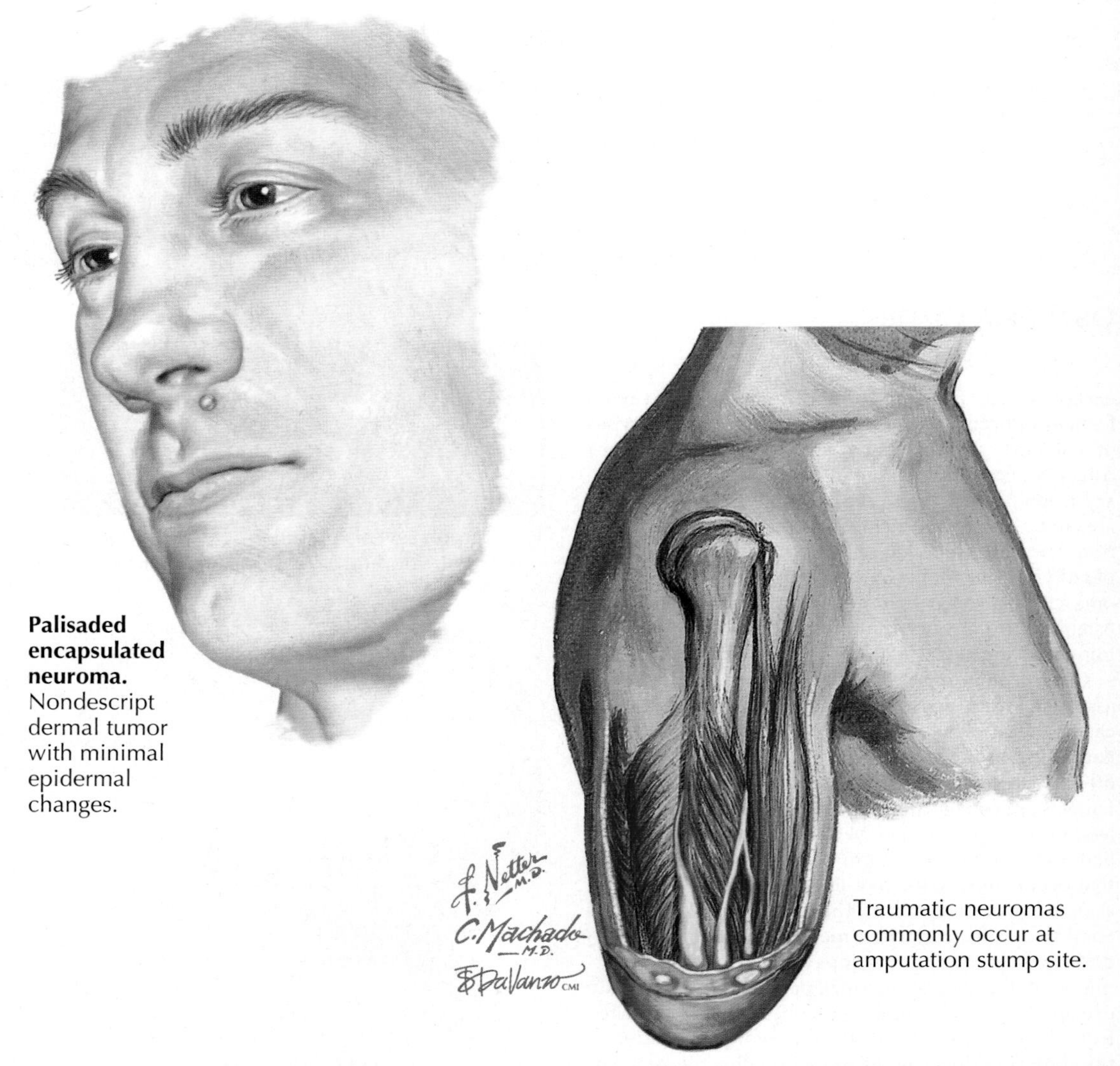

Palisaded encapsulated neuroma. Nondescript dermal tumor with minimal epidermal changes.

Traumatic neuromas commonly occur at amputation stump site.

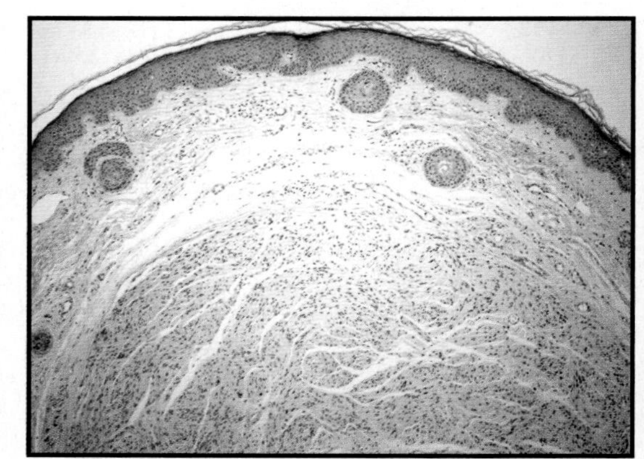

Low power. Well-circumscribed dermal tumor of spindle cells.

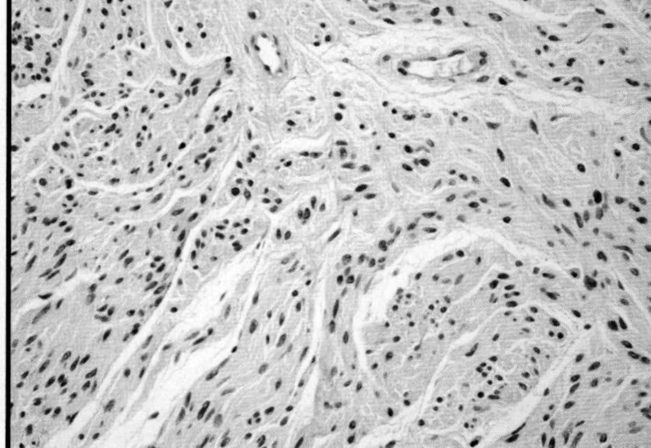

High power. Close-up of the fascicles that make up the tumor.

PILAR CYST (TRICHILEMMAL CYST)

Pilar cysts are relatively common benign growths that occur most frequently on the scalp. They go by many names, including wen, trichilemmal cyst, and isthmus-catagen cyst. Most are solitary, but it is not uncommon to see multiple pilar cysts in a single individual. Their appearance is similar to that of epidermal inclusion cysts, but the pathogenesis is completely different. There is a malignant counterpart called a metastasizing proliferating trichilemmal cyst. The malignant transformation of a pilar cyst is exceedingly rare. Subsets of these growths are inherited.

Clinical Findings: Pilar cysts can be mistaken for epidermal inclusion cysts. The main clinical differentiating points are that pilar cysts do not have an overlying central punctum, and they tend to be a bit firmer to the touch. These cysts occur more commonly in adults, and they tend to affect women more often than men. They typically manifest as slowly growing, firm dermal nodules with no overlying epidermal changes and no central punctum. These cysts do not drain, as epidermal cysts sometimes do. They also rarely get inflamed and are for the most part asymptomatic. Patients present to the clinician because of an enlarging nodule. As opposed to the epidermal inclusion cyst, which essentially has no malignant potential, the pilar cyst does have a small malignant potential. This risk is very low.

Some families show an autosomal dominant inheritance pattern. The gene defect has been determined to be the tumor suppressor gene *phospholipase C delta 1 (PLDC1)* and has been mapped to chromosome 3. Most patients with the hereditary version of this condition have solitary lesions. Numerous lesions are infrequently encountered in the inherited form.

Pathogenesis: Pilar cysts are also called trichilemmal cysts because they are derived from the outer root sheath of the hair follicle, which undergoes trichilemmal keratinization. This form of keratinization is unique in that there is no granular layer. The hereditary version of this disease was originally thought to be caused by a defect in the gene encoding β-catenin. This has been disproven, and the familial gene has been mapped to the short arm of chromosome 3. Somatic mutation in the *PLDC1* gene, which encodes a tumor suppressor gene, has been found to be pathogenic. These cysts are believed to be derived from the isthmus of anagen-type hairs. They are formed from deeper elements of the hair shaft apparatus than the more superficially located elements responsible for epidermal inclusion cyst formation.

Histology: Pilar cysts are composed of compact layers of stratified squamous epithelium without a granular cell layer. The cysts are found within the dermis, and the overlying epidermis is unaffected. These cysts show an absence of intercellular adhesion molecules. The cysts can become calcified or ossified. The cysts have a unique peripheral rim of keratinocyte nuclei, which is very helpful in classifying them. The central aspect of the cyst contains homogenous pale, eosinophilic, compressed keratin.

Treatment: Simple surgical excision is curative. The recurrence rate is minimal. These cysts typically are removed very easily after excision through the overlying skin into the cyst wall. The cyst almost always "pops" out with slight lateral pressure, and only a small incision is needed. After removal, care needs to be taken to decrease the amount of dead space left to avoid seroma formation. This can be prevented by removing some of the redundant overlying epidermis and suturing the deeper tissues together to close the space left by the removed cyst.

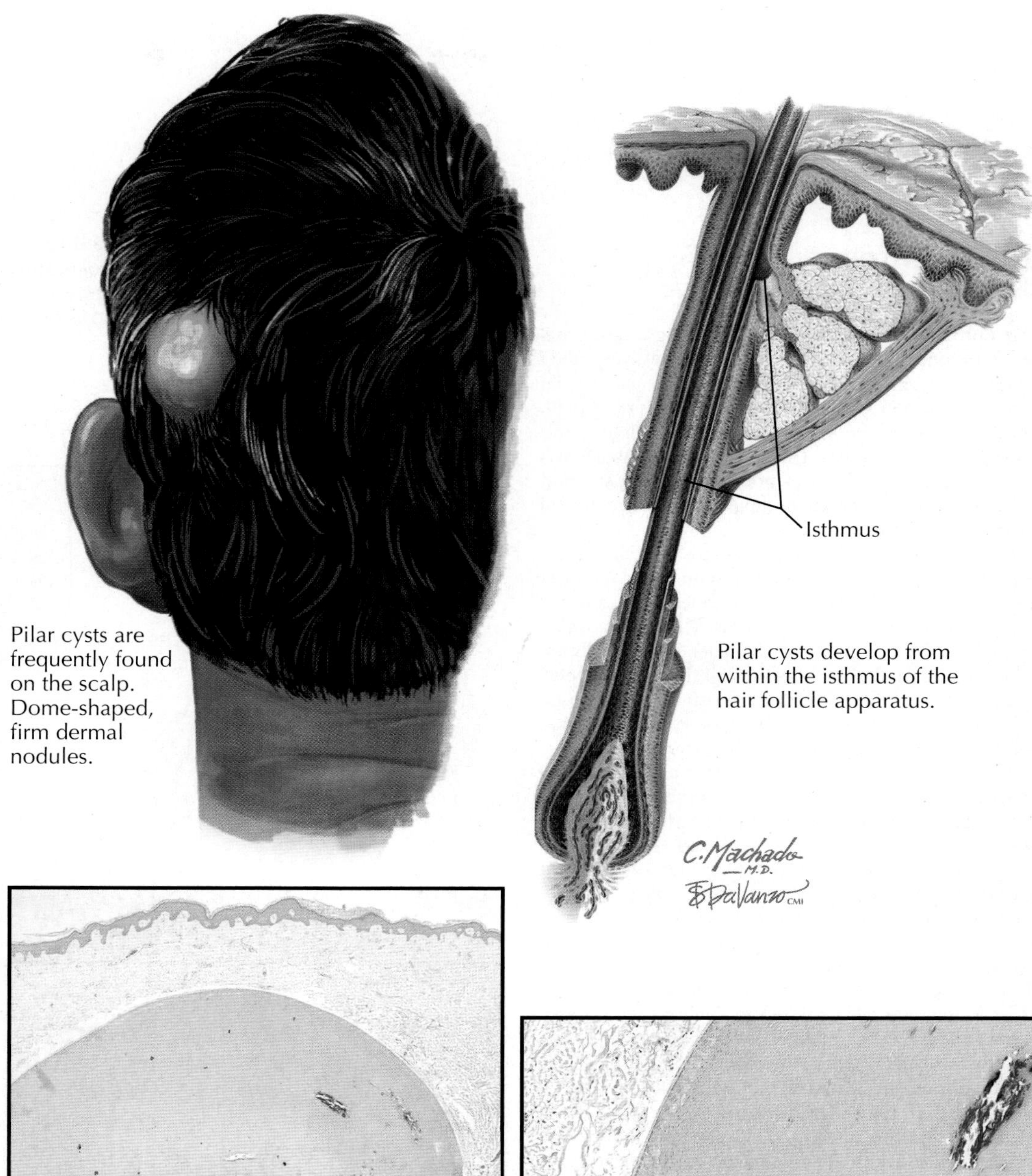

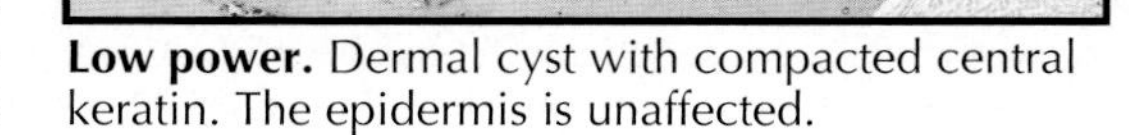

Low power. Dermal cyst with compacted central keratin. The epidermis is unaffected.

High power. The epithelial lining does not contain a granular cell layer and is composed of stratified squamous epithelium.

Porokeratosis

Disseminated superficial actinic porokeratosis (DSAP). Thin patches with a thin rim of epidermal hyperkeratosis on sun-exposed skin.

Types of Porokeratosis
▶ Disseminated superficial actinic porokeratosis (DSAP) ▶ Porokeratosis palmaris et plantaris disseminata ▶ Linear porokeratosis ▶ Punctate porokeratosis ▶ Porokeratosis of Mibelli (solitary porokeratosis)

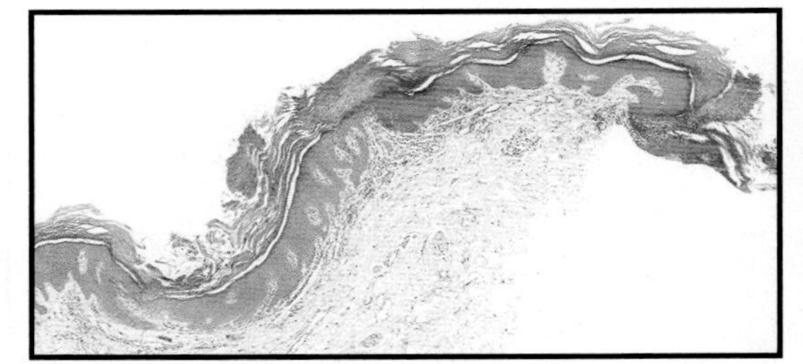

Low power. An atrophic epidermis with a scant amount of dermal inflammation is seen. A peripherally located cornoid lamella is appreciated.

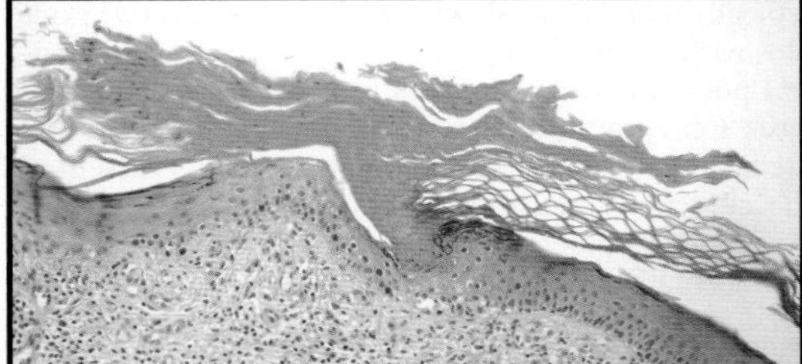

High power. The cornoid lamella is made of compacted stratum corneum. It overlies an area that has lost its granular cell layer. The cornoid lamella is oriented with its distal ends pointing inward.

The porokeratoses are a group of benign epidermal proliferations. The most common and best-described clinical variants include disseminated superficial actinic porokeratosis (DSAP), porokeratosis of Mibelli, porokeratosis palmaris et plantaris disseminata, and punctuate porokeratosis. The underlying disease state is the same for all variants, as are the characteristic and diagnostic histopathologic findings. Many other clinical variants are infrequently seen.

Clinical Findings: Porokeratoses are typically inherited in an autosomal dominant fashion. They manifest beginning in the third to fourth decades of life and are more common in sun-exposed areas. The lesions can be minute to a few centimeters in diameter. They usually are 1- to 2-cm, thin, flesh-colored to slightly pink or hyperpigmented patches with a characteristic hyperkeratotic surrounding rim. This rim encompasses the entire lesion and is almost pathognomonic for porokeratosis.

The DSAP form is the most common and most easily recognized clinical variant. Patients present with a family history of similar skin growths. The lesions are almost entirely located in sun-exposed regions of the body. Patients who have had more ultraviolet light exposure over their lifetime are more likely to have multiple and more noticeable lesions. Most porokeratoses are asymptomatic, and patients typically present because of the appearance of the lesions and the fact that they continue to develop more lesions over time. Most lesions are flesh colored to slightly pink or red. Some can be frankly inflamed, with redness and crusting. Transformation into squamous cell carcinoma has been reported, and patients should be counseled to be reevaluated if they develop growths or ulcerations within the porokeratosis. The lesions of DSAP are much more likely to affect the skin on the extremities than the facial skin.

The porokeratosis of Mibelli is a solitary lesion or a group of lesions with a linear array that have an identical morphology of a thin patch with a thin hyperkeratotic rim. They may occur anywhere on the body.

Porokeratosis palmaris et plantaris disseminata is a unique variant that affects the skin of the palms and soles initially and then can disseminate into a generalized pattern. The lesions of the palms and soles can be tender. This variant is also inherited in an autosomal dominant manner. The lesions begin on the palms and soles during the third to fourth decades of life and slowly spread to other areas of the skin in a generalized pattern.

Punctate porokeratosis of the palms and soles is a rare clinical variant localized to the palms and soles. The lesions tend to be 0.5 to 1 cm in diameter and have a well-defined rim of hyperkeratosis. Occasionally, they can be mistaken for plantar warts.

Pathogenesis: The pathogenesis of porokeratosis, no matter which variant, is believed to be an abnormality of keratinocyte proliferation. A clonal expansion of the abnormal keratinocytes leads to development of the expanding rim of hyperkeratotic tissue. This rim of hyperkeratosis is recognized histopathologically as the cornoid lamella. No genetic defect has been identified. Porokeratosis is more commonly found in patients taking chronic immunosuppressive medications (e.g., after solid organ transplantation) and in those infected with human immunodeficiency virus. This is indirect evidence that chronic immunosuppression may lead to a lack of tumor surveillance and the development of porokeratosis.

Histology: On biopsy, the hallmark of porokeratosis is recognition of the cornoid lamella. The cornoid lamella is the pathologic representation of the hyperkeratotic peripheral rim of tissue seen on clinical examination. The cornoid lamella is positioned at an angle away from the center of the lesion. The granular cell layer underneath the cornoid lamella is often absent or severely thinned. The appearance of the center of the lesion is dependent on the clinical variant seen. The area can be atrophic or acanthotic. It is not uncommon to see an inflammatory infiltrate underneath the lesion composed predominantly of lymphocytes.

Treatment: Treatment is difficult and often unsuccessful for widespread areas such as those involved in DSAP. Sun protection and sunscreen use are recommended. Solitary lesions can be removed surgically. Multiple disseminated lesions can be ablated with carbon dioxide laser ablation, 5-fluorouracil, or dermabrasion. These therapies are not always effective and may be associated with scarring. It is imperative to continue to monitor these patients with routine skin examinations because porokeratoses have the potential for malignant degeneration.

Pyogenic granuloma of the gingiva may be seen more frequently during pregnancy. This is occasionally termed granuloma gravidarum.

Pyogenic granuloma on the thumb with the characteristic collarette of scale

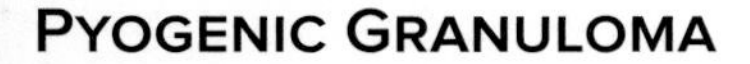

Pyogenic Granuloma

Pyogenic granulomas are common benign skin tumors. They frequently occur after trauma and can be induced by certain classes of medications. Pyogenic granulomas are vascular tumors or proliferations of vascular tissue. They occur in all races, and there is no age or sex predilection, although they are more commonly seen in pregnancy.

Clinical Findings: Patients often present with a bleeding papule or nodule that is beefy red and has a collarette of scale. Pyogenic granulomas are friable and bleed easily when manipulated. There is often a preceding history of trauma. The lesions are usually small (5 mm) papules, but some have been reported to be 1 to 2 cm in diameter. These benign growths can also occur on the mucosa, sometimes in a periungual position. They can be tender and occasionally can become superinfected. A characteristic finding is the "band-aid" sign. This sign represents the surrounding skin findings of a contact dermatitis caused by the frequent use of bandages to cover the pyogenic granuloma because of its propensity to bleed, sometimes profusely. Pyogenic granulomas are more common during pregnancy and can be seen on the gingival mucosa. The most frequent oral location of involvement is the gingival mucosa. They rarely resolve spontaneously. The differential diagnosis is usually between pyogenic granuloma and other vascular-appearing tumors including metastatic carcinoma, particularly renal cell carcinoma, bacillary angiomatosis, and amelanotic melanoma. Pyogenic granulomas are almost always removed, and the diagnosis is confirmed by histopathologic evaluation.

Oral retinoid medications are the most frequent therapeutics shown to induce pyogenic granulomas.

Pathogenesis: Pyogenic granulomas are thought to arise after trauma or secondary to medications and to be caused by a hyperplastic proliferation of vascular tissue. Chronic localized trauma can cause the release of vascular growth factors that may induce the proliferation. Pyogenic granulomas have not been shown to have any genetic inheritance pattern and are considered to be sporadic. The exact mechanism of formation is not well understood. The fact that they are more commonly seen in pregnancy suggests that certain hormonal regulations play a role in the formation of these tumors.

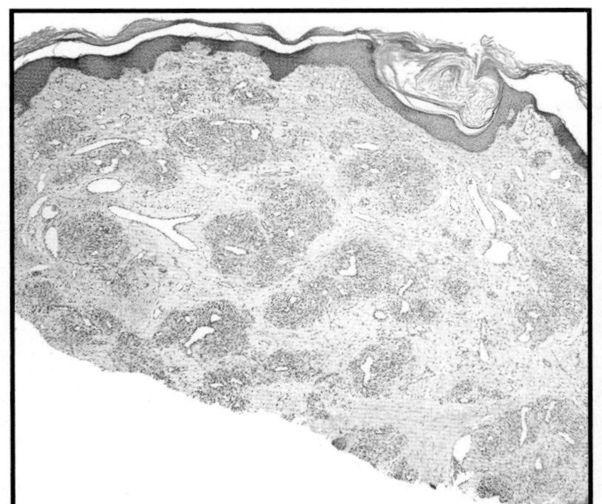

Low power. Multiple lobules of blood vessels are seen separated by a thin fibrous connective tissue.

High power. Proliferation of capillary vessels is prominent in the center of the tumor lobules.

Histology: Pyogenic granulomas are also known as lobular capillary hemangiomas. This is an excellent descriptive name. The lesion is an exophytic growth that has a lobular configuration to its growth pattern. The tumor is typically well circumscribed and surrounded by a collarette of hyperplastic epithelium. Multiple capillary loops are found within each of the tumor lobules. Strands of fibrous tissue divide the tumor into individual lobules of varying size. Many of these lesions show evidence of surface ulceration resulting from thinning of the overlying epidermis. The cells involved are bland appearing.

Treatment: Most pyogenic granulomas resolve after shave removal and curettage with cautery of the base of the lesion. These tumors do have a propensity to recur, and an elliptical excision is occasionally required for removal. Application of silver nitrate and laser ablation with a pulsed dye laser have been used successfully. If the pyogenic granulomas are drug induced, stopping the offending medication is sometimes effective in resolving them. However, many cases of medication-induced pyogenic granulomas require some method of surgical removal.

Reticulohistiocytoma

Reticulohistiocytomas, also called solitary epithelioid histiocytomas, are conglomerations of large eosinophilic histiocytes within the dermis. The cytoplasm of these cells has been described as "glassy" in appearance. Reticulohistiocytomas are a subset of the histiocytoses group of diseases. In contrast to the other histiocytoses, patients with reticulohistiocytoma have normal lipid levels.

Reticulohistiocytomas can occur as a solitary growth or as multiple growths in a condition known as multicentric reticulohistiocytosis. The solitary variant is more often seen. On histopathologic examination, the two clinical variants are identical in nature. Multicentric reticulohistiocytosis is a rare disease with systemic involvement. It can often be a marker of internal malignancy, and patients have severe arthritis.

Clinical Findings: Solitary lesions are typically small, firm dermal nodules ranging from 1 to 2 cm in diameter. They are usually asymptomatic. Their coloration may vary, but most often they are slightly pink to red-brown. They are found most commonly on the head and neck region of the body but have been described in all locations. They occur with similar frequency in males and females and have no age or race predilection.

Multicentric reticulohistiocytosis is unique in that it occurs in an older population, with a higher percentage of females affected. The number of lesions is in the hundreds to thousands. The multiple reticulohistiocytomas found in this condition are most often localized to the dorsal aspect of the hands and to the face. A distinctive finding is that of small papules along the lateral and proximal nail folds. This finding has been described as "coral beading," and it is highly specific for multicentric reticulohistiocytosis. These patients also have severe arthropathy; this diagnosis should trigger investigation for an underlying malignancy. The arthropathy almost always affects the interphalangeal joints, particularly the distal interphalangeal joints. Multicentric reticulohistiocytosis is believed to be a paraneoplastic condition in up to 25% of the cases. The type of malignancy is variable, with no predominant type more prevalent than any other. For this reason, age-appropriate cancer screening is recommended. In about one-third of patients with multicentric reticulohistiocytosis, the joint symptoms precede the growths; in one-third, they appear at the same time; and in one-third, the patients develop only clinically minor or no arthropathy. This arthropathy is a severe inflammatory arthropathy that is symmetric and polyarticular. Mutilating arthritis may develop, sometimes very quickly. Early recognition and treatment have helped decrease the progression into severe mutilating arthritis. This truly is a multisystem organ disease. Many patients have cardiac involvement, and almost all organ systems have been reported to be affected, some with fatal outcomes.

Pathogenesis: Multicentric reticulohistiocytosis and solitary reticulohistiocytoma are believed to represent a rare disorder of histiocytes. The cause of the histiocytic proliferation is unknown.

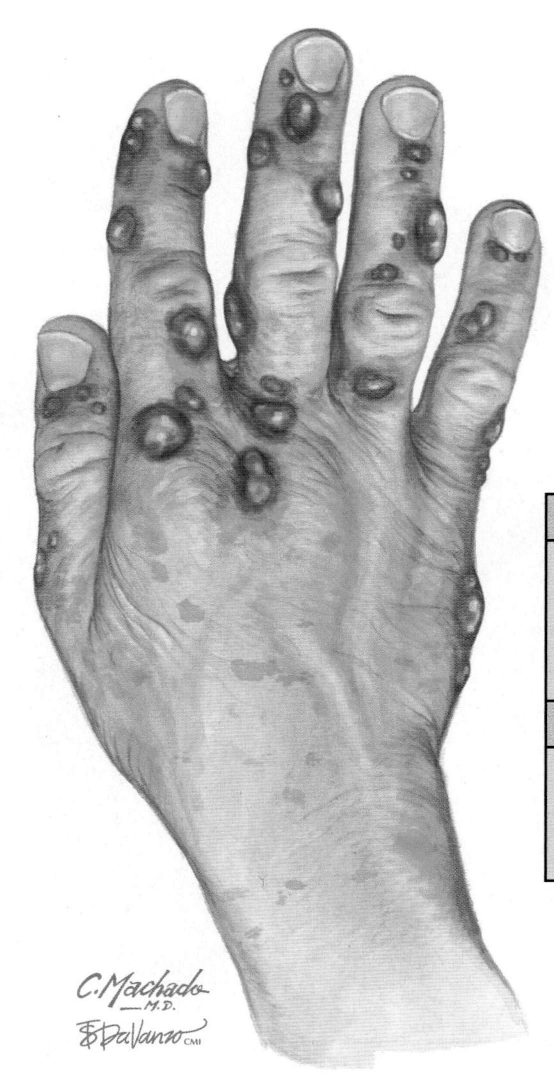

Multicentric reticulohistiocytomas. Coral red papules on the fingers. Can be associated with severe disabling arthritis.

Reticulohistiocytoma Involvement
▶ Inflammatory arthritis (hands, knees, shoulders) ▶ Lungs ▶ Bone marrow ▶ Eyes ▶ Heart

Associated Autoimmune Diseases and Malignancy	
▶ Systemic lupus erythematosus	▶ Lymphoma
▶ Breast cancer	▶ Lung cancer
▶ Colon cancer	
▶ Primary biliary cirrhosis	

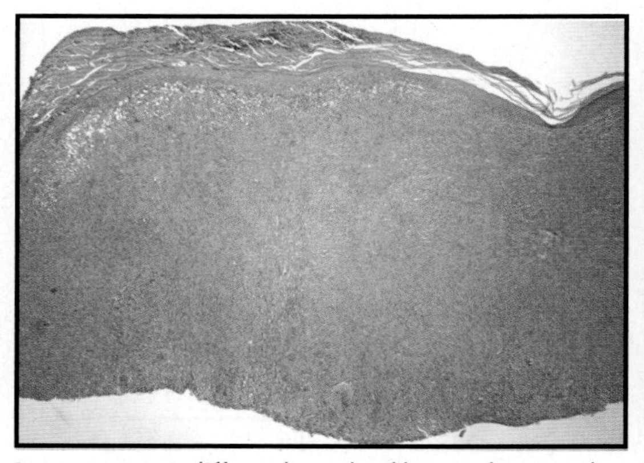

Low power. A diffuse dermal infiltrate of "ground-glass" histiocytes

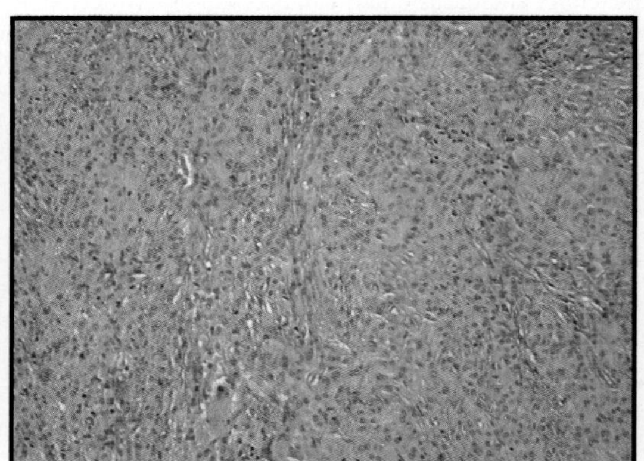

High power. A few multinucleated giant cells are seen within the tumor.

Histology: The tumor shows a well-circumscribed dermal infiltrate without a capsule. The infiltrate is composed almost entirely of histiocytes with a "ground glass" appearance of the cytoplasm. Multinucleate giant cells are always seen. They contain more than three nuclei, which can be arranged in many variations. The cells stain with the immunohistochemical stains CD45 and CD68 but do not stain with S100. On electron microscopy, no Langerhans cells are found in the infiltrate.

Treatment: Solitary reticulohistiocytomas are cured with a simple elliptical excision. They rarely recur. Patients with multicentric reticulohistiocytosis require systemic therapy. Screening and constant vigilance for an underlying malignancy are required in all cases. Corticosteroids, methotrexate, hydroxychloroquine, and cyclophosphamide have all been used. Anti–tumor necrosis factor agents have been used. The goals are to prevent or suppress the arthropathy and to screen for malignancy.

Seborrheic Keratosis

One of the most commonly encountered of all benign skin growths is seborrheic keratosis. These growths come in all sizes and shapes and invariably can be found on any human older than 40 years. They commonly begin in the fourth decade of life and tend to increase in number over the life span. They have no malignant potential but are often brought to the attention of physicians because they can mimic other skin growths, most importantly malignant melanoma.

Clinical Findings: Seborrheic keratoses are found equally in males and females, and they are seen in all races. They begin to manifest in the third to fifth decades of life and continue to increase in number thereafter. They come in various sizes and shapes. Some are quite small, whereas others can be 5 to 6 cm in diameter. They occur almost exclusively in sun-exposed regions of the body. The classic description is that of a 1- to 2-cm plaque with a waxy “stuck-on” appearance and small horn cysts. Most commonly flesh colored, they can also be tan, brown, or almost black, which results in occasionally being mistaken for melanoma. Most individuals have a few scattered keratoses, but not infrequently a patient may have thousands of these skin growths.

Many clinical variants of seborrheic keratosis can be seen. Stucco keratoses are small (1–5 mm), gray-tan papules with a stuck-on appearance or thin patches on the lower extremities. Dermatosis papulosis is a condition in which multiple seborrheic keratoses occur on the face and neck. This condition has a definite autosomal dominant inheritance pattern.

Some seborrheic keratoses are smooth surfaced, but more commonly they have a pebbly or dry, rough surface. They have a characteristic stuck-on appearance, and in some instances they are easily removed by gently peeling from one side. These growths can easily become irritated or inflamed. The resulting pain, itching, or bleeding often brings the patient to medical treatment.

The Leser-Trélat sign is the rapid onset of multiple seborrheic keratoses associated with an underlying internal malignancy. This sign has not been validated and is not a reliable indicator of an internal malignancy.

Pathogenesis: The formation of this benign epidermal tumor is not fully understood. It is caused by a proliferation of keratinocytes within the epidermis. The location in sun-exposed skin and the increasing number of lesions with increasing age have led some to believe they are caused by a local suppression of the immune system that results in epidermal proliferations. A definitive inheritance pattern has not been discovered, but these keratoses show some genetic predisposition. Chromosomal analysis of these tumors has not revealed any chromosomal defects. A link with the human papillomavirus has been proposed but has yet to be proven.

Histology: There is a well-circumscribed proliferation of keratinocytes. They have an exophytic growth pattern. The keratinocytes show acanthosis and hyperkeratosis. Marked papillomatosis is also commonly encountered. Two types of cysts are seen within the seborrheic keratosis. The horn cyst develops within the epidermis and is made of a keratin-filled cystic space with a surrounding granular cell layer. A pseudohorn cyst is formed by an invagination of the stratum corneum into the underlying epidermis. Multiple histologic subtypes have been described.

Treatment: These keratoses require no therapy. If they become inflamed or irritated, a simple shave biopsy removal is curative. Cryotherapy and curettage are often used to treat these benign skin growths, and both are extremely effective. After cryotherapy treatment, a blister usually forms at the base of the seborrheic keratosis, and within a day or two the keratosis falls off. Another extremely effective method of removal that can be done in the office is cryotherapy followed by a light curettage; this also allows for histologic evaluation. Occasionally, dark brown or black seborrheic keratoses can mimic melanoma; in other cases, a melanoma may arise adjacent to a seborrheic keratosis and mislead the clinician. When in doubt whether the growth could be a melanoma, a biopsy is required. This allows for pathologic confirmation of the diagnosis.

Seborrheic keratosis (close-up)

Low power. Acanthotic epidermis with overlying orthokeratosis.

Multiple seborrheic keratosis lesions

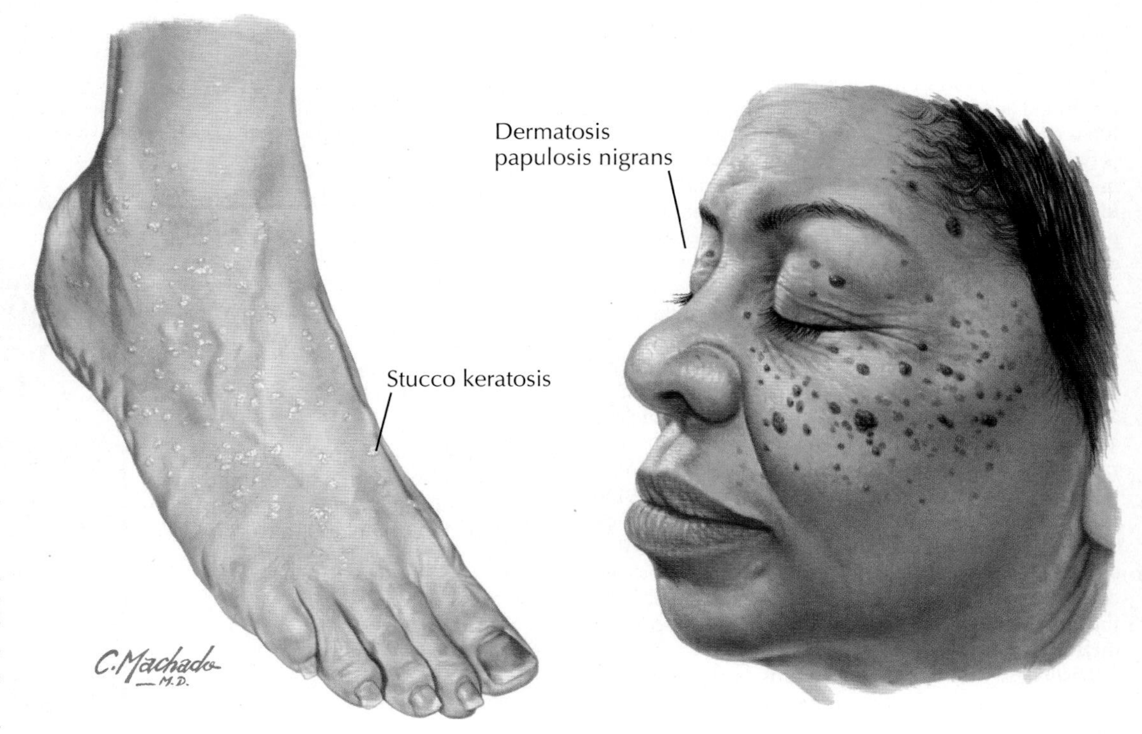

SPITZ NEVUS

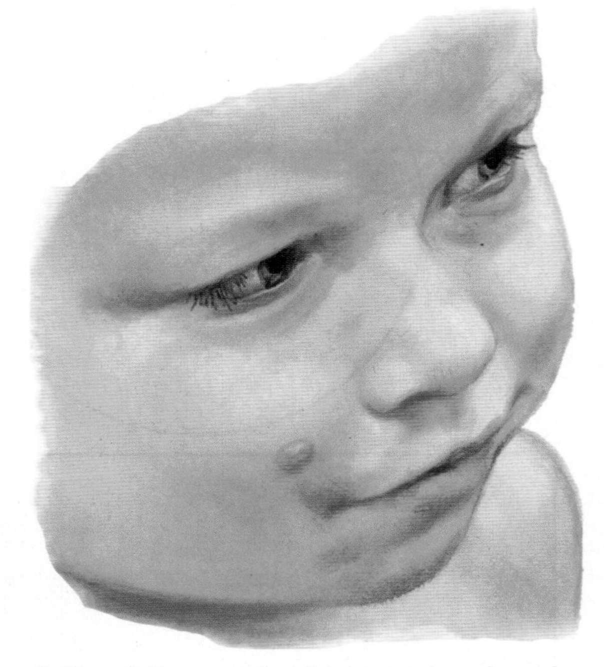

Solitary Spitz nevus. Reddish-brown dermal papule.

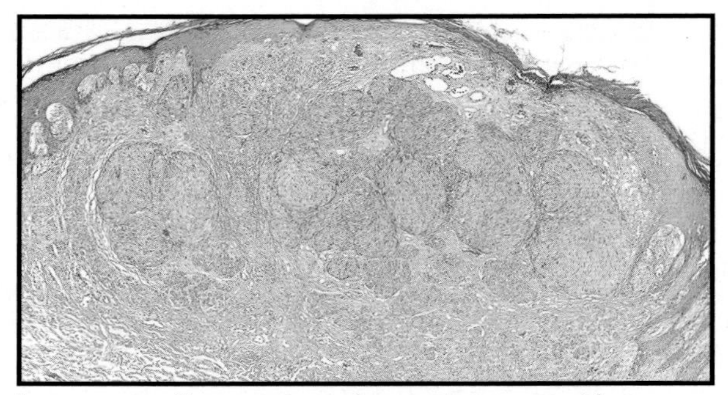

Low power. Symmetric melanocytic tumor with maturation of the melanocytes.

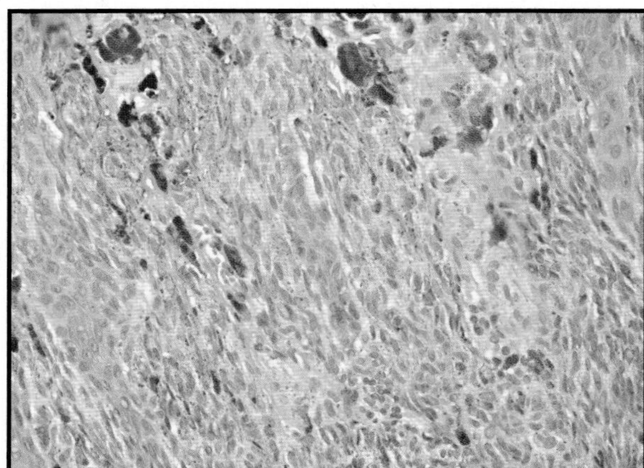

High power. Bland-appearing melanocytes predominate. A uniformity of cell size is seen, and no mitotic figures are appreciated. Melanophages are present.

Spitz nevi are acquired nevi that occur most commonly in children. The classic Spitz nevus is a benign growth with minimal malignant potential. The Spitz nevus is also known as a spindle cell nevus. In the past, they were also referred to as benign juvenile melanoma, but that name should be avoided because the term melanoma should only be used to describe malignant tumors. The difficulty with these melanocytic growths is that they do not always have the classic appearance and can be difficult to differentiate from melanoma. This is especially true in the adult population, where Spitz nevi are uncommon. For this reason, the terms atypical Spitzoid melanocytic lesion, atypical Spitz nevus, and Spitzoid tumor of undetermined potential have made their way into the dermatology lexicon to describe these difficult-to-classify cases.

Clinical Findings: The classic Spitz nevus occurs in childhood and has a characteristic reddish-brown color. It has even coloration and regular symmetric borders. It is typically dome shaped and smooth. It occurs equally in boys and girls and is more commonly found in White individuals. The most common location has been reported to be the lower limb. The size is variable, but they are usually 5 to 10 mm in diameter. Spitz nevi are almost always solitary, but multiple Spitz nevi in an agminated pattern have been described. The clinical differential diagnosis of a Spitz nevus includes the common acquired nevus, pilomatricoma, dermatofibroma, adnexal tumors, and juvenile xanthogranuloma. Most Spitz nevi are asymptomatic and are brought to the clinician's attention as an incidental finding. Classic Spitz nevi rarely, if ever, spontaneously bleed or change in color.

Pathogenesis: The Spitz nevus is a melanocytic lesion derived from spindle-shaped or epithelioid melanocytes. The initiating factors of this melanocytic proliferation are unknown. They are unique melanocytic lesions, and their pathogenesis is likely to be entirely different from that of congenital melanocytic or common acquired melanocytic nevi.

Histology: The classic Spitz nevus is symmetrically shaped, without shouldering. It shows the proper benign maturation of melanocytes from top to bottom of the lesion. The melanocytes do not show pagetoid spread (single melanocytes) within the epidermis. Spitz nevi melanocytes in general have a spindle shape or epithelioid morphology. Another helpful finding is the presence of eosinophilic Kamino bodies. These can be either solitary or coalescing into large globules. Kamino bodies are found in juxtaposition to the basement membrane zone and are composed of elements of the basement membrane, specifically type IV collagen. There is no immunohistochemical stain that can definitively differentiate a Spitz nevus from melanoma. As alluded to earlier, the classic Spitz nevus is usually a straightforward diagnosis. However, many difficult-to-classify melanocytic lesions have overlapping features of Spitz nevus and melanoma and can be exceedingly challenging diagnostically. In these cases, genetic evaluation of the tumors has been used to further classify these tumors as benign or malignant. Fluorescent in situ hybridization and comparative genomic hybridization have been the most commonly used tests.

Treatment: Complete excision for a classic Spitz nevus is curative and allows for a complete histologic evaluation. Indeterminate lesions should be reexcised with conservative margins to ensure they have been completely removed. Spitz nevi in adults should be excised to allow for complete histopathologic examination. Unclassifiable or difficult-to-classify melanocytic tumors with features of both Spitz nevus and melanoma are best treated as if they were melanoma. As genetic evaluation of these tumors becomes more refined, it will become more important in the diagnosis of these nevi. The Breslow depth should be used to plan for appropriate therapy.

MALIGNANT GROWTHS

ADNEXAL CARCINOMA

Adnexal carcinomas are a diverse group of malignant skin tumors derived from the various components of the skin appendageal structures. These tumors are extremely rare and comprise less than 1% of all skin cancers diagnosed annually. They are difficult to diagnosis clinically because they mimic the more common types of skin cancer, particularly basal cell carcinoma (BCC) and squamous cell carcinoma (SCC). A skin biopsy is required for the diagnosis because adnexal carcinomas can only be diagnosed with certainty after histologic examination. These various tumors are believed to be derived from unique components of the hair follicle, sebaceous gland, apocrine gland, or eccrine gland epithelium. They are thought to arise most commonly de novo but can also arise from a preexisting benign precursor. An example is an eccrine porocarcinoma developing within an eccrine poroma.

Clinical Findings: These tumors are very rare, and they are unlikely to be considered in the differential diagnosis when evaluating an undiagnosed skin growth. There are few clues to their origin, which makes diagnosis of these cancerous tumors almost impossible based on clinical findings alone. Most manifest as a solitary papule, plaque, or dermal nodule. These tumors tend to be asymptomatic, but pruritus, bleeding, and pain may be present. These tumors are most frequently located on the head and neck region but can occur anywhere.

Diagnosis of these tumors requires tissue sampling. Punch, deep shave, and excisional biopsies are the best methods to obtain tissue for histologic examination because they provide a large enough piece of tissue to evaluate. A punch biopsy is especially important to help differentiate microcystic adnexal carcinoma from a benign syringoma. The latter is very superficial in nature, whereas the microcystic adnexal carcinoma displays a deep infiltrative growth pattern that will not be appreciated with a superficial shave biopsy.

Pathogenesis: The pathogenesis of these tumors is poorly understood. In contrast to BCC and SCC, they are unlikely to be caused by ultraviolet light exposure. The rarity of the tumors makes them difficult to study. There is some evidence that the incidence of adnexal carcinomas is increasing, especially for eccrine porocarcinomas. The exact reasons for this are not fully understood. There appears to be no genetic inheritance to these malignant tumors, with the lone exception of the sebaceous carcinoma. Sebaceous carcinoma can be seen in Muir-Torre syndrome, which is inherited in an autosomal dominant pattern.

Histology: Each tumor is unique histologically. The tumors can be subdivided according to the type of epithelium from which they are derived: sebaceous, hair follicle, eccrine, or apocrine. The pathologist is able to differentiate these tumors based on certain criteria. These malignant tumors will show varying amounts of cellular atypia and an invasive growth pattern. They are usually poorly circumscribed with varying amounts of mitotic figures, necrosis, and abnormal-appearing cells. Various gland-like structures can be seen in some tumors, which can be helpful in making the diagnosis. Often, special immunohistochemical stains are used to help differentiate the subtypes of these tumors.

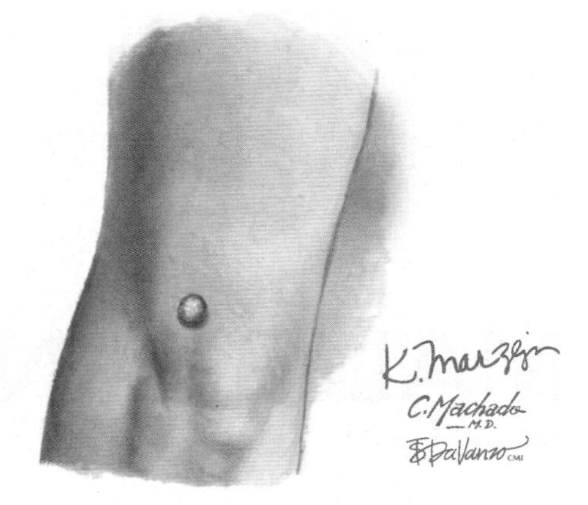

Eccrine porocarcinoma. Nondescript red papule or nodule. Ulceration may occur. A biopsy is required to diagnose this rare form of skin cancer.

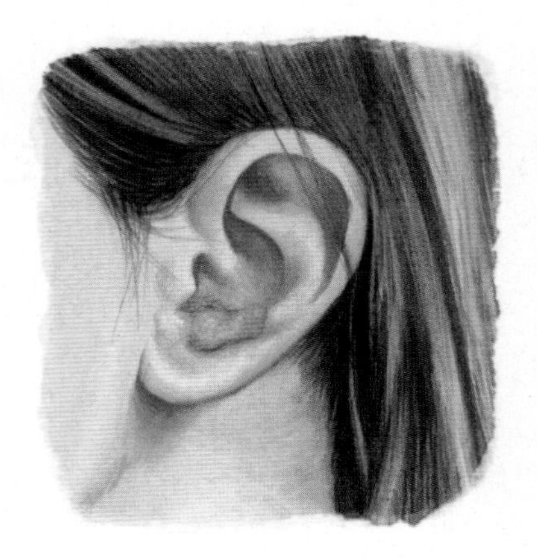

Spiradenocarcinoma, presenting as a plaque on the ear. Adnexal tumors are rare, and a biopsy for histologic evaluation is required for diagnosis.

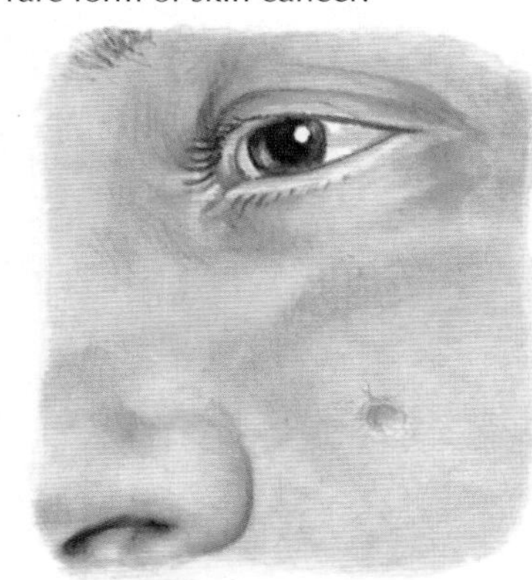

Microcystic adnexal carcinoma. Small plaque on cheek. Slow-growing tumor that can become quite large by the time of diagnosis.

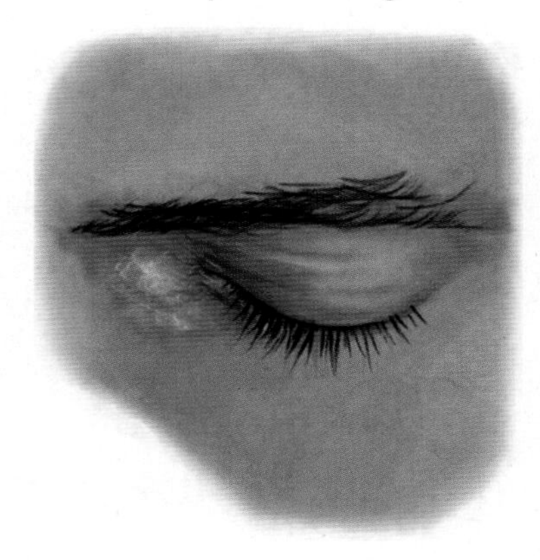

Sebaceous carcinoma. Yellowish patch often located around the eye, in this case near the medial canthus. These tumors may be seen in association with Muir-Torre syndrome.

Cutaneous Adnexal Tumors

Apocrine gland derived	Eccrine gland derived
Adenocarcinoma of Moll's glands	Adenoid cystic carcinoma
Apocrine carcinoma	Aggressive digital papillary adenocarcinoma
Ceruminous adenocarcinoma	Clear cell eccrine carcinoma
Cribriform apocrine carcinoma	Hidradenocarcinoma
Extramammary Paget disease	Eccrine ductal adenocarcinoma
Hair follicle derived	Eccrine porocarcinoma
Cutaneous adnexal carcinoma with follicular differentiation	Malignant chondroid syringoma
Cutaneous adnexal carcinoma not otherwise specified	Malignant cylindroma
Malignant proliferating trichilemmal tumor	Malignant eccrine spiradenoma
Pilomatrix carcinoma	Microcystic adnexal carcinoma
Trichilemmal carcinoma	Mucinous adenocystic carcinoma
Trichoblastic carcinoma	Mucoepidermoid carcinoma
Sebaceous gland derived	Polymorphous sweat gland carcinoma
Sebaceous carcinoma	Signet ring cell carcinoma of the eyelid
	Syringoadenocarcinoma papilliferum
	Syringoid eccrine carcinoma

Treatment: These tumors should all be surgically excised with clear surgical margins. The Mohs surgical technique has been used successfully to treat these tumors, as has a standard wide local excision. Sentinel node removal and evaluation are not routinely performed, but some clinicians advocate its use, especially in some of the more aggressive subtypes such as the eccrine porocarcinoma. Sentinel node removal and evaluation have not shown any survival benefit to date. Mohs surgery may lead to a decrease in recurrence rate and is tissue sparing. Because of the rare nature of these tumors and the lack of prospective randomized studies, it is difficult to determine the best removal method. For the same reasons, the ultimate prognosis and the recurrence rate of these tumors are unknown. After diagnosis and removal of these tumors, the patient should have long-term follow-up to evaluate for recurrence.

Adnexal tumors that have metastasized are treated with chemotherapy with or without radiotherapy. The prognosis is poor for patients who develop metastatic adnexal carcinoma.

Stewart-Treves syndrome. Plaque on chronic edematous arm. The chronic lymphedema is secondary to prior mastectomy and axillary lymph node dissection.

ANGIOSARCOMA

Angiosarcoma is a rare, aggressive, malignant tumor of vascular or lymphatic vessels. These tumors can be seen as a solitary finding or secondary to long-standing lymphedema, such as seen after radiation therapy or an axillary or inguinal lymph node dissection. This latter form tends to occur years after the radiation or surgical procedure. Soft tissue sarcomas are very rare and make up a small percentage of all malignancies reported.

Clinical Findings: Angiosarcomas are most common in the older male population. They have no race predilection. The tumors most commonly arise de novo in the head and neck region and can manifest in many fashions. These cancers often appear as a red to purple plaque with ill-defined borders. They can often look like a bruise, and the diagnosis can be delayed. The tumor continues to expand, forms satellite foci of involvement, and eventually ulcerates and bleeds. The scalp and face of older men are most commonly involved. Angiosarcoma has a propensity to involve sun-exposed areas of the face and scalp. The tumors typically show an aggressive growth pattern and tend to metastasize early in the course of disease.

Angiosarcomas can also arise in regions of previous long-standing lymphedema caused by radiation exposure or surgical procedures. Any procedure that can result in abnormal lymphatic drainage can lead to chronic lymphedema. It is believed that long-standing lymphedema can result in the development of angiosarcoma. Common surgical procedures that cause chronic lymphedema are radical mastectomies and lymph node dissections of the axilla or groin after a diagnosis of lymph node involvement by breast cancer or melanoma. Angiosarcomas arising in areas of chronic lymphedema were first described by Stewart and Treves and have been given the eponym Stewart-Treves syndrome. This type of angiosarcoma is highly aggressive and portends a poor outcome. Stewart-Treves angiosarcoma has been reported most commonly in women who have undergone radical mastectomy or lymph node dissection for treatment of breast cancer. After years of chronic lymphedema in the ipsilateral limb, the patient may develop a reddish bruise-like area on the limb. This area slowly enlarges and develops plaque-like areas or nodules within the affected region. At this point, the diagnosis is often considered and then made by skin biopsy. These tumors tend to be large at diagnosis, which most likely accounts for the poor prognosis.

Radiation-induced angiosarcomas may occur at the site of the radiation therapy or as a result of long-standing chronic lymphedema if the radiation therapy interrupts the lymphatic drainage. These tumors also tend to be diagnosed after they have become quite large, which portends a poor prognosis. These tumors tend to occur 4 to 10 years after the initial radiation therapy.

Angiosarcoma arising from the scalp showing red indurated plaque with a central crust due to underlying ulceration of the tumor. These tumors can be very aggressive.

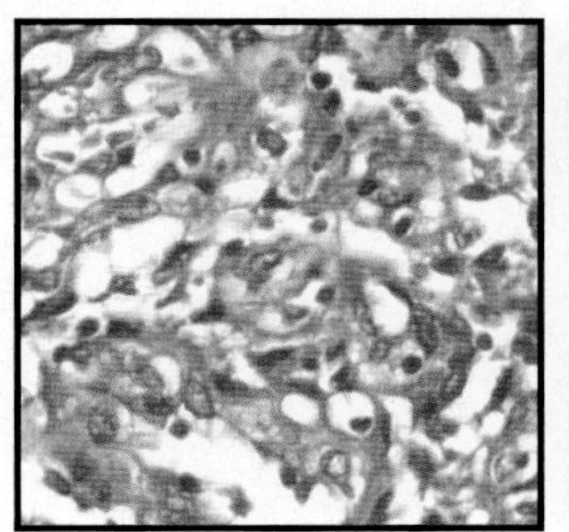

Hemangiopericytoma. Eccentric hyperchromatic nuclei of pericytic cells surrounding vascular spaces. (H&E stain)

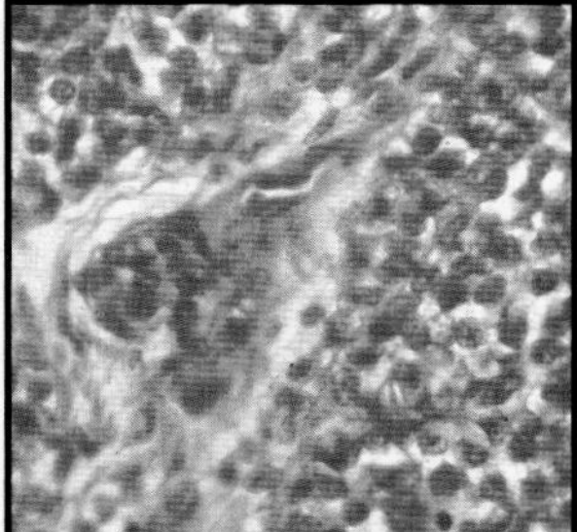

Hemangioendothelioma. Central hyperplastic capillary surrounded by malignant endothelial cells. (H&E stain)

Pathogenesis: Angiosarcomas are soft tissue tumors derived from the endothelial lining of small blood or lymphatic vessels. Some tumors are found to have elevated levels of vascular endothelial growth factor (VEGF), which is critical in the regulation of vessel growth. Loss of the tumor suppressor gene *TP53* has been shown in angiosarcomas without underlying lymphedema, and excessive expression of the *MYC* oncogene has been found in lymphedema-associated angiosarcomas. Other potential players in the pathogenesis of this tumor are mast cells, which cause an increase in stem cell factor; Fas and Fas ligand expression; and lack of the vascular endothelial cadherin protein. All these factors interact in an unknown way to induce tumorigenesis. The exact mechanism of formation of angiosarcoma is unknown. Radiation-induced angiosarcoma may result from a direct mutagenic effect of the radiation on the endothelial DNA. No relation with human herpesvirus-8 (HHV-8) infection has been proven.

Histology: All angiosarcomas share the same pathologic features. The tumor lobules are poorly circumscribed and have an infiltrative growth pattern. They contain large amounts of vascular tissue in a disorganized arrangement. The lining of the vascular spaces contains atypical-appearing endothelial cells. Mitoses are frequently encountered, as are intracytoplasmic lumina. The same tumor can contain well-differentiated and poorly differentiated regions.

Treatment: The standard treatment is wide local excision with the goal of obtaining clear margins. This is usually followed by postoperative radiation therapy. The 5-year survival rate is low (15%–20%). Metastatic or inoperable tumors can be treated palliatively with various chemotherapeutic regimens. The median survival in these cases is 3 to 6 months. Newer treatments targeting VEGF and VEGF receptors 1 to 3 have been developed and are being studied.

Basal Cell Carcinoma

Basal cell carcinoma (BCC) is the most common malignancy in humans. Its true incidence is unknown, but the number of BCCs diagnosed each year easily surpasses the number of all other malignancies combined. It is estimated to affect approximately 25% to 33% of the White population in the United States over their lifetime. The yearly number of BCCs diagnosed is quickly approaching 1 million. Thankfully, BCC rarely metastasizes or causes death. The real crisis it presents is in the significant morbidity and cost to the healthcare system. The vast majority of these lesions are located on the head and neck region and are of considerable cosmetic concern. The major morbidity involved is the significant disfigurement that these locally invading tumors can inflict.

Clinical Findings: The prototypical BCC is described as a pearly red papule with telangiectasias that has a rolled border and a central dell or ulceration. They occur with highest frequency in sun-exposed areas of the skin. Most BCCs start as a small red macule or papule and slowly enlarge over months to years. Once this occurs, the tumor may be friable and bleed easily with superficial trauma. The tumors most commonly range in size from 1 mm to 1 cm. However, neglected tumors can be enormous and have been reported to cover areas up to 60 cm^2 or more. They affect males and females with equal frequency. Basal cell carcinomas are more common in individuals with Fitzpatrick type I skin and decrease in frequency as one moves across the skin type spectrum. Fitzpatrick type VI skin has the lowest incidence of BCC, but these individuals still can develop these tumors. BCCs occur with an increasing frequency with age. They are uncommon in childhood, with the exception of the association of childhood BCCs with the nevoid BCC syndrome (also called basal cell nevus syndrome or Gorlin syndrome).

These tumors are most likely to occur (>80%) on the head and neck region. The trunk is the next most common area. The tumors are derived from follicular epithelium; therefore, the vermilion border, the palms of the hands and soles of the feet, and the glans theoretically should not develop BCCs because these areas are devoid of hair. However, they can be affected by direct extension from a neighboring tumor. These tumors rarely metastasize, and those that do are most often neglected large tumors or tumors in immunosuppressed patients. BCC most commonly metastasizes to regional lymph nodes and the lung.

Many clinical variants of BCC exist, including superficial, pigmented, nodular, and sclerotic or morpheaform variants. There are many other histologic variants. Clinically, a superficial BCC manifests as a very slowly enlarging, pink or red patch without elevation, induration, or ulceration. If left alone for a long enough period, it will develop areas of nodularity or ulceration. Nodular BCCs are probably the most common variant; they manifest as the classic pearly papule with telangiectasias and central ulceration. The pigmented variant can mimic melanoma and is often described as a speckled brown or black papule or plaque with or without ulceration. Early on, these types of BCCs can appear as pearly papules or plaques with minute flecks of brown or black pigmentation. Patients with the sclerotic or morpheaform version often have larger tumors at presentation because of their slow, inconspicuous growth pattern. These slow-growing tumors are almost skin colored and indurated and have ill-defined borders. They tend not to ulcerate until they have become large, which often delays the seeking of medical advice. These tumors can mimic the appearance of scar tissue, which can also hinder diagnosis. Eventually, the tumor enlarges enough to cause ulceration or superficial erosions, and the diagnosis is made. Sclerotic BCC is often much larger than the other variant types at the time of diagnosis.

The most important genetic syndrome associated with the development of BCC is the nevoid BCC syndrome. This syndrome is inherited in an autosomal dominant fashion and is caused by a defect in the *patched 1* gene (*PTCH1*). This gene is located on chromosome 9q22. It encodes a tumor suppressor protein that plays a role in inhibition of the sonic hedgehog signaling pathway. A defect in the patched protein allows uncontrolled signaling of the smoothened protein and an increase in various

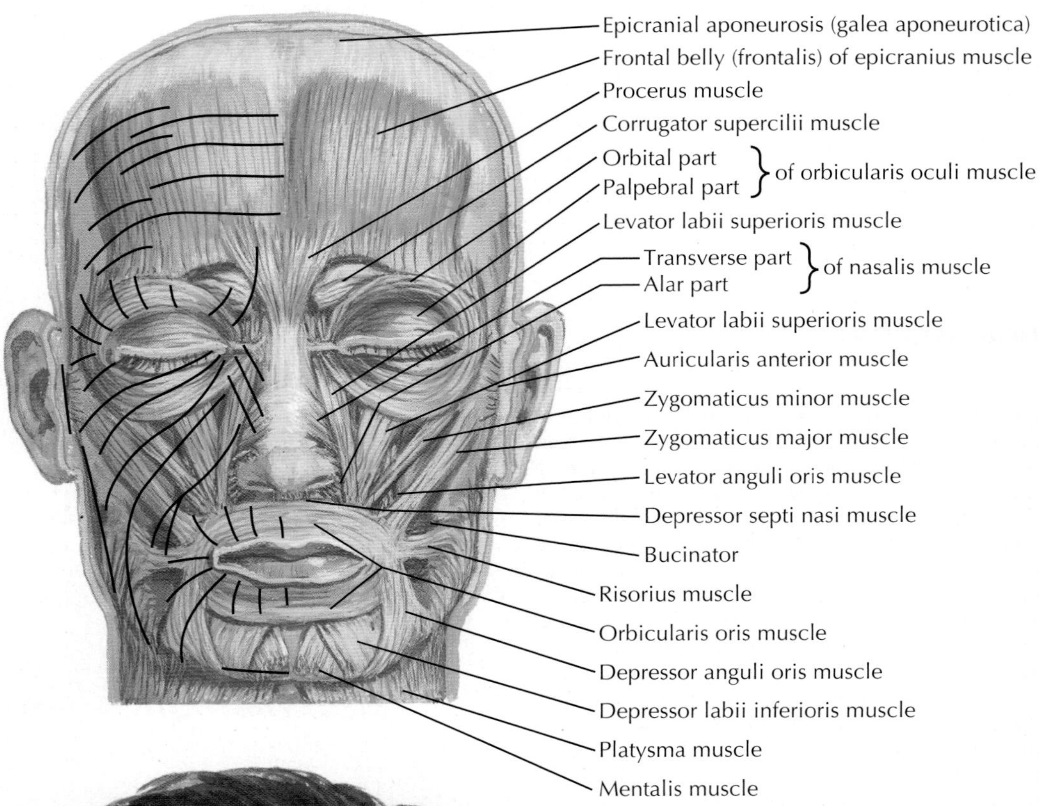

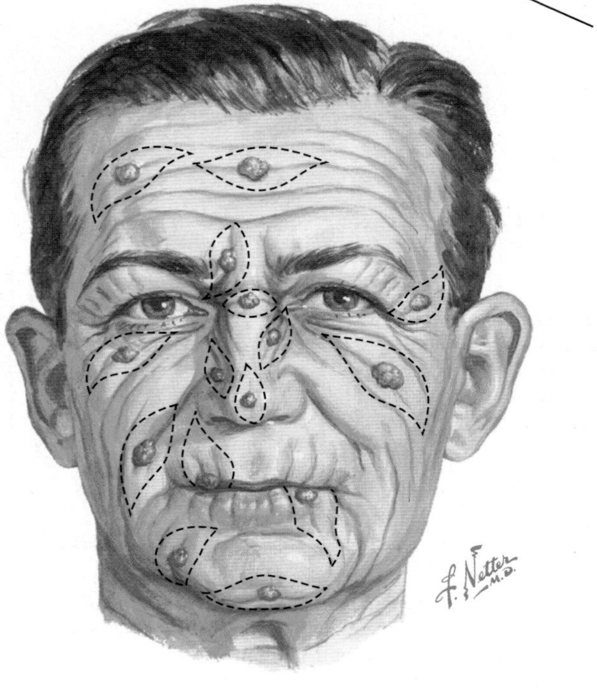

Course of wrinkle lines of skin is transverse to fiber direction of facial muscles. *Elliptical incisions* for removal of skin tumors conform to direction of wrinkle lines.

BASAL CELL CARCINOMA (Continued)

cell signaling pathways, ultimately culminating in the development of a BCC. Patients with nevoid BCC syndrome also may have odontogenic cysts of the jaw, palmar and plantar pitting, various bony abnormalities, and calcification of the falx cerebri. Frontal bossing, mental delay, and ovarian fibromas are only a few of the associated findings seen in this syndrome. Other rare syndromes in which BCCs can be seen include xeroderma pigmentosa, Bazex syndrome, and Rombo syndrome.

Pathogenesis: Risk factors associated with the development of BCC include cumulative exposure to ultraviolet radiation and ionizing radiation. In the past, arsenic exposure was a well-recognized cause of BCCs, and arsenic pollution is still a concern in some areas of the world. Since the advent of organ transplantation, there has been an increase in the development of skin cancers in immunosuppressed transplant organ recipients. The incidences of BCC, SCC, and melanoma are all increased in these chronically immunosuppressed patients. Mutations of various genes have also been implicated in the pathogenesis of BCCs, including *PTCH1*, *p53 (TP53)*, *sonic hedgehog (SHH)*, *smoothened (SMO)*, and the *glioma-associated oncogene homolog 1 (GLI1)*. However, it is still believed that most BCCs are sporadic in nature.

The greatest amount of information is known about the pathogenesis of BCC in nevoid BCC syndrome. The genetic defect in *PTCH1* allows uncontrolled signaling of the smoothened signaling pathway. This pathway initiates uncontrolled signaling of the *GLI1* transcription factors, which ultimately leads to uncontrolled cell proliferation.

Histology: Many histologic subtypes have been described, and a tumor can show evidence of more than one subtype. The most common subtypes are the nodular and superficial types. These tumors arise from the basaloid cells of the follicular epithelium. The tumor always shows an attachment to the overlying epidermis. The tumor extends off the epidermis as tumor lobules. These lobules are basophilic in nature and show clefting between the basophilic cells and the surrounding stroma. The cells have a characteristic peripheral palisading appearance. The cells in the center of the tumor lobules are disorganized. The ratio of nuclear to cytoplasmic volume in the tumor cells is greatly increased. Mitoses are present, and larger tumors usually have some evidence of overlying epidermal ulceration. The tumor is contiguous and does not show skip areas. The nodular form of this tumor extends into the dermis to varying degrees, and its depth of penetration is dependent on the length of time it has been present.

The superficial type is also quite common. The tumor does not extend into the underlying dermis but appears to be hanging off the bottom edge of the epidermis. It has not yet penetrated the dermal-epidermal barrier. There are numerous other histologic subtypes of BCC, including micronodular, adenoid, cystic, pigmented, infiltrative, and sclerosing varieties.

Treatment: Various surgical and medical options are available, and therapy should be based on the location and size of the tumor and the wishes of the patient. Tumors on the face are most often treated with Mohs micrographic surgery. This surgical technique allows for the highest cure rate and is tissue sparing, resulting in the smallest possible scar. It is more labor intensive than a routine elliptical excision. Most BCCs can be treated with an elliptical excision or electrodessication and curettage.

Medical therapy with imiquimod or 5-fluorouracil has also been shown to be useful in selected BCCs, usually the small, superficial type. Photodynamic therapy is effective and is performed by applying aminolevulinic acid to the skin tumor and then exposing the area to visible blue light. Oral inhibitors of the smoothened protein (vismodegib and sonidegib) have shown excellent results in patients with the nevoid BCC syndrome. These medications have good response rates but are associated with some side effects such as severe muscle cramping, hair loss, and loss of taste. These oral medications are typically used for BCCs that are too large for surgical resection, or in individuals who are fatigued from numerous surgical procedures. This is often the case in those with BCC syndrome who have had surgery after surgery to treat their numerous BCCs. Topical versions of the smoothened inhibitors are currently being studied in clinical trials.

CLINICAL AND HISTOLOGIC EVALUATION OF BASAL CELL CARCINOMA

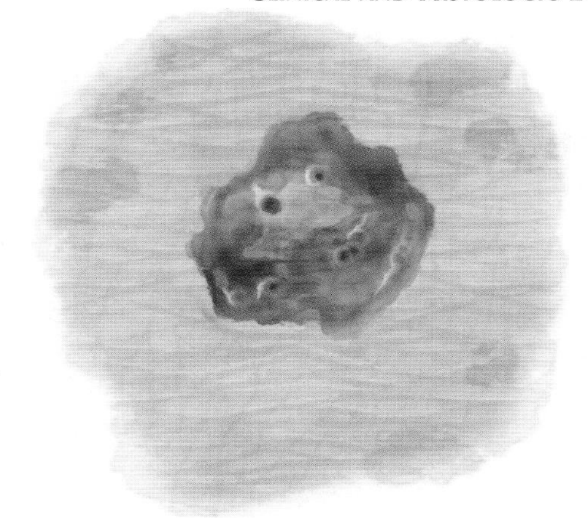

Superficial basal cell carcinoma. Slightly scaly pink to red patch. These tumors are slow growing and occur on chronically sun-exposed skin.

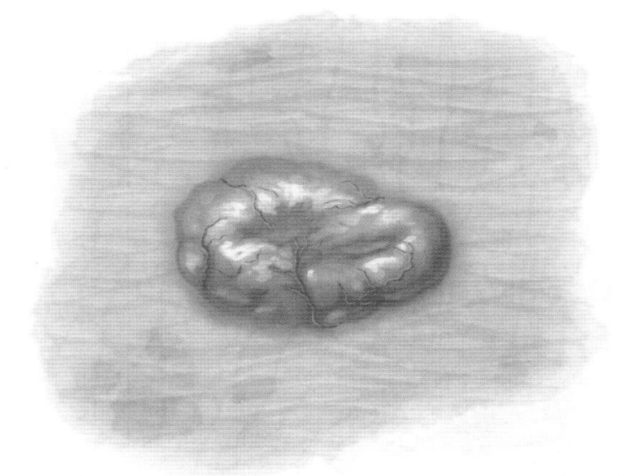

Nodular basal cell carcinoma. Pearly plaque with telangiectatic central ulceration and rolled border.

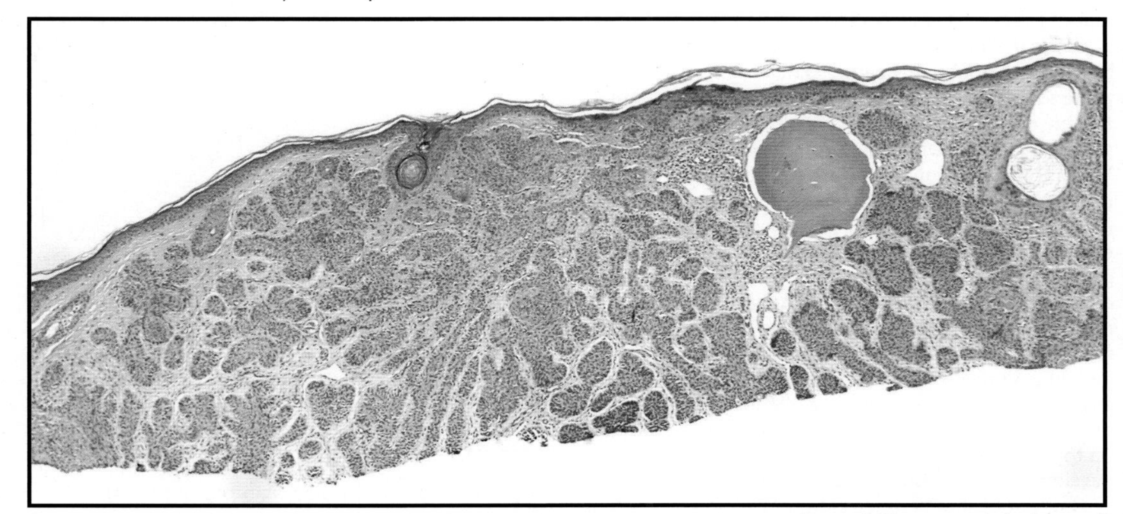

Basophilic tumor lobules and strands extending from the epidermis into the dermis

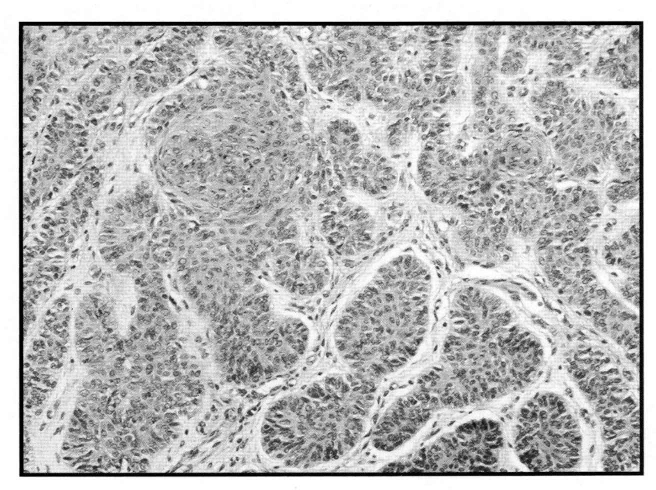

Basophilic tumor lobules within the dermis showing slight retraction artifact and peripheral palisading

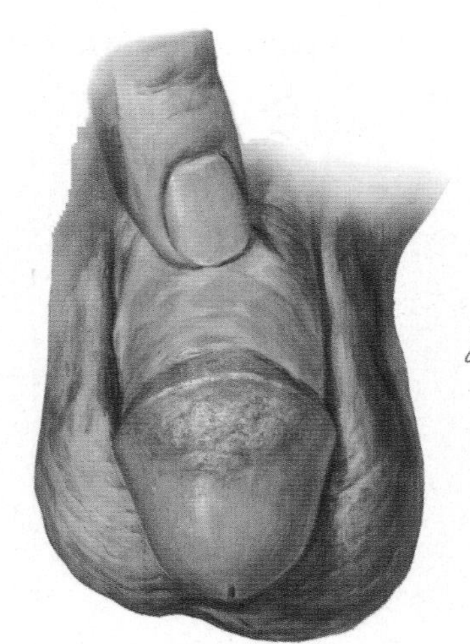

Erythroplasia of Queyrat

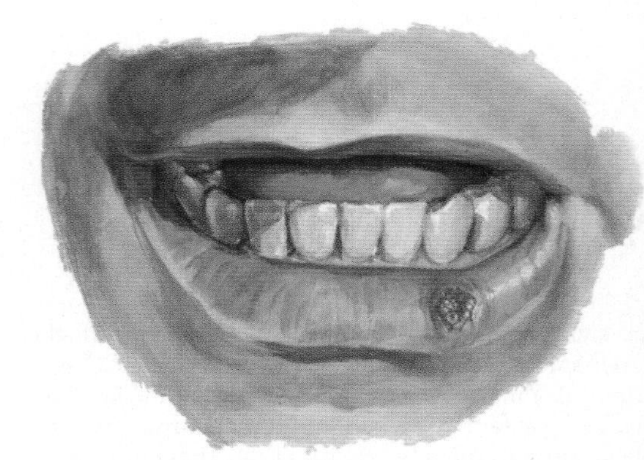

Early carcinoma of lip. Squamous cell carcinoma in situ is common on the lower lip.

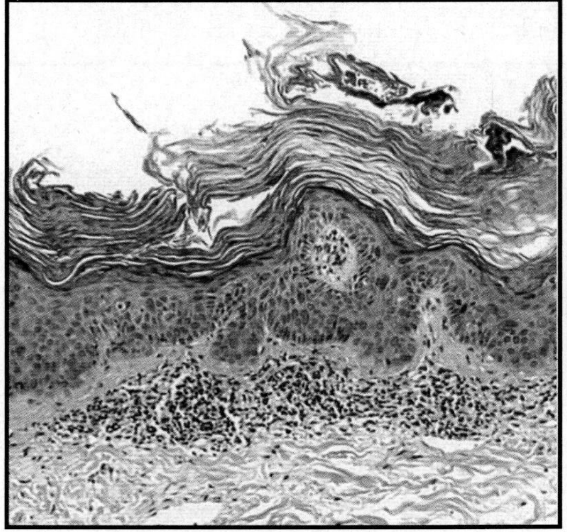

Bowen disease (squamous cell carcinoma in situ) showing full-thickness atypia of the epidermal keratinocytes. Note that the tumor does not invade the dermis.

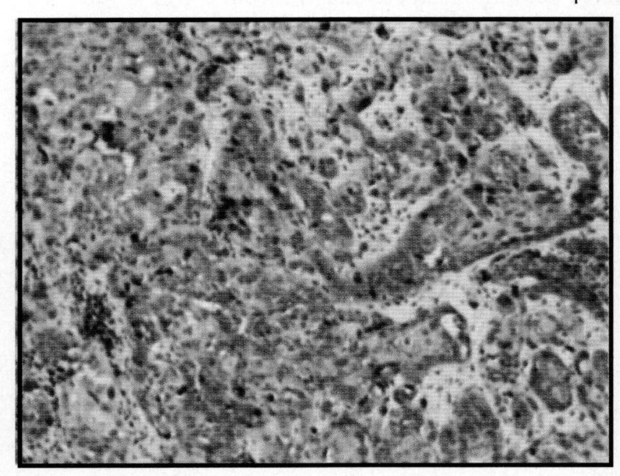

Squamous cell carcinoma. Tumor invading the dermis.

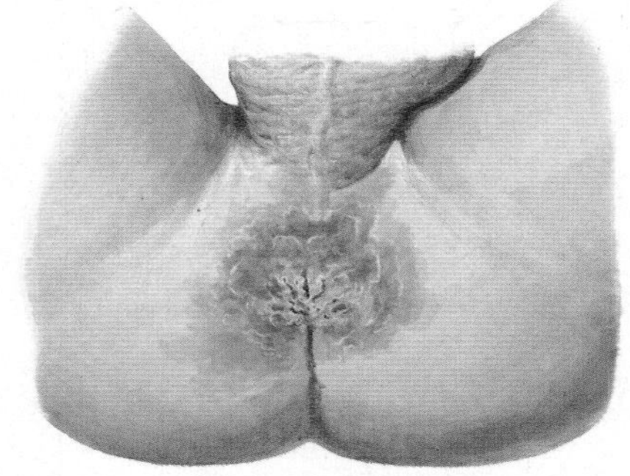

Perianal Bowen disease can have an insidious onset and be misdiagnosed as tinea or dermatitis. Biopsy of any rash not responding to therapy should be a consideration for the treating clinician.

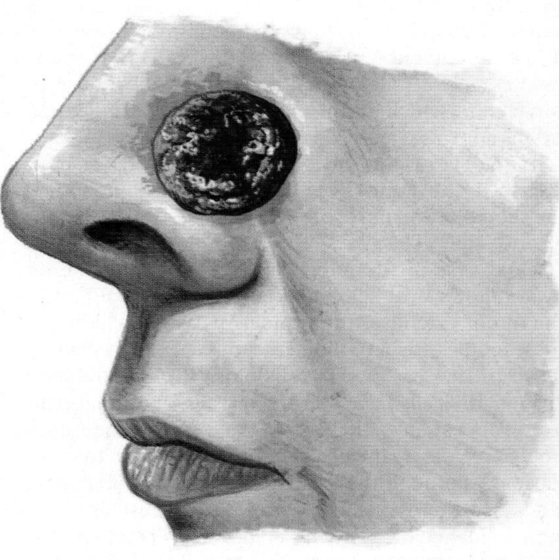

Large crateriform squamous cell carcinoma. These tumors can be locally invasive and destructive. On occasion they can also metastasize.

Bowen Disease

Bowen disease is a variant of cutaneous SCC in situ that occurs on non–sun-exposed regions of the body. That strict definition is not always followed, and the term Bowen disease is often used interchangeably with SCC in situ. SCC in situ is often derived from its precursor lesion, actinic keratosis. Actinic keratosis is differentiated from SCC in situ and Bowen disease by its lack of full-thickness keratinocyte atypia, which is the hallmark of Bowen disease and SCC in situ.

Clinical Findings: Bowen disease can occur on hair-bearing and non–hair-bearing skin, and the clinical appearance in various locations can be entirely different. Bowen disease on hair-bearing skin often starts as a pink to red, well-demarcated patch with adherent scale. Women are most commonly affected, and it occurs later in life. Multiple lesions can occur, but it is far more common as a solitary finding. Erythroplasia of Queyrat is a regional variant of Bowen disease that occurs on the glans penis. These lesions tend to be glistening red with crusting. The area is often well circumscribed. The diagnosis is often delayed because the lesion is easily confused with balanitis, dermatitis, psoriasis, or a cutaneous fungal infection. A biopsy should be performed on any nonhealing lesion or rash in the genital region that does not respond to therapy. It has been estimated that up to 5% of untreated Bowen disease lesions eventually develop an invasive component.

The relationship between Bowen disease and internal malignancy has come under scrutiny; if one exists, it is likely a consequence of arsenic ingestion. Patients with a history of arsenic ingestion are at a higher risk of developing Bowen disease and internal malignancy. Now that arsenic exposure is limited in most areas of the world, the association between Bowen disease and internal malignancy is thought to be unlikely.

Most SCCs in situ are found on sun-exposed areas of the skin and develop directly from an adjacent actinic keratosis. Some SCCs in situ eventually develop into an invasive form of SCC. This is clinically evident by increased thickness, crusting, bleeding, and pain associated with the lesion.

Pathogenesis: Exposure to arsenic and other carcinogens has been implicated in the development of Bowen disease. Certainly, ultraviolet radiation and other forms of radiation play a role in its pathogenesis. Human papillomavirus (HPV) has been implicated in causing many forms of SCC. The oncogenic viral types 16, 18, 31, and 33 are notorious for causing mutagenesis and malignancy in cervical and some other genital SCCs. HPV vaccines may decrease the incidence of these tumors dramatically in the future. HPV can cause cellular transformations to occur and is directly responsible for tumorigenesis.

Histology: Bowen disease shows full-thickness atypia of the keratinocytes within the epidermis. No dermal invasion is present. The underlying dermis may show a lymphocytic perivascular infiltrate. The atypia of the keratinocytes extends down to involve the hair follicle

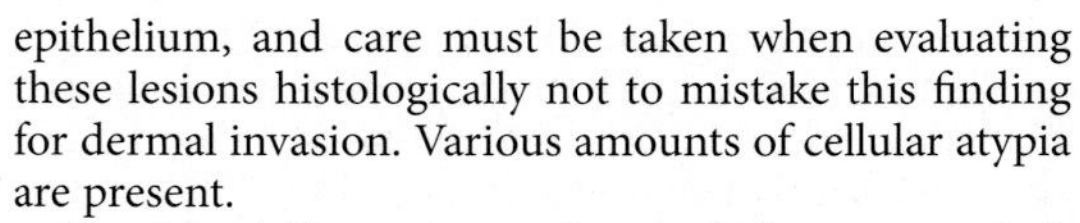

epithelium, and care must be taken when evaluating these lesions histologically not to mistake this finding for dermal invasion. Various amounts of cellular atypia are present.

Treatment: Treatment can be surgical or nonsurgical. The choice depends on various factors, most importantly the location and size of the lesion. Some tumors are best treated surgically, whereas others are best treated medically.

Simple excision or electrodessication and curettage are highly effective treatments. Cryotherapy is another destructive method that can be selectively used with good success. Medical therapies include the application of 5-fluorouracil, imiquimod, or 5-aminolevulinic acid followed by exposure to blue light (photodynamic therapy). These all have been reported to be successful with excellent cosmetic results. The risk of recurrence is between 3% and 10% depending on the type of therapy used.

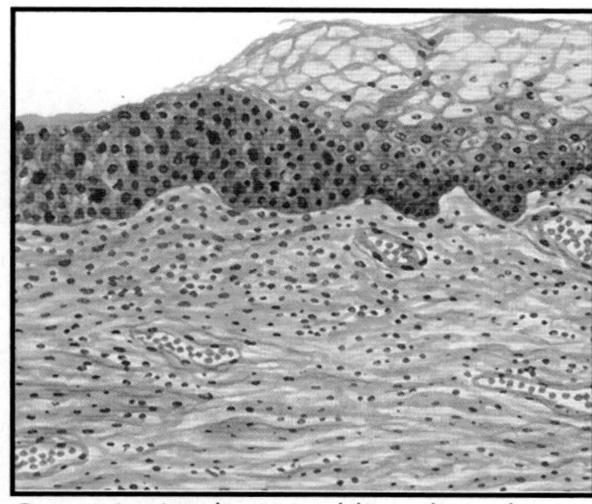
Cancer in situ showing oblique line of transition

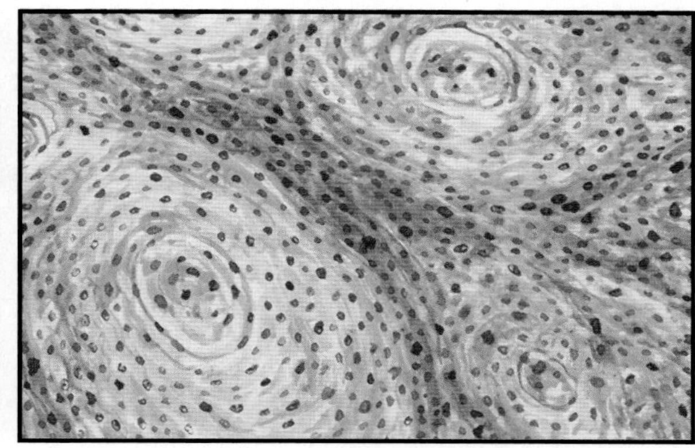
Squamous cell cancer showing pearl formation

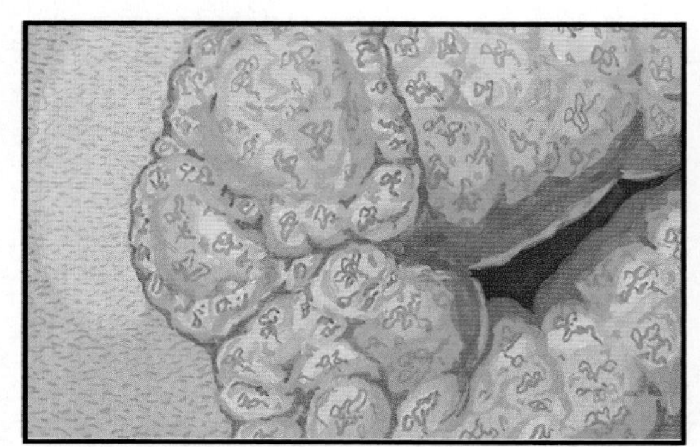
Papilloma of cervix. Some papillomas may predispose to cervical malignancy.

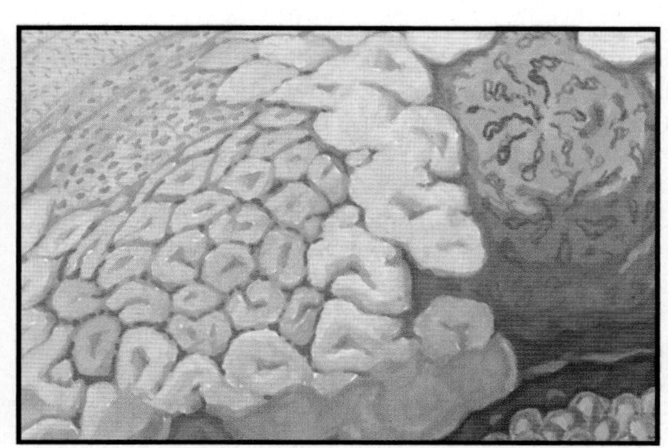
Changes suggestive of carcinoma in situ. Abnormal vasculature with leukoplakia, mosaicism, and punctation.

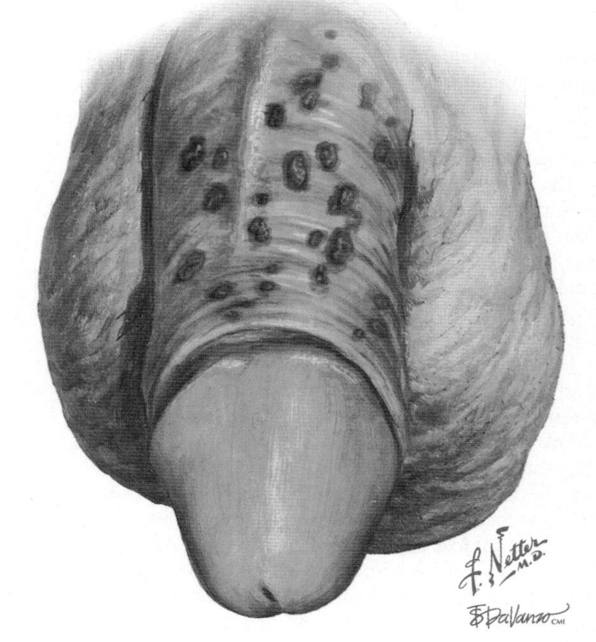

Bowenoid papulosis. Slightly hyperpigmented papules on the shaft of the penis.

Bowenoid Papulosis

Bowenoid papulosis is considered a special variant of SCC in situ that is caused by HPV and is located predominantly in the genital region, particularly on the penile shaft. As with other HPV-induced genital skin cancers, HPV 16, 18, 31, and 33 are the more common viral types, although many other subtypes have been found in these lesions. Bowenoid papulosis is considered by some to be a precancerous lesion with a low risk of developing invasive properties and by others as a true SCC in situ. This lesion does have a low risk of invasive transformation; if it is treated, the prognosis is excellent. It is believed that approximately 1% of all bowenoid papulosis lesions develop into invasive SCC.

Clinical Findings: Bowenoid papulosis is most commonly found in men in the third through sixth decades of life. There is no racial preference. It is believed to be more common in patients who have had multiple sexual partners because of their increased risk for exposure to HPV. It is too soon to determine whether vaccination against HPV has resulted in any changes in the incidence of bowenoid papulosis. In theory, widespread use of the HPV vaccine should decrease the incidence of bowenoid papulosis. In males, the lesions are most commonly found on the shaft of the penis; in females, they are found on the vulva. They are typically well-circumscribed, slightly hyperpigmented macules and papules that occasionally coalesce into larger plaques. Minimal surface change is noted. They are often found in association with genital warts and can be difficult to distinguish from small genital warts. The cause of bowenoid papulosis is thought to be transformation of the keratinocyte caused by HPV; lesions of bowenoid papulosis shed HPV and are contagious.

The lesions are rarely symptomatic and are usually brought to a physician's attention because of the patient's concern for genital warts. For undefined reasons, circumcision appears to help prevent penile cancer. It has been theorized that uncircumcised males are at higher risk for penile carcinoma because of retention of smegma and chronic maceration, which can provide a portal for HPV infection, in conjunction with chronic low-grade inflammation.

Pathogenesis: Almost all lesions of bowenoid papulosis have evidence of HPV. HPV subtype 16 is by far the most predominant HPV type found in bowenoid papulosis. Cells of the genital region that are chronically infected with HPV express various proteins that are critical in the transformation into cancer. The best-studied HPV oncoproteins, E6 and E7, can disrupt normal cell signaling in the p16 (TP16) and retinoblastoma pathways. This disruption can lead to a loss of control of cell signaling and loss of normal apoptosis. These alterations eventually result in loss of the normal cell processes and the development of cancer.

Histology: The histology is almost the same as that of SCC in situ. There is full-thickness atypia of the epidermis with involvement of the adnexal structures and a well-intact basement membrane zone. Varying amounts of epidermal acanthosis and hyperkeratosis are seen. The cells are often enlarged and pleomorphic with visible mitoses. Evidence of HPV infection is almost universally seen as cells mimicking vacuolated koilocyte cells. Special techniques such as polymerase chain reaction can be used to look for HPV subtyping. Because bowenoid papulosis occurs in non–sun-damaged skin, the histologic evidence of chronic sun exposure is not seen.

Treatment: After biopsy has ruled out an invasive component to this tumor, the main treatment of bowenoid papulosis is to clinically remove the areas of involvement. The importance of decreasing HPV transmission to the patient's sexual partners must be addressed. Condoms should be used at all times to help decrease the risk of transmission. Topical therapy with 5-fluorouracil or imiquimod or photodynamic therapy have been advocated as the first-line therapy. Surgical treatment with electrocautery, cryotherapy, or laser ablation or surgical excision has also been reported to be successful. Both patients and their sexual partners should be seen for routine follow-up examinations.

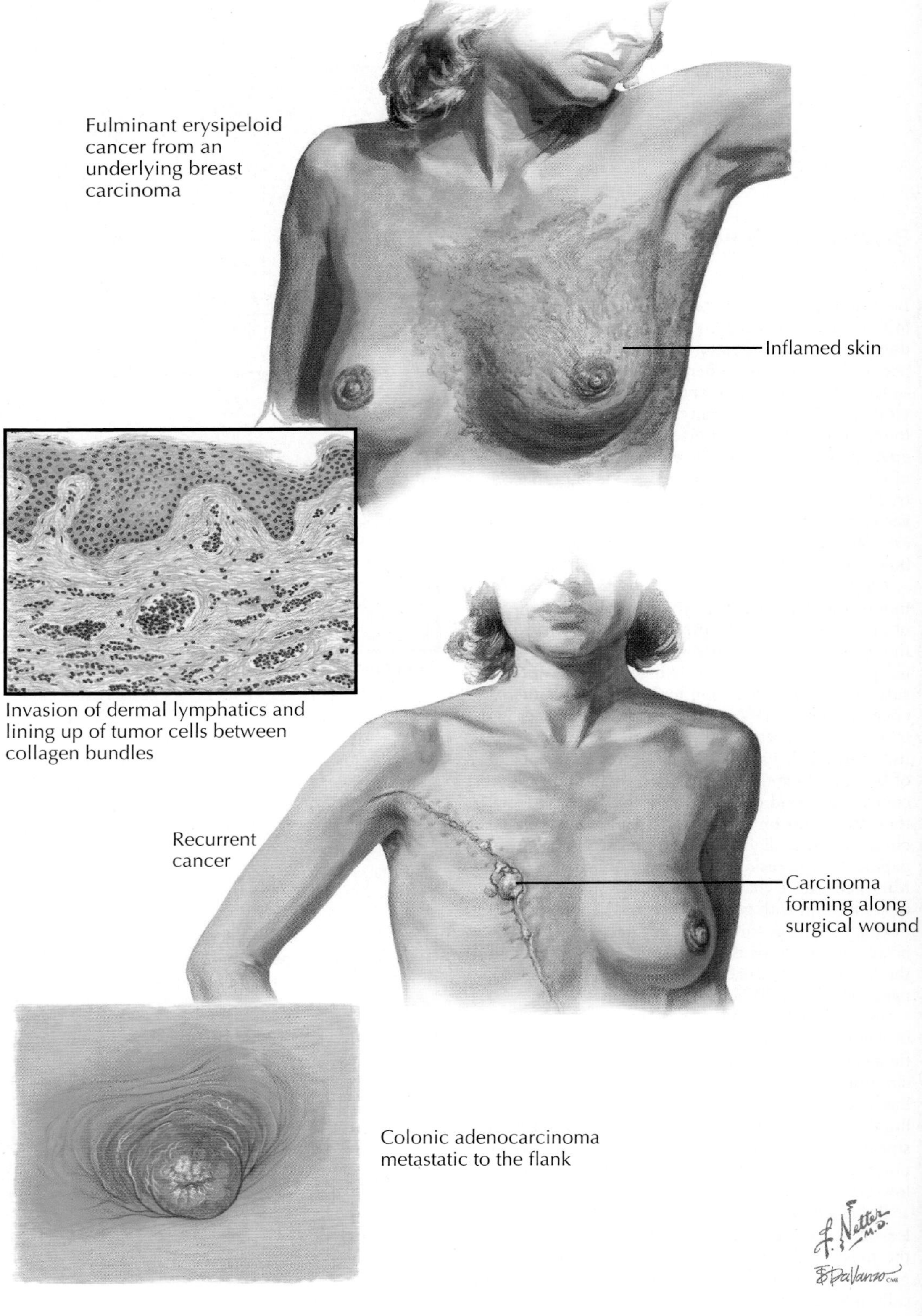

Cutaneous Metastases

Metastasis to the skin is an uncommon presentation of internal malignancy. Cutaneous metastases are far more likely to be seen in a patient with a diagnosis of previously metastatic disease. The frequency of cutaneous metastasis depends on the primary tumor. Almost all types of internal malignancy have been reported to metastasize to the skin; however, a few types of cancers account for the bulk of cutaneous metastases. The distribution of the metastases also depends on the original tumor. The most common form of skin metastasis is from an underlying, previously metastatic melanoma.

Clinical Findings: Most cutaneous metastases manifest as slowly enlarging dermal nodules. They are almost always firm and have been shown to vary in coloration. Some nodules eventually develop necrosis, ulcerate, and spontaneously bleed. Skin metastasis can occur as a direct extension from an underlying malignancy or as a remote focus of tumor deposition. Although skin metastasis often arises in the vicinity of the underlying primary malignancy, the location of tumor metastasis is not a reliable means of predicting the primary source. The scalp is a common site, probably because of its rich vascular supply.

The Sister Mary Joseph nodule is a name given to a periumbilical skin metastasis from an underlying abdominal malignancy. This is a rare presentation that was first described by an astute nun at St. Mary's Hospital at the Mayo Clinic. It has been described to occur most commonly with ovarian carcinoma, gastric carcinoma, and colonic carcinoma.

Melanoma metastases are usually pigmented and tend to occur in groups. Cutaneous metastasis from melanoma can manifest with the rapid onset of multiple black papules and macules that continue to erupt. They can also develop deeper in the skin and appear as firm flesh-colored papules and nodules. As the tumors progress, patients can develop a generalized melanosis. This is an almost universally fatal sign that occurs late in the course of disease. It is believed to be caused by the systemic production of melanin with deposition in the skin. Leukemia cutis is a unique form of cutaneous metastasis and can present as red dermal papules and nodules.

Breast carcinoma is another form of malignancy that frequently metastasizes to the skin. Breast carcinoma tends to affect the skin within the local region of the breast by direct extension. Renal cell carcinoma has a propensity to form ulcerated red vascular-like metastasis on the skin of the scalp.

Pathogenesis: Why some tumors metastasize to the skin is unknown. It is a complex biologic process that depends on many variables. Metastases are likely to depend on size, the ability to invade surrounding tissues (including blood and lymphatic vessels), and the ability to grow at distant sites far removed from the original tumor. This is an intricate process that depends on the production of multiple growth factors and evasion of the patient's immune system.

Histology: The diagnosis of cutaneous metastasis is almost always made by the pathologist after histologic review. Each tumor is unique, and the histologic picture depends on the primary tumor.

Treatment: Solitary cutaneous metastases can be surgically excised. The risk of recurrence is high, and adjunctive chemotherapy and radiotherapy should be considered. Palliative surgical excision can be undertaken for any cutaneous metastases that are painful, ulcerated, or inhibiting the patient's ability to function. The prognosis for patients with cutaneous metastasis is poor. The overall survival rate for multiple cutaneous metastases has been reported to be 3 to 6 months, but the length of survival is increasing, depending on the underlying primary tumor type, as a result of improved treatments.

Fulminant erysipeloid cancer from an underlying breast carcinoma

Inflamed skin

Invasion of dermal lymphatics and lining up of tumor cells between collagen bundles

Recurrent cancer

Carcinoma forming along surgical wound

Colonic adenocarcinoma metastatic to the flank

Dermatofibrosarcoma Protuberans

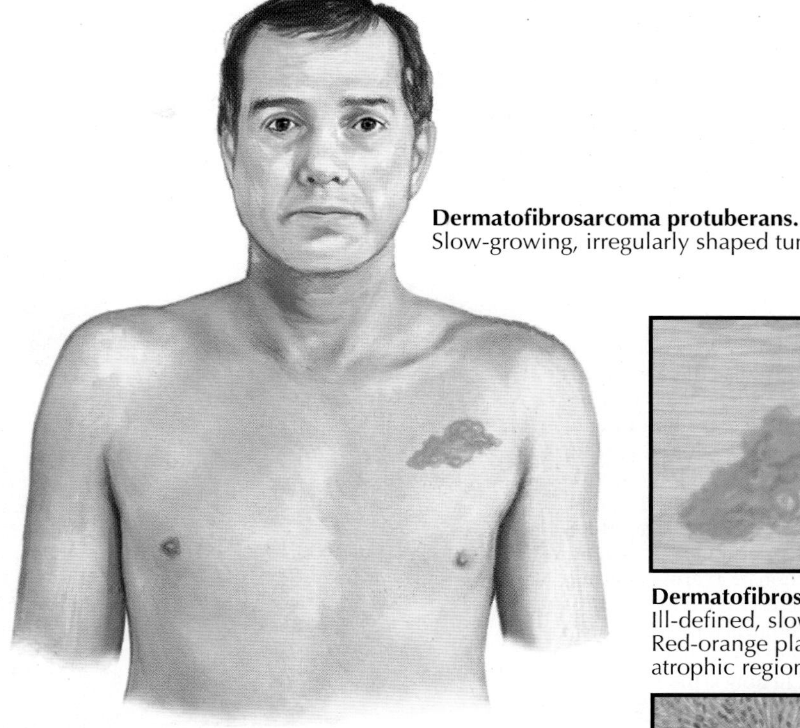

Dermatofibrosarcoma protuberans. Slow-growing, irregularly shaped tumor.

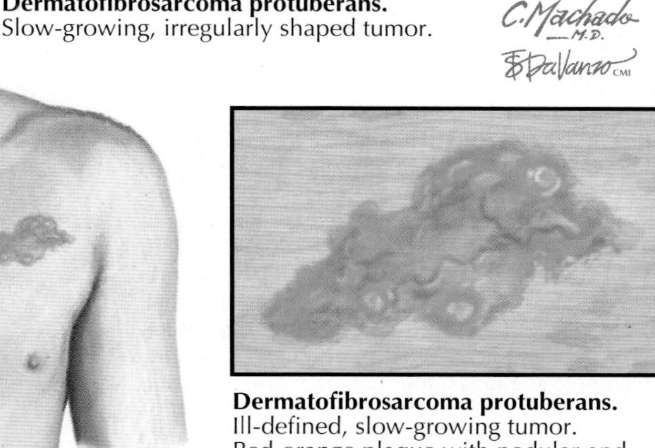

Dermatofibrosarcoma protuberans. Ill-defined, slow-growing tumor. Red-orange plaque with nodular and atrophic regions.

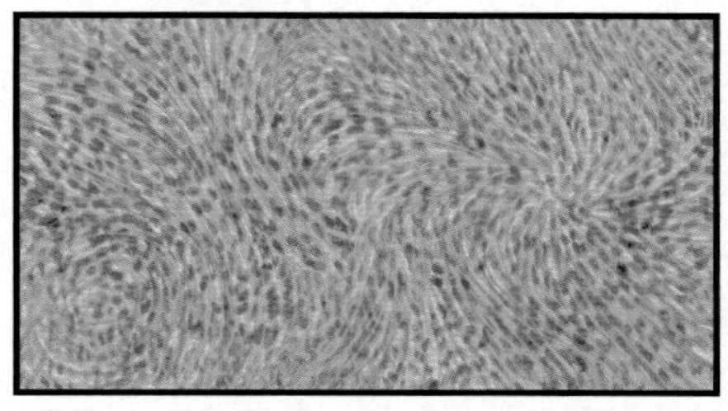

High power. Malignant spindle cells make up the bulk of the tumor.

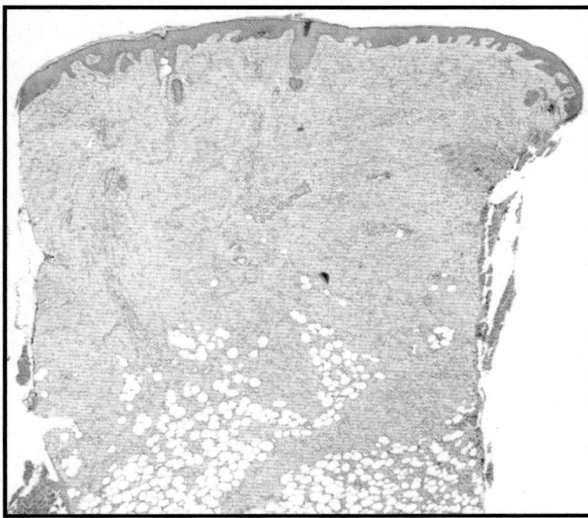

Low power. The tumor is seen invading the underlying subcutaneous tissue. The storiform pattern is seen throughout the dermal portions of the tumor.

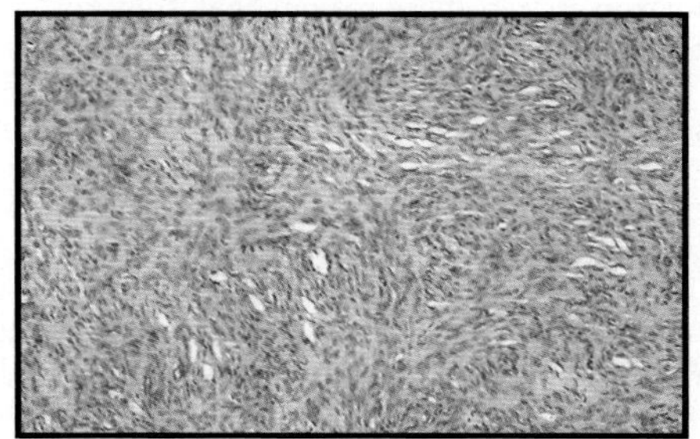

Medium power. The storiform or cartwheel-arranged cells.

Dermatofibrosarcoma protuberans is a rare cutaneous malignancy that is locally aggressive. The tumor is derived from the dermal fibroblast, and it is not believed to arise from previously existing dermatofibromas. Dermatofibrosarcoma protuberans rarely metastasizes, but it has a distinctive tendency to recur locally.

Clinical Findings: Dermatofibrosarcoma protuberans is a slow-growing, locally aggressive malignancy of the skin. These tumors are low-grade sarcomas and make up approximately 1% of all soft tissue sarcomas. The tumor is found with a higher incidence in darker-skinned individuals and affects women more than men, although the difference between the sexes is very small. Most tumors grow so slowly that the patient is not aware of their presence for many months to years. The tumor starts off as a slight, flesh-colored thickness to the skin. Over time, the tumor enlarges and has a pink to slightly red or red-brown coloration. It slowly infiltrates the surrounding tissue, particularly the subcutaneous tissue. If the tumor is allowed to grow long enough, the malignancy will grow into the fat and then back upward in the skin to develop satellite nodules surrounding the original plaque. This is often the reason a patient seeks medical care. The tumor tends to grow slowly for years, but it can hit a phase of rapid growth. This rapid growth phase allows the tumor to grow in a vertical direction; hence the term protuberans. If medical care is not undertaken, the tumor will to continue to invade the deeper structures, eventually invading underlying tissue, including fascia, muscle, and bone.

Dermatofibrosarcoma protuberans is, for the most part, asymptomatic in its initial phases. As it enlarges, the patient may notice an itching sensation or, less frequently, a burning sensation or pain. As the tumor enlarges, patients often notice tightness of the skin or a thickening sensation; however, this development is so slow that most patients ignore it for many more months or even years. The differential diagnosis is often between dermatofibrosarcoma protuberans and a keloid or hypertrophic scar. The atrophic variant can often be confused with morphea. One clue to the diagnosis of dermatofibrosarcoma is the loss of hair follicles within the tumor region. The adnexal structures are crowded out by the ever-expanding tumor. If the tumor is allowed to enlarge enough, it will begin to outgrow its blood supply, and ulceration and erosions develop thereafter. The tumors have ill-defined borders, and determining the extent of the tumor clinically can be challenging or impossible. A punch biopsy of the tumor leads to the appropriate pathologic diagnosis. Metastatic disease is uncommon; however, local recurrence after surgical excision remains an issue.

Pathogenesis: The exact pathogenesis is unknown. By genetic chromosomal tissue analysis, these tumors have been found to have a reciprocal translocation, t(17;22)(q22;q13.1), which is believed to be pathogenic in causing the tumor. The exact reason for this translocation is unknown. The translocation causes fusion of the *platelet-derived growth factor B-chain (PDGFB)* gene with the *collagen type I* α*1 (COL1A1)* gene. This translocation directly causes *PDGFB* to be under control of *COL1A1*. *PDGFB* is then overexpressed and drives a continuous stimulation of its tyrosine kinase receptor.

Histology: Dermatofibrosarcoma protuberans shows an infiltrative growth pattern. It invades the subcutaneous fat tissue. The tumor cells can be seen encasing adipocytes. The tumor is poorly circumscribed, and its borders can be difficult to distinguish from normal dermis. The tumor itself is made of fibroblasts arranged in a storiform pattern. These tumors stain positively with the CD34 immunohistochemical stain and are negative for factor XIII. These two stains are often used to differentiate dermatofibrosarcoma protuberans from the benign dermatofibroma, which has the opposite staining pattern. The stromolysein-3 stain is also used to help differentiate the two tumors; it is positive in cases of dermatofibroma and negative in cases of dermatofibrosarcoma protuberans. Cytogenetic alterations can also be examined by various techniques.

Treatment: Because of the ill-defined nature of the tumors and their often large size at diagnosis, Mohs surgery or a wide local excision with 2- to 3-cm margins is often undertaken and are the best approaches. Postoperative localized radiotherapy has been used to help decrease the recurrence rate. Imatinib, a tyrosine kinase inhibitor, has shown promise in dermatofibrosarcoma protuberans as a treatment before surgery (neoadjuvant) to help shrink large or inoperable tumors. There has also been anecdotal success with the use of imatinib in metastatic disease. Newer tyrosine kinase inhibitors are being studied in patients resistant to imatinib.

MAMMARY AND EXTRAMAMMARY PAGET DISEASE

Extramammary Paget disease is a rare malignant tumor that typically occurs in areas with a high density of apocrine glands. It is most commonly an isolated finding but can also be a marker for an underlying visceral malignancy of the gastrointestinal or genitourinary tract. Paget disease is an intraepidermal adenocarcinoma confined to the breast; it is commonly associated with an underlying breast malignancy.

Clinical Findings: Extramammary Paget disease is most often found in the groin or axilla. These two areas have the highest density of apocrine glands. It is believed that extramammary Paget disease has an apocrine origin. There is no race predilection. These tumors most commonly occur in the fifth to seventh decades of life. Women are more often affected than men. The diagnosis of this tumor is often delayed because of its bland eczematous appearance. It is often misdiagnosed as a fungal infection or a form of dermatitis. Only after the area has not responded to therapy is the diagnosis considered and confirmed by skin biopsy.

The tumor is slow growing and is typically a red-pink patch with a glistening surface. Itching is the most common complaint, but patients also report pain, burning, stinging, and bleeding. The area is sore to the touch, and there are areas of pinpoint bleeding with friction. The red, glistening surface often has small white patches. This has been described as a "strawberries and cream" appearance and is characteristic of extramammary Paget disease. As the cancer progresses, erosions develop within the tumor, and ulcerations occasionally form. The clinical differential diagnosis is often among Paget disease, eczematous dermatitis, inverse psoriasis, and dermatophyte infection. A skin biopsy is required for any rash in these regions that does not respond to therapy.

The tumor is often a solitary finding; however, it can be seen in conjunction with an underlying carcinoma, most commonly adenocarcinoma of the gastrointestinal or genitourinary tract. Rectal adenocarcinoma has been the most frequently reported underlying tumor. The percentage of tumors associated with an underlying malignancy is not known but is estimated to be low. Appropriate screening tests must be performed to evaluate for these associations. Usually, the underlying tumor is diagnosed before the extramammary Paget disease, or at the same time.

Pathogenesis: The exact mechanism of malignant transformation is unknown. Two leading theories exist as to the origin of the tumor. The first is that the tumor represents an intraepidermal adenocarcinoma of apocrine gland origin. The second theory is that an underlying adenocarcinoma spreads to the skin and forms an epidermal component that manifests as extramammary Paget disease. Although most believe this tumor to be of apocrine origin, controversy surrounds this theory and the exact cell of origin is still unknown. There are no known predisposing factors.

Histology: The histology is diagnostic of the disease; however, the pathologic appearance often mimics that of melanoma in situ or SCC. There are a plethora of pale-staining Paget cells scattered throughout the entire epidermis. This type of pagetoid spread of cells is often seen in melanoma. The cells can be clustered together and can have the appearance of forming glandular structures. Immunohistochemical staining is often used to differentiate melanoma and SCC from extramammary Paget disease. Extramammary Paget disease is unique in that it stains positively with carcinoembryonic antigen, some low-molecular-weight cytokeratins, and gross cystic disease fluid protein. It does not stain with S100, HMB-45, or melanin A. The staining pattern with cytokeratins 7 and 20 has been used with some success to predict an underlying adenocarcinoma; however, routine use of these tests is not clinically useful.

Treatment: The prognosis for extramammary Paget disease depends on the stage of the tumor. Disease that is localized to the skin has an excellent prognosis. The treatment of choice is Mohs surgery or wide local excision. The risk of recurrence is high, and lifelong clinical follow-up is required. The prognosis for disease associated with an underlying adenocarcinoma depends on the stage of the underlying tumor. Lesions associated with an underlying malignancy have a worse prognosis. Metastatic disease has a poor prognosis, and various chemotherapeutic regimens have been tried with and without radiotherapy.

Eczematous type of Paget disease

Ulcerating type of Paget disease

Extramammary Paget disease. Glistening red plaque with superficial adherent white patches

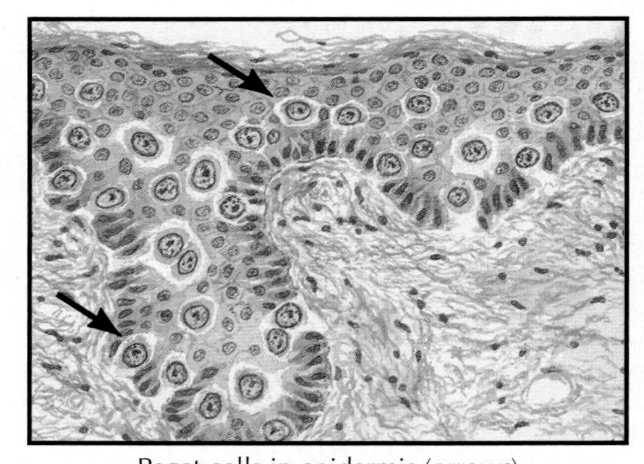

Paget cells in epidermis (*arrows*)

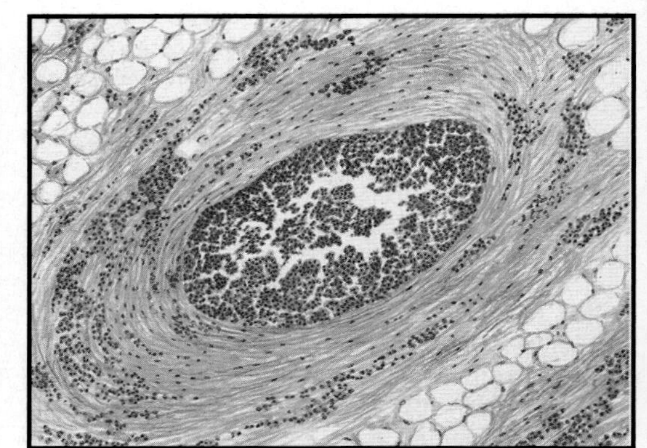

Duct invasion

KAPOSI SARCOMA

Kaposi sarcoma is a rare malignancy of endothelial cells seen in several unique settings. The classic variant is seen in older patients, most commonly individuals living in the region surrounding the Mediterranean Sea. Kaposi sarcoma associated with human immunodeficiency virus (HIV) infection or with acquired immunodeficiency syndrome (AIDS) is seen predominantly in men, and the tumor is thought to be caused by HHV-8. There is also a variant seen in chronically immunosuppressed patients, such as those who have undergone solid organ transplantation. The African cutaneous variant of Kaposi sarcoma is seen in younger men in their third or fourth decade of life. Kaposi sarcoma is a locally aggressive tumor that rarely has a fatal outcome. The one exception is the very rare African lymphadenopathic form, which is distinct from the more common African cutaneous form.

Clinical Findings: The tumors are very similar in appearance across the subtypes of clinical settings. They usually appear as pink-red to purple macules, papules, plaques, or nodules. In the classic form of Kaposi sarcoma, the tumors are most often found on the lower extremities of older men. Some tumors in this setting remain unchanged for years, causing few to no issues, and the patient often dies of other causes. Occasionally, the tumors grow and ulcerate, causing pain and bleeding. The disseminated form of classic Kaposi sarcoma can be very aggressive, and patients require systemic chemotherapy.

AIDS-associated Kaposi sarcoma is the most common form of the disease. It is most often seen in younger men. In comparison with the classic form, this form usually manifests as purple macules, plaques, and nodules on the head and neck, trunk, and upper extremities. This is an AIDS-defining illness. Patients with AIDS-associated Kaposi sarcoma are at a higher risk for internal organ involvement. The small bowel has been reported to be the internal organ most commonly affected by Kaposi sarcoma, but it can affect any organ system. Since the advent of multidrug therapy for HIV infection, the incidence of AIDS-associated Kaposi sarcoma has decreased dramatically.

Tropical African cutaneous Kaposi sarcoma is most often seen in younger men. The clinical findings are not much different from those of the classic form. These patients are much more likely to experience severe lower extremity edema. The tumor also has a higher incidence of bone invasion than the other types. The main difference between the classic and the African forms of Kaposi sarcoma is the age at onset. The aggressive form of African Kaposi sarcoma occurs in childhood and is often fatal because of its aggressive ability to metastasize. The lymph nodes are often involved before the skin is. Why the African forms act so differently from each other is poorly understood.

Pathogenesis: The pathogenesis of the classic and African forms of Kaposi sarcoma is unknown. The endothelial cell is believed to be the cell of origin. Matrix metalloproteinases 2 and 9 have been shown to increase angiogenesis and increase the tissue invasion of the affected endothelial cells. Kaposi sarcoma associated with AIDS or other immunosuppressive states is believed to be caused by the action of HHV-8 in a genetically predisposed individual. HHV-8 is thought to cause dysregulation of the immune response in the afflicted endothelial cells, allowing them to proliferate uncontrolled by normal immune functions.

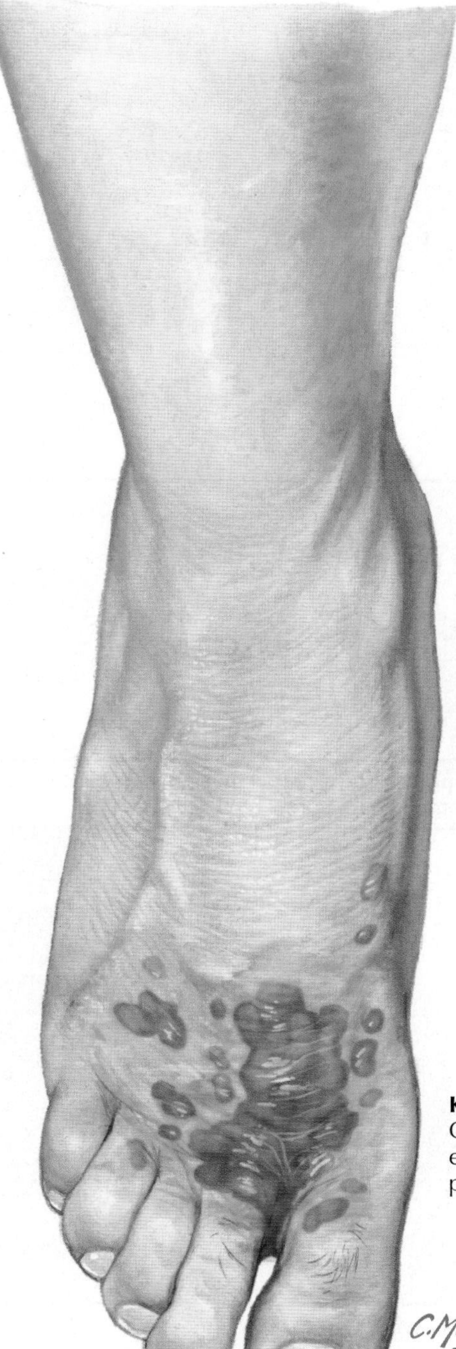

Kaposi sarcoma. Classic presentation on the lower extremity as purplish papules, plaques, and nodules.

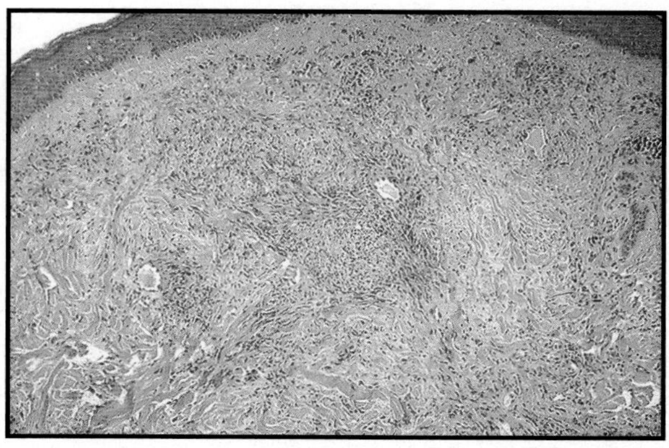

Low power. An abnormal proliferation of blood vessels with slit-like spaces and extravasation of red blood cells.

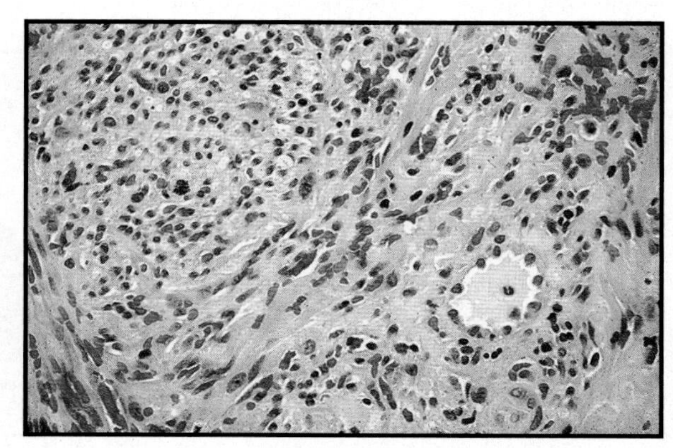

High power. Plump endothelial cells with multiple abnormal-appearing blood vessels in a disorganized pattern. Multiple extravasated red blood cells are appreciated.

Histology: Biopsies of Kaposi sarcoma show many characteristic findings. The promontory sign is often seen; it is represented by plump endothelial cells jutting into the lumen of the capillary vessel. Many slit-like spaces are also seen. These spaces represent poorly formed blood vessels, which have thin walls and are easily compressed. They are filled with red blood cells. The tumor in general is very vascular, with a predominance of vascular spaces and a large amount of red blood cell extravasation into the surrounding dermis.

Treatment: For classic Kaposi sarcoma, the mainstay of therapy has been localized radiation treatment. Many other treatments have been advocated, including topical alitretinoin, imiquimod, intralesional vincristine, interferon, immunotherapy checkpoint inhibitors, and antivirals. Treatment of the underlying HIV infection is often helpful in treating individuals with HIV-associated Kaposi sarcoma. Systemic chemotherapy for disseminated and aggressive forms is indicated and is usually based on a regimen of either vinblastine, paclitaxel, bleomycin, or pegylated liposomal doxorubicin.

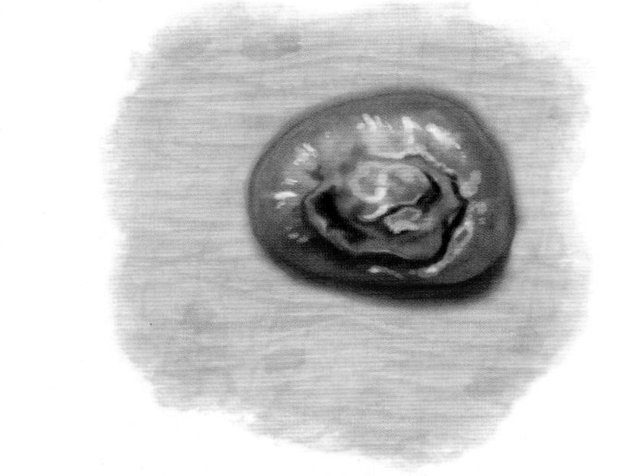

Solitary keratoacanthoma. Typical keratoacanthomas manifest as crateriform nodules with hyperkeratosis on sun-exposed skin.

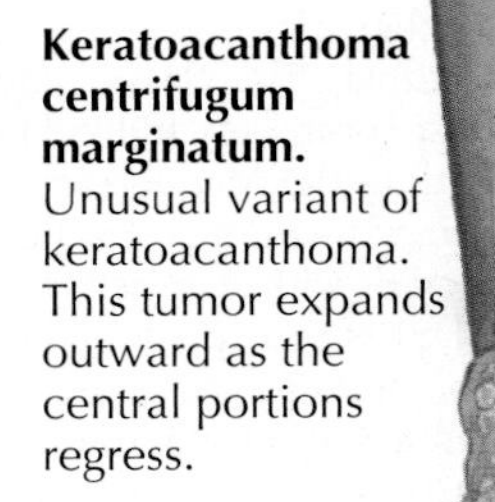

Keratoacanthoma centrifugum marginatum. Unusual variant of keratoacanthoma. This tumor expands outward as the central portions regress.

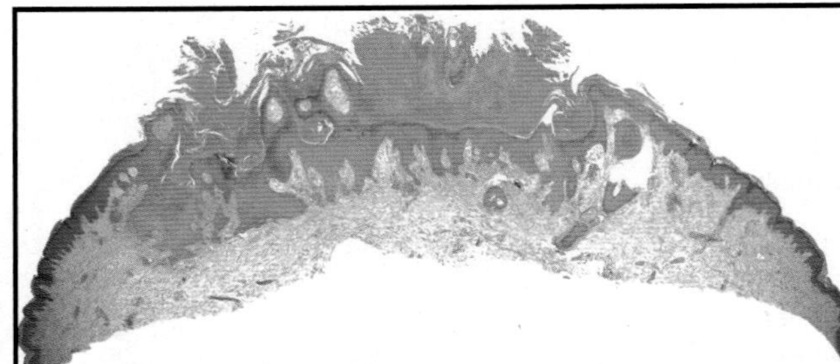

Low power. Cup-shaped invagination of the epidermis, with a central keratin core.

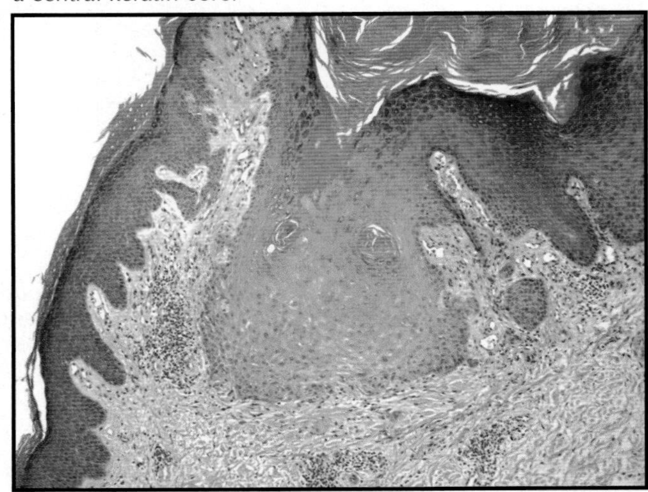

High power. Atypical keratinocytes are seen throughout the epidermis.

KERATOACANTHOMA

Keratoacanthoma is a rapidly growing malignant tumor of the skin that is derived from the keratinocyte. The tumor is believed to be a subset of SCC of the skin, but its natural history and morphology are distinct enough to merit a separate discussion. Most keratoacanthomas are solitary, but many rare variants have been well documented. These variants include Ferguson-Smith, Witten-Zak, and Grzybowski syndromes.

Clinical Findings: The classic solitary keratoacanthoma starts as a small, flesh-colored, tender papule that rapidly enlarges to form a crateriform nodule with a central keratin plug. This is the most common variant of keratoacanthoma. The tumor is unique in that, if left alone, the keratoacanthoma will spontaneously resolve after a few weeks to months. The nonclassic form of keratoacanthoma does not spontaneously resolve, and it is advisable to treat these tumors because a high percentage will continue to enlarge. If left alone, these tumors can behave aggressively, with local invasion as well as distant metastasis. The most common area of metastasis is the regional lymph nodes. This almost exclusively occurs in sun-exposed regions of the body. The peak age at onset is in the fifth to sixth decades of life. These tumors are more common in White individuals, and there is slight male preponderance.

Many unique variants of keratoacanthomas exist. Keratoacanthoma centrifugum marginatum is one variant that manifests with an ever-expanding ridge of neoplastic tissue. As the tumor enlarges, it can become an enormous plaque, often more than 20 cm in diameter, with a peculiar raised border. These tumors can be massive and can encompass a large portion of a limb. This subtype presents a therapeutic challenge.

Multiple keratoacanthomas occur rarely and have been divided into three distinct subtypes. Grzybowski syndrome consists of multiple keratoacanthomas erupting in a generalized distribution, almost always in an adult. The Ferguson-Smith form consists of multiple keratoacanthomas occurring in an autosomal dominant fashion. The keratoacanthomas are uniform in appearance and also form in a generalized pattern. The onset is in childhood, and the tumors have a higher chance of spontaneously resolving. Witten-Zak syndrome also has an autosomal dominant inheritance pattern. The tumors are more variable in size and configuration than in the Ferguson-Smith subtype. The onset of this type is also in childhood.

Pathogenesis: The exact pathogenesis is unknown; however, the tumor has a keratinocyte cell origin. There is more evidence for the keratinocytes derived from hair follicle epithelium as the primary cell responsible for the formation of this tumor. Keratoacanthomas have an increased incidence in patients with long-term ultraviolet exposure and in the chronically immunosuppressed. The classic keratoacanthoma is described as a self-resolving tumor. The reason that some of these tumors undergo autoinvolution is unknown. Some evidence suggests that the tumors, like hair follicles, are under a preset growth and involution control system. The hair follicle grows to a certain point, after which a signal stops the growth, the follicle is shed, and a new hair shaft is formed. The growth and involution of keratoacanthomas may be analogous to the turnover of hair follicles. Keratoacanthomas are also seen with an increased incidence in Muir-Torre syndrome. The genetic defect in these patients may play a role in the pathogenesis of keratoacanthomas.

Histology: The tumor is typically a cup-shaped exophytic nodule with a prominent keratin-filled plug. The borders of the tumor are well circumscribed, and the tumor is symmetric. Neutrophilic abscesses within the outer layers of the involved epidermis are a characteristic finding. The keratinocytes that make up the bulk of the tumor have a glassy cytoplasm with large amounts of glycogen. Other unique findings in this tumor are the presence of plasma cells and eosinophils and the elimination of elastic fibers through the overlying epidermis.

Treatment: After a keratoacanthoma has been biopsied, the treatment of choice is surgical removal. This can be done with a standard elliptical excision or with Mohs micrographic surgery. Intralesional methotrexate, 5-fluorouracil, and oral retinoids have been used in refractory cases and in individuals who cannot tolerate surgery. The familial forms of keratoacanthoma often require long-term retinoid therapy to keep the tumors at bay.

MUCOCUTANEOUS MALIGNANT MELANOMA

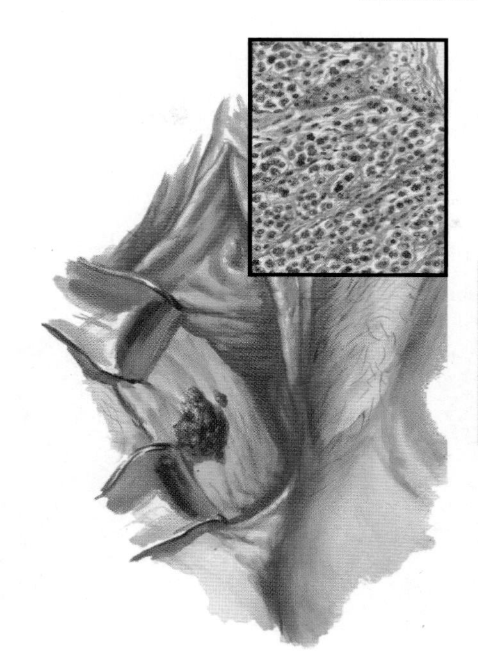

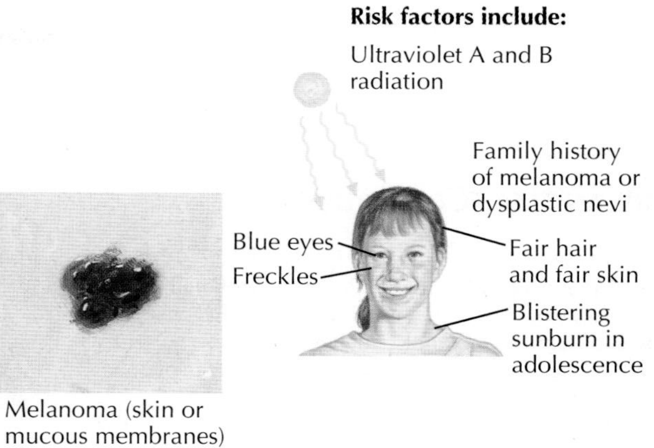

Clinical considerations

Typical clinical appearance of melanoma exhibiting features of "ABCDE" mnemonic

A) Asymmetry
B) Border irregularity
C) Color variation
D) Diameter >6 mm
E) Evolving or changing

Wide local excision of melanoma is based on the thickness of the tumor. A 1-cm border is recommended for lesions <2 mm thick and a 2-cm border for lesions >2 mm thick.

Excisions of lesions

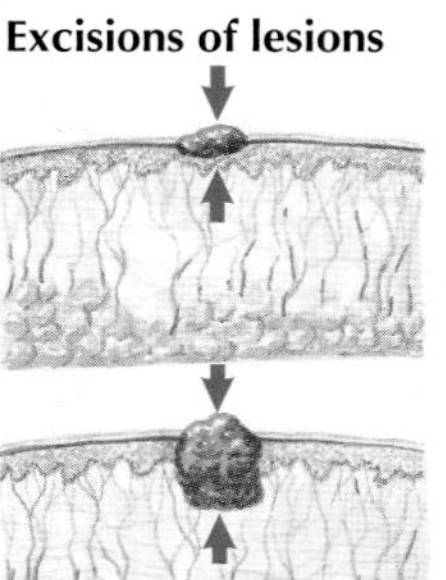

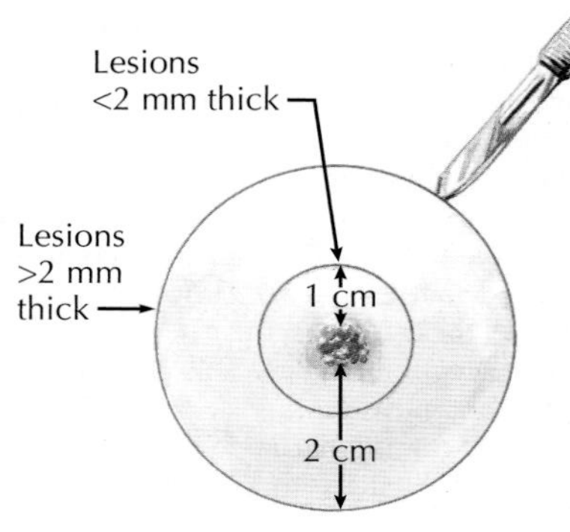

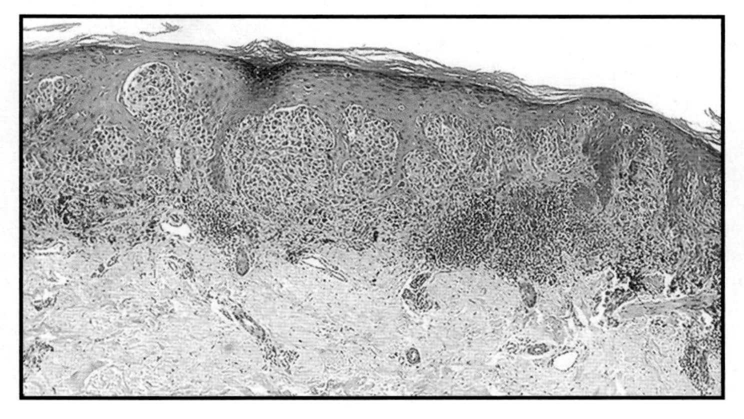

Melanoma with a Breslow depth of 0.7 mm. Dermal invasion is evident, and the tumor shows an abnormal proliferation of melanocytes within the epidermis.

MELANOMA

Malignant melanoma is one of the few types of cancers that has continued to increase in incidence over the past century. Currently, the lifetime risk of melanoma in the United States is 1 in 63; this is projected to continue to increase over the next few decades. The risk is 1 in 32 White, 1 in 167 in Hispanic, and 1 in 1000 in Black individuals. However, the mortality rate has dropped as a result of early detection, surgical intervention, and immunotherapy. According to cancer registries, melanoma ranks fifth in incidence for men and sixth for women. Melanoma is the most common cancer in women aged 25 to 30 years. Approximately 200,000 cases of melanoma (invasive and in situ) were diagnosed in the United States in 2021, and approximately 7600 people died from complications directly related to melanoma.

Clinical Findings: Melanoma follows a characteristic growth pattern. The tumor arises de novo from previously normal skin in approximately 60% of cases and from preexisting melanocytic nevi in the remaining 40%. Melanoma is uncommon in children, the one exception being melanoma arising from giant congenital nevi. The incidence of melanoma peaks in the third decade of life and remains fairly stable over the next 5 decades. There is no sex predilection. Melanoma is more common in White individuals. There are regional variances in distribution of melanoma. The back is more commonly involved in men, and the posterior lower legs are more common in women. Melanoma has been described to occur in any region of the skin. Melanoma has also been shown to develop within the retinal melanocytes, causing retinal melanoma.

Melanoma has been described using the ABCDE mnemonic: **a**symmetric, irregular **b**order, variation in **c**olor, **d**iameter greater than 6 mm, and **e**volving or changing. These are rough guidelines intended to be used by the lay public to increase awareness and as a method to screen for melanoma; they are not diagnostic. Some melanomas have all ABCDE characteristics, and some have only one or two. Some variants of melanoma do not follow the ABCDE rules.

There are four main variants of melanoma. The most common is the superficial spreading type, followed by the nodular type. Lentigo maligna melanoma and acral lentiginous melanoma are the remaining types. Rare variants are also seen, including the amelanotic type and the nevoid type. Superficial spreading melanoma is the most common variant. It manifests as a slowly enlarging, irregularly shaped macule with variegation in color. If not recognized and removed, it will continue to enlarge and develop a vertical growth component with metastatic potential. Nodular lesions grow quickly and can be relatively large at the time of diagnosis. Melanoma that has entered its vertical growth phase has developed the ability to metastasize.

Acral lentiginous melanoma has long been thought to portend a poor prognosis: most likely not because of the subtype, but because this type of melanoma is often diagnosed later in the course of its development. The lesions are often located on the soles, toes, or hands. Patients are often unaware of their presence, and they can mimic a subungual hematoma or bruise. This form of melanoma is more commonly seen in Black persons.

Lentigo maligna melanoma is most often seen on the face of patients in the fifth to seventh decades of life, especially in those with a considerable sun exposure history. This type of melanoma can be difficult to treat because of its ill-defined nature and has a propensity for local recurrence. The borders of the lentigo maligna melanoma are ill defined, and it is difficult to distinguish the background normal sun-damaged melanocytes from the tumor cells.

Amelanotic melanoma is the most difficult of all melanomas to diagnosis. These tumors often appear as slowly enlarging pink patches or plaques with no pigment. They are commonly misdiagnosed as dermatitis or tinea infections, and the diagnosis is often delayed. They can also resemble actinic keratoses. The lack of pigment takes away the clinician's most important diagnostic clue. These tumors are often biopsied because they have not gone away after being treated for something entirely different or after they have developed a papule or nodule. At that point, they are still most commonly thought to be BCCs or SCCs; rarely does the clinician include amelanotic melanoma in

MELANOMA (Continued)

the differential diagnosis. Patients with albinism or xeroderma pigmentosum are at a higher risk for development of amelanotic melanoma. These patients need to be screened routinely, and any suspicious lesions should be biopsied.

Pathogenesis: No single gene defect explains the development of all melanomas. The most plausible theory is that a melanocyte within the epidermis is damaged by some external event, such as chronic ultraviolet exposure, or by some internal event, such as the spontaneous mutation of a key gene in the regulation of cell proliferation or apoptosis. After this event has occurred, the abnormal melanocyte proliferates within the epidermis, starting as an in situ variant of melanoma. After time, the clonal melanoma cells begin to coalesce and form nests of melanoma cells. They then continue to proliferate and enlarge until the clinical features are evident. The tumor first enters a radial growth phase and eventually develops a vertical growth phase with metastatic potential.

Approximately 10% of melanomas are considered an inherited familial form. Although no single gene explains all these tumors, the *p16* gene *(TP16)* is likely the main susceptibility gene. This gene, when mutated, increases an individual's risk for melanoma as well as pancreatic carcinoma. *TP16* is a tumor suppressor gene that is inherited in an autosomal dominant fashion. Genetic testing for this gene is commercially available.

Histology: The diagnosis by histology of melanoma is based on multiple criteria, including symmetry, melanocyte atypia, mitosis, distribution of the melanocytes within the epidermis, lack of maturation of melanocytes as they extend deeper into the dermis, circumscription, and architectural disorder. Melanoma is believed to begin with an in situ portion, followed by an upward spread of single melanocytes within the epidermis, termed pagetoid spread. If no epidermal component of melanoma is seen, the possibility of a metastatic focus is entertained.

Treatment: Pigmented skin lesions believed to be a melanoma should be biopsied promptly. The best method is an excisional biopsy using a small (1- to 2-mm) margin of normal skin. This allows for the diagnosis and an accurate measurement of the Breslow depth, which is the distance from the granular cell layer to the base of the tumor. This depth is considered the most important prognostic indicator for melanoma.

Therapy for melanoma is based on the Breslow thickness, the presence of ulceration, and the mitotic rate of the primary tumor. The standard of care is to perform a wide local excision with varying margins of skin based on the criteria described previously. Melanoma in situ is treated surgically by wide local excision with 5-mm margins. Surgical margins are determined by the Breslow depth of the tumor. Sentinel lymph node sampling is routinely performed in the care of patients with invasive melanoma and aids in staging of the disease. If the patient has a positive sentinel lymph node biopsy, staging is performed based on positron emission tomography/computed tomography scanning and magnetic resonance imaging of the brain. Patients with stage III disease, metastatic disease to local lymph nodes, are treated with adjuvant therapy; they are no longer treated with lymph node dissection because it has not been shown to improve mortality rates. The National Comprehensive Cancer Network/National Cancer Institute has published standardized guidelines for clinicians.

METASTATIC MELANOMA

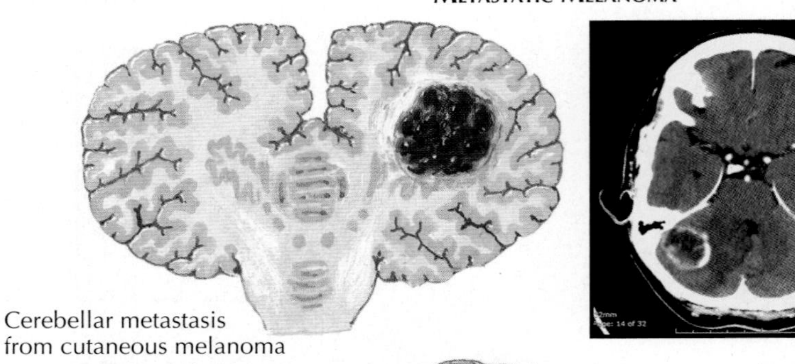
Cerebellar metastasis from cutaneous melanoma

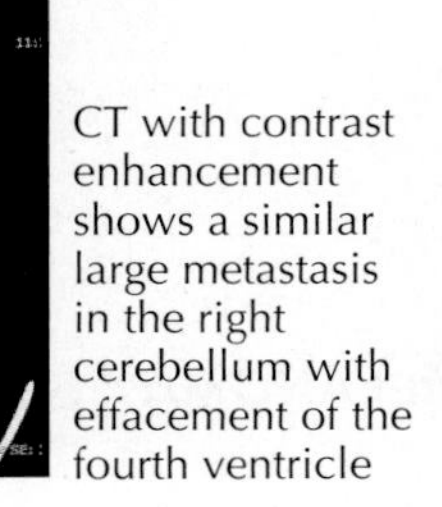
CT with contrast enhancement shows a similar large metastasis in the right cerebellum with effacement of the fourth ventricle

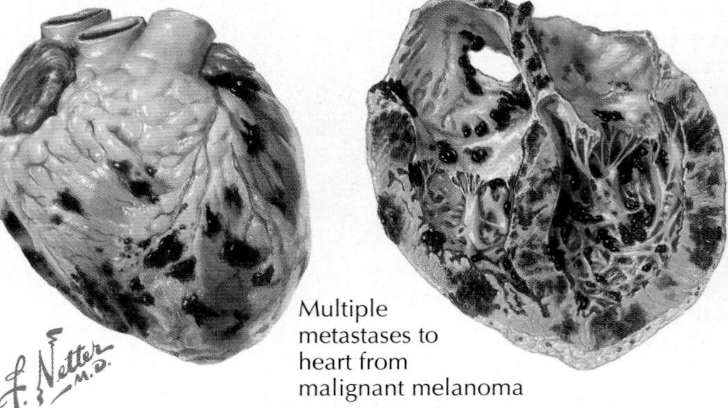
Multiple metastases to heart from malignant melanoma

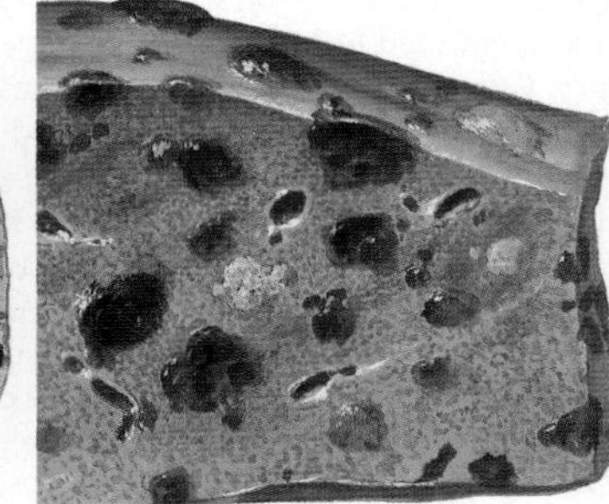
Malignant melanoma metastases to the liver

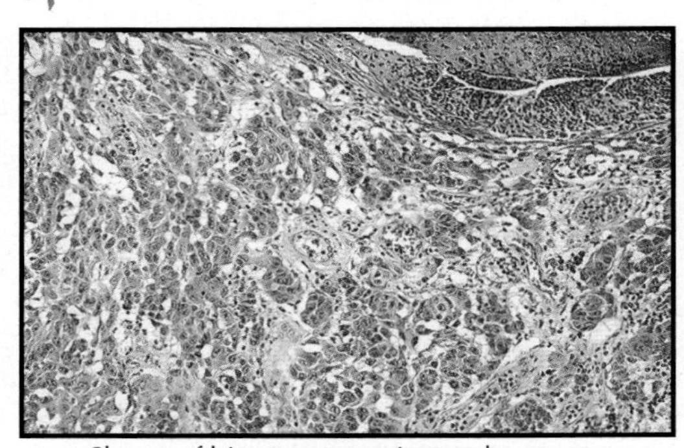
Sheets of bizarre-appearing melanocytes

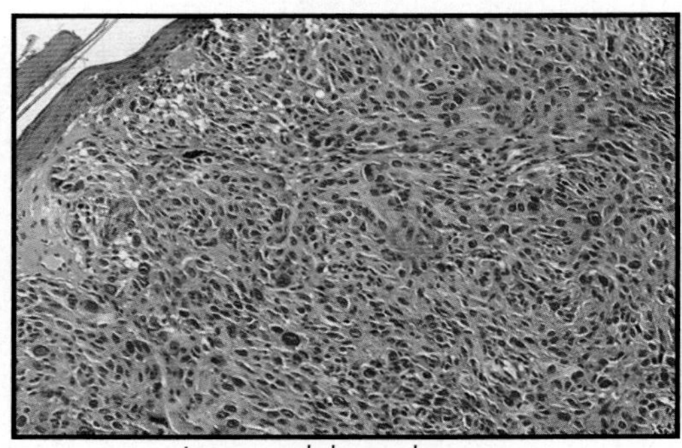
Large nodular melanoma

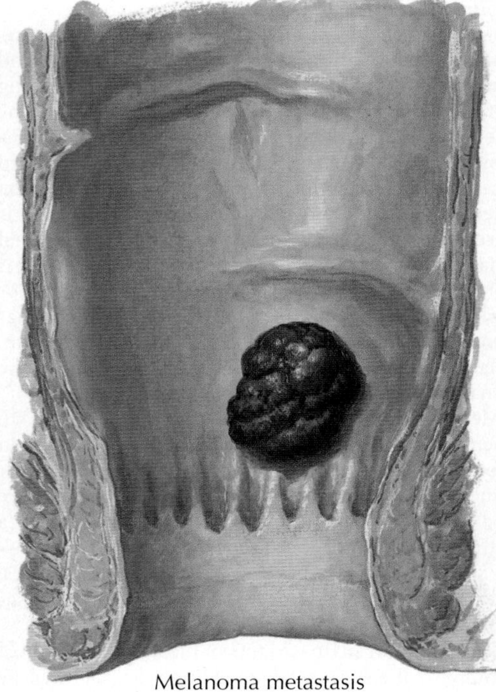
Melanoma metastasis to the large intestine

MELANOMA THERAPEUTICS

Over the past decade, the number of therapies that have been developed and made available for the treatment of metastatic melanoma has increased dramatically. Prior to 2010, the main treatments for metastatic melanoma included dacarbazine (or similar nonspecific alkylating agents), interleukin-2 (IL-2), and interferon. Over the past 10+ years, three main classes of medications have been developed, including immunotherapies, targeted cell therapies, and the injectable class of medications for treatment of metastatic melanoma.

Survival rates for metastatic melanoma had stayed consistently low before the advent of these newer medications. Dacarbazine and IL-2–based therapeutic regimens were both poorly tolerated and showed only small survival benefits. High-dose IL-2 therapy is

MELANOMA (Continued)

poorly tolerated because of its severe side effects and can only be given after admission to an intensive care unit or similarly capable oncology unit because of the severe and predicable side effects. These include hypotension, renal insufficiency, severe rigors, and other flu-like symptoms. These treatments were the mainstay of therapy for 20 to 30 years and, although they did not work as well as anticipated, they paved the way for the development of newer medications. Scientists used the information gained from the use of existing medications to enhance their knowledge on the immunologic basis of treating metastatic melanoma and better their understanding of chemoresistance.

Improvements in molecular analysis and enhanced understanding of the functions of the immune system have been the drivers in the discovery and application of the newer classes of medications. Improved molecular techniques have determined various genomic alterations in tumor-specific tissues. Once tumor-specific alterations in *BRAF* were determined, this allowed the protein B-Raf to be used as a target for potential therapy. B-Raf inhibitors were one of the first of these new therapeutics to be developed. These medications have shown high response rates, but they tend not to be durable. Photosensitivity and the development of numerous warts and cutaneous SCCs were two unique and common side effects. The MEK protein works in conjunction with B-Raf. This synergistic blocking of the MEK protein improved response rates and overall survival compared with dacarbazine. The combination of these medications also dramatically decreased the development of cutaneous SCC. These medications are now almost exclusively used in combination.

Interferon and IL-2 were some of the first agents used as immunotherapies. They are nonspecific enhancers of immune function. They have very broad functionality, and enhancement can lead to many unwanted side effects. As scientists' understanding of the immune system deepened, they began targeting highly specific cell-to-cell interactions by blocking or enhancing cell surface molecule signaling pathways. The programmed cell death receptor-1 (PD-1) and programmed cell death receptor ligand-1 (PD-L1) are two such cell surface molecules that have been specifically targeted to treat metastatic melanoma and other cancers. PD-1 is a cell surface molecule on immune-surveilling T cells. Interaction with its normal ligand PD-L1 causes the T cell to downregulate and become quiescent. This essentially turns off any potential immune-response. This interaction has been termed an immune checkpoint. If the T cell encounters a cell with a proper PD-L1 to interact with its PD-1 receptor, the T cell is turned off. Inhibitors of these receptors and ligands have been developed. When the interaction of PD-1 and PD-L1 is blocked, the T cell is turned into an active state. The active T cells become available to kill tumor cells. Another receptor, CTLA-4, works in a similar fashion.

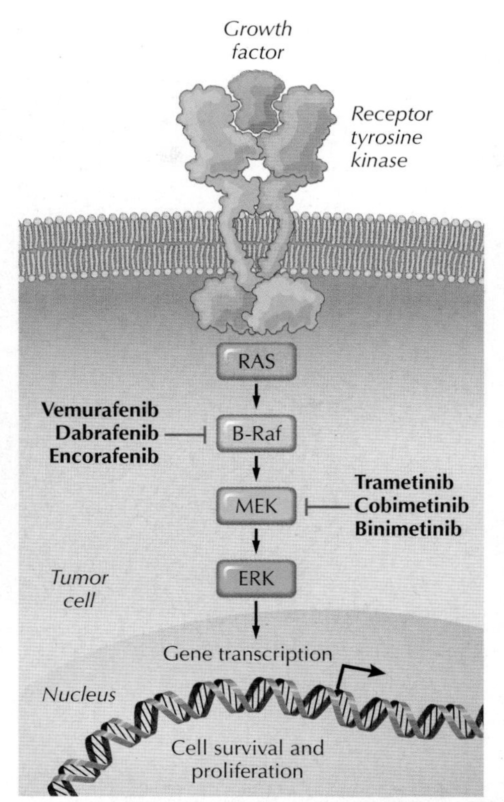

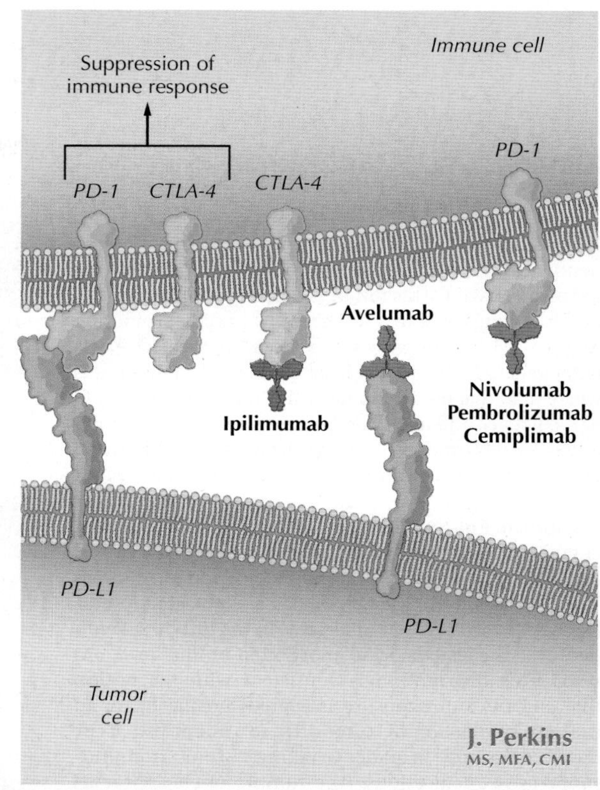

Treatments Available for Metastatic Melanoma	
Immunotherapies	Nonselective immune enhancement • IL-2 • Interferon PD-1 inhibitors • Pembrolizumab • Nivolumab CTLA-4 inhibitor • Ipilimumab
Targeted Cell Therapies	B-Raf inhibitors • Vemurafenib • Dabrafenib • Encorafenib MEK inhibitors • Trametinib • Cobimetinib • Binimetinib
Injectable Therapy	Talimogene laherparepvec (T-VEC)
Alkylating Agents	Dacarbazine

These immunotherapies essentially act by allowing the body's own immune system to fight off any foreign cells recognized by the T cells. These medications have been shown to dramatically improve overall survival and disease-free survival compared with dacarbazine. Combination of a PD-1 inhibitor and a CTLA-4 inhibitor has shown excellent results, with a nearly 50% 5-year survival rate. This is a rate that was unimaginable in 2000. These medications are generally well tolerated, but they are not without side effects. One of the most frequent side effects is interface dermatitis. Drug-induced vitiligo and pruritis are also frequently encountered. Interestingly, the development of cutaneous adverse events is a marker for better clinical response rates. More serious side effects include the induction of autoimmunity. Severe autoimmune colitis, thyroiditis, adrenal insufficiency, and other endocrinopathies can be seen. PD inhibitors have now supplanted interferon as the treatment of choice for the adjuvant treatment of melanoma.

Talimogene laherparepvec is a genetically modified herpesvirus injected directly into a metastatic focus of melanoma. The modified virus replicates within the tumor cells, eventually causing tumor lysis. The virus has also been modified to express granulocyte–macrophage colony-stimulating factor, which is believed to induce an antitumor immune response.

Merkel Cell Carcinoma

Merkel cell carcinoma is an uncommonly encountered neuroendocrine malignant skin tumor that has an aggressive behavior. This tumor is derived from specialized nerve endings within the skin. The tumor-promoting Merkel cell polyomavirus has been implicated in its pathogenesis. The prognosis of Merkel cell carcinoma is worse than that of melanoma. This tumor has a high rate of recurrence and often has spread to the regional lymph nodes by the time of diagnosis. Immunotherapies have changed the treatment strategies and have increased survival.

Clinical Findings: Merkel cell carcinoma is a rare cutaneous malignancy with an estimated incidence of 1 in 200,000. Merkel cell carcinoma is more common in White individuals. The tumor has a slight male predilection. The average age at onset is in the fifth to seventh decades. The lesions occur most often on the head and neck. This distribution is consistent with the notion that chronic sun exposure is a predisposing factor in the development of this tumor. These tumors also occur more commonly in patients taking chronic immunosuppressive medications. The tumors often appear as red-purple papules or plaques that quickly increase in size. They can also appear as rapidly enlarging nodules. On occasion, the tumor ulcerates. The clinical differential diagnosis is often between Merkel cell carcinoma and BCC, inflamed cyst, SCC, or an adnexal tumor. These tumors are so rare that they are infrequently considered in the original differential diagnosis.

It has been estimated that up to 50% of all patients diagnosed with a Merkel cell carcinoma will develop lymph node metastasis. Other notable areas of metastasis include the skin, lungs, and liver. The staging of this tumor is based on its size (<2 cm or >2 cm), the involvement of regional lymph nodes, and the presence of metastasis. Patients with higher stage disease have a progressively worse prognosis. The 5-year survival rate for local stage I or II disease is 65% to 75% and approximately 50% to 60% for stage III (lymph node involvement). Patients with metastatic disease (stage IV) have a 5-year survival rate of about 30%. This dramatic increase in survival for individuals with metastatic disease can most certainly be attributed to the use of checkpoint inhibitor immunotherapy. Grouping all stages together, 20% to 30% of patients diagnosed with Merkel cell carcinoma will die of their disease.

Pathogenesis: Merkel cell carcinoma is derived from a specialized cutaneous nerve ending. The normal Merkel cells function in mechanoreception of the skin. Merkel cells, like melanocytes, are embryologically derived from the neural crest tissue. Chronic immunosuppression is believed to be one of the largest risk factors. Patients taking immunosuppressive medications after organ transplantation are at much higher risk than age-matched controls. Chronic sun exposure and its effect on downregulating local immunity in the skin have also been theorized to play an etiologic role. The Merkel cell polyomavirus has been studied to assess its role in the development of Merkel cell carcinoma.

Polyomaviruses are similar in nature and structure to the better-known papillomaviruses. There are at least five polyomaviruses that cause human disease. Most of them affect patients who are chronically immunosuppressed at a higher rate than healthy matched controls. Researchers have implicated the Merkel cell polyomavirus as a potential cause of Merkel cell carcinoma. This virus has been isolated from a high percentage of Merkel cell tumors, but not from all of them. It is likely to be a player in the pathogenesis of a subset of patients with Merkel cell carcinoma, but it is unlikely to be the only explanation. The discovery of this virus may lead to therapeutic options in the future. Following serum antibody polyomavirus levels in individuals with Merkel cell carcinoma can help assess for and discover early cases of recurrence.

Histology: Merkel cell carcinoma is a neuroendocrine tumor. The tumor is composed of small, uniformly shaped, basophilic-staining cells. The tumor is poorly circumscribed and grows in an infiltrative pattern between dermal collagen bundles and subcutaneous fat lobules. The cells have a characteristic nuclear chromatin pattern. These tumors can be stained with various immunohistochemical stains. The most helpful one is cytokeratin 20. It has a characteristic, if not pathognomonic, perinuclear dot staining pattern.

Treatment: Surgical excision with wide (2- to 3-cm) margins is still the standard therapeutic treatment. Sentinel node sampling has been helpful in staging. Patients with localized disease often undergo postoperative irradiation of the surgical site. Adjuvant immunotherapy is more frequently performed with the immune checkpoint inhibitor immunotherapies (nivolumab and pembrolizumab). Patients with widespread metastatic disease are treated with immunotherapy, with cisplatin-based chemotherapeutic regimens used in cases of immunotherapy failure.

Merkel cell carcinoma. Pink-red papule on the cheek. These tumors may arise quickly and have an accelerated growth rate.

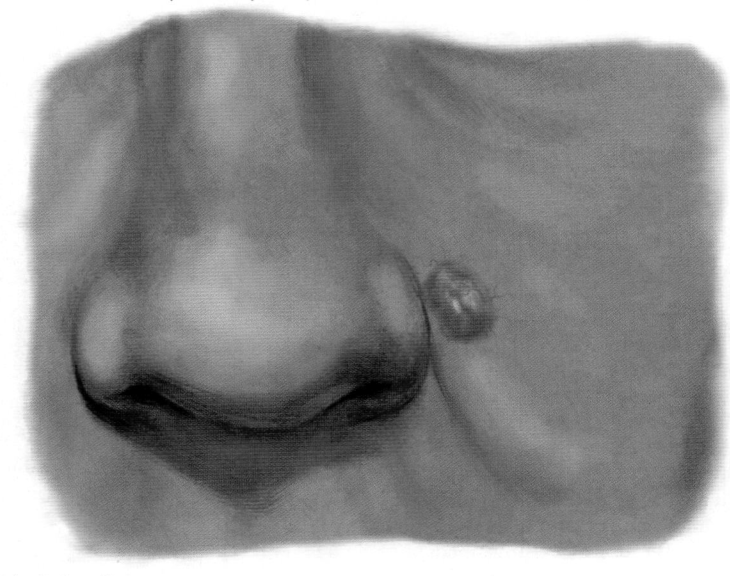

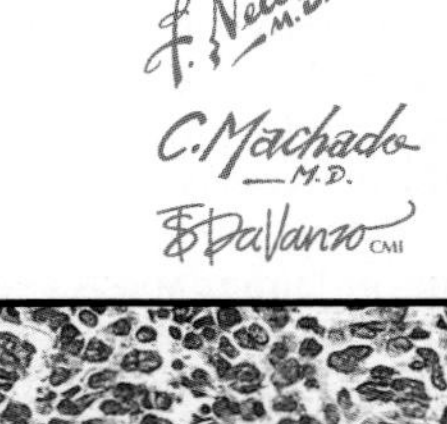

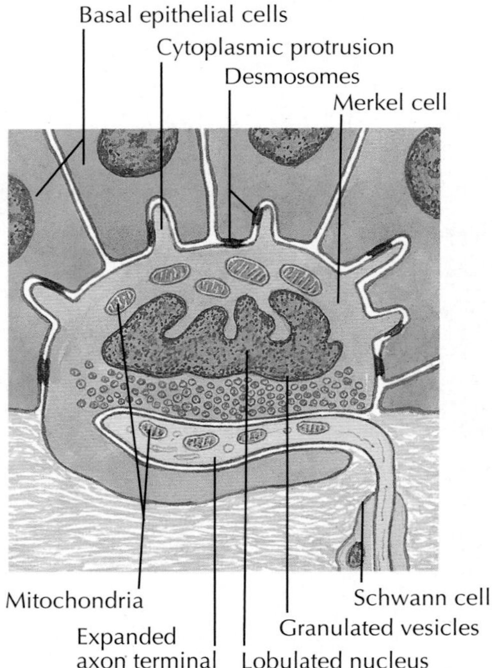

Detail of a Merkel disc nerve ending

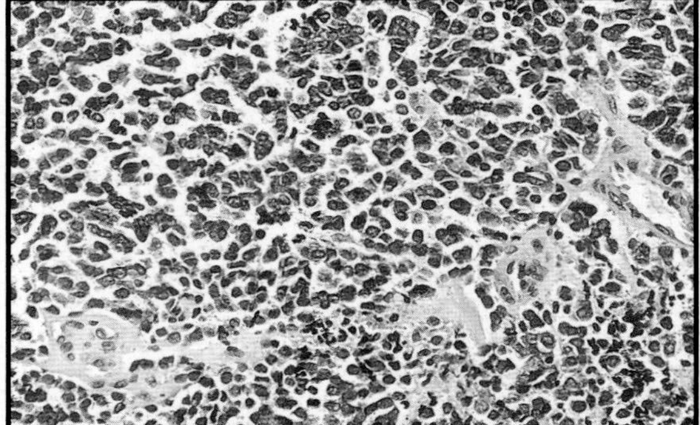

Uniform basophilic-appearing Merkel cells. Merkel cell carcinoma is classified as a small blue cell tumor. (H&E stain)

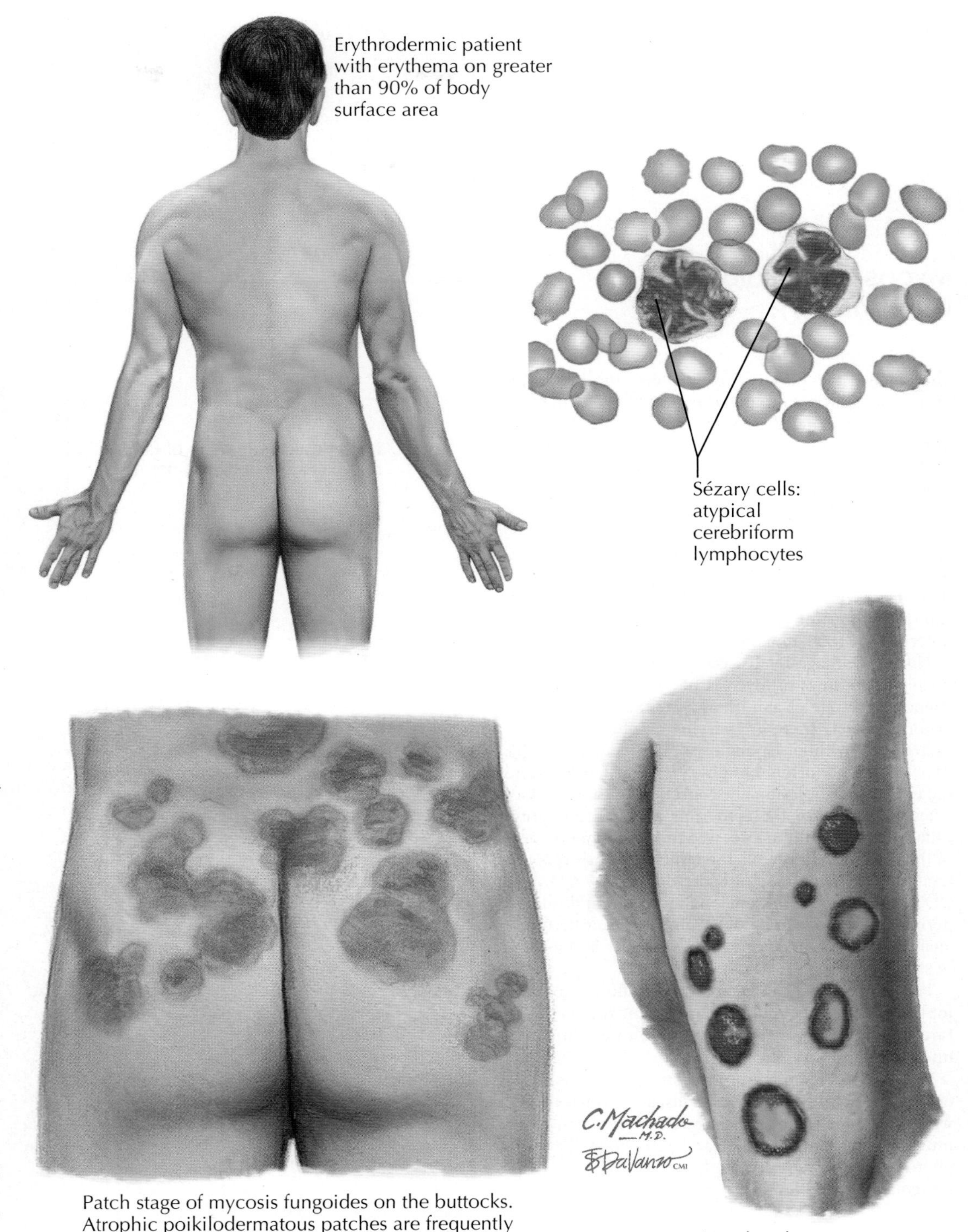

Patch stage of mycosis fungoides on the buttocks. Atrophic poikilodermatous patches are frequently encountered on the buttocks.

Annular plaques

MYCOSIS FUNGOIDES

Mycosis fungoides is the most common form of cutaneous T-cell lymphoma. The cutaneous T-cell lymphomas are an assorted group of cancers with varying genotypes and phenotypes. Mycosis fungoides is a rare form of cancer, but it is the most frequent form of cutaneous lymphoma. Mycosis fungoides is predominantly a disease of abnormal $CD4^+$ lymphocytes that have become malignant and have moved into the skin, causing the characteristic lesions. Advances with immunophenotyping and gene rearrangement studies have helped characterize the disease and are used for diagnostic and prognostic purposes. Altogether, mycosis fungoides is a rare condition afflicting approximately 6 in 1 million individuals.

Clinical Findings: Mycosis fungoides often manifests as a slowly progressing rash that occurs in double-covered areas such as the groin and breast skin. The buttocks are a very common area of involvement. There is a 2:1 male predominance. Mycosis fungoides is seen in all races, with a predominance in those of African ancestry compared with White or Asian populations. It is infrequently encountered in children. Mycosis fungoides is staged based on its appearance, the body surface area (BSA) involved, and the involvement of lymph nodes, blood, and other organ systems. The most common stage of mycosis fungoides is stage IA.

Stage IA mycosis fungoides carries an excellent prognosis, with most patients living a normal life span and dying from another cause. Stage IA disease is typically described as patches of involvement totaling less than 10% of the BSA and no lymph node involvement. The rash of stage IA disease appears as thin, atrophic patches on the buttocks, breasts, or inner thighs or other locations. There are often areas of poikiloderma (hyperpigmentation and hypopigmentation as well as telangiectasias and atrophy). The atrophic skin displays varying amounts of fine wrinkling and xerosis and has a somewhat transparent appearance due to the thinning of the skin. The rash is often asymptomatic early on, but pruritus can be problematic for some, especially with more involved disease. The diagnosis of mycosis fungoides is based on clinical and pathologic findings.

Patch-stage mycosis fungoides can go undiagnosed for years to decades because of its indolent nature and often bland appearance. It often appears as psoriasis, or a nonspecific form of dermatitis, and initial biopsies are often nonspecific. The application of topical steroids before a skin biopsy is obtained may alter the histologic picture enough to make the diagnosis of mycosis fungoides impossible. Often, serial biopsies over years are required until one shows the characteristic features of mycosis fungoides. It is best to biopsy a previously untreated area. In addition to being a very slow-developing cancer, mycosis fungoides may start as a form of dermatitis and over many years transform into a malignant $CD4^+$ process.

At the other end of the spectrum is Sézary syndrome. This is an erythrodermic variant of mycosis fungoides with peripheral blood involvement. Circulating Sézary cells are the hallmark of this syndrome. Sézary cells are enlarged lymphocytes with cerebriform nuclei. The cerebriform nuclei can best be appreciated under electron microscopy. It is considered a leukemic phase of mycosis fungoides. Sézary syndrome has a poor prognosis.

There are many varying stages of disease between these two extremes. The morphology of cutaneous lymphoma changes from patches to plaques to nodules or tumors. Varying amounts of ulceration may be present. The natural history of progression of mycosis fungoides is variable and difficult to predict clinically. The most accurate way to predict the course is based on the type of involvement and the BSA involved.

Histologic Analysis of Cutaneous T-cell Lymphoma

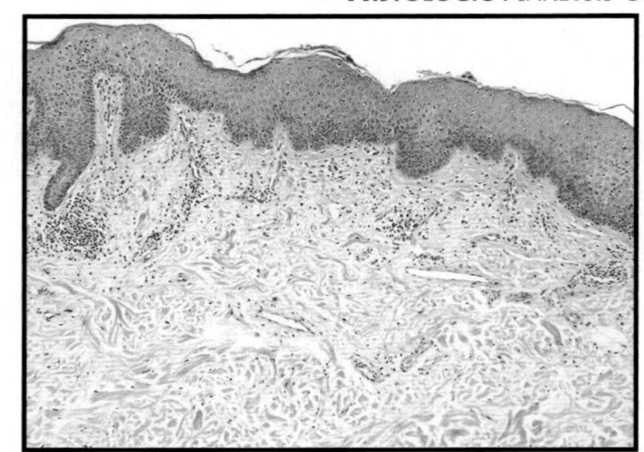

Low power. Lichenoid infiltrate of lymphocytes with epidermotropism.

Mycosis Fungoides (Continued)

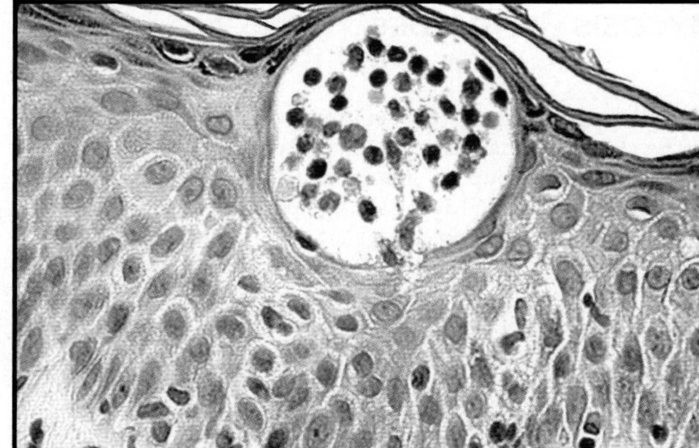

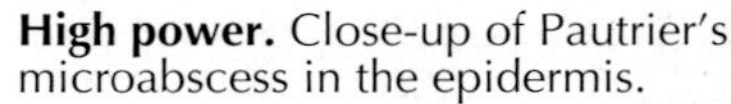

High power. Close-up of Pautrier's microabscess in the epidermis.

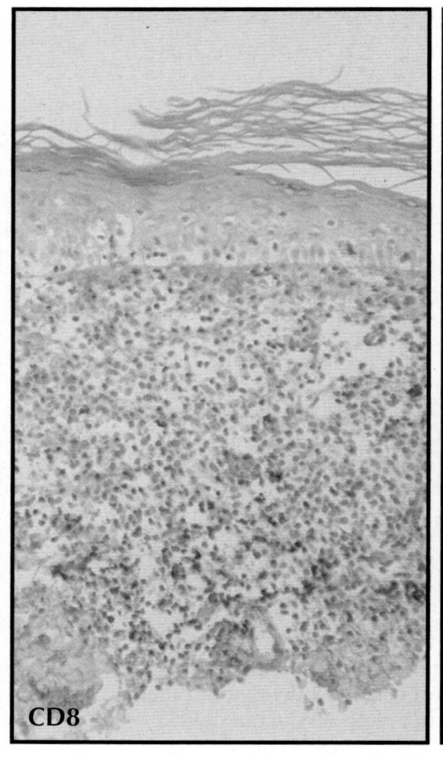

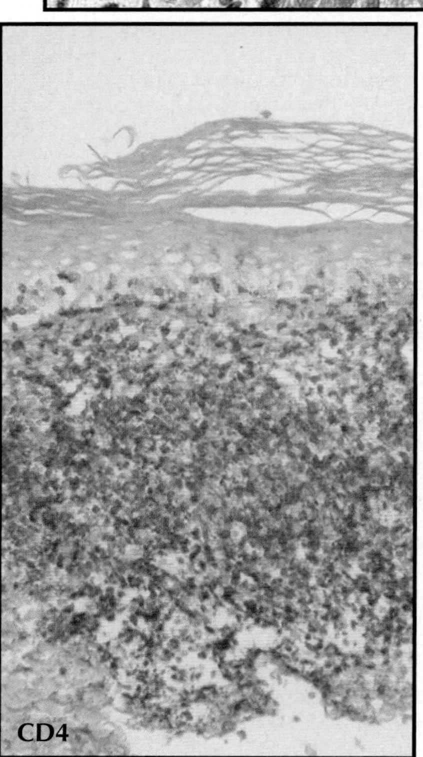

CD8 and CD4 stains showing a predominance of CD4 cells in the infiltrate

The smaller the BSA of involvement, the better the prognosis. A worse prognosis is seen with the nodular form as opposed to the plaque type or the patch form of mycosis fungoides.

Pathogenesis: The etiology of mycosis fungoides is unknown. The pathomechanism that causes the responsible lymphocytes to transform into malignant cells is also unknown. Significant work has explored various causes, including retroviruses, environmental insults, gene deletions, and chronic antigen stimulation. However, the exact mechanism of malignant transformation for this disease, which was originally described in 1806, remains unresolved.

Histology: Stage IA disease shows the characteristic histologic findings of mycosis fungoides. There is a lichenoid infiltrate of abnormal lymphocytes with cerebriform nuclei. There are varying amounts of epidermotropism without spongiosis. The epidermotropic cells are the abnormal lymphocytes that have entered the epidermis. Occasionally, collections of the lymphocytes occur within the epidermis as small groupings called Pautrier's microabscesses. Immunophenotyping of the cells present reveals the infiltrate to be predominantly $CD4^+$ lymphocytes with a loss of the CD7 and CD26 surface molecules. Clonality of the infiltrate, or peripheral blood, can be determined by Southern blot analysis. The presence or lack of clonality is not diagnostic, however.

Peripheral blood can be analyzed by flow cytometry for the presence of circulating lymphoma cells. This is a rare finding in low-stage disease and a near-universal finding in Sézary syndrome.

Treatment: Treatment of mycosis fungoides is based on the stage of disease. Stage IA disease is often treated with a combination of topical corticosteroids, nitrogen mustard ointment, narrow-band ultraviolet B (UVB) phototherapy, or psoralen + ultraviolet A (PUVA) phototherapy. As the BSA of involvement increases, the use of creams becomes difficult. Phototherapy is often used for those with widespread patch disease.

Isolated tumors respond well to local radiotherapy. Systemic treatments are also often used. Systemic agents include methotrexate, pralatrexate, romidepsin, retinoids (bexarotene, acitretin, and isotretinoin), and interferon, both α and γ types. Extracorporeal photophoresis has been used for all stages of mycosis fungoides, especially Sézary syndrome. The patient is given intravenous psoralen and then has peripheral blood removed and separated into its components. The white blood cells are isolated, exposed to UVA light, and then returned to the patient. The exposed leukocytes that have been damaged by the psoralen and UVA are believed to induce a vaccine-like immunologic response.

Total skin electron beam therapy can be used in special cases. Denileukin diftitox is an approved therapy for refractory disease. This drug is created by fusion of the IL-2 molecule and the diphtheria toxin. Cells that express the CD25 molecule (IL-2 receptor) are selectively killed by this medication. Denileukin diftitox can cause severe side effects and should be administered only by specialists adept at its use. Many new medications are being used with variable success in the treatment of mycosis fungoides, including an anti-CD52 monoclonal antibody, alemtuzumab. Mogamulizumab, an anti-CCR4 antibody, has shown efficacy in individuals with Sézary syndrome. Various investigational medications are being studied. Bone marrow transplantation is another option for life-threatening refractory disease.

Despite the many therapies available, no treatment has been shown to dramatically increase survival in patients with mycosis fungoides. It is therefore inadvisable to treat stage IA disease with a medication that has acute, potentially life-threatening side effects.

SEBACEOUS CARCINOMA

Sebaceous carcinoma is a rare malignant tumor of the sebaceous gland. These tumors are most frequently seen on the eyelids. They are most commonly found as solitary tumors but may be seen as a part of Muir-Torre syndrome. Muir-Torre syndrome is caused by a genetic abnormality in the tumor suppressor genes *MSH2* and *MLH1* and is associated with multiple sebaceous tumors, both benign and malignant. The syndrome is also associated with a high incidence of internal gastrointestinal and genitourinary malignancies.

Clinical Findings: These tumors are most commonly found on the eyelid skin and the eyelid margin because the periocular skin contains many types of modified sebaceous glands, including the meibomian glands and the glands of Zeis. Many other less common modified sebaceous glands exist, including the caruncle glands and the multiple sebaceous glands associated with the hairs of the periocular skin. It is believed that most sebaceous carcinomas arise from the meibomian glands, with the glands of Zeis the second most common site of origin. The meibomian glands are modified sebaceous glands located within the tarsal plate of the upper and lower eyelids.

Sebaceous carcinoma has been reported to occur in all areas of the body, but the vast majority occur on the eyelids, with the next most common area being the rest of the head and neck region, probably because the density of sebaceous glands is higher in these regions. The tumors typically start as small subcutaneous nodules or thickenings of the skin. They are initially asymptomatic and can be mistaken for a stye or chalazion. The tumor almost always has a slight yellowish coloration, which, together with the characteristic periocular location, can help with the diagnosis. The major differentiating factor is that styes and chalazions are very acute in onset, are painful, and resolve within a few weeks. Sebaceous carcinoma is a slow-growing tumor that persists and continues to enlarge, eventually causing erosions and ulceration. Once this occurs, the tumor becomes painful and can easily bleed with superficial trauma. The clinical differential diagnosis is often between sebaceous carcinoma and BCC or SCC.

Sebaceous carcinomas occur with a higher incidence in the older female population. There is a predilection for White individuals and for patients receiving chronic immunosuppressive therapy. Patients with Muir-Torre syndrome are at dramatically higher risk for sebaceous carcinoma compared with age-matched controls. Previous radiation therapy for the treatment of facial or ocular tumors has also been shown to be a predisposing factor for the development of sebaceous carcinoma.

As the tumors enlarge, they exhibit an aggressive local growth pattern. They can rapidly enlarge and metastasize to regional lymph node basins.

Pathogenesis: Solitary sebaceous carcinomas arise from sebaceous glands, but the exact pathomechanism is not understood. Many risk factors have been determined, but how these translate into tumor development is still being studied. More is known about the sebaceous tumors associated with Muir-Torre syndrome. This syndrome is caused by a genetic defect in the mismatch repair genes. The syndrome is inherited in an autosomal dominant fashion. The genes that are abnormal in this syndrome are responsible for microsatellite instability within the cells of the sebaceous carcinomas and may lead directly to malignant transformation of the benign sebaceous gland.

Histology: These tumors are derived from sebaceous glands and show a high degree of infiltrative growth. The tumor deeply invades the subcutaneous tissue; in the periocular area, it often invades the underlying muscle tissue. The lesions are poorly circumscribed, and mitoses are frequently seen. The tumor cells are large basaloid cells that show areas of mature sebocyte differentiation and areas that are poorly differentiated.

Treatment: The tumors are locally aggressive and have a high rate of regional lymph node metastasis. The treatment of choice is surgical removal, either with Mohs micrographic surgery or with a wide local excision, making sure to get clear tumor margins. These tumors have a high risk of recurrence, and clinical follow-up is required. The use of postoperative radiotherapy is warranted in specific cases. Patients with metastatic disease may benefit from a combination of radiotherapy, immunotherapy, and systemic chemotherapy.

Levator palpebrae superioris muscle
Orbital septum
Superior tarsal (Müller's) muscle (smooth)
Superior conjunctival fornix
Orbicularis oculi muscle (palpebral part)
Superior tarsus
Meibomian glands of the tarsal plate
Glands of Zeis (sebaceous glands)
Eyelashes (cilia)
Openings of tarsal glands
Inferior tarsus
Orbicularis oculi muscle (palpebral part)
Inferior conjunctival fornix
Orbital septum
Sclera
Bulbar conjunctiva
Palpebral conjunctiva
Cornea
Lens
Anterior chamber
Iris
Posterior chamber

Sebaceous carcinoma most frequently arises from the meibomian glands or the glands of Zeis.

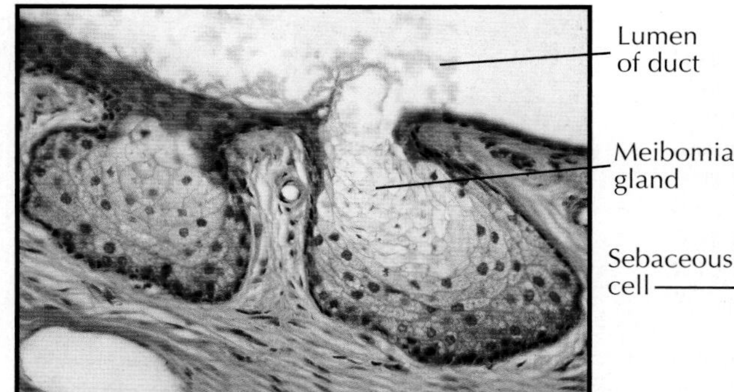

Two alveoli of a meibomian sebaceous gland arranged in a row. The left one seems to discharge secretory product directly onto the surface into a straight opening duct. Secretory epithelial cells of the alveoli look foamy and washed out because of high lipid content.*

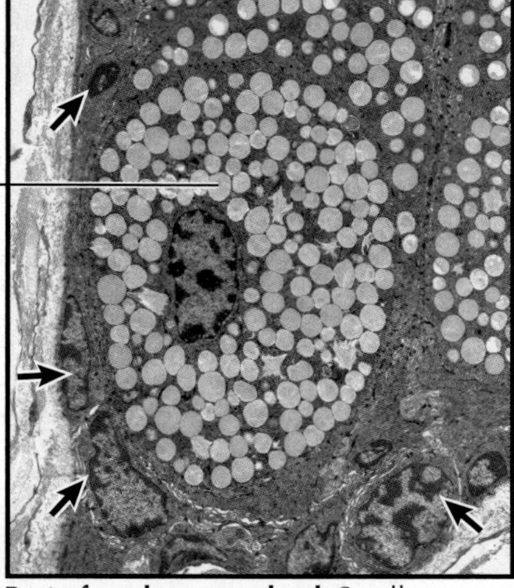

Part of a sebaceous gland. Small nucleated cells with euchromatic nuclei (*arrows*) in the periphery of the gland serve as proliferating stem cells. A thin basement membrane covers them externally. A large sebaceous cell in the center contains many prominent lipid droplets, which surround a central nucleus. The cells ultimately break down and add their contents to oily secretory product. Sebum reduces water loss from the skin surface and lubricates hair. It may also protect skin from infection with bacteria.*

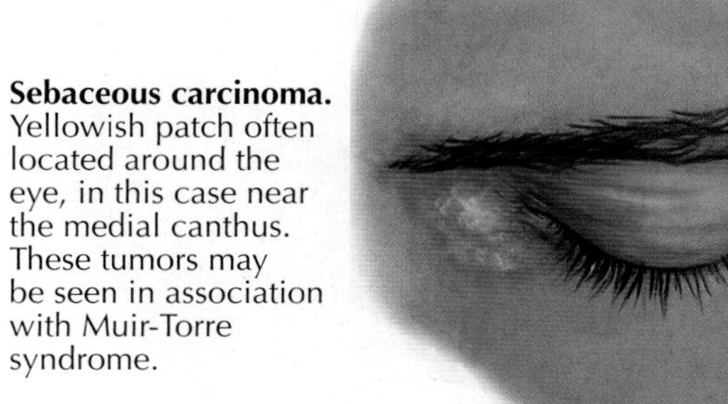

Sebaceous carcinoma. Yellowish patch often located around the eye, in this case near the medial canthus. These tumors may be seen in association with Muir-Torre syndrome.

**Micrographs reprinted with permission from Ovalle W, Nahirney P.* Netter's Essential Histology. *Philadelphia: Saunders; 2008.*

Genital Squamous Cell Carcinoma

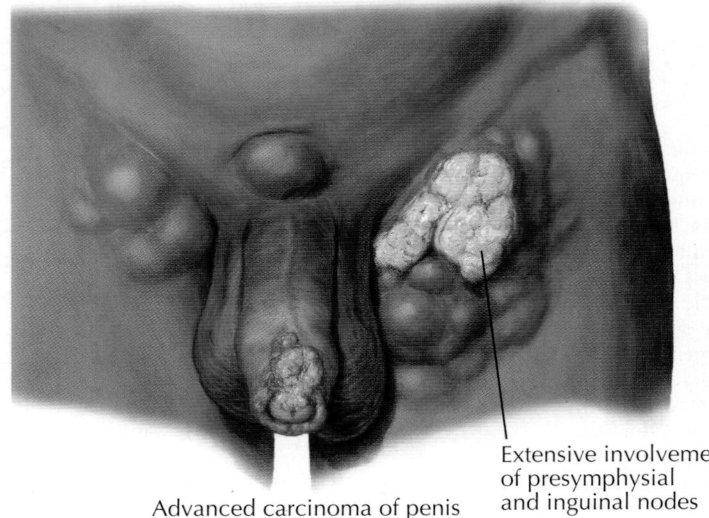
Advanced carcinoma of penis

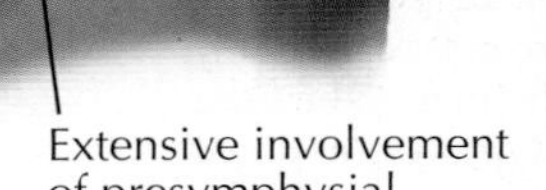

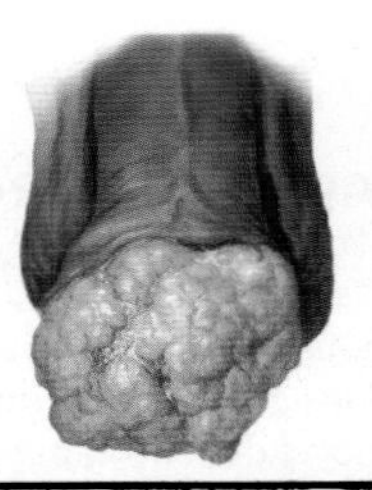

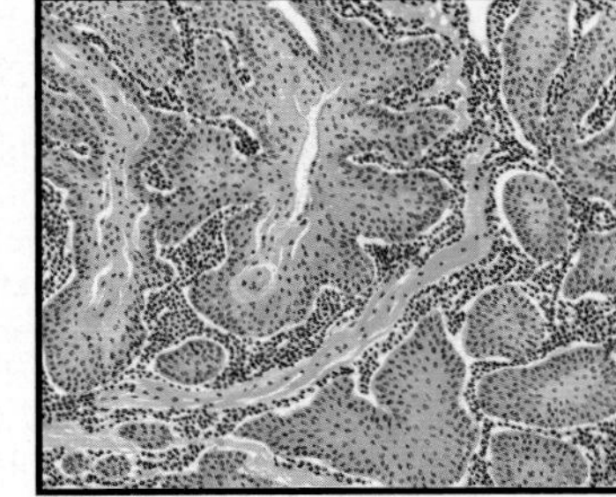
Squamous cell carcinoma of penis, histology

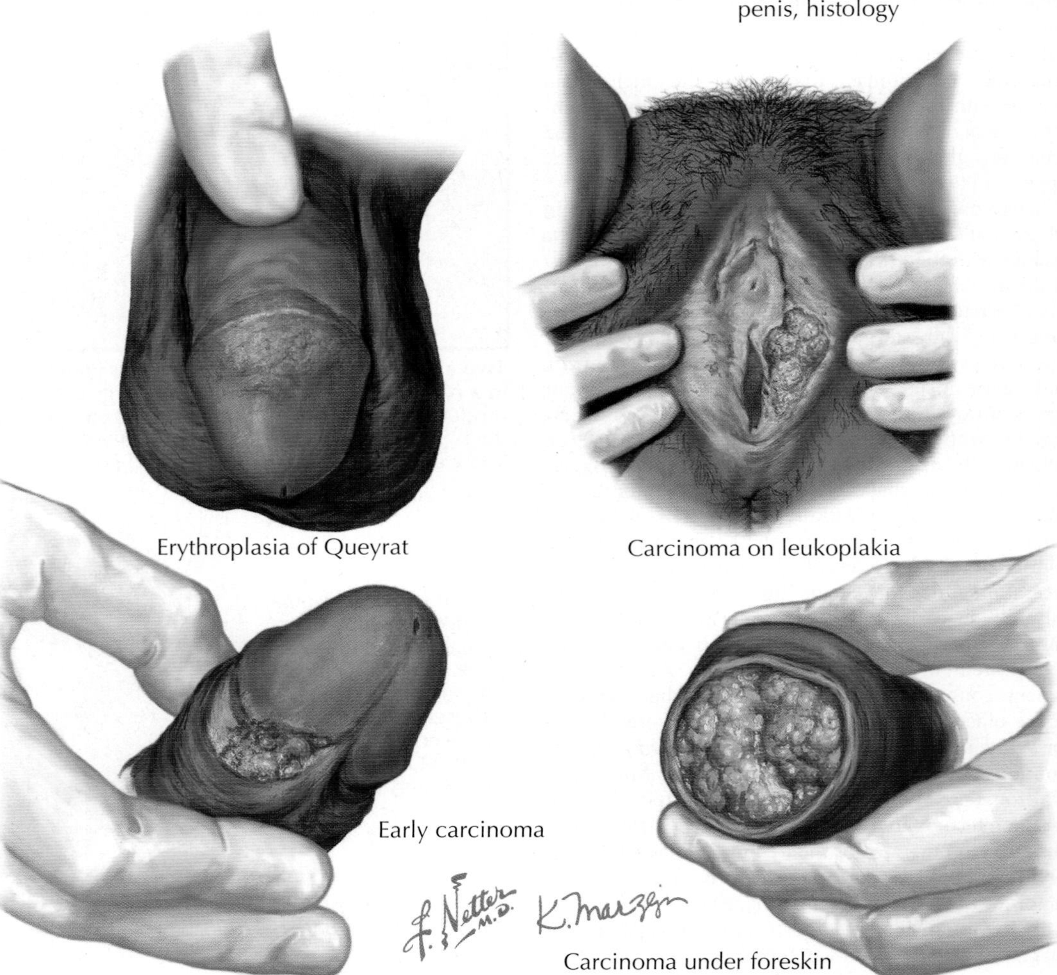

Squamous Cell Carcinoma

Squamous cell carcinoma (SCC) of the skin is the second most common skin cancer after BCC. Together, these two types of carcinoma are known as nonmelanoma skin cancer. SCC accounts for approximately 20% of all skin cancers diagnosed in the United States. SCC can come in many variants, including in situ and invasive types. Bowen disease, bowenoid papulosis, and erythroplasia of Queyrat are all unique forms of SCC in situ. Another unique subtype of SCC is the keratoacanthoma. Invasive SCC is defined by invasion through the basement membrane zone into the dermis. SCC has the ability to metastasize; the most common area of metastasis is the local draining lymph nodes. Most forms of cutaneous SCC occur in chronically sun-damaged skin, and they are often preceded by extremely common premalignant actinic keratosis.

Clinical Findings: SCC of the skin is most commonly located on the head and neck region and on the dorsal hands and forearms. These areas receive the most ultraviolet sun exposure over a lifetime. This type of skin cancer is more common in White and older individuals. It is more prevalent in the fifth to eighth decades of life. The incidence of SCC increases with each decade of life. This form of nonmelanoma skin cancer is definitively linked to the amount of sun exposure received over a lifetime. Fair-skinned individuals are most commonly affected. There is a slight male predilection. Other risk factors include arsenic exposure, HPV infection, prior PUVA therapy, chronic scarring, chronic immunosuppression, and radiation exposure. Organ transplant recipients taking chronic immunosuppressive medications often develop SCC. Their skin cancers also tend to occur on the head and neck and on the arms, but they also have a higher percentage of tumors developing on the trunk and other non–sun-exposed regions.

SCCs of the skin can occur with various morphologies. They can start as thin patches or plaques. There is usually a thickened, adherent scale on the surface of the tumor. Variable amounts of ulceration are seen. As the tumors enlarge, they can take on a nodular configuration. The nodules are firm and can be deeply seated within the dermis. Most SCCs are derived from a preexisting actinic keratosis. Patients often have chronically sun-damaged skin with poikilodermatous changes and multiple lentigines and actinic keratoses. Approximately 1% of actinic keratoses per year develop into SCC.

Subungual SCC is a difficult diagnosis to make without a biopsy. It is often preceded by HPV infection, and the area has often been treated for long periods as a wart. HPV is a predisposing factor, and with time a small percentage of these warts transform into SCC. This development is usually associated with a subtle change in morphology. There tends to be more nail destruction and a slow enlargement over time in the face of standard wart therapy. Prompt biopsy and diagnosis can be critical in sparing the patient an amputation of the affected digit.

A few chronic dermatoses can predispose to the development of SCC, including lichen sclerosis et atrophicus, disseminated superficial actinic porokeratosis, warts, discoid lupus, long-standing ulcers, and scars. Many genetic diseases can predispose to the development of SCC; two of the best recognized ones are epidermodysplasia verruciformis and xeroderma pigmentosum.

Pathogenesis: SCC is related to cumulative UV light exposure. UVB light appears to be the most important action spectrum in the development of SCC. UVB is much more potent than UVA light. UVB can damage keratinocyte DNA by causing pyrimidine dimers and other DNA mutations. The damaged DNA leads to

Squamous Cell Carcinoma (Continued)

errors in translation and transcription and ultimately can lead to cancer. *TP53* is one of the most frequently mutated genes. This gene encodes a protein that is important in cell cycle arrest, which allows for DNA damage repair and apoptosis of damaged cells. If *TP53* is dysfunctional, this critical cell cycle arrest period is bypassed and the cell is allowed to replicate without the normal DNA repair mechanisms acting on the damaged DNA. This ultimately leads to unregulated cell division and cancer.

Histology: Actinic keratosis shows partial-thickness atypia of the lower portions of the epidermis. The adnexal structures are spared. SCC in situ shows full-thickness atypia of the epidermis that also affects the adnexal epithelium.

SCC is derived from the keratinocytes. The pathologic findings are characterized by full-thickness atypia of the epidermis and invasion of the abnormal squamous epithelium into the dermis. Variable numbers of mitoses are seen, as well as invasion into the underlying subcutaneous tissue. Horn pearls are often seen throughout the tumor. The tumors are often described as being well, moderately, or poorly differentiated. Many histologic subtypes of SCC have been reported, including clear cell, spindle cell, verrucous, basosquamous, and adenosquamous cell carcinomas.

Treatment: Actinic keratoses can be treated in myriad ways. Cryotherapy with liquid nitrogen is very effective and can be used repeatedly. If this fails to clear the area, or if the actinic keratoses are numerous, 5-fluorouracil (5-FU), imiquimod, or photodynamic therapy is initiated. The two medication creams work, respectively, by directly killing the affected cells or by causing the immune system to attack and kill the affected cells. Photodynamic therapy works by directly killing the abnormal skin cells. They are all highly effective. The disadvantage is that they cause an inflammatory response that can be severe as well as erythema, crusting, and weeping during the period of application, usually 1 month or longer.

The treatment for SCC in situ is often electrodessication and curettage or simple elliptical excision. 5-FU cream is also effective but leads to a higher rate of recurrence than the traditional surgical methods. 5-FU is appropriate as a first-line agent for bowenoid papulosis. If residual areas are left at follow-up, surgical removal is indicated. Occasionally, large areas of SCC in situ on the face are treated by Mohs microsurgery. Photodynamic therapy is becoming more commonly used in the treatment of SCC in situ.

Invasive SCC should be treated surgically, with Mohs surgery for lesions on the face or recurrent lesions; standard elliptical excision is adequate for most invasive SCCs. Some small, well-differentiated SCCs have been treated successfully with electrodessication and curettage. The metastatic rate for well-differentiated cutaneous SCC is low, but certain locations have a higher rate of metastasis. These areas include the lip, the ear, and areas of chronic scarring or ulceration in which the tumors develop. Recurrent SCCs, those larger than 2 cm in diameter, those that are poorly differentiated, and those developing in patients taking chronic immunosuppressive medications pose a higher risk for the development of metastatic disease. Patients with chronic lymphocytic leukemia are at much higher risk for metastases; the reason is unknown but is thought to be related to the immunosuppression resulting from disease. The most common areas for metastasis are the local lymph nodes and lung.

Metastatic SCC of the skin should be treated with checkpoint inhibitor immunotherapy with adjunctive radiotherapy and/or chemotherapy. However, these therapies have not shown a clear survival benefit, and the key to treatment ultimately lies in the prevention of metastasis.

Clinical and Histologic Evaluation of Sun-Induced Squamous Cell Carcinoma

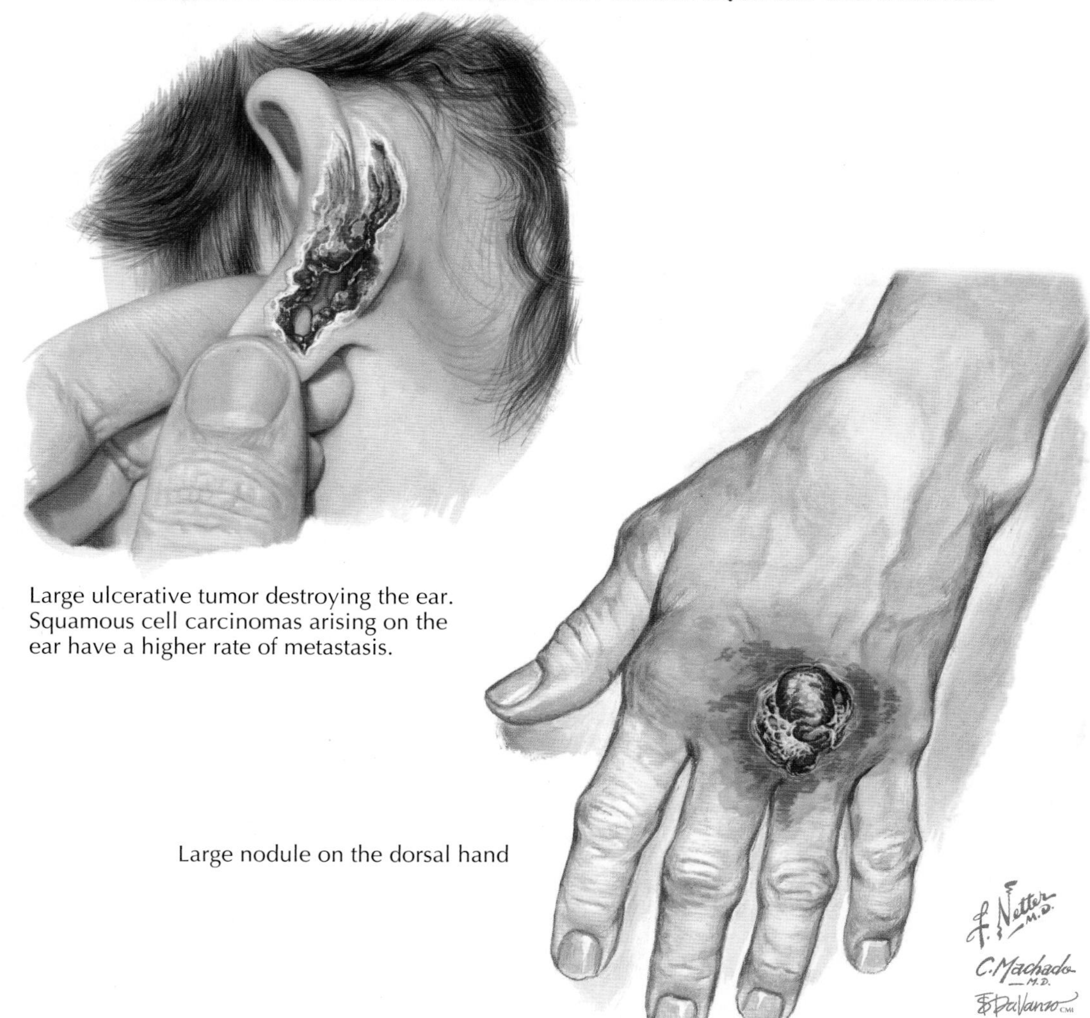

Large ulcerative tumor destroying the ear. Squamous cell carcinomas arising on the ear have a higher rate of metastasis.

Large nodule on the dorsal hand

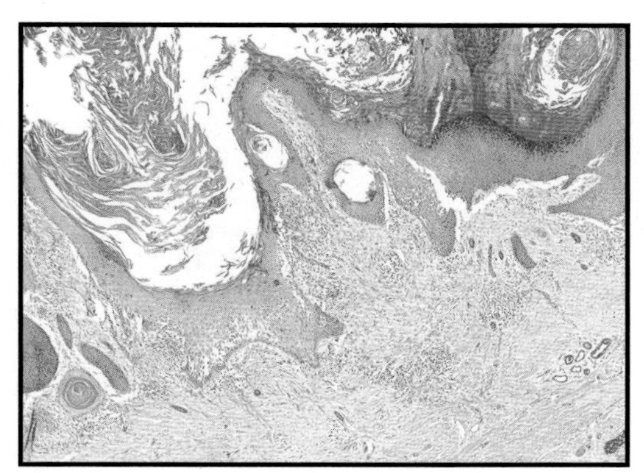

Low power. Atypical squamous epithelium invading the dermis. This tumor is poorly circumscribed.

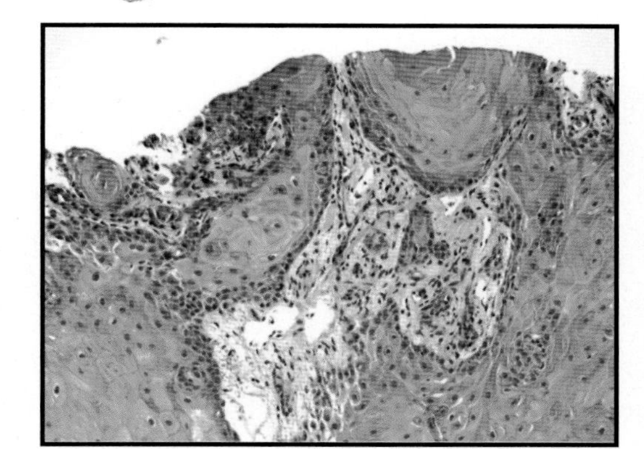

High power. Atypical keratinocytes, mitotic figures, and horn pearl formation.

SECTION 4

RASHES

ACANTHOSIS NIGRICANS

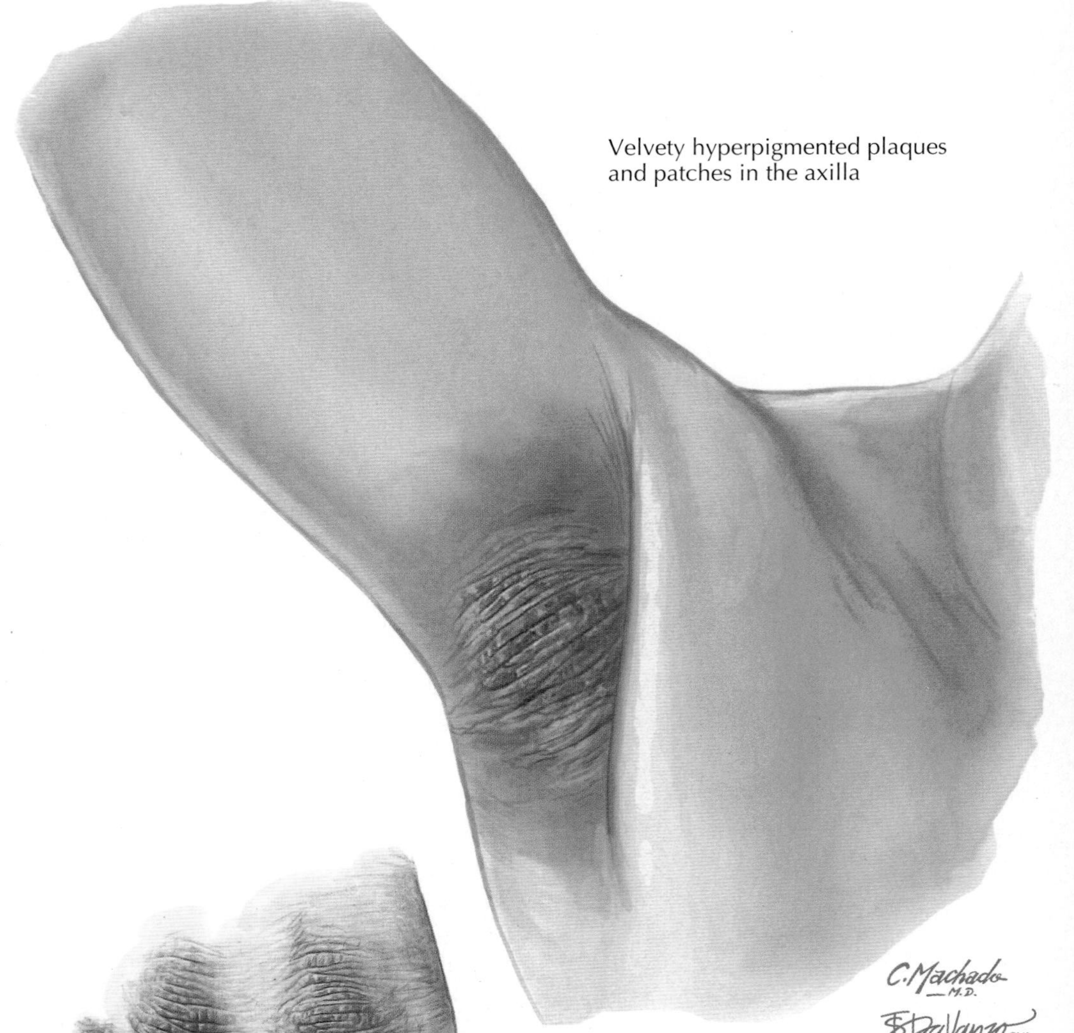

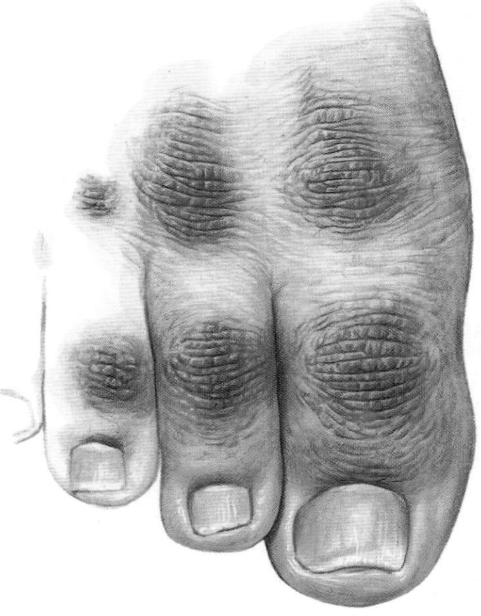

Acanthosis nigricans is a commonly encountered skin dermatosis that can be seen in various clinical scenarios. It is overwhelmingly associated with obesity but can occur secondary to medications, endocrine disorders such as the HAIR-AN syndrome (**h**yper**a**ndrogenism, **i**nsulin **r**esistance, and **a**canthosis **n**igricans), diabetes, and internal malignancies. This last association is clinically distinctive and manifests in a unique manner.

Clinical Findings: Classic cases of acanthosis nigricans affect the nape of the neck, the axillae, and the groin regions. Native Americans and African Americans are at a significantly increased risk for development of acanthosis nigricans. It is most frequently seen in adults. The slow, insidious onset of patches and plaques with a velvety, hyperpigmented, thickened, rough surface is characteristic. Maceration with a malodorous smell is often noted in the intertriginous regions. The patients are for the most part asymptomatic, although some report intermittent pruritus. The clinical findings in association with obesity are enough to make the diagnosis. A thorough history should be taken to rule out a medication-induced form of acanthosis nigricans. The only routine laboratory testing performed is screening for occult diabetes. Patients with obesity are at higher risk for diabetes later in life, and lifelong follow-up and screening by their primary care physician are required.

Many medications have been shown to induce acanthosis nigricans, including niacin, glucocorticoids, insulin, and some birth control pills. The medication most commonly associated with acanthosis nigricans is niacin. Most cases resolve or improve greatly with discontinuation of the medication. The appearance is often identical to that of classic acanthosis nigricans, but the history is suggestive, with the timing of rash onset related to the introduction of the causative medication.

Malignancy-associated acanthosis nigricans is often widespread and involves unique areas, including the mucous membranes, palms, and soles. This form has a rapid onset and affects different areas of the body than the classic form of acanthosis nigricans. The palms and soles are often involved, and the face can be affected. Any case of rapid onset of acanthosis nigricans in a widespread distribution, often in a nonobese individual, warrants proper evaluation to rule out an internal malignancy. Referral to a gastroenterologist and an internist for cancer screening is of utmost importance.

A few endocrine disorders can be associated with acanthosis nigricans, most frequently diabetes mellitus and the HAIR-AN syndrome.

There is a rare familial form of acanthosis nigricans inherited in an autosomal dominant fashion.

Pathogenesis: The skin thickening and clinical findings are possibly caused by an increase in insulin-like growth factor receptor, fibroblast growth factor receptor, and epidermal growth factor receptor and their subsequent effects on the skin. Hyperinsulinemia in overweight individuals has been shown to activate insulin-like growth factor receptors. The reason it affects certain regions preferentially is unknown. Malignancy-associated acanthosis nigricans is believed to be caused by a cytokine or growth factor directly secreted by the tumor, possibly in the fibroblast growth factor receptor class of molecules. The tumor causes the clinical findings by secreting these substances. Acanthosis nigricans is believed to be a paraneoplastic process in these cases. Medication-induced acanthosis nigricans is poorly understood but is possibly related to the medication's local effects on the skin in genetically predisposed individuals.

Histology: Epidermal hyperplasia, acanthosis, and papillomatosis are present. There is minimal to no inflammatory infiltrate, and the reticular dermis is essentially normal in appearance. Papillomatosis is caused by a thickened papillary dermis expanding into the epidermis. Extensive hyperkeratosis with a mild excess of melanin production likely explains the hyperpigmentation seen in acanthosis nigricans.

Treatment: Treatment is often difficult unless the afflicted individual makes a conscious effort to achieve an ideal body weight and excellent control of their diabetes. This is the only likely scenario in which the skin findings of acanthosis nigricans will resolve. Temporizing methods of therapy include the use of keratolytic agents such as lactic acid or urea to help thin the plaques and make them less noticeable. These agents are difficult to use in the axillae because of stinging. The topical use of retinoid creams and vitamin D analogs has also been successful. Destructive laser therapies and chemical peels have been used with varying success.

Treatment of malignancy-associated acanthosis nigricans is directed at the underlying malignancy. Removal of the tumor may result in complete resolution of the skin disease.

Velvety hyperpigmented plaques and patches in the axilla

C. Machado M.D.
DalVanzo CMI

Acanthosis nigricans. Hyperpigmented plaques on the dorsal foot with accentuation of the skin lines.

ACNE

Acne is an almost universal finding in teenagers across the globe. Acne vulgaris is the most common form of acne; it affects almost every human at some point in their lifetime. Many cases are mild and do not cause any significant disease. Most acne vulgaris is seen in the postpubertal years. Many clinical variants exist, and excellent therapeutic modalities are available.

Clinical Findings: Acne vulgaris typically begins soon after puberty. It has no racial or sex preference, although males may develop more severe cases of the disease. The first sign of acne development is the formation of microcomedones, both open and closed. Open comedones, known as *blackheads*, appear as small (0.5–1 mm), dilated skin pores filled with a dark material (oxidized keratin). This material can be easily expressed with lateral pressure or with the help of a comedone extractor. The closed comedone, known as a *whitehead*, is a small (0.5–1 mm), whitish to skin-colored papule. Comedones are believed to be the precursor lesion to the other lesions of acne. As acne progresses, red inflammatory, slightly tender papules develop, along with a variable number of pustules. The pustules are centered on the hair follicle. More severe cases of acne, such as nodulocystic acne, show inflammatory nodules as well as cyst formation. These nodules and cysts can become large (2–3 cm in diameter) and cause considerable pain. They often heal with scarring of the skin.

The face, back, upper chest, and shoulders are the predominant areas of involvement, most likely because of the higher density of sebaceous glands and the role of the sebaceous gland in the development of acne. Acne is a relentless condition: as one lesion heals, another develops simultaneously. Females often report a flare of their acne 1 week before menstruation, denoting hormonal influence. Acne has many clinical variants.

Adult female acne is typically seen in women between 25 and 45 years of age. They often report that they had minimal to no acne during adolescence. This form of acne is found predominantly on the cheeks, perioral region, and jaw line, and it manifests as deep-seated papules, nodules, and cysts. There is a pronounced flare around the time of menstruation.

Neonatal and infantile acne are self-limited types seen frequently in this population. Neonatal acne may be seen a day or two after delivery; it is caused by transplacental passage of maternal hormones. It resolves without therapy and seems to be more prevalent in male newborns. Infantile acne is seen after the first few months of life. Most cases show a few transient papules, comedones, and pustules. Most self-resolve, although a few cases last into adolescence.

Acne cosmetica and acne medicamentosa are similar forms of acne thought to be caused or exacerbated by cosmetics and facial medications. Cessation of these products usually is enough for the patient to see significant improvement. Most products implicated in this form of acne are oily in nature; they cause follicular plugging, which allows acne production.

Acne excoriée is a form of acne that is made worse by chronic picking or manipulation of the acneiform lesions. This often leads to scarring and a worsening of the clinical appearance. It is often coexistent with an underlying anxiety disorder, obsessive compulsive disorder, or depression.

Rare forms of acne include acne fulminans, acne conglobata, and acne aestivalis. Acne fulminans is seen almost exclusively in teenage boys. It is a form of severe cystic nodular acne that heals with severe, disfiguring scarring. The cysts and nodules can easily rupture and break down, leaving multiple ulcerations. This is associated with systemic symptoms including fever, arthralgias and arthritis, and myalgias. A peripheral leukocytosis is often seen on laboratory examination. Lytic bone lesions can be seen, with the clavicle the most commonly affected bone. This may be preceded by localized pain over the bony involvement. *Acne conglobata* refers to severe cystic acne, which is seen mostly in young males. Patients often have multiple cysts that can be interconnected with sinus tracts. The areas involved are very painful and heal with severe scarring. This form of acne occurs in the same locations as acne vulgaris. Acne conglobata has been seen in association with hidradenitis

ACNE VULGARIS

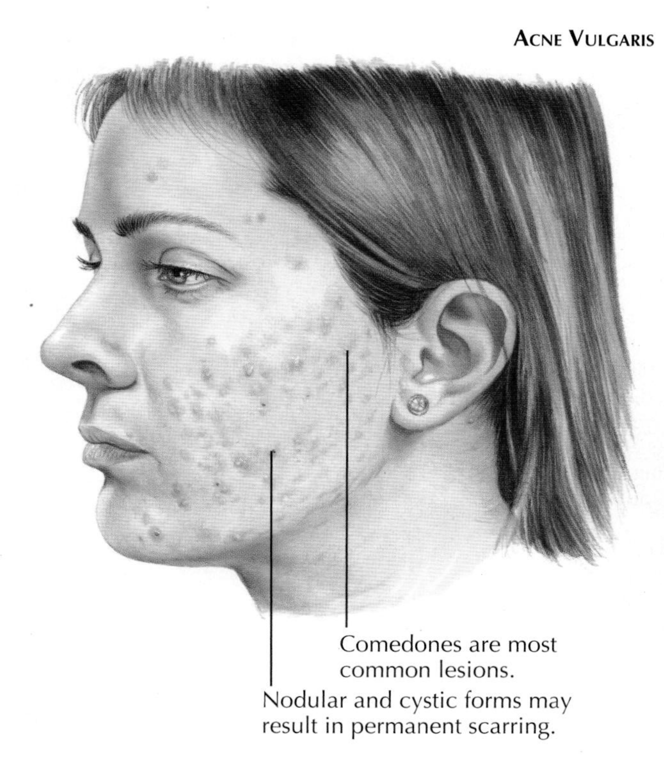

Forehead, nose, cheeks, and chest are commonly involved in acne.

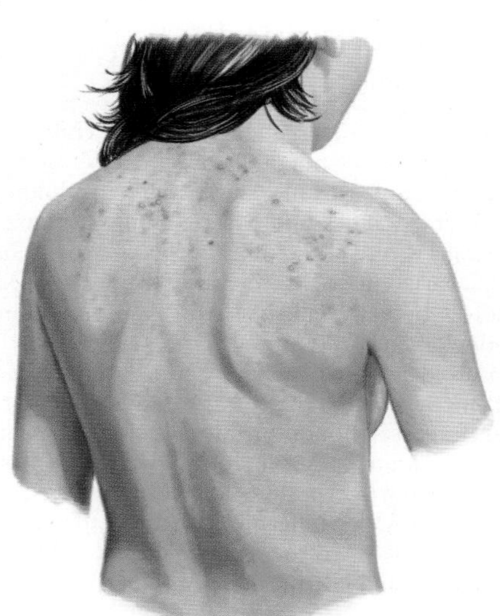

Papules, pustules, comedones, postinflammatory hyperpigmentation, and mild scarring are seen here. The upper back is commonly involved in acne.

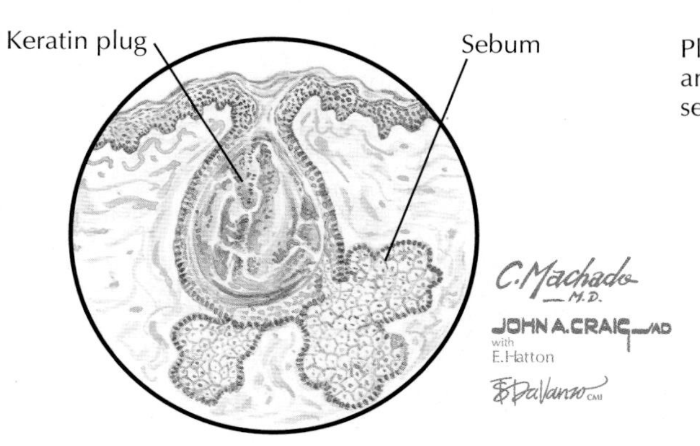

Section of closed comedone (whitehead) showing keratin plug and accumulated sebum in sebaceous glands

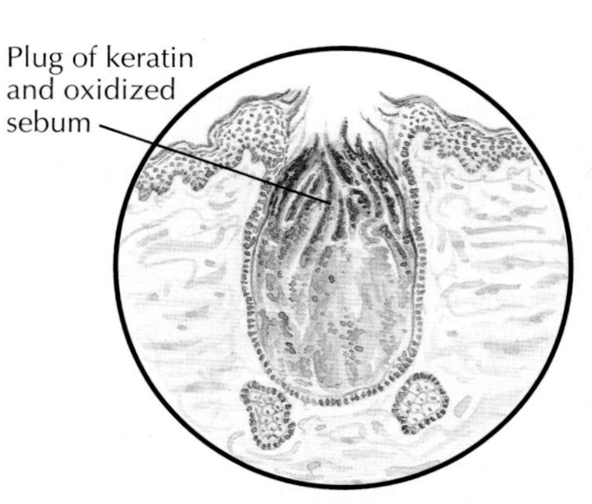

Section of open comedone (blackhead) showing plug of keratin and oxidized sebum

ACNE (Continued)

suppurativa, and some consider these conditions to be in the same spectrum of disease processes. Acne conglobata may run a chronic course well into adulthood, with persistent nodules and cysts coming and going. Acne aestivalis is one of the rarest forms of acne. It has a seasonal variation to its course. It begins in spring and resolves by early fall. It is a disease predominantly of adult women.

Steroid-induced acne occurs secondary to the chronic use of oral or intravenous (IV) steroids. It manifests as a monomorphic eruption of inflammatory papules. Many other medications can be associated with acneiform eruptions, including iodides, isoniazid, lithium, and the epidermal growth factor inhibitors.

Chloracne is a rare form of acne caused by exposure to halogenated chemicals, most commonly as an accidental exposure to dioxin. Open comedones are the predominant morphology seen.

Pathogenesis: Acne is believed to have a multifactorial basis. Follicular keratinization appears to be faulty, and the keratinocyte adhesions do not separate as quickly as they should, leading to a follicular plug and microcomedone formation. Excessive sebaceous gland production also plays a role and is probably mediated by hormonal influences. If the sebaceous gland material is produced in an amount sufficient to cause rupture of the comedone, the contents spill into the dermis, causing an inflammatory response; clinically, this is manifested by inflammatory papules, nodules, and cysts. The third player in the pathogenesis is the gram-negative anaerobic bacteria *Propionibacterium acnes*. This bacterium is believed to cause an activation of the immune system and results in an inflammatory infiltrate. Rare causes of acne include adrenal gland disorders that can cause virilization. These tumors are rare and often are associated with a sudden onset of acne, hirsutism, and irregular menstrual cycles. Any state of hyperandrogenism can cause acne or make preexisting acne worse. The most common cause is polycystic ovarian syndrome in women. Less commonly, a Sertoli-Leydig cell tumor can lead to a hyperandrogenic state and resultant acne.

Histology: Biopsies of acne are not required for diagnosis. A biopsy specimen from an inflammatory acne papule shows a folliculocentric lesion with a dense inflammatory infiltrate. The follicular epithelium has signs of spongiosis. Foreign body giant cells, plasma cells, neutrophils, and lymphocytes are all seen in varying degrees. Comedones show compacted corneocytes within the sebaceous gland lumen.

Treatment: Treatment for acne vulgaris is multidimensional. A combination approach is often used, with a keratolytic and antibacterial agent, such as benzyl peroxide, with tretinoin (a medication that increases differentiation and maturation of keratinocytes) and an antibiotic. The antibiotics are used for their antiinflammatory and antibacterial properties. The antibiotic may be given in a topical or oral form. More severe acne, cystic acne, acne conglobata, and acne fulminans require the systemic use of isotretinoin to prevent severe scarring. Isotretinoin is given for 5 to 6 months. Significant precautions need to be taken because this medication is a well-known teratogen. Prednisone is often advocated for severe cases of cystic acne. It is typically used transiently, when first beginning therapy with isotretinoin, to help decrease some of the severe inflammation. It should not be used for long periods.

Many other treatment options exist, including topical agents such as azelaic acid, adapalene, tazarotene, trifarotene, dapsone, clascoterone, salicylic acid, and topical antibiotics. Oral medications include spironolactone, contraceptive pills, and multiple antibiotics. The first two medications are especially helpful in the treatment of adult female acne. They work on the hormonal influence on acne and are highly successful in this type of patient. All of the medications used for acne have potential side effects, and treatment must be tailored to the individual. Comedone extraction, intralesional triamcinolone, and photodynamic therapy have shown some success in treating acne. Laser resurfacing, chemical peels, and use of artificial fillers should be reserved for the treatment of scarring after the inflammatory acne has been controlled.

ACNE VARIANTS

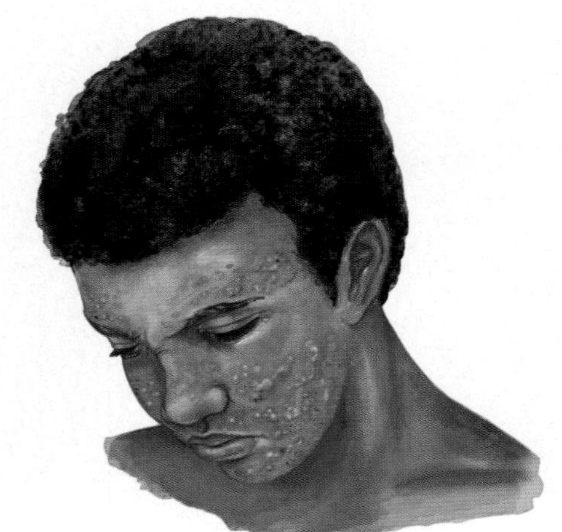

Acne conglobata. Severe cystic, scarring, nodular acne lesions that can be exquisitely tender. Associated with disfiguring scarring and psychological distress. Almost always treated with isotretinoin.

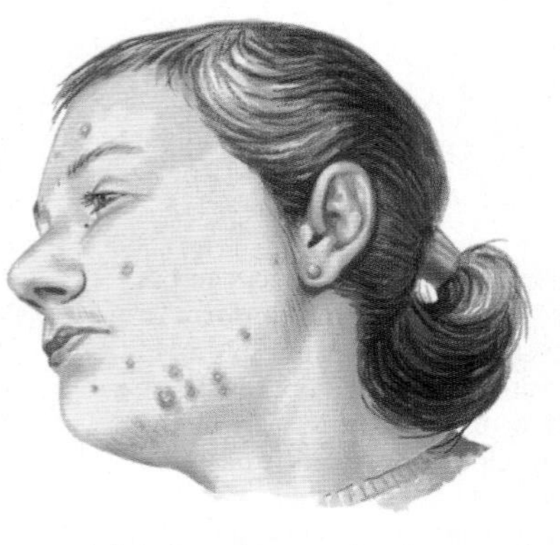

Adult female acne is characterized by acneiform papules and pustules along the jaw line.

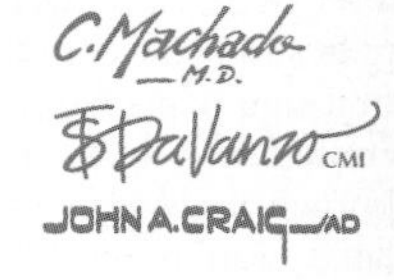

Sertoli-Leydig cell tumor

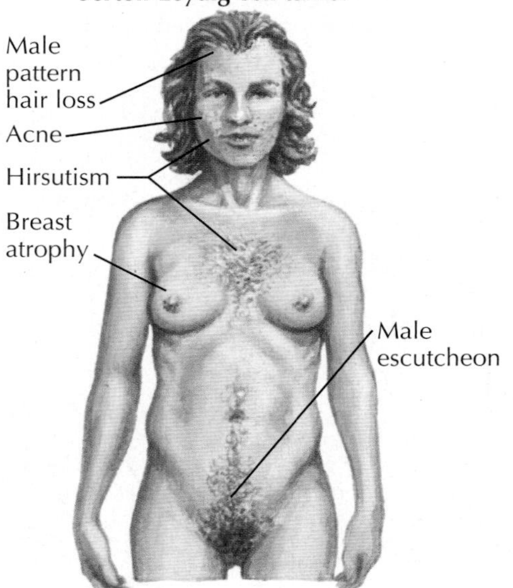

Excessive androgen production results in loss of female secondary sex characteristics.

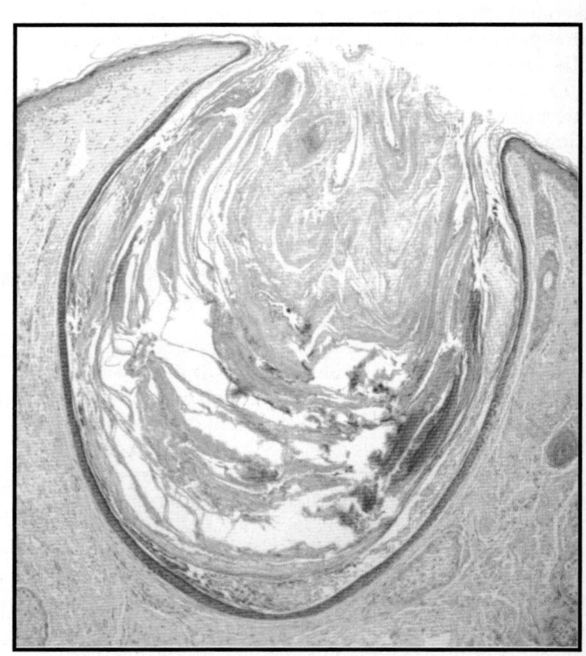

Open comedone is a common finding in patients with acne. Compact keratin fills the comedone cavity.

Acne Keloidalis Nuchae

Acne keloidalis nuchae is a fairly common form of inflammatory, scarring alopecia that typically occurs on the posterior occipital scalp. There is a variable clinical spectrum of disease, ranging from very minor cases to severe scarring alopecia. The condition has psychosocial implications and is difficult to treat effectively. It is diagnosed clinically, and biopsies are rarely needed.

Clinical Findings: Acne keloidalis nuchae begins on the posterior scalp or nape of the neck as tiny, follicular, flesh-colored to red papules. The papules enlarge to form plaques, which coalesce into larger plaques. Ultimately, in severe cases, the entire posterior scalp is involved. Early in the disease, no hair loss is appreciated. As the disease progresses, the hair follicles become scarred down and crowded out by the encroaching fibrosis, resulting in a variable amount of scarring alopecia.

This condition is most commonly seen in young adult Black men. It was originally believed to be caused by close shaving of the hair and the subsequent inflammation caused by the newly regrowing hair as it pierces the epidermis. The curly nature of the hair follicle was believed to be one of the most important factors. This theory of the pathophysiology of the disease has been questioned, and the cause of the condition is not as simple as once theorized.

The plaques, if left untreated, eventually form thickened scar tissue resembling the appearance of a keloid scar. The scarring alopecia is permanent, and the patient is left with a considerable cosmetic issue. Severe cases of this condition can cause psychological issues, as can almost any form of severe alopecia.

Pathogenesis: As mentioned above, acne keloidalis was believed to be caused by a close haircut that set off an inflammatory reaction. It has now been determined that this is an oversimplification of the disease state. A complex combination of inflammation, hormonal factors, infection, and trauma in an individual with a genetic predisposition likely comprises the lead pathogenetic factors.

Histology: Early disease often appears as a dense, mixed inflammatory infiltrate around the hair follicle and adnexal structures with plasma cells present. It appears similar to folliculitis. As the hair follicles rupture, the contents spill into the dermis and set off a dermal inflammatory reaction. There is overlying epidermal hyperplasia and acanthosis. Occasional pustule formation is seen and is composed of pools of neutrophils.

Late disease is very similar to the pathology of a keloid. There is a lack of adnexal structures and fibrosis throughout the dermis. Hair follicles are absent.

Treatment: Therapy for mild disease requires a multifaceted approach. If only a few papules are present with minimal hair loss, a combination of a topical antibiotic and an oral antibiotic can be used for their anti-inflammatory effects. The most commonly used oral antibiotics are in the tetracycline class. The topical antibiotic most often prescribed is clindamycin. Strict hair care regimens are required to help decrease the trauma to the skin. Shaving of the scalp should be avoided, and haircuts with shears should also be minimized, because the shears can cause microtrauma to the skin and potentially induce the process and scarring formation. Cutting the hair to a length of 3 to 5 mm is a reasonable approach that minimizes trauma to the skin. Topical retinoids such as tretinoin and tazarotene have been used with varying results. They are theorized to help the follicular epithelium mature and help correct the abnormal keratinization of the epidermis. Intralesional triamcinolone injections into the papules and plaques can also be an effective method of treating mild disease.

Severe disease is rarely responsive to medical therapy. Surgical options remain the best therapeutic choice. The goal is to remove the abnormal skin and close the wound under as little tension as possible. If the tension is too great, it is best to leave the wound open to granulate and heal by secondary intention. The scar that results is often better appearing than the thick, plaque-like scar that it is replacing. Laser and radiation therapy have been used with success and should be considered in severe cases.

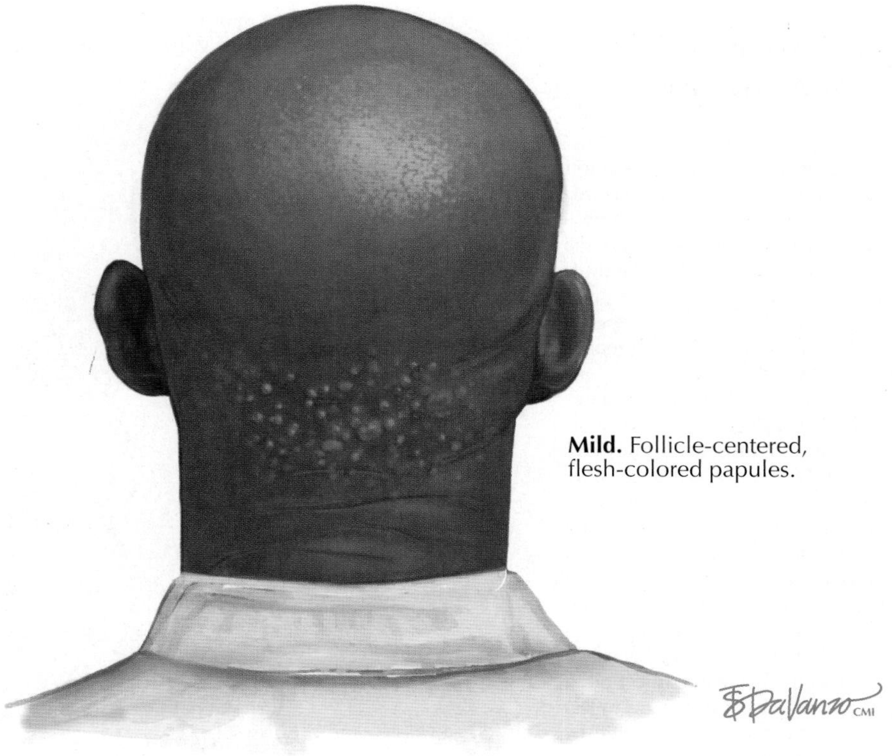

Mild. Follicle-centered, flesh-colored papules.

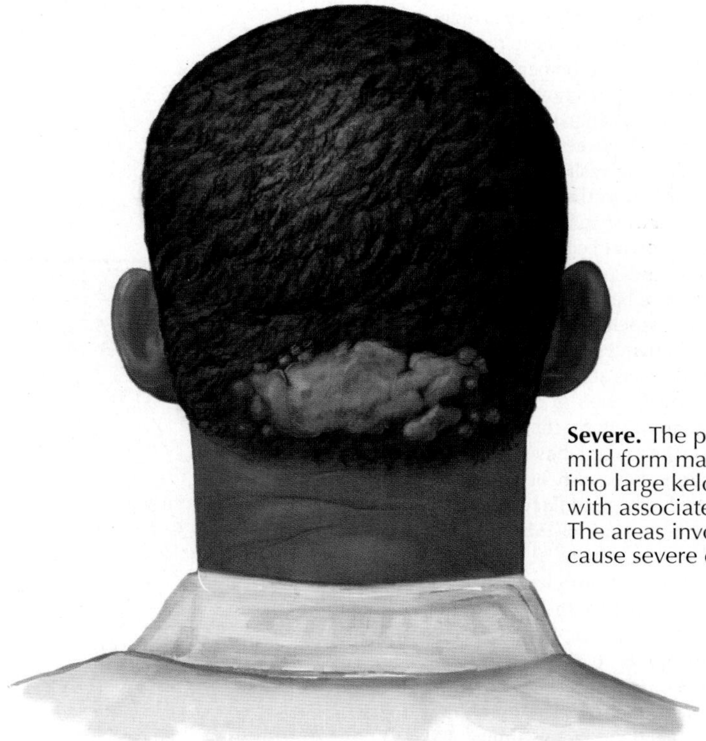

Severe. The papules of the mild form may coalesce into large keloidal plaques with associated hair loss. The areas involved can cause severe disfigurement.

ACUTE FEBRILE NEUTROPHILIC DERMATOSIS (SWEET SYNDROME)

Acute febrile neutrophilic dermatosis is an uncommon rash that is most often idiopathic but can be seen secondary to an underlying inflammatory bowel disease, infection, medication, or malignancy. The diagnosis is made by fulfilling a constellation of criteria. Both clinical findings and pathology results are required to make the diagnosis in a patient with a consistent history. Three types of Sweet disease have been described: drug induced, malignancy associated, and classic Sweet disease.

Clinical Findings: Acute febrile neutrophilic dermatosis is often associated with a preceding infection. The infection can be located anywhere but most commonly is in the upper respiratory system. Females appear to be more likely to be afflicted, and there is no race predilection. Patients present with fever and the rapid onset of painful papules and plaques. Because the papules can look as if they are fluid filled, they are given the descriptive term *juicy papules*. They can occur anywhere on the body and can be mistaken for a varicella infection. Patients also have neutrophilia and possibly arthritis and arthralgias. If this condition is associated with a preceding infection, it is usually self-limited and heals without scarring unless the papules and plaques are excoriated or ulcerated by scratching. Variable amounts of pruritus and pain are associated with this skin disease. When evaluating a patient with this condition, a thorough history is required. A skin biopsy must be performed. A chest radiograph, throat culture, and urinalysis should be performed to assess for the possibility of bacterial infection.

Lymphoproliferative malignancies have also been seen in association with Sweet syndrome. The malignancy often precedes the rash, and the skin disease is believed to be a reaction to the underlying malignancy. It is important to obtain specimens from these patients for histologic evaluation and culture for aerobic, anaerobic, mycobacterial, and fungal organisms. The main differential diagnosis is between an infection and Sweet syndrome in cases associated with a malignancy. The most common malignancy associated with acute febrile neutrophilic dermatosis is acute myelogenous leukemia. The prognosis in these cases is directly related to the underlying malignancy. Often, the skin disease continues to recur unless the malignancy is put into remission.

A few medications have also been shown to induce Sweet syndrome, including granulocyte colony-stimulating factor (G-CSF), azathioprine, all-*trans*retinoic acid, tetracyclines, and oral contraceptives.

Pathogenesis: The pathomechanism of Sweet syndrome is theorized to involve the secretion of a neutrophilic chemoattractant factor, which causes massive quantities of neutrophils to migrate into the skin. An enhanced T helper-1 (Th1) response is seen in Sweet syndrome with the associated Th1 cytokines, interleukin (IL)-2, tumor necrosis factor-alpha (TNF-α), and interferon-gamma (IFN-γ). The exact molecule responsible for the recruitment of neutrophils into the skin is unknown. Reports of exogenous use of G-CSF have led to the theory that it is responsible for the chemoattraction of neutrophils. Other chemoattractants are possible players in the pathogenesis, including IL-8. Genetic susceptibly is an active area of research.

Histology: Histologic examination shows massive dermal edema with a dense infiltrate composed entirely of neutrophils. Varying amounts of leukocytoclasis are present. Subepidermal bulla formation is possible because of the extensive dermal edema. Special stains for microorganisms must be negative to exclude an infectious process; these must be backed up with cultures to help disprove an infection because the histologic picture can mimic an infectious process.

Treatment: Treatment should be directed at the causative agent if an underlying infection is found. Supportive care is needed for those with postinfectious Sweet syndrome. Topical and oral steroids can dramatically shorten the course of the disease.

Sweet syndrome that develops as a paraneoplastic process secondary to underlying leukemia should be treated with oral or IV steroids once an infectious process has been ruled out. This can result in a rapid response, but it is short-lived once the steroids are removed. True remission occurs only if the cancer is treated and put into remission. Medication-induced cases resolve once the medication has been removed.

Classic Sweet syndrome can be treated with oral steroids. Many second-line therapies are available. Dapsone and colchicine have been used frequently with good success. Potassium iodide, doxycycline, and clofazimine have also been reported to be successful. Numerous case reports on the use of immunosuppressants and biologic medications have been published.

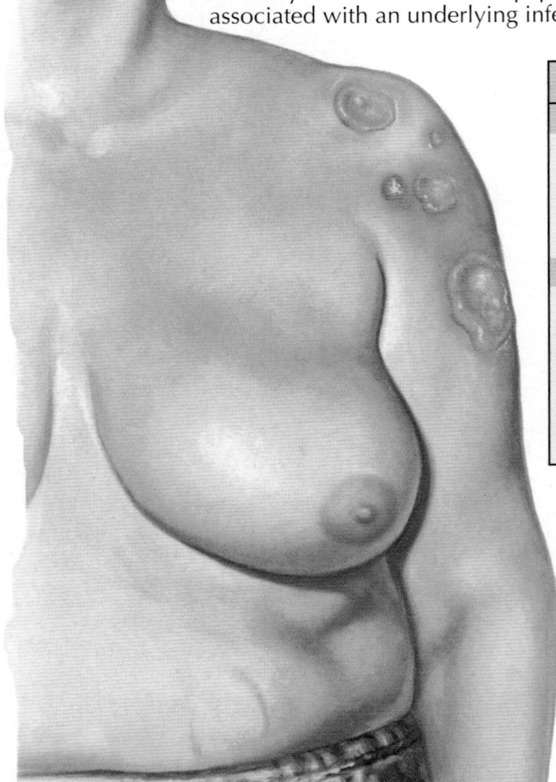

Sweet syndrome. Edematous papules and plaques, often associated with an underlying infection or systemic illness

Diagnostic Criteria for Sweet Syndrome*
Major criteria
▶ Abrupt onset of rash—various morphologies
▶ Histologic evaluation shows diffuse neutrophilic infiltrate with papillary edema
Minor criteria
▶ Preceding infection or pregnancy or malignancy
▶ Fever >38°C
▶ Sedimentation rate >20 or elevated C-reactive protein level or leukocytosis with left shift
▶ Rapid resolution with systemic steroids

*For the diagnosis, both major criteria and one minor criterion must be present. Adapted from Odom RB, James WD, Berger T. *Andrews' Diseases of the Skin: Clinical Dermatology*. 10th ed. Philadelphia: Saunders; 2006.

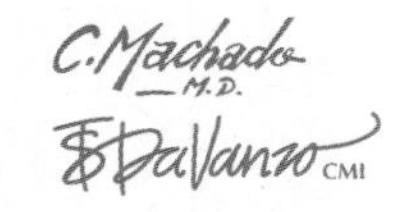

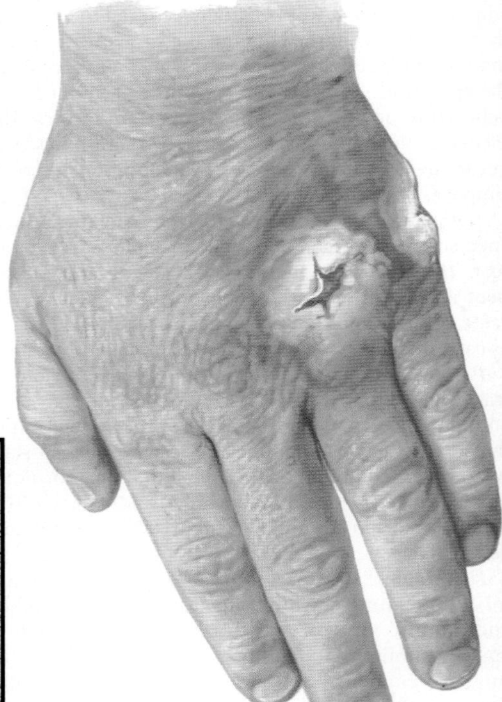

Sweet syndrome on the dorsal hand. This can be difficult to differentiate from pyoderma gangrenosum.

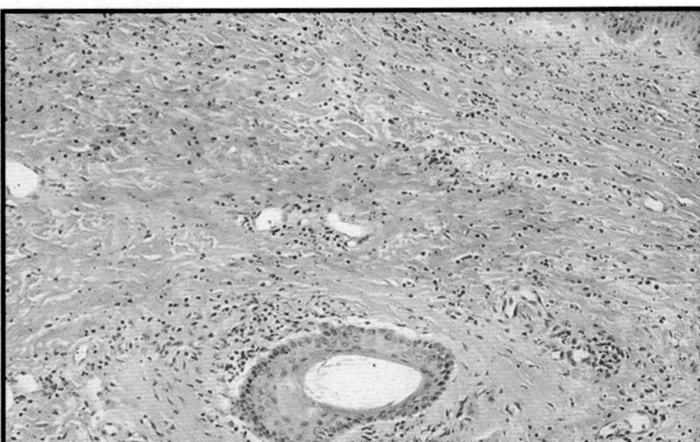

Diffuse neutrophilic infiltrate throughout the dermis

Morphology of Allergic Contact Dermatitis

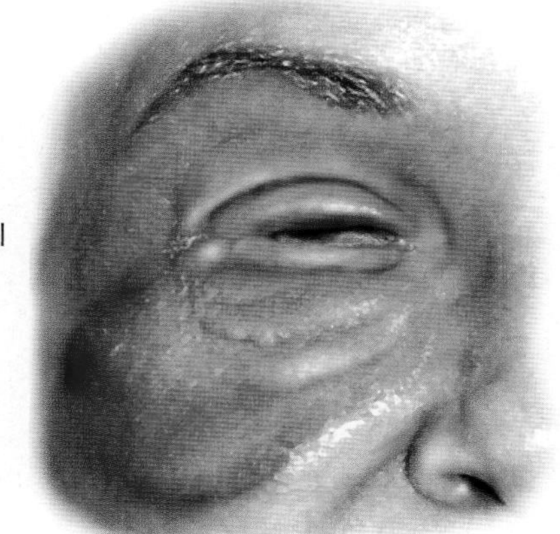

Eyelid dermatitis (red eczematous patches). Potential allergens include fragrances, thimerosal, neomycin, and various preservatives.

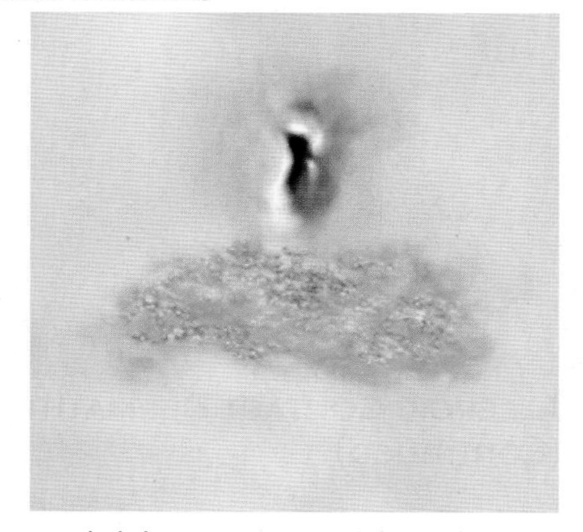

Nickel dermatitis (around the umbilicus) caused by metal snaps

Poison ivy–induced allergic contact dermatitis, with the characteristic linear areas of involvement

Plaque of dermatitis caused by the repeated use of neomycin-containing ointment on a superficial cut

C. Machado M.D.
J. Chovan

Allergic contact dermatitis of the hands is a frequent form of occupationally induced contact allergy.

Allergic Contact Dermatitis

Allergic contact dermatitis is one of the most frequently encountered causes of skin disease. It can be seen in recreational and occupational settings. It is responsible for a large proportion of occupationally induced skin disease and lost work hours. Mechanics, machinists, agricultural workers, and healthcare workers are frequently affected by occupational allergic contact dermatitis. Urushiol from the sap of poison ivy, oak, or sumac plants is the most common cause of allergic contact dermatitis in the United States. The clinical morphology, distribution of the rash, and results from skin patch testing are used to make the diagnosis. Fragrances and preservatives found in personal care products are a frequent cause of allergic contact dermatitis. Patch testing is performed when the causative agent is unknown. Nickel has been the most frequent cause of positive patch testing in the world for years. Urushiol is not tested clinically because nearly 100% of the population reacts to this chemical. Without patch testing it is impossible to determine the causative allergen.

Clinical Findings: Allergic contact dermatitis can manifest in a multitude of ways. The acute form may show linear streaks of juicy papules and vesicles. Variable amounts of surrounding erythema and edema can be seen. Edema is much more common in the loose skin around the eyelids and facial region. Chronic allergic contact dermatitis can manifest with red-pink patches and plaques with varying amounts of lichenification. There are localized forms and generalized forms. One of the unique forms of allergic contact dermatitis is the scattered generalized form. Pruritus is an almost universal finding, and it can be so severe as to cause excoriations and small ulcerations.

The prototype of allergic contact dermatitis is the reaction to the poison ivy family of plants *(Toxicodendron).* After contact with any portion of the plant, urushiol resin is absorbed into the skin and initiates the immune system response, which leads to an allergic contact dermatitis. The dose and the duration of contact with the allergen are important influences on the severity of the rash that develops. Between 3 and 14 days after exposure, the patient notices linear juicy papules and vesicles forming at the sites of contact. The most commonly affected areas are the extremities. Airborne contact dermatitis may be seen from burning of wood with the poison ivy vine present. These reactions are usually seen on skin that was not covered with clothing, and they can be very severe on the face and eyelids, often causing massive swelling and impeding vision.

The location of the dermatitis can be used as a clue to the diagnosis. A nurse with hand dermatitis may be allergic to a component of the gloves being worn occupationally. A child with a lichenified rash around the umbilicus may be allergic to a metal component of a snap or zipper on their clothing. The most common culprit in these cases is nickel. Finger dermatitis may be caused by the application of acrylic nails or nail polish. Allergic contact dermatitis can also be seen within the oral cavity, most commonly adjacent to dental amalgams or prostheses. Oral allergic contact dermatitis can mimic oral lichen planus. Lichen planus is usually widespread and affects the mucosa and gingiva both adjacent to and distant from any dental restorations.

The diagnosis in all of these cases can be made based on patch testing. Chambers loaded with specific concentrations and amounts of known allergens are applied to the back of the individual. The patches are left on for 48 hours and then removed. After an hour, the first reading is made based on the reaction seen under the chamber. Elevation of the skin or vesiculation is considered a positive reaction. The presence of only macular erythema should be interpreted cautiously but can be considered a positive result in certain situations.

ALLERGIC CONTACT DERMATITIS (Continued)

Pustular reactions are considered irritant reactions and are not relevant. The patient must come back for a final reading 3 to 7 days after application of the patches. This is the most critical reading and gives the most valuable information.

Pathogenesis: Much is known about the mechanism of allergic contact dermatitis. This form of dermatitis requires a sensitization and elicitation phase for development. During the sensitization phase, the patient is exposed for the first time to the antigen. The antigen is absorbed through the skin and is phagocytosed by an antigen-presenting cell within the epidermis. The antigen-presenting cell internalizes the antigen and processes it within its lysosomal apparatus. The processed antigen is then sent to the cell surface and expressed on a human leukocyte antigen (HLA) molecule. The antigen-presenting cell migrates to the local draining lymph node and presents the antigen in association with the HLA molecule to T cells. The T cells recognize each individual antigen and proliferate locally, resulting in a clone of lymphocytes that recognize that specific antigen; these lymphocytes then remain ready for when the patient comes in contact with the same antigen in the future.

During the elicitation phase, the patient is reexposed to the antigen. The antigen-presenting cells again process the antigen and present it to the newly cloned lymphocytes, which migrate back to the skin and cause the clinical findings of edema, spongiosis, vesicles, and bullae. If the antigen is exposed in a chronic manner, the findings will be less acute in nature, and the typical findings of a chronic dermatitis are seen.

This entire process is dependent on the size and permeability of the antigen, the recognition and processing of the antigen by the antigen-presenting cell, and the complex interactions among multiple T and B cells. Antigen-presenting cells and B cells are required for activation of the T cells and propagation of the allergic contact dermatitis.

Histology: The initial finding in acute allergic contact dermatitis is spongiosis of the epidermis with an associated superficial and deep lymphocytic infiltrate with scattered eosinophils. As the rash progresses, the spongiosis can worsen, and intraepidermal vesicles start to form. The vesicles may eventually coalesce into large bullae.

Chronic allergic dermatitis usually shows acanthosis with spongiosis and eosinophils within the infiltrate. A superficial and deep perivascular lymphocytic infiltrate is seen. Excoriations can also be appreciated.

Treatment: Acute localized allergic contact dermatitis can be treated with a potent topical steroid and strict avoidance of the offending agent. Oral sedating antihistamines work better for the pruritus than their nonsedating counterparts do. Soaks that help dry the dermatitis are helpful and include aluminum acetate (Domeboro solution). Because the most common culprit is the poison ivy plant, time should be taken to explain to the patient the appearance and nature of this plant. As a good rule of thumb, if a plant has three leaves, it could be poison ivy: "Leaves of three, let it be." Allergic contact dermatitis that is widespread or that affects the eyelids, hands, or groin region can be treated with a tapering dose of oral corticosteroid over a 2- to 3-week period. If the steroid is tapered too quickly, the patient may experience a poststeroid flare of their dermatitis, which can be resistant to further corticosteroid therapy.

Patients who do not respond to these measures should undergo patch testing to determine whether another antigen is causing or provoking the dermatitis. Without the use of patch testing, the allergen will remain unknown and the dermatitis will persist. Not infrequently, patients are found to be allergic to a fragrance or preservative that is an ingredient in one of their personal care products. Once they stop using the product, the dermatitis finally resolves.

PATCH TESTING AND TYPE IV HYPERSENSITIVITY FOR ALLERGIC CONTACT DERMATITIS

Patch test

Patch test placement

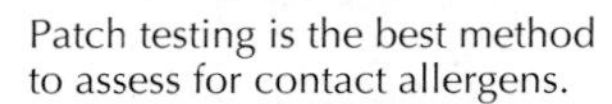

Patch testing is the best method to assess for contact allergens.

Positive patch test

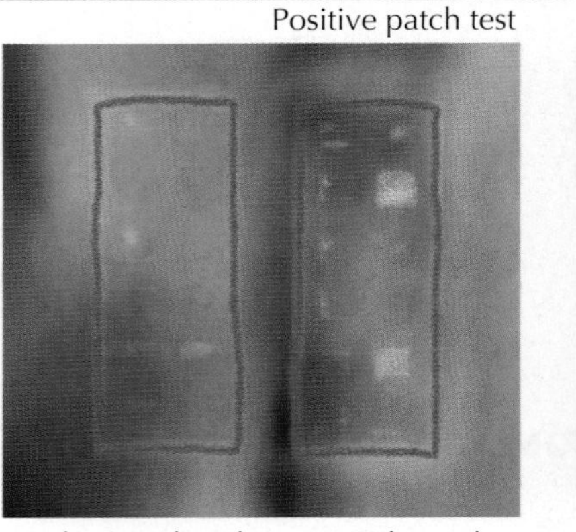

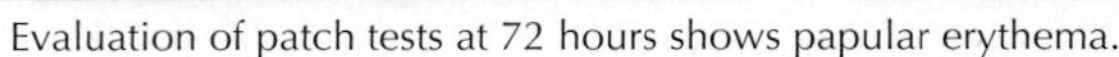

Evaluation of patch tests at 72 hours shows papular erythema.

Type IV (cell-mediated, delayed/hypersensitivity, contact dermatitis) reactions

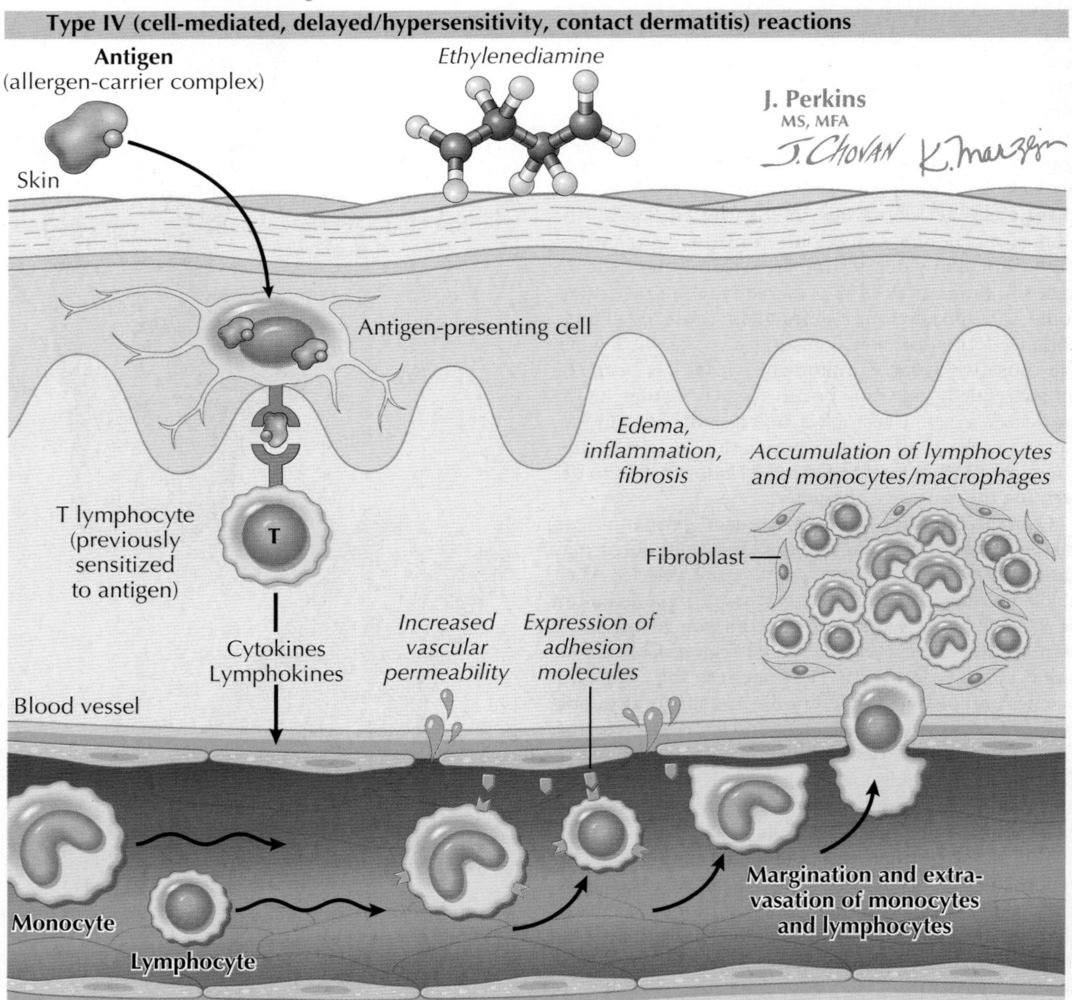

Atopic Dermatitis

Atopic dermatitis is one of the most common dermatoses of childhood. It typically manifests in early life, often before 5 years of age, and can have varying degrees of expression. It is frequently associated with asthma and allergies. Most children eventually improve over time, with many cases resolving in late childhood. Adults who had childhood atopic dermatitis relate having higher rates of skin irritation, dryness, and intermittent dermatitis. Atopic dermatitis has been estimated to affect up to 15% of all children and 1% to 3% of adults, and its prevalence has been steadily increasing. Patients frequently have a family history of atopic dermatitis, asthma, or skin sensitivity. Atopic dermatitis has been shown to have a significant effect on an afflicted individual's quality of life and has been found to affect school and job performance.

Clinical Findings: Atopic dermatitis typically begins early in life. There is no racial predilection. The clinical course is often chronic, with a waxing and waning nature. Infants a few months old may initially present with pruritic, red, eczematous patches on the cheeks and extremities as well as the trunk. The itching is typically severe and causes the child to excoriate the skin, which can lead to secondary skin infections. The skin of patients with atopic dermatitis is abnormally dry and is sensitive to heat and sweating. These children have difficulty sleeping because of the severe pruritus associated with the rash. During flares of the dermatitis, patients may develop weeping patches and plaques that are extremely pruritic and occasionally painful. With time, the patches begin to localize to flexural regions, particularly the antecubital and popliteal fossae. Severely afflicted children may have widespread disease. Patients with atopic dermatitis are more prone to react to contact and systemic allergens. Sensitivity to contact allergens is likely a consequence of the frequent use of topical medicaments and the broken skin barrier. This combination leads to increased exposure to foreign antigens that are capable of inducing allergic contact dermatitis. One should suspect coexisting contact dermatitis if a patient who is doing well experiences a flare for no apparent reason or if a patient continues to get worse despite aggressive topical or oral therapy. Laboratory testing commonly shows eosinophilia and an elevated immunoglobulin E (IgE) level. No lab tests can make the diagnosis.

Secondary infection is common in atopic dermatitis. It may manifest with the appearance of honey-colored, crusted patches in the excoriated regions, which indicates impetigo. It may also manifest as multiple follicle-based pustules, representing folliculitis, or as deep red, tender macules, indicating a deeper soft tissue infection. The rate of methicillin-resistant *Staphylococcus aureus* infection has increased in patients with atopic dermatitis at the same rate as in the general public. The rate of colonization of patients with atopic dermatitis is much higher than in normal controls, most likely because of the disruption of the underlying epidermis. Colonization in certain situations may lead to infection. Acquisition of a widespread herpesvirus infection can have severe and potentially life-threatening consequences. Patients with atopic dermatitis are much more prone than others to develop eczema herpeticum. The extensive areas of abnormal, broken skin provide the perfect environment for the development of this widespread viral infection. For this reason, some live attenuated smallpox vaccinations are contraindicated in individuals with atopic dermatitis.

Most childhood atopic dermatitis improves or resolves spontaneously over time. It is estimated that 10% of cases will resolve by the age of 1 year, 50% by 5 years, 70% by 7 years, and so on. A small percentage of children with atopic dermatitis continue with the rash into adulthood. These cases tend to be chronic in nature and last for the patient's lifetime.

Pathogenesis: The cause of atopic dermatitis is unknown, but there are two main theories: inside-out and outside-in. The first proposes that immunologic interactions lead to a skin barrier defect, and the latter proposes that a skin barrier defect leads to

Infants and Children with Atopic Dermatitis

Infants with atopic dermatitis

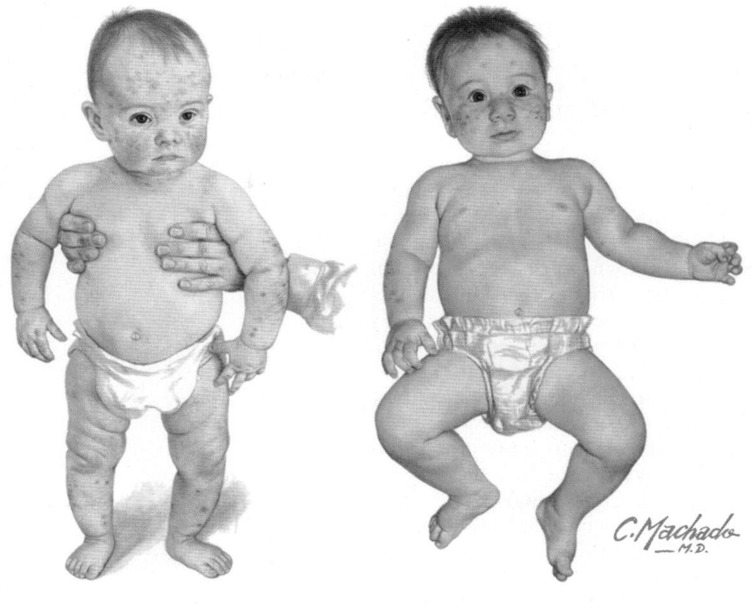

Child with atopic dermatitis

Frontal view

Dorsal view

Lymphadenopathy in a child with atopic dermatitis

Atopic Dermatitis (Continued)

immunologic activation. It is most likely a combination of the two. Individuals with *filaggrin (FLG)* gene mutations have been shown to have higher rates of atopic dermatitis. Many exacerbating factors have been found. They include anything that irritates the skin, such as heat, sweating, stress, many chemicals, and various types of clothing. Atopic dermatitis is believed to be caused by an aberrant T-cell (Th2) response in the skin with elevated levels of Th2 cytokines. Interleukin-4 (IL-4), IL-5, and IL-13 are abnormally elevated. These cytokines are responsible for eosinophil production and recruitment and for IgE production. The concentrations of the Th1 cytokines (IL-12 and interferon-α) are below average in these patients. The reason for this response is unknown. Ultimately, the barrier of the epidermis is disrupted; this is evident by the increase in transepidermal water loss, which can be measured.

Histology: A nonspecific lymphocytic infiltrate is seen, with associated exocytosis of lymphocytes into the epidermis with widespread spongiosis. Varying degrees of acanthosis and parakeratosis are seen. Often, bacterial elements are seen on the surface of the skin. Small intraepidermal vesicles may develop secondary to the massive spongiosis. Excoriations are frequently seen.

Treatment: Therapy consists of patient and family education about the natural history of the disease and the episodic waxing and waning. Bathing regimens must be thoroughly explained, and the use of soap should be discouraged. The patient should take shorter baths in lukewarm water, followed immediately by moisturization and application of topical steroid medications as appropriate. The intermittent use of moisturizers is also helpful. The use of topical immunomodulators, alternating with topical corticosteroids or alone, decreases the atrophogenic side effects of the topical corticosteroids. On occasion, oral steroids may be needed to calm the inflammation and give the patient some well-needed, albeit temporary, relief. Antipruritic agents are almost always required and include both topical antipruritic and oral antihistamines.

Most children do not need to avoid particular foods. If any question exists as to whether a food is potentially exacerbating the dermatitis, an allergist may be consulted to perform specific food allergy testing.

Prompt recognition of any bacterial or viral infection should lead to therapy that is not delayed. Impetigo, molluscum contagiosum, and eczema herpeticum are the three infections most commonly associated with atopic dermatitis. Of these, eczema herpeticum is the most important, and its recognition depends on a strong index of suspicion in any child with atopic dermatitis and new onset of a widespread, blistering rash. The differential diagnosis is varicella. A Tzanck test can help diagnose the condition but cannot differentiate herpes simplex virus from varicella zoster virus. A viral culture or direct immunofluorescence antibody staining of blister fluid is required for differentiation.

Treatment of atopic dermatitis has been profoundly changed with the introduction of dupilumab. Dupilumab is a subcutaneously administered medication that inhibits both IL-4 and IL-13. These interleukins are elevated in individuals with atopic dermatitis and have been shown to drive the skin inflammation. Inhibiting their function has been shown to dramatically improve atopic dermatitis. Tralokinumab has been introduced, and it works by inhibiting IL-13. The Janus kinase inhibitor class of medications has also been shown to be efficacious in atopic dermatitis.

Occasionally in children and more commonly in adults, other systemic therapies are used to keep the dermatitis under control. Some patients respond to ultraviolet phototherapy, but most are not able to tolerate the warmth and sweating induced by the phototherapy unit. Oral immunosuppressants that have been used include cyclosporine, azathioprine, and mycophenolate mofetil. These medications have severe potential side effects and should be administered only by experienced clinicians. Routine laboratory testing is required with all of these medications.

Adolescents and Adults with Atopic Dermatitis

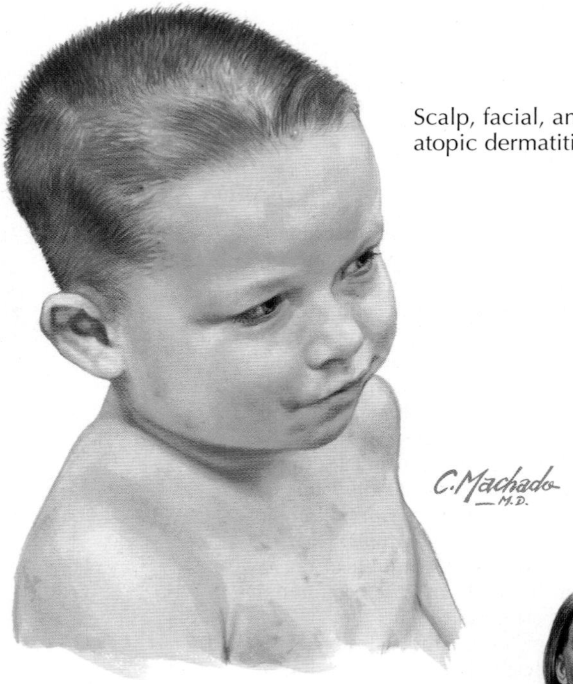

Scalp, facial, and truncal atopic dermatitis in a child

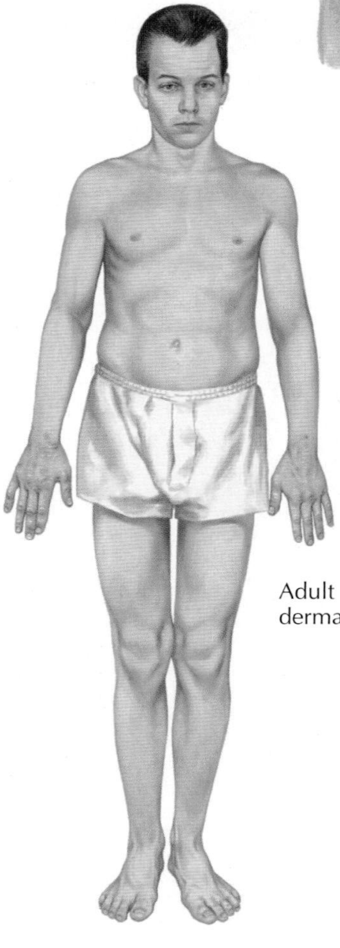

C. Machado M.D.

Adult patient with atopic dermatitis

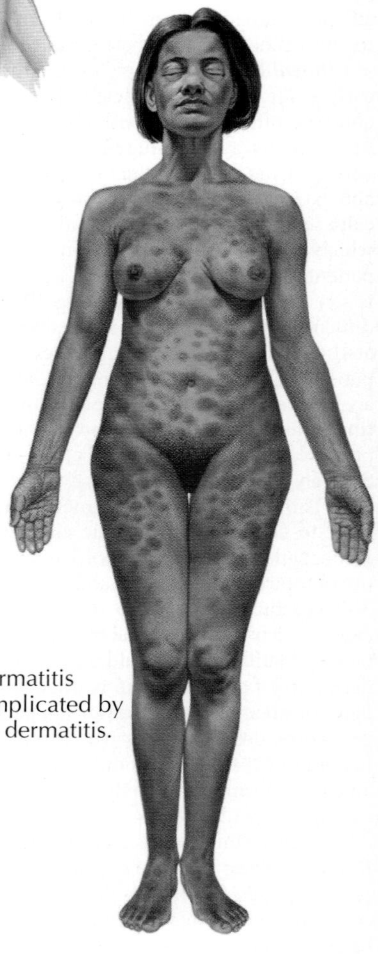

Adult atopic dermatitis can also be complicated by allergic contact dermatitis.

AUTOINFLAMMATORY SYNDROMES

The autoinflammatory syndromes are a rare group of diseases for which the specific causes have been determined. The diseases in this category include hyperimmunoglobulin D (hyper-IgD) syndrome (HIDS); the cryopyrinopathies; familial Mediterranean fever (FMF); cyclic neutropenia; deficiency of the IL-1 receptor antagonist (DIRA); deficiency of the IL-36 receptor antagonist (DITRA); pyogenic arthritis, pyoderma gangrenosum, and acne (PAPA); periodic fever, aphthous stomatitis, pharyngitis, and adenopathy (PAPFA); Schnitzler syndrome; and TNF receptor–associated periodic syndrome (TRAPS). The cryopyrinopathies are a group of conditions composed of Muckle-Wells syndrome, familial cold autoinflammatory syndrome (FCAS), neonatal-onset multisystem inflammatory disease (NOMID), and chronic infantile neurologic cutaneous and articular syndrome (CINCA). These groupings were first proposed in the 1990s to bring together a collection of inflammatory disorders that are distinct in nature and pathophysiology from other forms of allergic, autoimmune, and immunodeficiency syndromes. Patients with these autoinflammatory diseases lack autoreactive immune cells (T and B cells) and autoantibodies. The identification of specific defective genes and the roles played by those genes in the development of these disorders has been critical in increasing understanding of these diverse diseases. The common link in these conditions is that they all represent abnormalities of the innate immune system.

Clinical Findings: HIDS is inherited in an autosomal recessive fashion. Patients present with fever, arthralgias, abdominal pain, cervical adenopathy, and aphthous ulcers. Skin findings are consistent with a cutaneous vasculitis with palpable purpura and purpuric macules and nodules. Patients develop attacks of these symptoms with some evidence of periodicity. The attacks can last from 3 to 7 days, and typically the first attack occurs within the first year of life. As the child ages, the frequency and severity of the attacks lessen. No reliable trigger has been found that initiates the attacks, and patients are completely normal between attack episodes.

Within the group of cryopyrinopathies, the distinctions among Muckle-Wells syndrome, FCAS, NOMID, and CINCA are not clear, and many believe that they represent a phenotypic expression spectrum of the same condition. These very rare syndromes are all inherited in an autosomal dominant fashion. Patients present with recurrent fevers, arthralgias, myalgias, and varying degrees of ophthalmic involvement with conjunctivitis and anterior uveitis. The skin findings are typically generalized and consist of red, edematous papules and plaques. The rash can appear urticarial but is less pruritic. The attack episodes almost always last less than 24 hours. The trigger for FCAS is cold exposure, but the other conditions have no known precipitating factors. Twenty-five percent of patients with Muckle-Wells syndrome develop amyloidosis later in life, which may lead to chronic renal failure. The other conditions also have been reported to lead to amyloidosis but much less commonly than Muckle-Wells syndrome. NOMID tends to be the most severe of the cryopyrinopathies. Patients with NOMID can develop aseptic meningitis and varying degrees of intellectual disability along with hepatosplenomegaly. These patients can develop a characteristic overgrowth of cartilage around the knee that is quite noticeable on physical examination.

FMF is inherited in an autosomal dominant fashion. It is the most common of all autoinflammatory syndromes. Patients experience attacks of fever and abdominal pain along with monoarthritis. Occasionally, pleuritis and pericarditis are also present. The skin findings consist of an erysipelas-like rash occurring almost exclusively on the lower extremities. Lesions of palpable purpura may also be present, indicating a cutaneous vasculitis. The attacks usually last less than 3 days, with a variable length of time between attacks. Some adults develop renal dysfunction because of amyloidosis.

TRAPS is inherited in an autosomal dominant pattern and also can occur sporadically. Patients develop attacks early in childhood, which consist of fever, abdominal pain, conjunctivitis, arthralgias, and migratory myalgias. The attacks last longer than in the other autoinflammatory syndromes. Each attack may last from days to weeks, with frequent recurrences. Attacks may be precipitated by varying amounts of stress, both physical and emotional. Again, the development of renal amyloidosis in adulthood has

PATHOPHYSIOLOGY OF AUTOINFLAMMATORY SYNDROMES

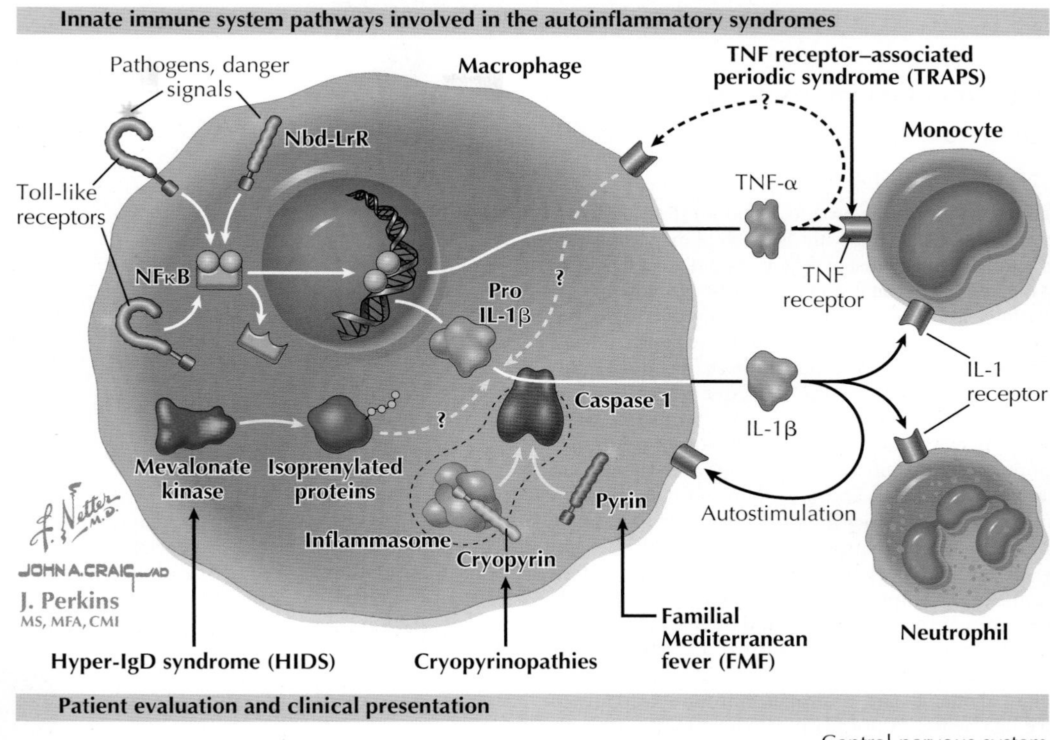

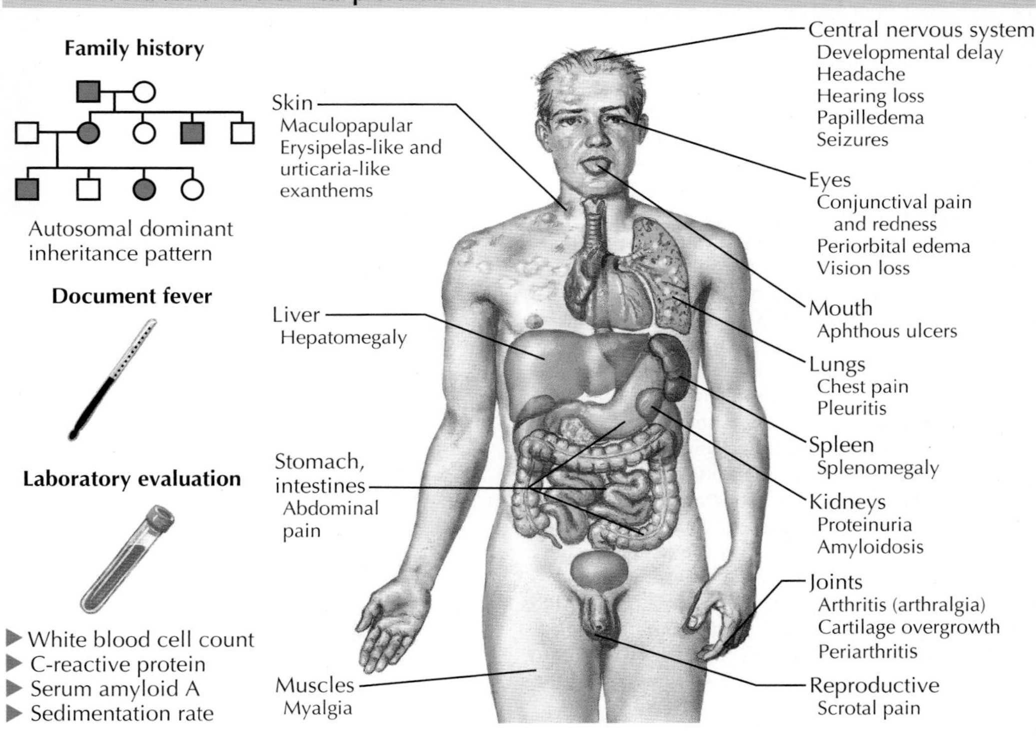

Clinical Manifestations of Autoinflammatory Syndromes

Cutaneous findings

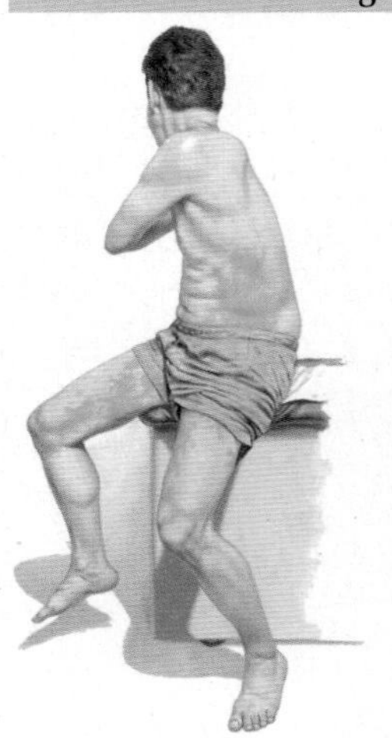

Classic TRAPS rash that migrates in a centrifugal pattern

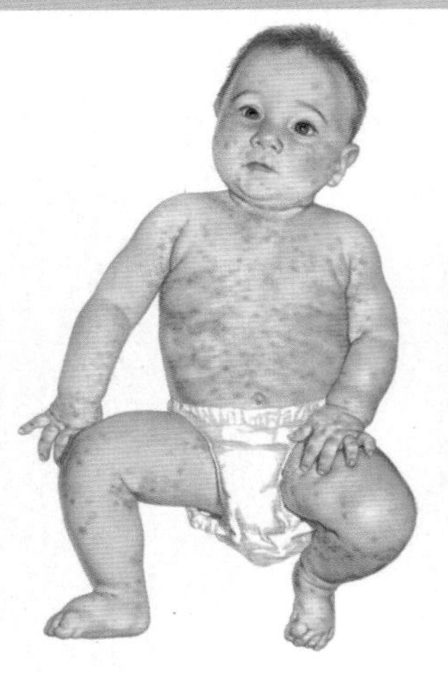

The rash in HIDS can be variable, including maculopapular and urticarial forms.

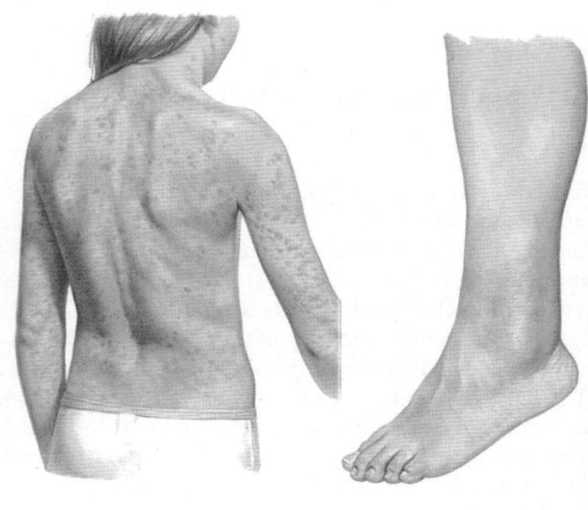

Typical appearance of urticaria-like rash of the cryopyrinopathies

Typical appearance of erysipelas-like FMF rash, often on lower extremities

Joint and central nervous system findings

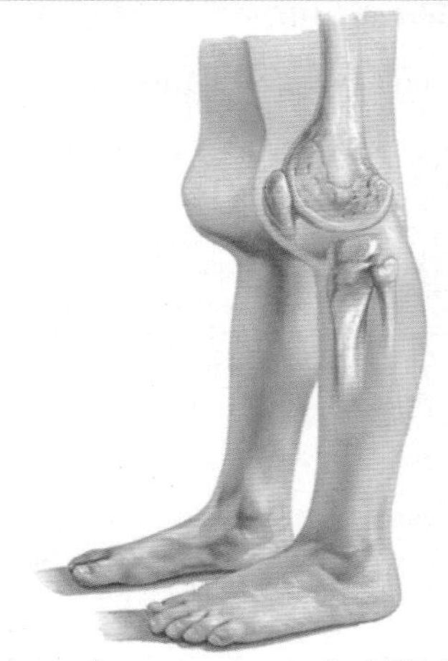

Joint enlargement seen in NOMID

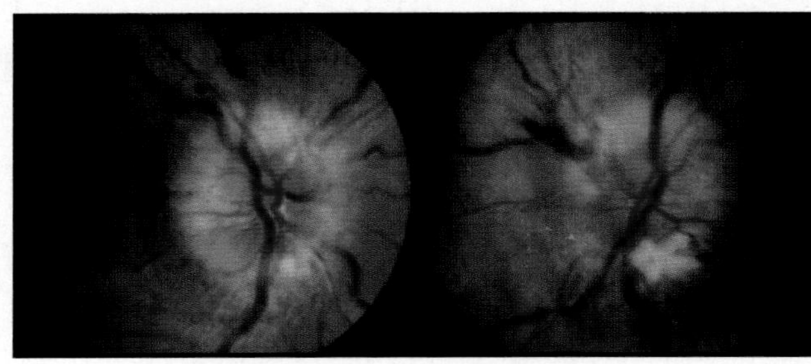

Optic fundus with papilledema

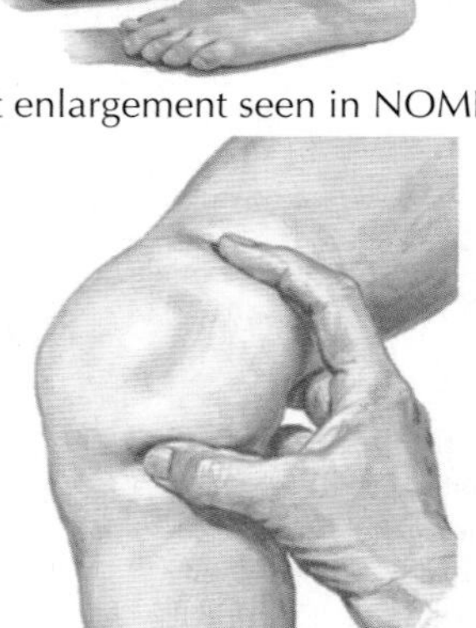

Arthritis/periarthritis

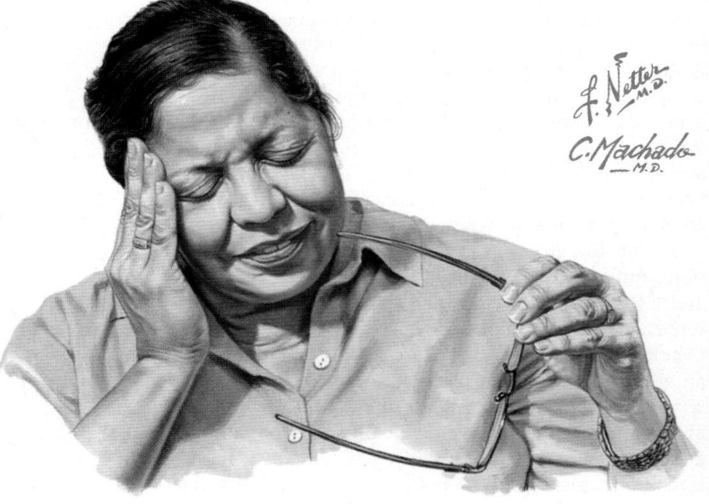

Headache

Autoinflammatory Syndromes (Continued)

profound effects on the prognosis and is estimated to occur in 10% of patients with TRAPS. Skin findings are characteristic and consist of migratory, pink to red patches and macules. Periorbital swelling may be prominent.

Pathogenesis: Remarkable success has been achieved in deciphering the pathogenesis of these disease states, which are all interconnected through the innate immune system. Many of the defective genes and the proteins that they encode have been determined. These proteins play a critical role in regulation of the innate immune system's inflammatory response. If they are defective, they cause varying amounts of dysregulation of neutrophils and other inflammatory cells. The innate immune system is nonspecific in nature and does not rely on antibody production. Various innate pattern recognition receptors (e.g., toll-like receptors) are able to recognize foreign molecules and directly activate the innate immune system. The normal activation of the innate immune system allows prompt recognition of foreign elements and a proper immune reaction to those elements. Autoinflammatory conditions have been discovered to involve defects in various components of the innate immune system.

HIDS is caused by a mutation in the *MVK* gene, located on chromosome 12, which encodes the protein mevalonate kinase. This gene helps regulate cholesterol synthesis, but it is also important for production of precursors that will ultimately be isoprenylated. The lack of these isoprenylated proteins leads to dysregulation of IL-1β and ultimately to the clinical findings of HIDS. All of the cryopyrinopathies are caused by a genetic defect of the *NLRP3* gene located on chromosome 1. This gene, which is also called *CIAS1*, encodes the protein cryopyrin. The defect allows for a gain in function of the cryopyrin protein, which results in hyperactivity of the inflammasome. The inflammasome is a cytoplasmic soluble conglomeration of various proteins that is part of the innate immune system and is constantly identifying foreign material. Its stimulation ultimately increases the activity of the caspase 1 protein and the production of IL-1β. FMF has been found to be caused by a defect in the *MEFV* gene, which encodes the pyrin protein. Pyrin is also a regulator of the inflammasome, and defects in pyrin result in increased levels of IL-1β. TRAPS is caused by a defective gene on chromosome 12 named *TNFRSF1A*. This gene encodes the 55-kd TNF receptor. The defect leads to excessive signaling because of serum TNF activation of the receptor.

Histology: Each of the autoinflammatory skin lesions has a unique histology. The diagnosis cannot be made on the basis of histology alone, but histologic findings are used to rule out other conditions in the differential diagnosis and to help confirm the diagnosis of an autoinflammatory disease. Skin biopsies should be taken during acute attacks when a rash is present.

Cutaneous biopsy specimens from patients with HIDS typically show a neutrophilic vasculitis. Neutrophils are found throughout the dermis. Skin biopsy from patients with a cyropyrinopathy shows a neutrophilic perivascular infiltrate associated with diffuse dermal edema. NOMID and CINCA also exhibit a perivascular infiltrate of lymphocytes scattered within the neutrophilic infiltrate. FMF skin biopsies show a diffuse population of dermal neutrophils. TRAPS skin biopsies are nondescript and show a bland lymphocytic infiltrate in a dermal perivascular location. Biopsy of the periorbital edema shows a perivascular lymphocytic infiltrate and dermal edema.

Treatment: Therapy is specific to each syndrome. The molecular understanding of the pathogenesis has led to specific therapies. Because of their rarity, no randomized studies have been performed on the treatment of these conditions. HIDS has been successfully treated with nonsteroidal antiinflammatory drugs (NSAIDs), statin medications, and the IL-1 receptor antagonist anakinra. The cryopyrinopathies have been treated with cold avoidance in the case of FCAS, and NSAIDs, oral steroids, and anakinra; other immunosuppressants have also been tried. FMF has been treated with good success with colchicine, taking advantage of its antineutrophil effect. TRAPS has been successfully treated with etanercept or anakinra. Etanercept is believed to remove the soluble TNF that is responsible for activating the mutated receptor.

BROWN RECLUSE SPIDERS AND SCABIES MITES

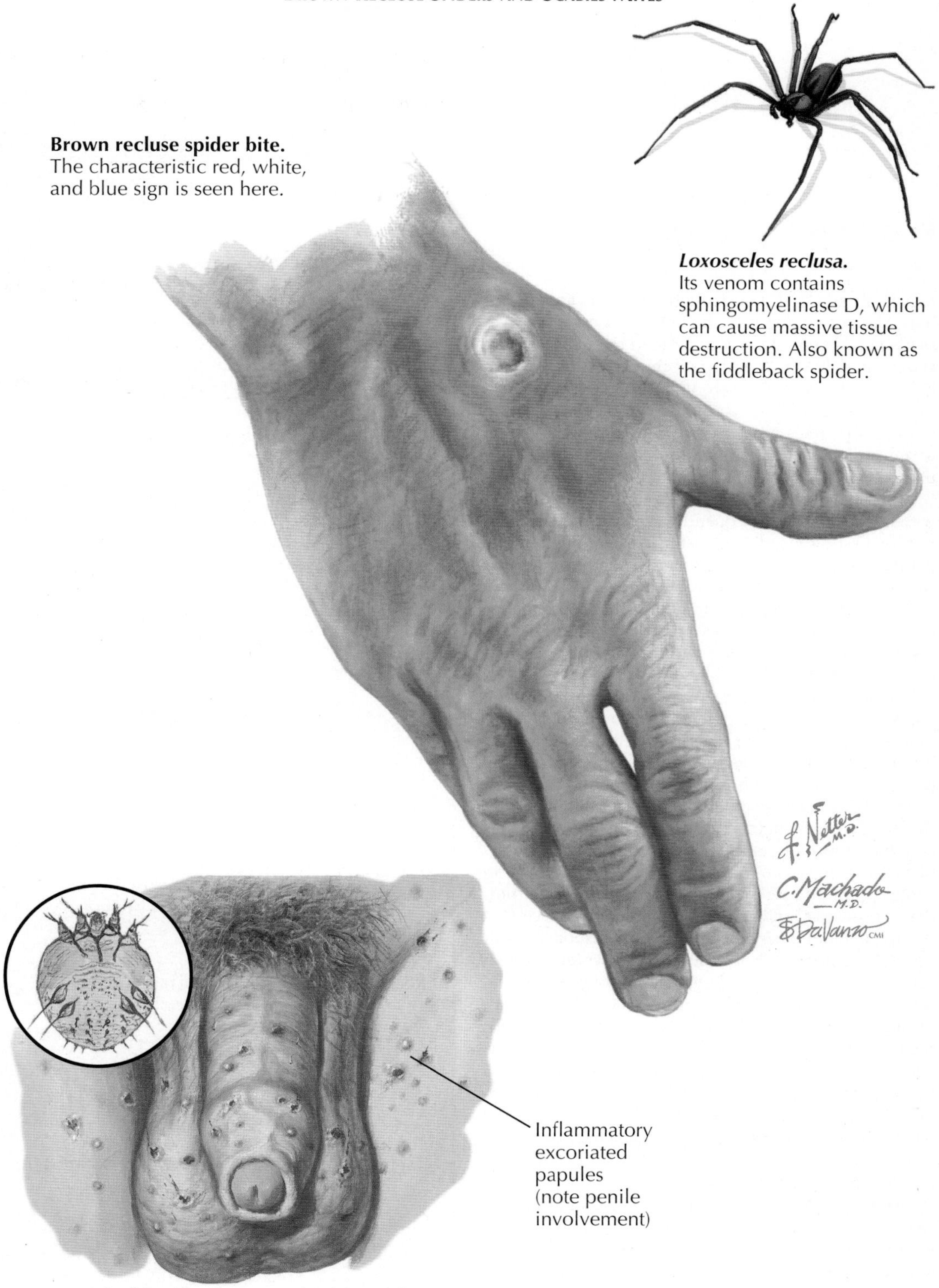

Brown recluse spider bite. The characteristic red, white, and blue sign is seen here.

Loxosceles reclusa. Its venom contains sphingomyelinase D, which can cause massive tissue destruction. Also known as the fiddleback spider.

Inflammatory excoriated papules (note penile involvement)

Scabies (*Sarcoptes scabiei*) in *circle*

BUG BITES

Human skin is exposed to the environment on a continual basis and encounters multiple threats, including arthropods of many varieties. Each species of arthropod can inflict its own type of damage to the skin; some bites are mild and barely noticeable, whereas others can be life-threatening. The most common bites are those of mosquitoes, fleas, bedbugs, mites, ticks, and spiders. These bites cause direct damage to the skin, and the organisms may have the ability to transmit infectious diseases such as Lyme disease, leishmaniasis, and rickettsial diseases, to name a few.

Clinical Findings: In northern climates, mosquitoes are prominent insects in the spring, summer, and early fall seasons. In warmer climates, they can be seen year-round. Their bite is often not noticed until after the mosquito has flown away. The recently bitten person is left with a pruritic urticarial papule that typically resolves by itself within an hour or so. Some individuals are prone to severe bite reactions and develop warm, red papules and nodules that can last for a week or two and can be associated with regional lymphadenopathy. Mosquitoes are a nuisance for the most part, but in some areas of the world they are the major vectors for transmission of malaria and encephalitis viruses. Sand flies (Phlebotominae family) can cause similar skin reactions. In certain regions of the globe, they are the major vector for leishmaniasis.

Fleas have been around since before the beginning of human civilization and in the Middle Ages were responsible for helping transmit the bubonic plague, which killed millions of people. Fleas are most commonly seen in households with pets. Individuals can be bitten after the pet transfers the fleas to bedding, carpeting, or clothing. Characteristic bites occur in groups of three, referred to as "breakfast, lunch, and dinner." Flea eggs can lie dormant for years, only to reactivate in response to movement and vibration that indicate a meal is likely to be nearby. Many flea bites occur around the ankles of adults; the fleas jump from the carpeting to the ankles, take their meal, and leave. The typical skin lesion is a small papule with a central punctum. It is self-resolving. Fleas have been known to carry organisms responsible for infectious diseases, including *Yersinia pestis* (bubonic plague) and *Rickettsia typhi* (murine typhus).

Bedbugs *(Cimex lectularius)* have made a resurgence in the United States. They are ubiquitous insects that can live in any area of the country. Households, hotels, and other sleeping quarters become infested with colonies of bedbugs. They emerge in the night, typically 1 to 2 hours before dawn, and search for a blood meal. They find their victim asleep and feed for a few minutes before retreating back to the nest. The nest is almost never in the bed; it is most likely to be located within the baseboard molding or floorboards. In the morning, the afflicted individual awakens with one to hundreds of bites. Most are small papules with a central punctum. Depending on the species of bedbug, a more inflammatory response may occur, causing vesiculation and bullae. Bedbugs have been reported to transmit hepatitis B virus.

Encounters with the large mite family of organisms are more likely to occur in the summer months in Northern latitudes but can occur at any time of the year in the southern regions. The term *chigger* refers to the larval phase of the Trombiculidae family of mites; it is one of the most common and well-recognized causes of human bites. Chiggers are red mites—so small that they are not felt, and they bite quickly. They usually leave pinpoint red papules that can be numerous and can cause severe pruritus. Many other mites are present in the environment and can cause similar reactions.

Most ticks bite and feed for up to 24 hours before falling off after obtaining their blood meal. They can leave a tick bite granuloma, which is a small red papule with a central punctum, at the site of the bite. Many methods have been used to remove ticks; most can result in more skin damage than the actual tick bite. These methods include burning the end of the tick with a cigarette or a

Bug Bites (Continued)

match, an approach that is more likely to cause a skin burn than it is to remove the tick. The best method of removal is to grab the tick as close to the surface of the skin as possible and gently pull in a direction perpendicular to the skin. If the mouthparts are left embedded in the skin, a small punch biopsy can be performed to remove the remaining parts. Ticks are well known to transmit many infectious diseases, including Lyme disease and Rocky Mountain spotted fever.

Most spider bites are caused by jumping spiders. As with all spiders, bites frequently occur after the spider's web or nesting location is disturbed. The bites can be painful and can leave erythema and a papule or nodular reaction. On occasion, these bites develop secondary cellulitis. Two spiders are unique in their potential to cause severe human disease: the black widow spider *(Latrodectus mactans)* and the brown recluse spider *(Loxosceles reclusa)*.

The black widow spider is a web-weaving spider that paralyzes its prey with a potent neurotoxin called *latrotoxin*. The venom causes massive release of acetylcholine from nerve endings. In humans, this can lead to pain, fever, and symptoms of an acute abdomen.

The brown recluse spider is a solitary stalking spider that lives in dark, hidden locations. It is not aggressive and typically bites only when a human accidentally disturbs its location. The toxin released in its venom contains a mixture of sphingomyelinase D, hyaluronidases, proteases, and esterases. Sphingomyelinase D is the major component believed to be responsible for most of the tissue damage caused by the spider's bite. It can cause severe pain and aggregation of platelets and red blood cells, resulting in intravascular clotting with resultant necrosis of the skin. The characteristic pattern seen on the skin is a central bluish region with necrosis and coagulation, a surrounding vasoconstricted area that appears to be blanched white, and a peripheral rim of erythema. This has been termed the "red, white, and blue" sign of a brown recluse bite. Some bites can progress rapidly and cause severe necrosis of the skin requiring surgical debridement.

Histology: Most bite reactions are not biopsied because they are typically diagnosed clinically. The histologic findings for most bug bites are very similar. There is a superficial and deep inflammatory infiltrate with many eosinophils. Superficial necrosis of the epidermis may be seen at the site of the bite. Occasionally, tick mouth parts are located in the biopsy specimen. Brown recluse spider bites show intravascular thrombosis and necrosis of the skin.

Treatment: The treatment of most bites is supportive. Pruritus can be treated with a potent topical corticosteroid and an oral antihistamine. Avoidance is the most important preventive measure. Areas of standing water provide breeding grounds for mosquitoes and should be drained routinely. Pets should be groomed and treated with preventive tick and flea medications. Flea and bedbug infestations should be treated by a professional exterminator. Proper use of bug repellant sprays containing DEET (*N*,*N*-diethyl-*m*-toluamide) and staying in the center of wooded trails can help decrease one's chance of being bitten. In endemic areas, any patient with a deer tick bite that has lasted longer than 24 hours should be considered for prophylactic therapy for Lyme disease.

Narcotics (for pain control) and anivenom have been used to treat black widow spider bites and have been helpful. The antivenom, given via IV, is derived from horse serum, and there is a risk of an allergic reaction in susceptible patients. Brown recluse spider bites have been treated with many agents, including dapsone, to try to mitigate some of the inflammation-induced skin damage. A horse-derived antivenom for brown recluse spider bites is available in some countries in Central and South America. Recognition and avoidance of these spiders are critical.

Arthropods and Diseases They Carry

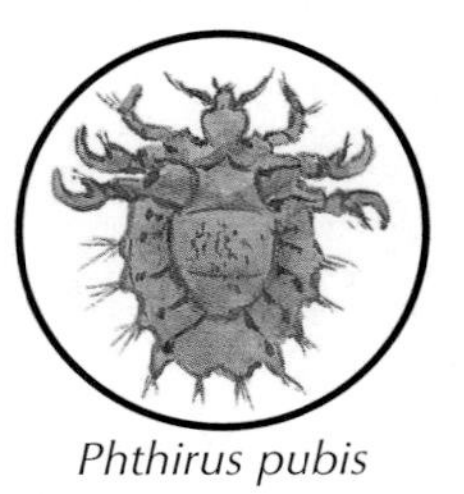

Phthirus pubis

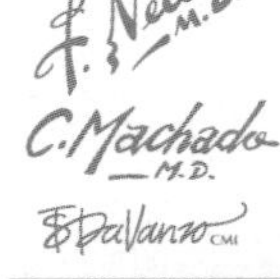

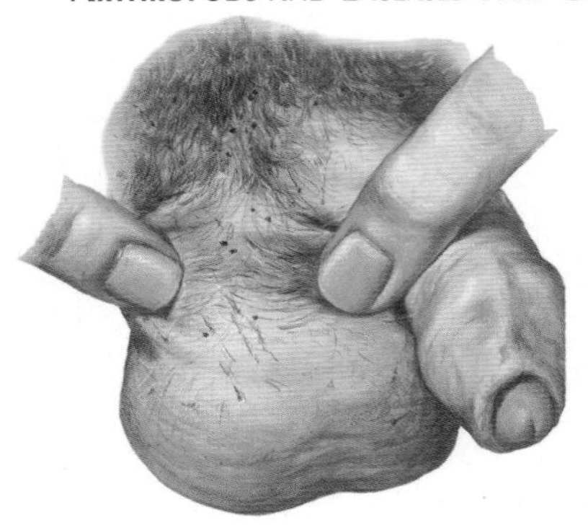

Pediculosis pubis (exposure of pediculi in hair)

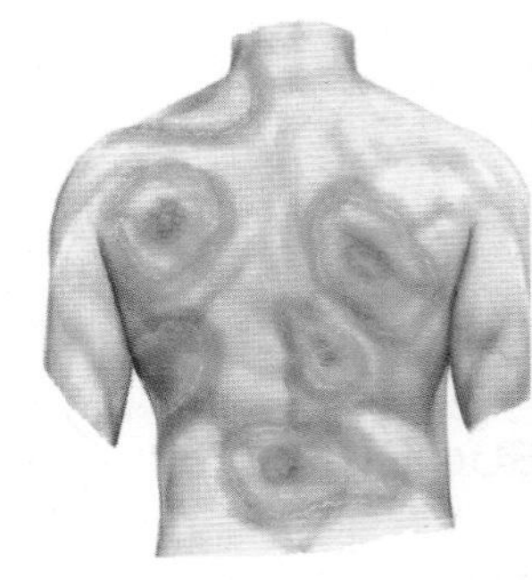

Deer ticks that carry Lyme disease can cause erythema migrans (bull's-eye rash)

Arthropod	Disease it transmits	Appearance
Blackfly	Onchocerciasis	
Deer tick	Lyme disease, anaplasmosis, babesiosis	
Flea	Plague	
Lice	Typhus	
Lone star tick	Tularemia, anaplasmosis	
Mosquito	Malaria, yellow fever, dengue, encephalitis, West Nile virus	
Reduviid bug	Chagas disease	
Sandfly	Leishmaniasis	
Tsetse fly	African trypanosomiasis	
Wood tick	Rocky Mountain spotted fever	

CALCIPHYLAXIS

Calciphylaxis (calcific uremic arteriolopathy) results from deposition of calcium in the tunica media portion of the small vessel walls in association with proliferation of the intimal layer of endothelial cells. It is almost always associated with end-stage renal disease, especially in patients undergoing chronic dialysis (either peritoneal dialysis or hemodialysis). Those undergoing peritoneal dialysis are at higher risk. It has been reported to occur in up to 5% of patients who have been on dialysis for longer than 1 year. Calciphylaxis typically manifests as nonhealing skin ulcers located in adipose-rich areas of the trunk and thighs, but the lesions can occur anywhere. They are believed to be caused by an abnormal ratio of calcium and phosphorus, which leads to the abnormal deposition within the tunica media of small blood vessels. This eventually results in thrombosis and ulceration of the overlying skin. Calciphylaxis has a poor prognosis, and there are few well-studied therapies. It is estimated that individuals diagnosed with calciphylaxis have an average overall survival of less than 1 year.

Clinical Findings: Calciphylaxis is almost exclusively seen in patients with chronic end-stage renal disease. Most patients have been on one form of dialysis for at least 1 year by the time of presentation. The initial presenting sign is that of a tender, dusky red to purple macule that quickly ulcerates. A livedo pattern can be seen on the extremities. The ulcerations have a ragged border and develop a thick black necrotic eschar. The ulcers tend to increase in size, and new areas appear before older ulcers have any opportunity to heal. Ulcerations begin proximally and tend to follow the path of the underlying affected blood vessel. The skin surrounding the ulcerations is often thickened and stiff. The most prominent location of ulcerations is within the adipose-rich areas of the trunk and thighs, especially the abdomen and mammary regions. Patients often report that ulcerations form in areas of trauma. The main differential diagnosis is between an infectious cause and calciphylaxis. Skin biopsies and cultures can be performed to differentiate the two. Skin biopsies are diagnostic. Radiographs of the region often show calcification of the small vessels, which can be used to support the diagnosis. Patients who develop calciphylaxis have a poor prognosis, with the mortality rate reaching 80% in some series. For some unknown reason, those with truncal disease tend to survive longer than those with distal extremity disease. Complications caused by the chronic severe ulcerations (e.g., infection, sepsis) are the main cause of mortality.

Laboratory findings often show an elevated calcium × phosphorus product. A calcium × phosphorus product greater than 70 mg^2/dL^2 appears to be an independent risk factor for development of calciphylaxis. Other risk factors are obesity, hyperparathyroidism, diabetes, and the use of warfarin. Elevated parathyroid hormone (PTH) levels are often found in association with calciphylaxis. The exact role that PTH plays is unknown, but it has been reported that parathyroidectomy, a standard treatment for calciphylaxis in the past, is not an effective means of therapy and is only done in refractory cases. PTH may play a role in starting the disease, but it does not appear to be necessary to exacerbate or cause continuation of calciphylaxis.

Although most commonly seen in areas of high fat content (abdomen, breast), all areas of the skin may be involved in calciphylaxis. Almost all cases are associated with underlying renal disease.

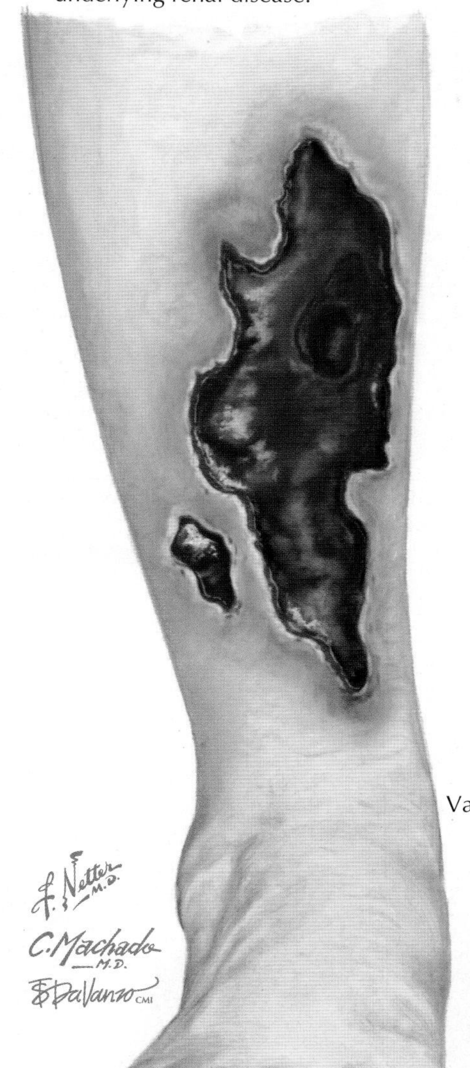

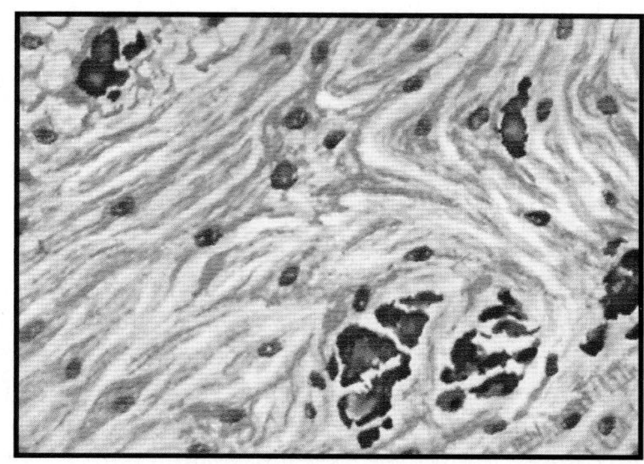

Calcium deposits in the conduction system of the heart, which may cause serious or fatal arrhythmias

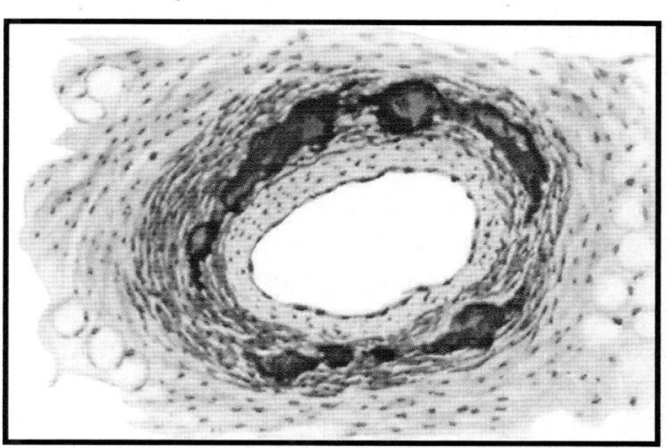

Medial calcification of small arteries and arterioles

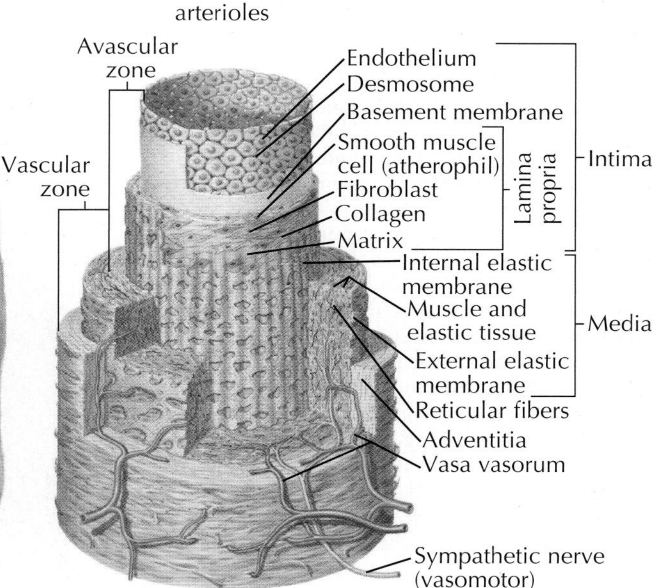

Wall of an artery: cutaway view

Pathogenesis: The exact mechanism of calcification of the tunica media of blood vessels in calciphylaxis is not completely understood. The fact that it is seen almost exclusively in patients undergoing chronic dialysis therapy has led to many theories on its origin. The final mechanism is a hardening of the vessel wall with calcification and intimal endothelial proliferation that leads to rapid and successive thrombosis and necrosis.

Histology: The main finding is of calcification of the medial section of the small blood vessels in and around the area of involvement. Thrombi within the vessel lumen are often observed. Intimal layer endothelial proliferation is prominent. The abnormal calcification can easily be seen on hematoxylin and eosin staining.

Treatment: Aggressive supportive care with analgesia and early treatment of superinfections are critical. Treating and removing risk factors is critically important. Surgical debridement of wounds is necessary to remove necrotic tissue that provides a portal for infection. Renal transplantation offers some hope for cure. Treatment with sodium thiosulfate has shown success, but this is not a universal cure. Bisphosphonate medications have also been used with limited success. Parathyroidectomy may help initially with the ulcerations, but it does not decrease mortality rate.

Cutaneous Lupus

Lupus erythematosus is a multisystem, idiopathic connective tissue disease that can have variable and unique clinical cutaneous findings. Cutaneous lupus may be considered as a spectrum of skin disease. Many variants have been described. Discoid lupus, subacute cutaneous lupus, tumid lupus, lupus panniculitis, neonatal lupus, lupus chilblains, and systemic lupus erythematosus (SLE) all have morphologically distinctive cutaneous findings. Lupus is a heterogeneous disease with a wide continuum of clinical involvement, from purely cutaneous disease to life-threatening SLE. The cutaneous findings are often the first presenting signs, and recognition of the skin manifestations can help make the diagnosis.

SLE is the most severe form of lupus. Its clinical course and outcome vary from mild forms to severe, life-threatening variants. In the most severe cases, the pulmonary, cardiac, neurologic, and connective tissue and integumentary systems are affected. Death may occur from complications of renal failure. Severe arthritis and skin findings are often present. SLE is diagnosed by fulfillment of criteria that have been established by the American College of Rheumatology. Variations in meeting these criteria are reflected in the differing clinical spectrum of disease.

Patients with lupus can have numerous laboratory abnormalities. These include anemia of chronic disease and an elevated erythrocyte sedimentation rate. Antinuclear antibodies (ANAs) are found in some subsets of lupus, with almost 100% of patients with the systemic form testing positive for ANAs. Many other, more specific antibodies are found in patients with SLE, including anti-Smith antibodies and anti–double-stranded DNA antibodies. Patients with renal disease often have hypertension, elevated protein levels in their urine, and an elevated creatinine level.

Clinical Findings: Many variants of cutaneous lupus exist, each with its own morphologic findings. Lupus is more common in women; it can be seen at any age but is most frequently observed in early adulthood. However, lupus is common enough that it is not infrequently seen in males. Neonatal lupus is a rare form that occurs in neonates born to mothers with lupus.

Discoid lupus is one of the easiest forms of cutaneous lupus to recognize. It is most commonly found on the head and neck region and tends to be present on the scalp and within the conchal bowl of the ear. Lesions are often found in patients with SLE. Discoid lupus may occur as an entirely separate disease with no other systemic or clinical findings of lupus. Ten percent to 20% of these patients eventually progress to the systemic form of lupus. Discoid lesions are exacerbated by sun exposure, more specifically by exposure to ultraviolet A (UVA) light. The lesions tend to have an annular configuration with varying amounts of scale. The lesions can produce alopecia, and there is almost always some amount of skin atrophy present. Follicular plugging is commonly seen in discoid lupus. It is noticed clinically as a dilation of the follicular orifices. Follicle plugs can also be seen by gently removing the scale from a discoid lesion. On close inspection of the inferior side of the scale, minute keratotic follicular plugs can be seen. This finding is specific for discoid lupus and has been termed the "carpet tack sign" because it resembles tiny outreaching tacks. This sign can be easily missed if the scale is removed too quickly or not inspected closely enough. Discoid lesions in darker-skinned individuals may also have varying amounts of hyperpigmentation. Patients will have some amount of erythema and hyperpigmentation on close inspection. Fortunately, most patients present with only a few discoid lesions and are diagnosed with localized discoid lupus. Those rare patients with widespread disease have generalized discoid lupus. This variant is rare, and such patients are much more likely than those with localized disease to meet the criteria for SLE at some point. The alopecia seen in discoid lupus is scarring in nature, and the hair that has been lost will not regrow even with aggressive therapy. Alopecia can be life-altering and can cause significant psychological morbidity.

Subacute cutaneous lupus erythematosus (SCLE) is seen in a subset of patients and has a higher incidence (>50%) of developing into full-blown SLE compared with other forms of cutaneous lupus. There are variants of subacute cutaneous lupus, with the annular form and the papulosquamous form being the most common and

Cutaneous Lupus Band Test

A. Erythematous malar rash

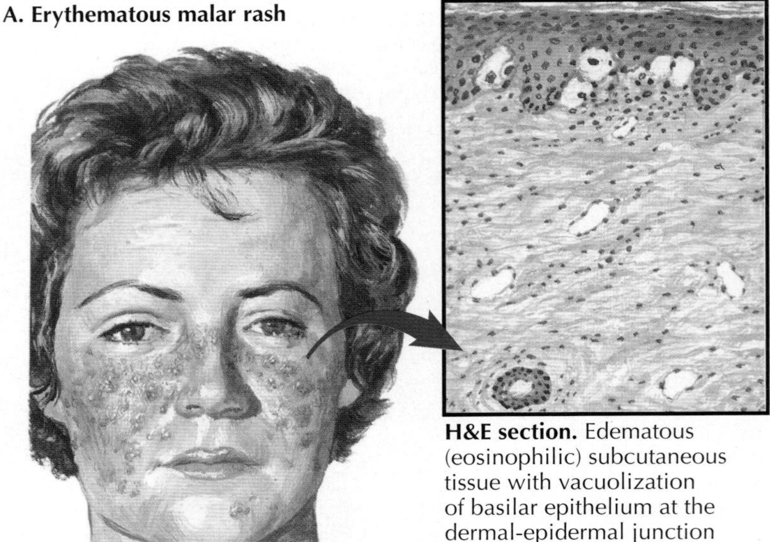

H&E section. Edematous (eosinophilic) subcutaneous tissue with vacuolization of basilar epithelium at the dermal-epidermal junction

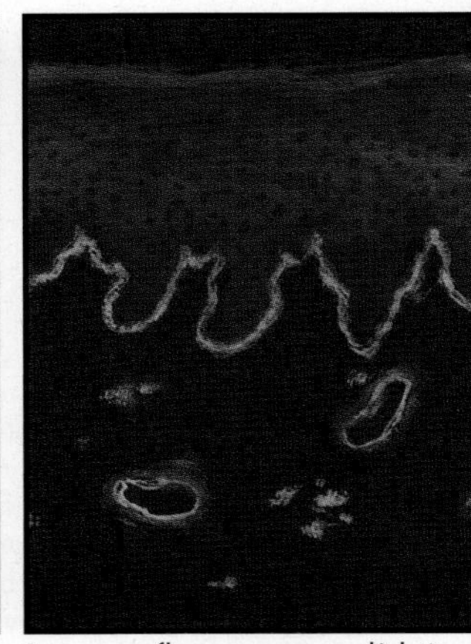

Immunofluorescence slide*: band-like granular deposit of gamma globulin and complement at the dermal-epidermal junction and in the walls of small dermal vessels

B. Normal-appearing (nonlesional and non–sun-exposed) skin of patient with lupus

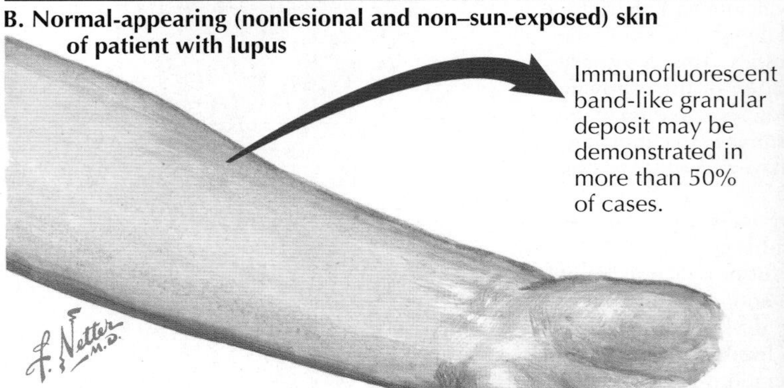

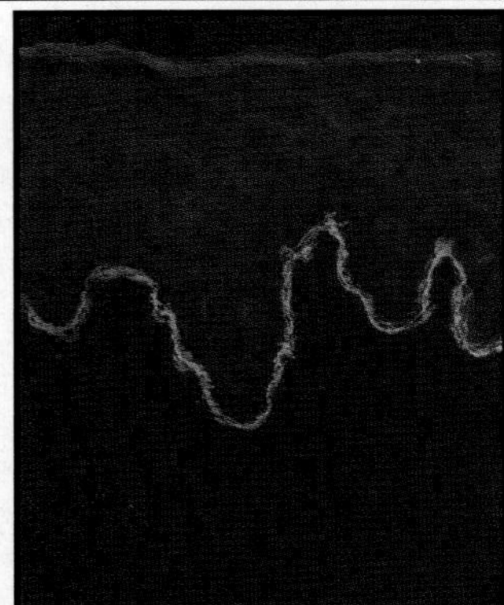

C. Discoid lupus

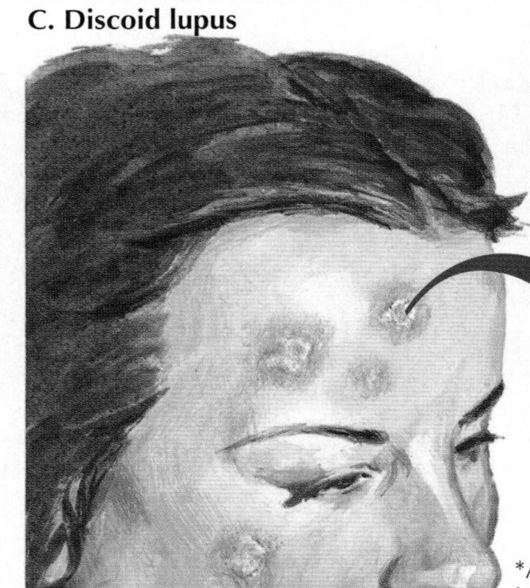

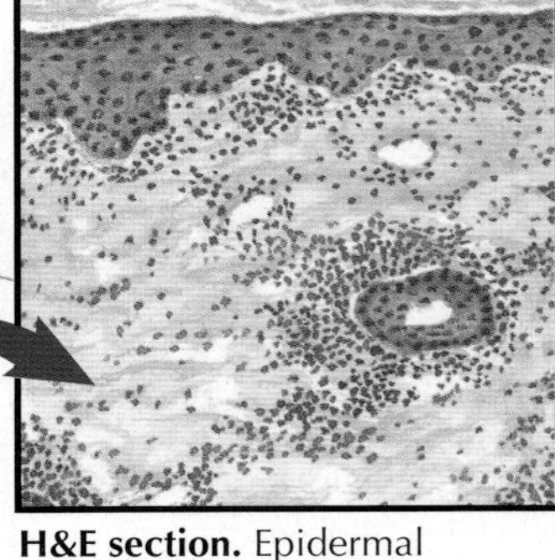

H&E section. Epidermal atrophy, hyalinization of dermis, chronic inflammation around hair follicles.

Granular deposits of immune complexes at the dermal-epidermal junction and within dermis

*All fluorescence slides were stained with fluorescein-labeled rabbit antihuman gamma globulin.

CUTANEOUS LUPUS (Continued)

most important to recognize. The annular form manifests with pink to red annular patches that slowly expand and coalesce into larger, interconnected polycyclic patches. They occur most commonly on sun-exposed skin of the face and upper trunk. The papulosquamous version also manifests in sun-exposed regions. It appears as smaller, pink-red patches with overlying scale. Both forms are exacerbated by sun exposure and are pruritic. They heal with no scarring. ANA positivity and anti-Ro/SSA are seen in more than 50% of individuals with SCLE.

Neonatal lupus is an uncommon form of lupus that can manifest with or without cutaneous findings. However, cutaneous findings are the most common clinical finding, occurring in more than 90% of cases. The most common scenario is a child born to a mother who has not yet been diagnosed with lupus. Neonatal lupus can manifest with varying degrees of congenital heart block, which is the most serious sequela. Some children require a pacemaker to control the arrhythmia. Thrombocytopenia is another frequent effect of neonatal lupus. Neonatal lupus is directly caused by the transplacental migration of anti-Ro/SSA antibodies and, to a lesser extent, anti-La/SSB antibodies. The antibodies are only transiently present because the newborn does not produce any new antibodies. Therefore neonatal lupus improves over time, and most children have no long-term difficulties. The cutaneous findings in neonatal lupus include pink to red patches or plaques, predominantly in a periorbital location. The rash resolves with time, and if any residual skin finding remains, they are fine telangiectasias in the location of the patches with fine atrophy. The telangiectasias and atrophy tend to improve as the child enters adulthood.

Lupus panniculitis (lupus profundus) is a rare cutaneous manifestation of lupus. It manifests as a tender dermal nodule, more commonly in women. A large percentage of patients with lupus panniculitis have been reported to develop SLE. The overlying skin may appear slightly erythematous to hyperpigmented, but there is no appreciable surface change. The dermal nodules tend to slowly enlarge with time. The diagnosis can be made only by biopsy because the clinical picture is not specific. Biopsies of these dermal nodules are best performed with an excisional technique to obtain sufficient tissue for diagnosis. The inflammation is entirely confined to the subcutaneous tissue. The histologic differential diagnosis of lupus panniculitis is often between lupus and cutaneous T-cell panniculitis. The diagnosis requires the use of both clinical and histologic information. The histologic evaluation often requires immunohistochemical staining to help differentiate the lesions from those of other mimickers. Lesions of lupus panniculitis often heal with atrophic scarring.

Tumid lupus is a rare clinical variant of cutaneous lupus that typically manifests as a red dermal plaque on a sun-exposed surface of the skin. Clinically, it can appear similar to polymorphous light eruption, lymphoma, pseudolymphoma, or Jessner lymphocytic infiltrate. The plaques are exacerbated by ultraviolet light exposure. They are frequently asymptomatic to slightly tender but rarely pruritic. They tend to wax and wane, with the worst outbreaks occurring in the springtime and remissions in the winter. Histologically, the infiltrate has been found to be more of a $CD4^+$ T-cell infiltrate.

SYSTEMIC MANIFESTATIONS OF SYSTEMIC LUPUS ERYTHEMATOSUS

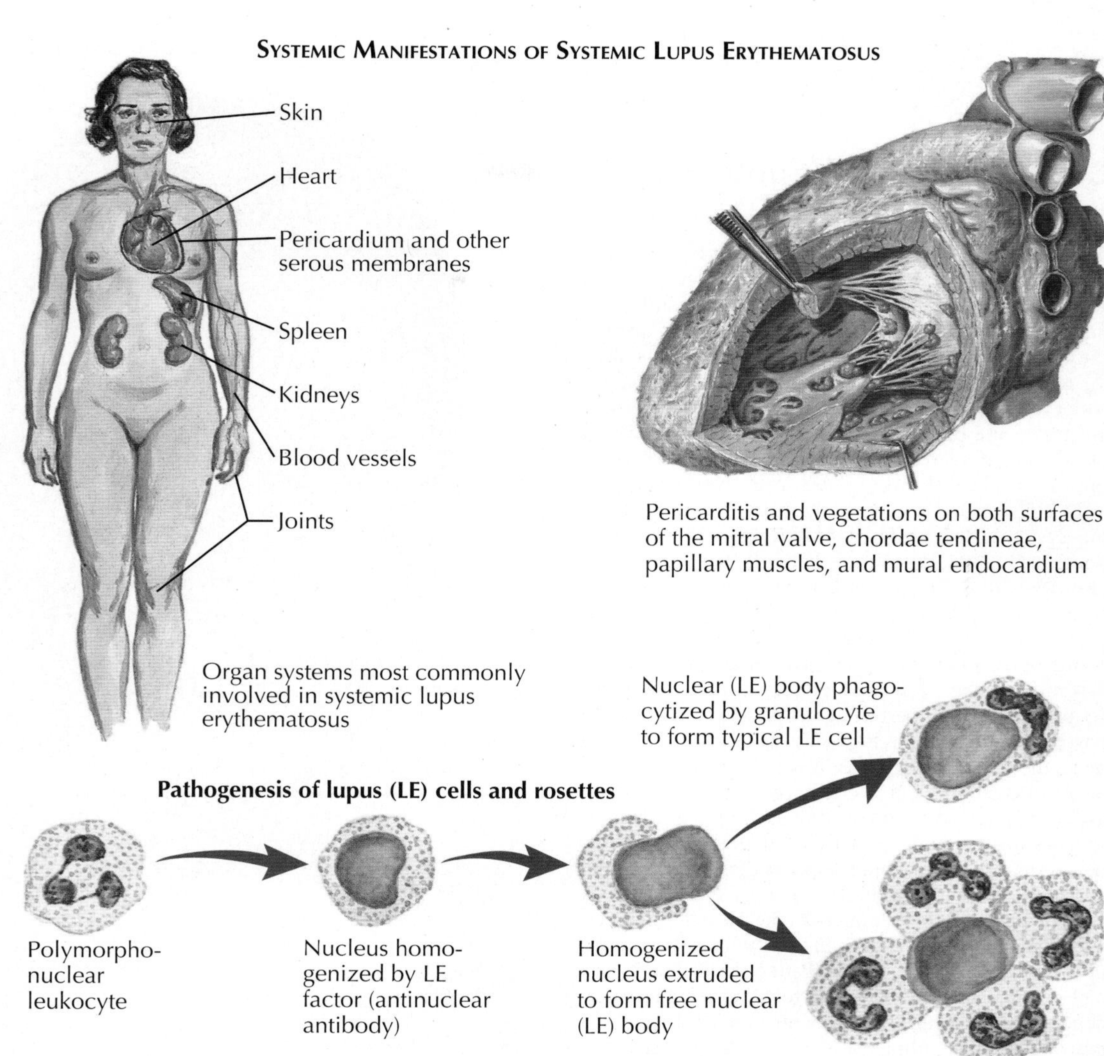

Organ systems most commonly involved in systemic lupus erythematosus

Pericarditis and vegetations on both surfaces of the mitral valve, chordae tendineae, papillary muscles, and mural endocardium

Pathogenesis of lupus (LE) cells and rosettes

Nuclear (LE) body phagocytized by granulocyte to form typical LE cell

Nuclear body encircled by granulocytes to form LE rosette

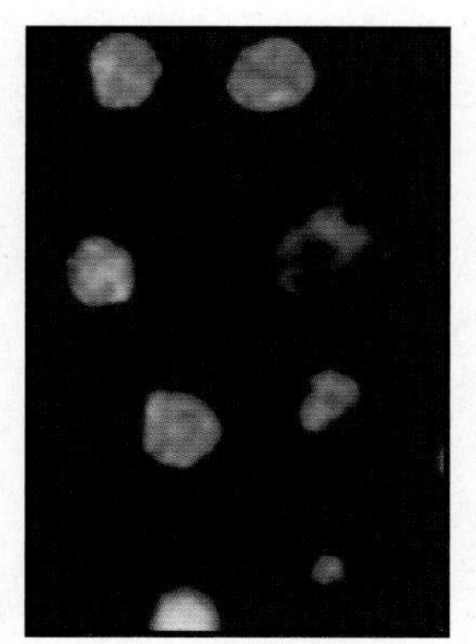

Antinuclear antibodies demonstrated by fluorescence

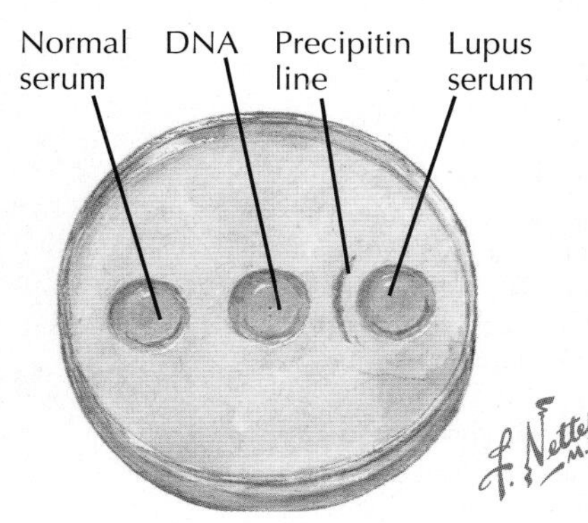

DNA antibodies demonstrated by precipitin test on agar plate

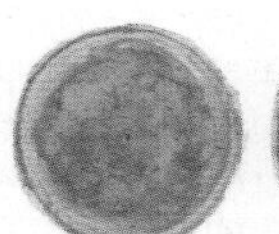

Hemagglutination of gamma globulin–coated red cells by SLE serum (tubes viewed from below). Latex agglutination test may also be done as for rheumatoid factor.

Lupus chilblains is a unique form of Raynaud phenomenon and is identical in clinical presentation to pernio. It may be that this is simply pernio occurring in a patient with lupus. Lupus chilblains and pernio typically manifest on the distal extremities, with the toes being the most commonly affected region. The patient develops tender, cold, purplish papules and plaques. The rash is exacerbated by cold and wet environments. Treatment includes keeping the regions dry and warm by avoiding cold and wet exposures. Patients diagnosed with pernio should undergo screening for lupus because a small percentage will be found to have lupus chilblains. Histologic evaluation of lupus chilblains shows a dense lymphocytic infiltrate with some areas of thrombosis of small vessels and a lymphocytic vasculitis.

The cutaneous findings seen in SLE are vast and can overlap with other forms of cutaneous lupus. Although the systemic findings are responsible for the morbidity and mortality, the cutaneous findings are often the presenting sign and can help make the diagnosis. The most

CUTANEOUS MANIFESTATIONS OF LUPUS

CUTANEOUS LUPUS (Continued)

important of the cutaneous skin findings in SLE is the malar rash. This rash manifests as a tender, pink-to-red plaque or patch on the cheeks and nose, mimicking the shape of a butterfly; hence it has been termed the butterfly rash of lupus. It is commonly mistaken for rosacea, and vice versa. Rosacea typically affects a wider area of skin and is associated with more telangiectasias and papulopustular lesions. The malar rash of lupus also spares the nasolabial fold, which is an important clinical finding and a discriminating objective discovery. It is typically more prominent during systemic flares of the underlying SLE, and patients can appear very ill. Patients are exquisitely photosensitive, and the rash is exacerbated by exposure to ultraviolet light.

Discoid lupus is also seen as a manifestation of systemic lupus, and it has the same clinical appearance as described earlier. Raynaud phenomenon is well described, and a high percentage of patients with SLE report those symptoms. Alopecia was long used to help make the diagnosis of lupus. It is no longer part of the diagnostic criteria, but it can have significant psychological effect on the patient. Nail and capillary nailfold changes can be seen. The true incidence of these findings is unknown. Nailfold telangiectasias and erythema are the two most common nail findings. Dermoscopy is an invaluable tool in helping evaluate the nailfolds. Nail pitting, ridging, and alterations in the color of the lunula have also been reported. Patients with lupus with nail changes have been found to have a higher incidence of mucosal ulcerations, which are another of the mucocutaneous findings of SLE. Livedo reticularis is a fishnet-like pattern found typically on the lower extremities; it is a nonspecific finding but has been commonly reported in lupus. It also occurs in many other skin and systemic diseases.

Pathogenesis: Scientists continue to unravel the pathologic basis of cutaneous lupus. Thus far no single mechanism has been discovered; cutaneous lupus is believed to be caused by a complex interaction between the environment (e.g., UV light, medications) and an individual's underlying immune system, leading to autoimmunity and autoantibody formation. The subtypes of cutaneous lupus likely have similar mechanisms of formation, but most certainly also have unique pathologic processes.

Histology: The histologic findings in all forms of lupus are similar, with specific forms having some unique findings. Most forms show an interface dermatitis with hydropic changes in the basilar layer of the epidermis. A superficial and deep periadnexal lymphocytic infiltrate is almost universally seen. Other connective tissue diseases (e.g., dermatomyositis) can have similar histologic findings. Discoid lupus may show scarring, atrophy, and follicular plugging along with these other findings. Lupus panniculitis is unique in that the inflammation is localized to the subcutaneous tissue. The diagnosis of lupus panniculitis is difficult and requires a host of special stains and clinical pathologic correlation.

Treatment: The treatment of cutaneous lupus is difficult and must be tailored to the patient and the specific form. Potent topical corticosteroids may work for a tiny lesion of discoid lupus, but they are not effective in lupus panniculitis. Universal treatment of cutaneous lupus requires sun protection and sunscreen use. Sun protection and sun avoidance work better than sunscreen. Any sunscreen used should be broad spectrum and specifically block in the UVA range, which is the most active form of ultraviolet light that exacerbates lupus. Smoking should be ceased immediately, and patients should be screened routinely by their family physician or rheumatologist for progression of the disease. Medications that are known to cause drug-induced lupus or exacerbate lupus should be discontinued.

Specific therapies for cutaneous lupus include oral prednisone and hydroxychloroquine or chloroquine as the typical first-line agents. If these are unsuccessful, quinacrine can be added. Other agents that have been reported to be effective include dapsone, isotretinoin, thalidomide, lenalidomide, mycophenolate mofetil, azathioprine, IV immunoglobulin (IVIG), and methotrexate. Targeting B-cell production of antibodies has been done with medications such as rituximab and belimumab. Janus kinase inhibitors have also shown some efficacy by decreasing IL-6 and IFN levels.

Neonatal lupus. Neonatal lupus is transient in nature and is caused by maternal antibodies that cross the placenta. Newborns are at risk for developing heart block. The cutaneous findings eventually resolve spontaneously.

Lupus erythematosus disseminatus

Lupus chilblains. Tender red to purple macules and papules on the feet. Exacerbated by cold and wet environments.

Cutis Laxa

Cutis laxa is an unusual skin disease with multisystem complications. It has highly characteristic cutaneous findings. Laxity of the skin is the hallmark of this disease. The skin becomes easily stretched, and there is little elastic rebound. As patients age, gravity alone can make the skin droop to a disfiguring degree. Some forms of cutis laxa are incompatible with life, and those affected die in infancy. Many variants of cutis laxa have been described. With the discovery of the responsible gene defects, the phenotypes of this disease seen clinically have been better defined on the genetic level. Acquired variants of cutis laxa have also been described.

Clinical Findings: Cutis laxa has no sex or racial predilection. The cutaneous hallmark of the disease is loose, hanging skin with a lack of elasticity. The skin is hyperextensible, meaning it can be pulled with little resistance; the normal return of the skin to its preexisting state is delayed. The skin in the axillae and groin folds is prominently affected, as is the facial skin. The face is said to take on a "hound dog" appearance. All skin is involved to varying degrees, but the effects are most noticeable in areas of the face and in the skin folds. The overlying epidermis is completely normal, and the adnexal structures are spared.

Internal manifestations are variable and are more common with the autosomal recessive forms of the disease. The pulmonary, cardiovascular, and gastrointestinal systems can be affected by fragmentation or loss of elastic tissue, leading to emphysema, aneurysms, and diverticula, respectively.

Those with the autosomal dominant form appear to have normal life spans, whereas those with the other variants have significantly shortened life spans secondary to severe systemic involvement.

Acquired cutis laxa can be caused by medications, infection, and lymphoproliferative neoplasms. It starts as an inflammatory skin rash that then develops loose skin and shows elastolysis on histology. It is most frequently seen on the trunk, sparing the acral regions. It can affect multiple organ systems.

Pathogenesis: Many modes of inheritance have been reported for cutis laxa, including autosomal recessive, autosomal dominant, and X-linked recessive forms. The X-linked form is now considered to be the same disease as Ehlers-Danlos syndrome IX. This form is caused by a defect in a copper-dependent adenosine triphosphatase protein found within the Golgi apparatus.

There are two autosomal recessive variants of cutis laxa. The autosomal recessive variant type I is extremely rare, and those afflicted typically die early in infancy from severe pulmonary and multisystem failure. This variant is caused by a defect in the *fibulin-5* gene *(FBLN5)*. The product of this gene is critical in producing functional elastic fibers. Its absence is incompatible with life. Type II autosomal recessive cutis laxa is more common. The genetic defect in type II cutis laxa has been determined to be a defect in the *ATPVOA2* or *ATPV1E1* genes. Patients with type II experience developmental delay and have varying amounts of joint laxity.

The most frequently seen form of cutis laxa is the autosomal dominant form, which is caused by a defect in the *elastin* gene *(ELN)*. Many different mutations in this gene have been described, and they lead to slightly different phenotypes of the disease.

All of these gene defects lead to abnormalities in the elastic fiber protein, resulting in elastolysis. Various defects lead to different irregularities in the elastic fibers, but the end result in all forms is seen clinically as cutis laxa.

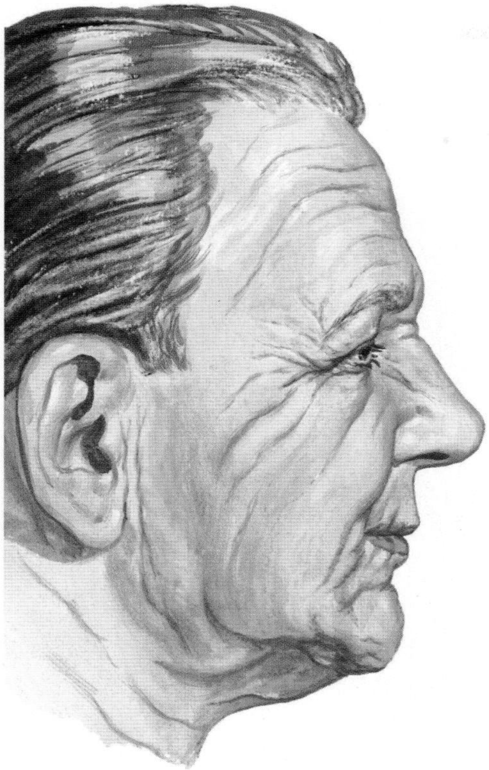

Cutis laxa. This rare disease is caused by the premature degeneration of elastic fibers. It manifests clinically with excessive sagging of the skin. The affected face may take on a "hound dog" appearance.

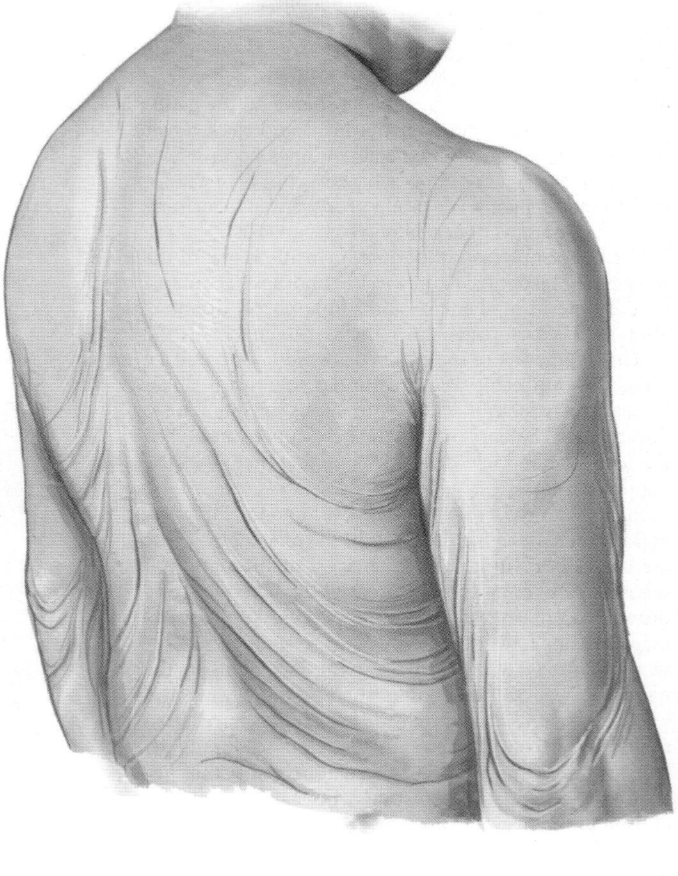

Cutis laxa is an inherited or acquired abnormality of elastic tissue. The skin becomes loose over time and hangs from the body. Large folds of redundant skin present on the trunk.

F. Netter M.D.
C. Machado M.D.
DaVanzo CMI

Histology: Histologic examination of skin biopsies from patients with cutis laxa reveals varying degrees of elastic fiber damage and/or loss. The best way to appreciate this is with special staining to highlight elastic tissue. In some cases, there is a complete loss of elastic fibers; in others, fragmented and reduced amounts of elastic tissue are seen.

Treatment: The main goal of therapy is to screen for underlying cardiac, neurologic, or gastrointestinal abnormalities for the possibility of aortic aneurysm, developmental delay, or gastrointestinal diverticula formation. Long-term surveillance is required. No medication can reverse the genetic defect, and no gene replacement therapy is yet available. Excessive skin can be surgically removed to improve functionality and cosmesis.

DERMATOMYOSITIS

Dermatomyositis is a chronic connective tissue disease that can be associated with an underlying internal malignancy. This connective tissue disease shares similarities with polymyositis, but the latter has no cutaneous findings. Up to one-third of patients with dermatomyositis have an underlying malignancy. The myositis is often prominent and manifests as tenderness and weakness of the proximal muscle groups. The pelvic and shoulder girdle muscles are the most commonly affected. Dermatomyositis sine myositis is a well-recognized variant that has only the cutaneous findings; evidence of muscle involvement is absent.

Clinical Findings: Dermatomyositis has a bimodal age of onset, with the most common form occurring in the female adult population, usually between the ages of 45 and 60 years, and a smaller peak in childhood at about 10 to 15 years of age. Black individuals have a higher incidence than any other race. Dermatomyositis has an insidious onset, with the development of proximal muscle weakness in association with various dermatologic findings. Skin findings start slowly and are nonspecific at first. Usually, there is some mild erythema on the hands and sun-exposed regions of the head and neck. Over time, the more typical cutaneous findings become evident. Pruritus is a common symptom, and patients not infrequently report severe scalp pruritus well before any signs or symptoms of dermatomyositis appear.

The heliotrope rash of dermatomyositis is one of the most easily recognized and specific findings. It is manifested by periorbital edema and a light purple discoloration of the periorbital skin. The skin is tender to the touch. Hyperemia of the nail beds and dilated capillary loops are noticeable and are similar to those seen in progressive systemic sclerosis or lupus erythematous. The dilated capillary loops are best appreciated with the use of a handheld dermatoscope that magnifies the region of interest.

Purplish to red, scaly papules develop on the dorsum of the hands overlying the joints of the phalanges. These are not Heberden nodes, which are a manifestation of osteoarthritis seen as dermal swellings overlying the distal interphalangeal joints. The papules seen in dermatomyositis have been termed *Gottron papules*. Gottron papules may be seen overlying any joint on the hands, as well as other joints such as the elbows and knees. The skin findings on the dorsal hands have led to the term "mechanic's hands." This refers to the ragged appearance of the hands in dermatomyositis; they resemble the hands of someone who has experienced chronic trauma, abrasions, and erosions.

The "shawl sign" is a cutaneous finding seen on the upper back and chest named for its location on the body. The skin has poikilodermatous macules and patches. The amount of skin atrophy varies, with telangiectasias, mottled hyperpigmentation and hypopigmentation, and erythema of the involved region.

Patients with dermatomyositis also report photosensitivity and notice a flare of their skin disease with ultraviolet light exposure. Children with dermatomyositis are much more prone to develop calcinosis cutis than their adult counterparts, and approximately 50% of all children with dermatomyositis develop this feature. Calcinosis cutis manifests as tender dermal nodules or plaques of calcification along the muscle fascia. Leukocytoclastic vasculitis also is seen much more frequently in juvenile dermatomyositis than in the adult form.

Dermatomyositis is a multisystem disorder. Diagnostic criteria have been established by the American College of Rheumatology. They are based on the presence of clinical, laboratory, and histologic findings. Not all patients have all aspects of the disease, and the diagnosis is based on the number of criteria fulfilled.

Inflammation of the proximal muscle groups has been well described. Patients often report difficulty in standing from a sitting position or in raising their hands above their heads. Patients have elevated serum concentrations of creatinine kinase, aldolase, and lactate dehydrogenase. This is indicative of muscle

MANIFESTATIONS OF DERMATOMYOSITIS

Weakness of central muscle groups evidenced by difficulty in climbing stairs, rising from chairs, and combing hair

Weakness of diaphragm and intercostal muscle causes respiratory insufficiency or failure.

Gottron papules. Erythematous or violaceous, scaly papules on dorsum of interphalangeal joints

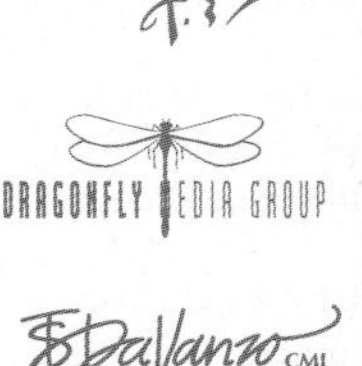

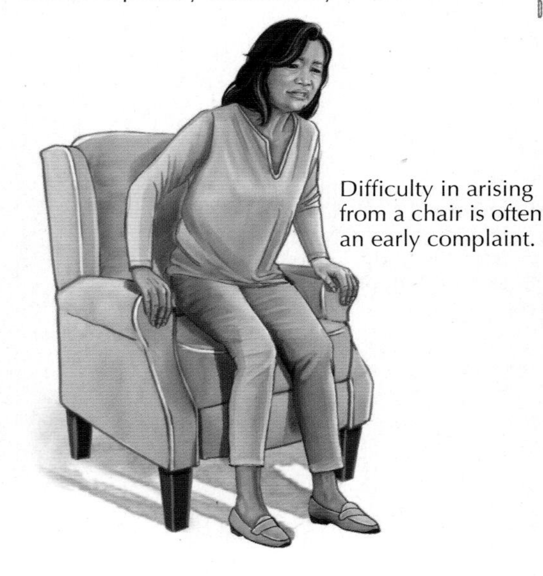

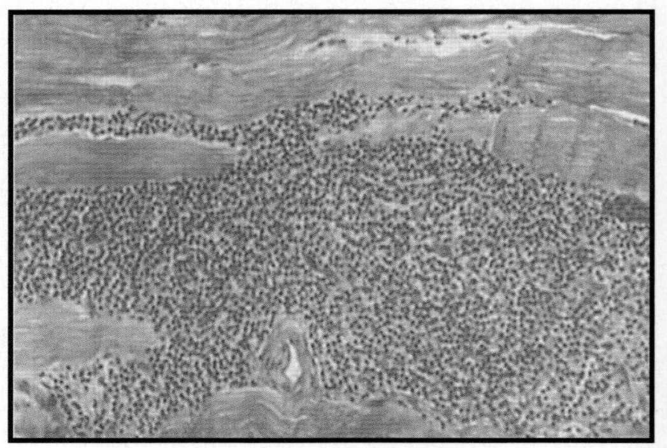

Longitudinal section of muscle showing intense inflammatory infiltration plus degeneration and disruption of muscle fibers

DERMATOMYOSITIS (Continued)

inflammation and breakdown. An electromyogram (EMG) can be used to evaluate the weakness and to differentiate a nerve origin from a muscle origin. Muscle biopsy, most commonly of the deltoid muscle, shows active inflammation on histologic examination.

This disease can rarely manifest with severe, diffuse interstitial pulmonary fibrosis. Patients with pulmonary fibrosis most often test positive for the anti-Jo1 antibody. Anti-Jo1 antibodies have been found to be targeted against the histidyl–transfer RNA synthetase protein. Overall, it is an uncommon finding except in patients with dermatomyositis with pulmonary disease. More than 75% of patients with dermatomyositis test positive for ANAs. Those with malignancy-associated dermatomyositis typically do not develop pulmonary fibrosis, and those with pulmonary fibrosis do not develop a malignancy.

The malignancy most commonly associated with dermatomyositis is ovarian cancer. Many other malignancies have been seen in association with dermatomyositis, including lymphoma and breast, lung, and gastric cancers. Malignancy is seen before the onset of the rash in about one-third of the cases, concurrently with the rash in one-third, and within 2 years after diagnosis of the dermatomyositis in one-third. After the diagnosis of dermatomyositis, it is imperative to search for an underlying malignancy and to perform age-appropriate cancer screening. Individuals with antibodies against TIF-1γ have been shown to be at a higher risk for malignancy. Childhood dermatomyositis is rarely associated with an underlying malignancy.

Individuals with dermatomyositis sine myositis have only cutaneous findings. This diagnosis should be reserved for individuals with no signs of muscle involvement as ruled out by lab testing, magnetic resonance imaging, EMG, and muscle biopsy. These individuals are more likely to have Mi-2 antibodies.

Many medications have been shown to cause drug-induced dermatomyositis. The most common class of medications is the statins. Prompt recognition and discontinuation of the offending agent is paramount.

Pathogenesis: The exact etiology of dermatomyositis is unknown. It has been theorized to occur secondary to abnormalities in the humoral immune system. The precise mechanism is under intense research.

Histology: Histologic examination of a skin biopsy specimen shows an interface lymphocytic dermatitis. Hydropic change is seen scattered along the basilar cell layer. The epidermis has varying degrees of atrophy. A superficial and deep periadnexal lymphocytic infiltrate is common. The presence of dermal mucin in abundance is another histologic clue to the diagnosis. A muscle biopsy often shows atrophy of the involved muscle with a dense lymphocytic infiltrate.

Treatment: There is no known cure for dermatomyositis, although some cases spontaneously remit. Cases associated with an underlying malignancy have been shown to go into full remission with cure of the underlying cancer. Relapse of dermatomyositis in these patients should prompt the clinician to search for a recurrence of the malignancy. Initial treatment is usually with prednisone, which acts as a nonspecific immunosuppressant. The addition of a steroid-sparing agent is almost always needed to avoid the long-term side effects of prednisone. Some patients require a smaller dose of prednisone along with a steroid-sparing agent to keep the disease at bay. Many steroid-sparing agents have been used, including hydroxychloroquine, quinacrine, cyclosporine, IVIG, rituximab, azathioprine, methotrexate, and Janus kinase inhibitors, all with variable success. Combination therapy is the norm.

The use of sun protection and sunscreen cannot be overemphasized. Topical corticosteroids help relieve the itching and decrease some of the redness. The treatment of juvenile dermatomyositis is similar. It is believed to have a better prognosis because few cases are associated with an underlying cancer. It is thought that early treatment of juvenile dermatomyositis decreases the risk of developing severe calcinosis cutis during the course of the disease.

CUTANEOUS AND LABORATORY FINDINGS IN DERMATOMYOSITIS

Head in flexed position due to proximal muscle weakness

Difficulty in swallowing due to esophageal weakness

Edema and heliotrope discoloration of eyelids; erythematous rash

Gottron papules. Erythematous, nodular eruption on fingers.

Atrophy of muscle fibers and lymphocyte infiltration (muscle biopsy)

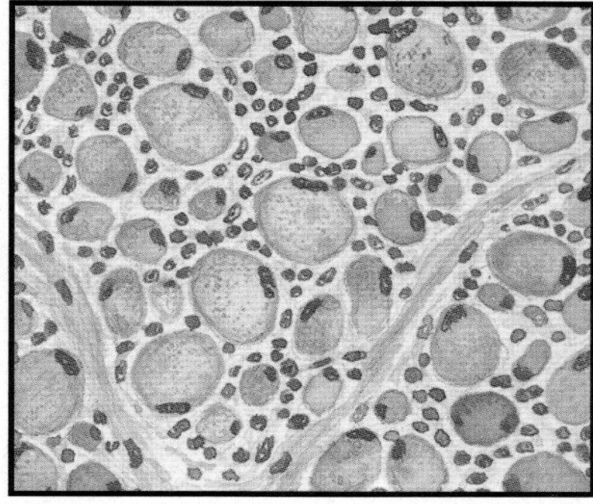

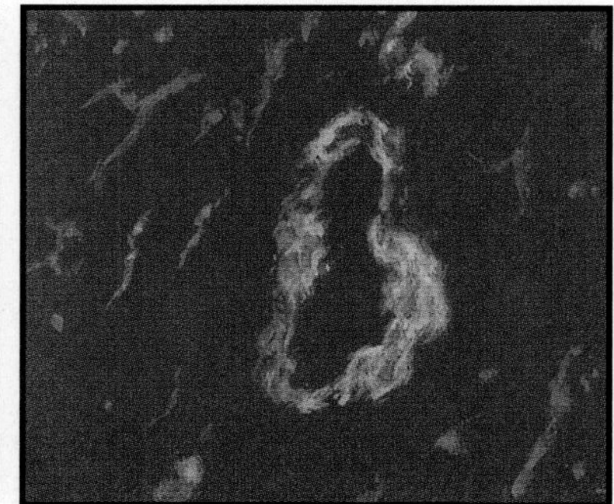

Immunoglobulin deposition in blood vessel of muscle (immunofluorescence)

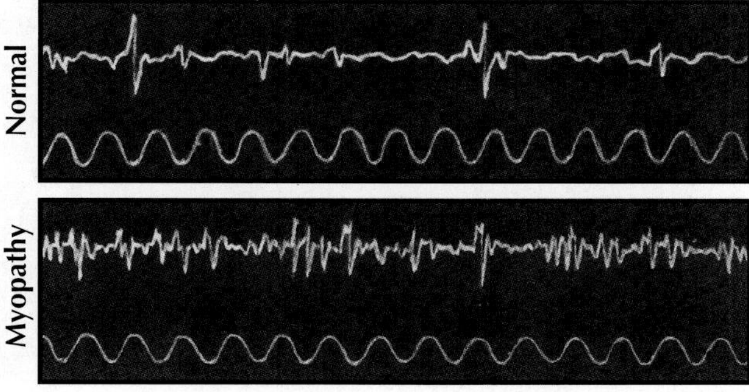

Electromyogram shows fibrillations

Laboratory findings

1. Nonspecific hypergammaglobulinemia; low incidence of antinuclear antibodies and rheumatoid factor
2. Elevated serum enzymes. creatine phosphokinase (CPK), aldolase, and aspartate amine transferase (AST, SGOT)
3. Elevated urinary creatine and myoglobulin levels

DISSEMINATED INTRAVASCULAR COAGULATION

Disseminated intravascular coagulation (DIC) is a serious, life-threatening condition of the blood clotting system that can be caused by myriad insults to the body. It has a grave prognosis unless caught and treated early in the course of disease. Skin manifestations occur early and continue to progress unless the patient recovers. The skin lesions may lead to gangrene and secondary infection, further worsening the prognosis. DIC is seen as an end-stage process, caused by the consumption of blood clotting factors, that results in uncontrolled clotting and bleeding occurring simultaneously.

Clinical Findings: DIC occurs in males and females with equal incidence and has no racial or ethnic predilection. DIC has a wide range of cutaneous findings. Patients are often gravely ill and hospitalized in a critical care setting. A small subset of patients with early DIC present with cutaneous findings. The remainder of patients are first diagnosed with DIC and eventually develop cutaneous manifestations. The initial cutaneous clinical appearance is that of small petechiae that enlarge and coalesce into large macules and plaques of erythema. Bleeding is often noted from IV sites. There may be a livedo reticularis pattern to the extremities. This fishnet-like appearance can be seen in other dermatologic conditions. The petechiae quickly convert to purpuric plaques. Ulceration, necrosis, and hemorrhagic blister formation are commonly seen in the areas of involvement. As the disease progresses, gangrene may develop in the affected areas as the blood flow to the skin is significantly decreased because of clotting of various components of the vascular system. Gangrene may lead to secondary infection. The finding of gangrene indicates a grave prognosis, and most of these patients do not survive. If DIC is treated aggressively and early, the survival rate is still only 40% to 50% at best.

Pathogenesis: DIC is a consumptive coagulopathy. The initial event that starts the reaction can be multifactorial. The most common causes of DIC are underlying malignancy (especially leukemia), severe traumatic events, sepsis, and obstetric complications. Rocky Mountain spotted fever and meningococcemia are two infections known to induce DIC. Each of these associated conditions has its own specific clinical setting. As DIC progresses, uncontrollable clotting and bleeding coexist, and patients often succumb to infection, thrombosis, or exsanguination. Thrombocytopenia is a common laboratory finding, as is an elevation of the bleeding time, prothrombin time, and partial thromboplastin time. Fibrinogen is consumed, leading to an increase in fibrin degradation metabolites.

DIC may be subdivided into predominantly hemorrhagic and predominantly thrombotic types, although overlapping features of both occur in all cases. An inciting event such as massive trauma or infection initiates the clotting cascade in which the clotting factors are used up (or lost, in cases of severe bleeding) faster than they can be replaced. This sets off a cascade of events within the clotting system that results in consumption of all the factors used in clotting, leading to thrombosis and hemorrhage.

Histology: Examination of skin biopsies shows necrosis of the overlying epidermis and parts of the dermis. Thrombosis of the small veins and arterioles is seen, as is widespread hemorrhage. In cases of sepsis-induced DIC, evidence of the causative organism may be found in the biopsy specimen.

Treatment: Treatment requires prompt recognition of the condition and immediate supportive care. Treatment of the underlying infection is a must, and in trauma-induced cases, bleeding must be stopped and coagulation factors replaced as they are lost. The main component of therapy is treatment of the underlying cause that has precipitated the DIC event. The treatment of DIC is complicated and should be undertaken in a critical care setting. Many agents are used to help decrease thrombosis and replace lost clotting factors. A fine balance must be maintained between clotting and thrombosis. Patients with severe DIC have a poor prognosis. The skin is best treated with excellent wound care as the patient is treated for their underlying medical conditions.

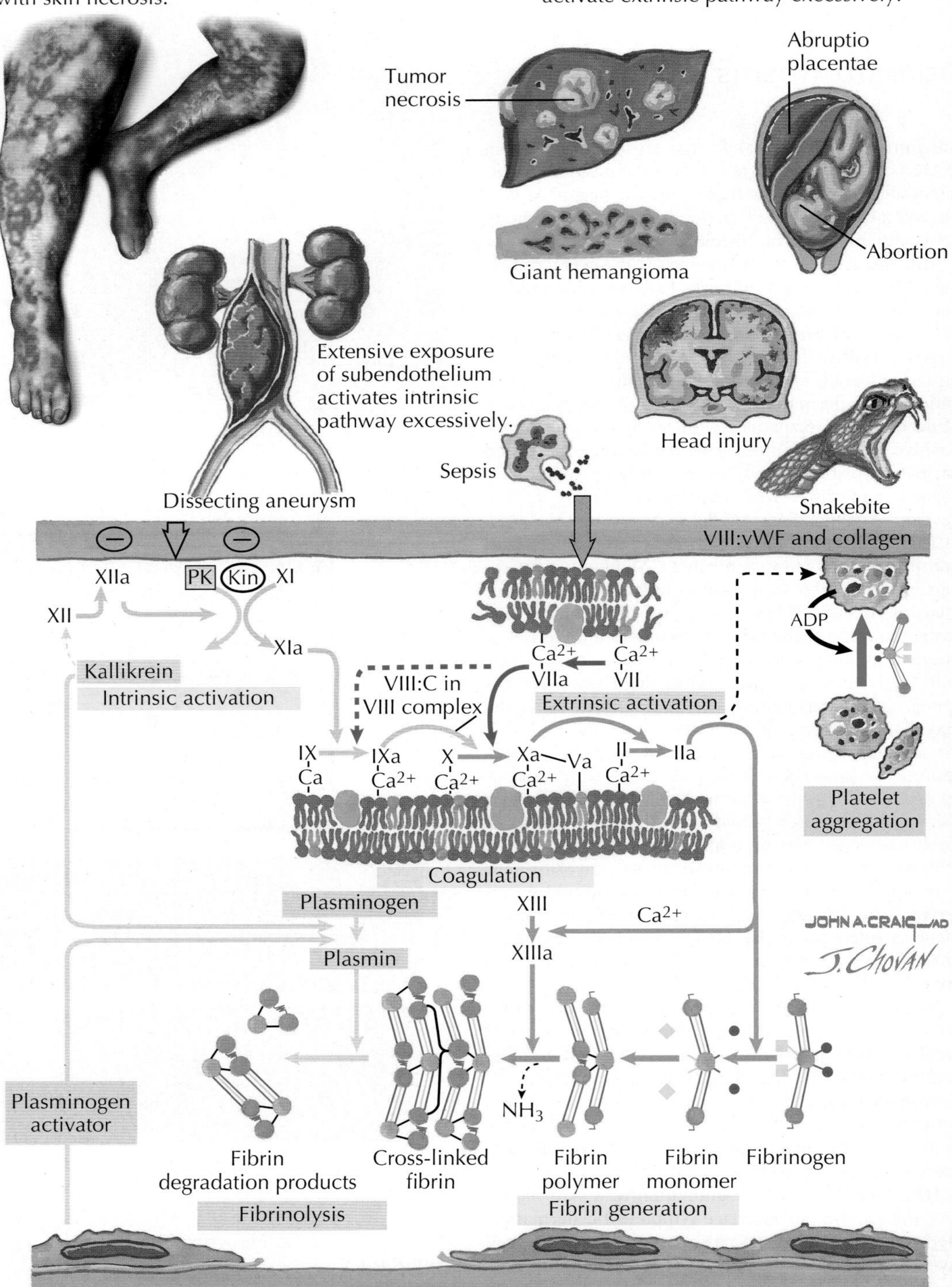

Elastosis Perforans Serpiginosa

Elastosis perforans serpiginosa is classified as a perforating skin disorder. This rare cutaneous eruption is believed to be caused by an abnormal expulsion of fragmented elastic fibers from the dermis. The elastic fibers penetrate the surface of the epidermis and manifest as an unusual serpiginous eruption. It has been seen as an isolated finding but also in association with many underlying conditions, including Down syndrome, Ehlers-Danlos syndrome, and Marfan syndrome.

Clinical Findings: Elastosis perforans serpiginosa is a rare cutaneous perforating skin disease. It is much more commonly seen in the young adult population, and it has a significant male predominance, with a ratio of 4:1 to 5:1. Elastosis perforans serpiginosa is seen equally in all races. The condition has been most often reported on the neck. The eruption typically begins as small red papules with an excoriated or slightly ulcerated surface. Initially, mild pruritus is the main symptom. The rash is seldom painful or uncomfortable. Over time, the papules coalesce into serpiginous, "wandering" eruptions. They can be annular or semicircular, often in bizarre configurations. The rash runs a waxing and waning course, but most cases resolve spontaneously with or without therapy. Resolution on average occurs within 6 months, but cases lasting up to 5 years have been reported in the literature. Most cases are solitary in nature. Patients with underlying Down syndrome may have only one lesion or widespread cutaneous involvement. It has been estimated that up to 1% of patients with Down syndrome will develop evidence of this rash over the course of their lifetime. Approximately 33% of cases of elastosis perforans serpiginosa are associated with an underlying disorder. An autosomal dominant pattern of inheritance has been described in a small number of cases, independent of any underlying conditions. The medication penicillamine has long been known to cause abnormalities of elastic fibers, and use of this medication has been shown to induce an eruption resembling elastosis perforans serpiginosa.

Individuals with underlying connective tissue disease such as Marfan syndrome, cutis laxa, and Ehlers-Danlos have been shown to have a higher incidence of elastosis perforans serpiginosa.

As the lesions progress, the epidermis ulcerates in pinpoint regions and the underlying fragmentized and abnormal elastic tissue extrudes. The areas may become more pruritic over time, and occasionally they are slightly tender. Most are asymptomatic. The appearance is most concerning for the patient and family members.

Pathogenesis: The cutaneous eruption is caused by the transepidermal extrusion of abnormally fragmented elastic fibers. The abnormal fibers perforate through the epidermis and cause the skin manifestations. The reason for the abnormality in the elastic fibers has yet to be determined, except in cases induced by penicillamine. Penicillamine has been shown to disrupt proper formation of elastic tissue. The abnormally formed fibers are then extruded from the dermis.

Histology: Abnormally fragmented eosinophilic elastic tissue can be appreciated on routine hematoxylin and eosin staining. Special elastic tissue stains can be used to better isolate and appreciate the elastic tissue. Examination of biopsy specimens shows an isolated area of acanthotic epidermis in which a passageway has formed. The passage begins in the superficial dermis and leads to the surface of the epidermis. This is filled with the abnormal elastic tissue, a few histiocytes, and an occasional giant cell. Early biopsies can show a cap of keratin overlying the passageway.

Treatment: Many therapies have been attempted, and their use is anecdotal at best. There have been no randomized, prospective, placebo-controlled trials for the treatment of this eruption. Many destructive modalities have been attempted with varying success. Cryotherapy has the most information to support its use, but ablative carbon dioxide lasers have also been used with good results. Topical retinoids and photodynamic therapy have been shown to be beneficial in case reports. No therapy is required because these eruptions almost always spontaneously remit.

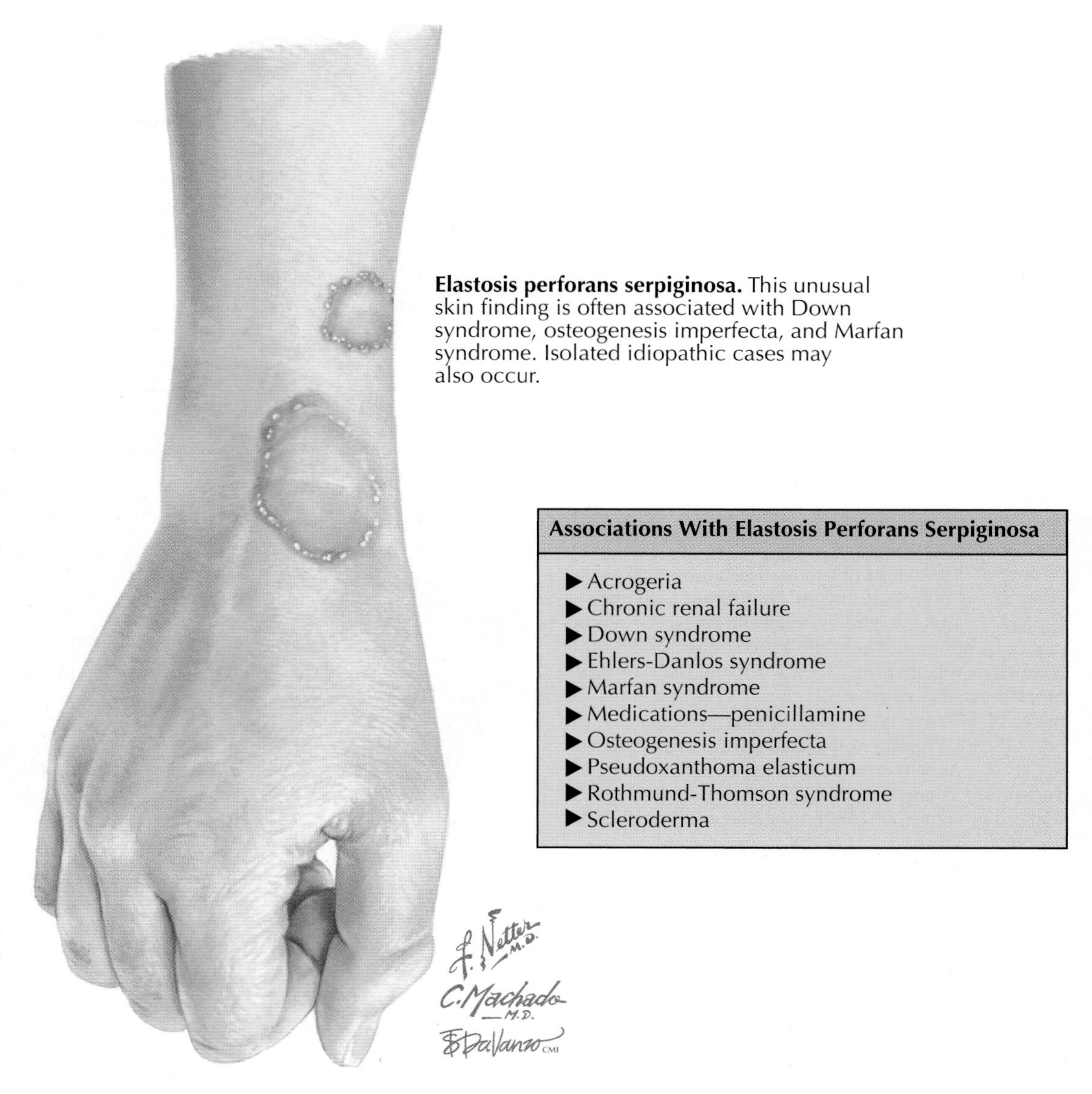

Elastosis perforans serpiginosa. This unusual skin finding is often associated with Down syndrome, osteogenesis imperfecta, and Marfan syndrome. Isolated idiopathic cases may also occur.

Associations With Elastosis Perforans Serpiginosa
▶ Acrogeria
▶ Chronic renal failure
▶ Down syndrome
▶ Ehlers-Danlos syndrome
▶ Marfan syndrome
▶ Medications—penicillamine
▶ Osteogenesis imperfecta
▶ Pseudoxanthoma elasticum
▶ Rothmund-Thomson syndrome
▶ Scleroderma

Dense connective tissue

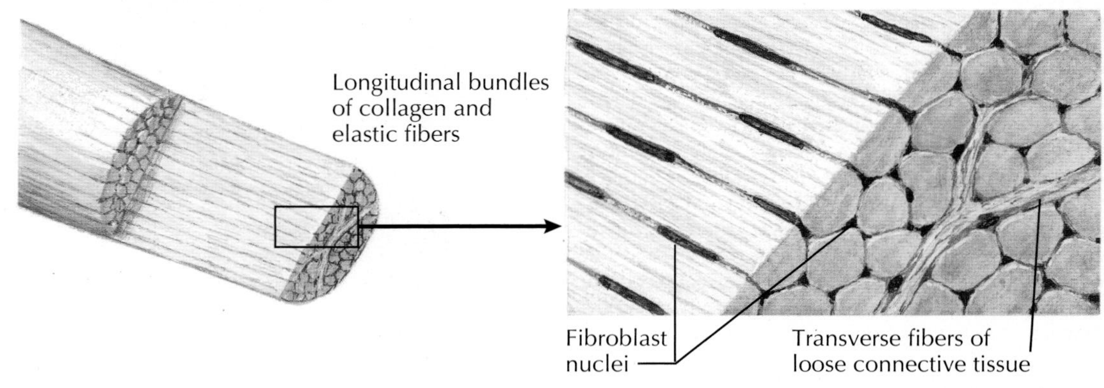

Congenital Hyperlipoproteinemia

Fasting total serum cholesterol mg/100 mL — Normal range

Fasting total serum phospholipid mg/100 mL — Normal range

Fasting total serum neutral fat mg/100 mL — or higher — Normal range

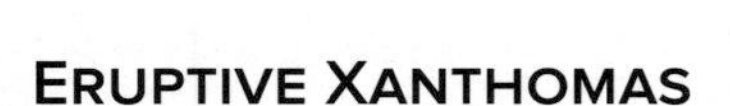

ERUPTIVE XANTHOMAS

Abnormal accumulation of triglycerides in various tissues, including the skin, may lead to the cutaneous finding of eruptive xanthomas. The xanthomatous diseases are a diverse group of conditions with unique clinical, laboratory, and systemic findings. An abnormality in lipid and cholesterol metabolism links these conditions together. Fatty acids provide the body with more than 40% of its daily energy requirements. The majority of fatty acids are supplied directly by the normal diet. Proteins and carbohydrates, when present in excess, can be converted to triglycerides to be stored as a future energy source. This process makes up the remaining source of free fatty acids and triglycerides supplied to the body.

Normal metabolism of triglycerides occurs through complex biochemical pathways. Triglycerides are converted into free fatty acids, which are broken down into acetyl-coenzyme A (acetyl-CoA). Acetyl-CoA then enters the Krebs cycle to be oxidized and turned into adenosine triphosphate (ATP), one of the main forms of energy used in cellular processes.

Ingested triglycerides are broken down into free fatty acids in the lumen of the intestine by bile acids. The free fatty acids are then transported across the gut lining as chylomicrons. This process is very rapid and occurs within 6 hours after eating. The chylomicrons are absorbed by many tissues and are converted back into free fatty acids and glycerol by the enzyme lipoprotein lipase. The free fatty acids can be converted to acetyl-CoA, converted to triglyceride, and stored as an energy source for later use or used to make various phospholipids. The storage of triglycerides for future energy use is ideal because it yields higher amounts of energy than either proteins or carbohydrates. Triglycerides can yield 9 kcal/g of energy, whereas proteins and carbohydrates produce about 4 kcal/g. This is an efficient means of storing energy. Abnormalities in the production, breakdown, or storage of triglycerides may lead to complications resulting in cutaneous and systemic findings.

Eruptive xanthomas are one of the cutaneous findings caused by an abnormality in lipid metabolism. They can be caused by various familial hyperlipoproteinemias (types I, III, and V), by medications, or as a complication of diabetes. The cutaneous findings are identical in all of these conditions. Eruptive xanthomas should not be confused with tuberoeruptive, tendinous, or planar xanthomas; those conditions have different biochemical bases and other unique systemic features. Treatment of eruptive xanthomas requires a team approach including endocrinology, cardiology, and dermatology specialists.

LPL or apo CII deficiency: eruptive xanthomas of cheek, chin, ear, and palate

Creamy serum

Hepatosplenomegaly

F. Netter M.D.

Paul Kim

Umbilicated eruptive xanthomas of buttocks, thighs, and scrotum. Yellowish papules with some slight surrounding erythema

Clinical Findings: Eruptive xanthomas have a rapid eruptive onset (hours to a few days). The most common location is the buttocks, but these eruptions can be seen anywhere on the body, including the mucous membranes. They have a predilection for the extensor surfaces of the skin. They appear as yellow to slightly red-orange, dome-shaped papules with an erythematous base. Patients often report mild pruritus, but occasionally describe a painful sensation when the lesions are palpated. Eruptive xanthomas are more commonly seen in adulthood. There are no racial or sex differences in incidence.

Patients diagnosed with eruptive xanthomas caused by a deficiency in the enzyme lipoprotein lipase are classified as having type I hyperlipoproteinemia. This is a rare form of hyperlipoproteinemia with onset in childhood. Systemic involvement is significant, with recurrent bouts of pancreatitis and hepatosplenomegaly. These patients have extremely elevated triglyceride and chylomicron levels but normal cholesterol levels. The eye may also be affected by lipemia retinalis. Lipemia retinalis can be seen only by funduscopic examination. Vision is typically normal, and the patient is unaware of any eye

ACQUIRED HYPERLIPOPROTEINEMIA

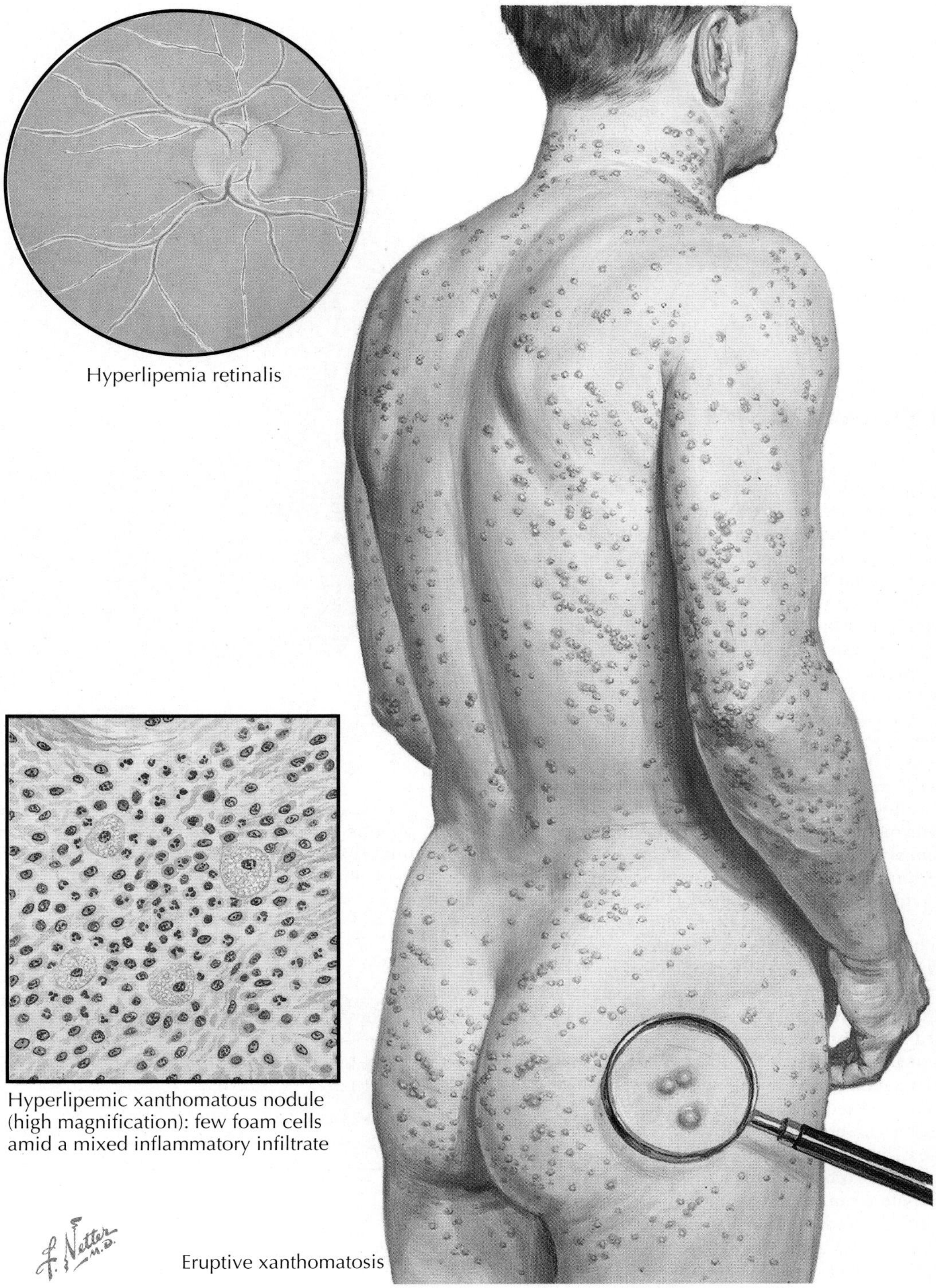

Hyperlipemia retinalis

Hyperlipemic xanthomatous nodule (high magnification): few foam cells amid a mixed inflammatory infiltrate

Eruptive xanthomatosis

ERUPTIVE XANTHOMAS (Continued)

abnormalities. The blood vessels within the eye have a creamy white color because of the excess lipid in the bloodstream. The arteries and veins are equally affected, and the only way to differentiate the two is by comparing the caliber of the vessel. The arterial light reflex is lost. The vessels appear flat, and the rest of the fundus is a uniform creamy color. Lipoprotein lipase enzyme activity can be measured, and this test is used to help diagnosis type I hyperlipoproteinemia. Eruptive xanthomas can also be seen as part of hyperlipoproteinemia type III (familial dysbetalipoproteinemia) and hyperlipoproteinemia type V. Type III is caused by a defect in the *APOE* gene, which encodes the apolipoprotein E protein. This protein is particularly important in clearing chylomicrons and intermediate-density lipoproteins.

Multiple medications have been implicated in the production of hypertriglyceridemia. They include isotretinoin, glucocorticoids, cyclosporine, olanzapine, protease inhibitors (especially ritonavir), and indomethacin. Alcohol abuse can also be a cause of hypertriglyceridemia. Patients presenting with eruptive xanthomas who are taking any of these medications should have the medication discontinued or another substituted and should be reevaluated after treatment.

Diabetes is the most common cause of hypertriglyceridemia and is probably also the most common cause of eruptive xanthomas. Insulin is required for normal functioning of the lipoprotein lipase enzyme. Patients with diabetes who are deficient in insulin have lower activity levels of lipoprotein lipase and increased levels of chylomicrons and triglycerides as a result.

On laboratory evaluation, the patient has triglyceride levels that are extremely elevated, in the range of 2000 mg/dL, sometimes even surpassing the laboratory's ability to quantify it. If a sample of blood is centrifuged for a few minutes, the white to creamy-colored triglycerides will become evident and will take up a considerable amount of the specimen. On occasion, there are so many triglycerides present that the blood sample is a light creamy color even before centrifugation.

Pathogenesis: The varying conditions that can manifest with eruptive xanthomas all have unique mechanisms of causing hypertriglyceridemia. The final common pathway in the pathogenesis of eruptive xanthomas is the presence of significantly elevated triglyceride levels in the bloodstream.

Histology: The histologic findings from biopsies of early lesions of eruptive xanthomas can mimic those of granuloma annulare. Neutrophils can be evident during the formation of an eruptive xanthoma. The neutrophilic infiltrate lessens and disappears once the lesion has had time to establish itself. The biopsy specimen should be taken from an established lesion (one that has been present for a day or two) so that more characteristic findings will be seen. Foam cells are present with a stippled cytoplasm. The number of foam cells is not as prominent as in tuberous or tendinous xanthomas. One unique finding is the presence of extracellular lipid, which is seen between bundles of collagen.

Treatment: The main goal of therapy is to return the triglyceride level back to a normal range. Medications that can cause hypertriglyceridemia should be discontinued. Underlying diabetes must be treated aggressively to get better control of glucose metabolism and insulin requirements. Patients with familial causes need to institute dietary changes (to avoid medium-chain triglycerides), increase their activity level, and take triglyceride-lowering medications. These medications can be used for all causes of hypertriglyceridemia. The medications most commonly used to lower triglyceride levels are niacin, fenofibrate, and gemfibrozil. Individuals are at increased risk of developing atherosclerosis and coronary heart disease as well as pancreatitis if not treated. The skin findings will spontaneously remit once the triglyceride level returns to the normal range.

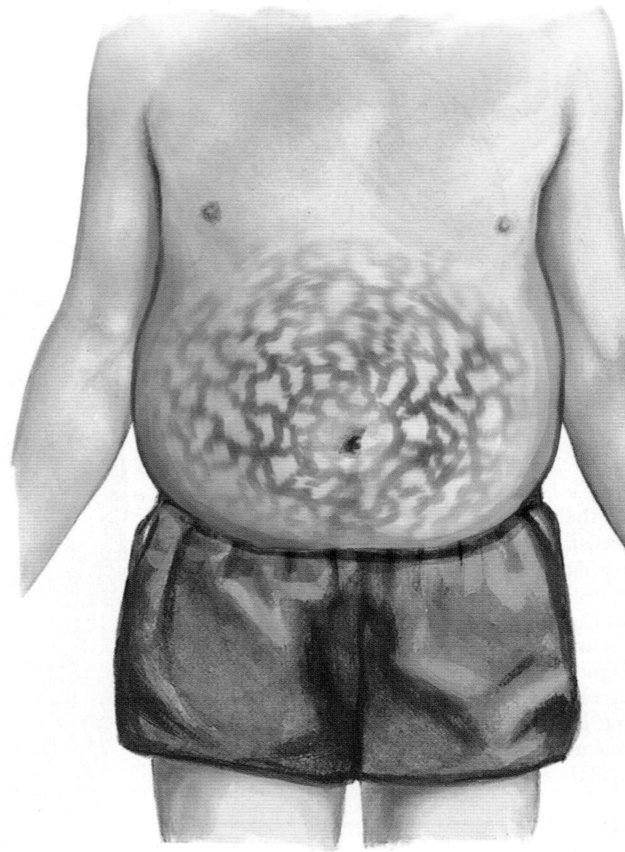

Erythema Ab Igne

Erythema ab igne is an unusual rash that can develop secondary to chronic exposure to an exogenous heat source. The name is derived from the Latin phrase meaning "redness from the fire." It has a clinically characteristic pattern. The differential diagnosis is limited. For unknown reasons, not all persons exposed to heat sources develop erythema ab igne. Many patients develop the rash without even knowing of its existence. Reported causes have included hot water bottles, heating blankets, heaters, and laptop computers. Essentially any exogenous heat source can precipitate this reaction. Erythema ab igne has also been called "roasted skin" or "toasted skin" syndrome. The exact temperature needed for the reaction to occur is unknown. It does not occur from hot tub use, most likely because the triggers of erythema ab igne are at temperatures higher than those of most hot tubs.

Clinical Findings: This condition can be seen in individuals of any race and sex. The initiating factor is an exogenous heat source that is in approximation or applied to the skin. The heat source exposure is typically chronic and repetitive. Patients often notice a fine, lacy, red-brown reticulated macule or patch. Occasionally, no inflammatory phase is noticed, only a reticulated hyperpigmentation of the skin. Some patients do not realize that the rash is located on skin in direct approximation to a heat source. The lower back is a commonly affected area, secondary to the use of heating blankets or bottles to help treat chronic lower back pain. There have been many reports of erythema ab igne from exposures to all sorts of heat sources. Laptop computers can release a substantial amount of energy as infrared radiation; long-term use of a laptop computer in direct approximation to the skin (e.g., anterior thighs) may cause erythema ab igne. The diagnosis is typically made by clinical examination and history. Patients often need to be asked whether they have been using a heating device or consistently using a laptop computer, because the correlation is not evident to them. The development of actinic keratosis or squamous cell carcinoma within the areas of erythema ab igne has rarely been reported.

Pathogenesis: Erythema ab igne is caused by the direct effects of heat on the skin. The temperature required has not been precisely defined, but the range of 43°C to 47°C seems to be most likely. In any case, repeated exposure to subthermal burning temperatures is required. More frequent and longer exposures seem to increase the risk of development. The exact mechanism by which the rash develops is unknown.

The abdomen, lower back, and legs are most frequently affected.

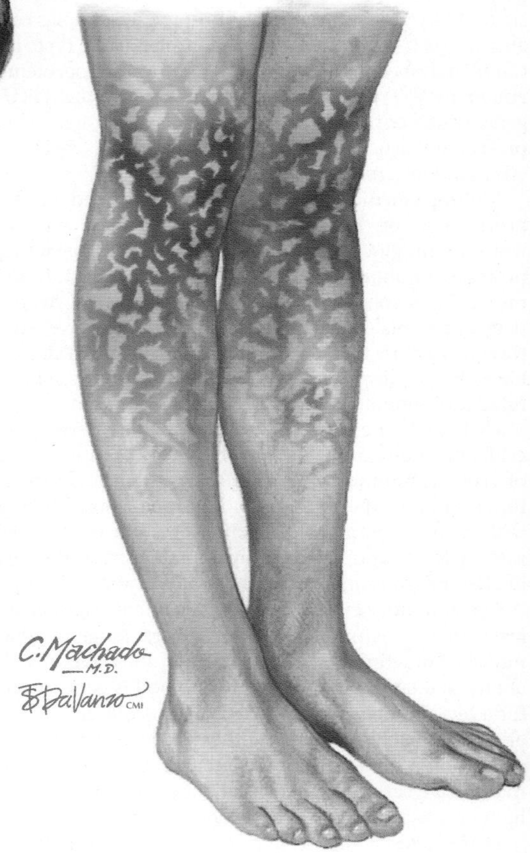

Also known as "toasted skin syndrome," erythema ab igne is caused by excessive heat transfer to the underlying skin. Hot water bottles and heating pads are most commonly implicated.

Common Etiologies of Erythema Ab Igne
▶ Heating blanket/pad ▶ Hot water bottles ▶ Localized heaters/radiators ▶ Laptop computers

C. Machado M.D.
DaVanzo CMI

Histology: The skin may be slightly atrophic, and elastotic tissue is seen within the dermis. Melanin and hemosiderin are often seen in the dermis. The rete ridges may be thinned. Some areas may show evidence of changes such as those seen in actinic keratosis. Vacuolar degeneration of the basal layer can be seen.

Treatment: The goal of therapy is to discover and remove the exogenous heat source. Once the heat source is removed, most rashes slowly fade away over months. Some of the hyperpigmented areas may persist, however. Use of emollient creams or Kligman's formulation has been reported. Kligman's formulation includes a retinoid, a steroid, and a skin bleaching cream. Laser therapy has also been used to decrease the pigmentary disturbance. Individuals with keratinocyte atypia may respond to topical tretinoin or 5-fluorouracil cream.

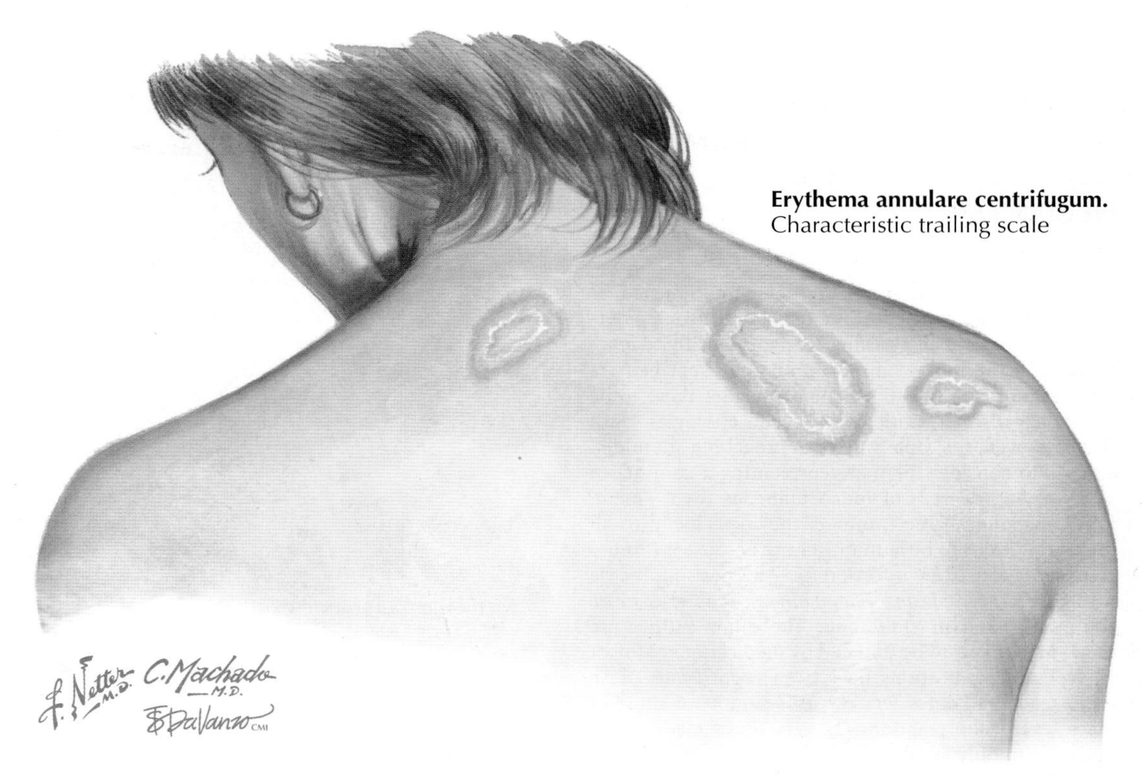

ERYTHEMA ANNULARE CENTRIFUGUM

Erythema annulare centrifugum (EAC) is an idiopathic rash classified with the gyrate erythema family. It is believed to be a cutaneous reaction to many unique antigenic stimuli, although no firm conclusion on the pathogenesis has been made. It has a characteristic clinical presentation that is easily recognized. The pathology of EAC is also characteristic and helps make the diagnosis by ruling out other conditions. EAC can be a marker of internal malignancy, but the vast majority of cases are not associated with an underlying malignancy.

Clinical Findings: EAC often manifests insidiously. It has been reported to occur at any age and has no sex or racial predilection. It is most frequently seen in the adult population. It has an unusual and peculiar morphology. The lesions start as small, pink urticarial papules that slowly expand. The patches of EAC are pink to red with a slowly expanding border. The peculiar and characteristic finding is the presence of a trailing scale. The leading edge of the rash advances and is followed by a few millimeters of fine trailing scale that continues to track the leading edge. As the rash expands outward, a central area of clearing forms. This central area is flesh colored. In tinea infections, in contrast, the scale represents the leading edge and travels in front of the expanding erythema. The main differential diagnosis includes erythema annulare centrifugum, tinea corporis, and mycosis fungoides. Potassium hydroxide (KOH) examination will rule out a dermatophyte, and a biopsy is required to differentiate EAC from mycosis fungoides.

EAC can be asymptomatic to severely pruritic. Most cases are mildly pruritic, but the most common complaint is of the unsightly appearance. Most lesions do not get larger than 10 cm in diameter. The trunk is most commonly involved, followed by the extremities. It is rarely seen on the face. Some areas may resolve while new areas are occurring.

Pathogenesis: The exact etiology of EAC is unknown. It is believed to be a reaction to many different antigenic stimuli. Research has suggested that EAC can be seen as a reaction pattern to an underlying tinea infection; this is thought to be a type IV hypersensitivity reaction. Many causes have been reported, including infections (fungal, bacterial, and viral) and medications. EAC has been reported in association with many different underlying malignancies and is named *paraneoplastic erythema annulare centrifugum eruption.*

Histology: Biopsies of EAC lesions should be taken from the advancing border. EAC has a superficial and deep perivascular lymphocytic infiltrate. The infiltrate has a highly characteristic "coat sleeve" appearance around the vessels. The lymphocytic infiltrate is concentrated immediately around the vessels in the dermis, and the lymphocytes appear to be coating the vessel walls. There is no true vasculitis present.

Treatment: EAC is almost always a self-limited process that spontaneously resolves. If an underlying infection is suspected, treatment and resolution of the infection have been shown to help resolve the rash. Malignancy-associated EAC is chronic in nature; it tends to resolve with treatment of the malignancy and to recur with relapses. Drug-induced EAC responds to discontinuation of the offending medication. Topical corticosteroids and/or antihistamines such as triamcinolone and diphenhydramine creams, respectively, may be used to help decrease the erythema and pruritus.

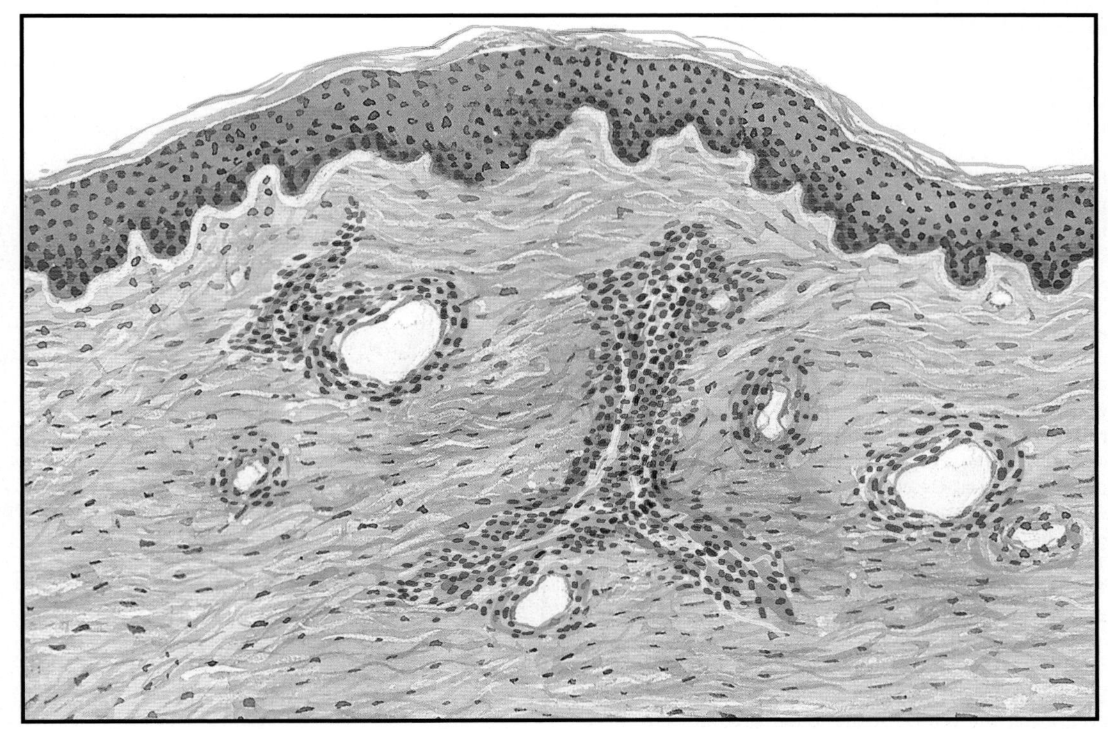

Histology of erythema annulare centrifugum shows tight perivascular infiltrates of lymphocytes, often referred to as "coat sleeving" of the vessels.

ERYTHEMA MULTIFORME, STEVENS-JOHNSON SYNDROME, AND TOXIC EPIDERMAL NECROLYSIS

Erythema multiforme minor, erythema multiforme major, Stevens-Johnson syndrome (SJS), and toxic epidermal necrolysis are all classified as hypersensitivity reactions, with the most common initiating event being a medication or an infection. Some consider these to be completely distinct entities with specific etiologies. Until that is proven, a simple way of approaching these diseases is to consider them as representing a continuum with varying degrees of mucocutaneous involvement. Erythema multiforme minor is the most likely of all these conditions to be a unique entity because it is more commonly caused by infection (e.g., herpes simplex virus [HSV], *Mycoplasma pneumoniae*). It is also more commonly seen in childhood. The other entities are much more likely to be initiated by medications. Almost all types of medications have been reported to cause these reactions, but a few classes account for most of these severe skin reactions. The classes of medications most commonly implicated are antibiotics (especially sulfa-based products), antiepileptics, allopurinol, antimalarials, highly active antiretroviral therapeutics, and NSAIDs.

Clinical Findings: There is no racial or ethnic predilection, and males and females are equally affected. For unknown reasons, patients with coexisting human immunodeficiency virus (HIV) infection are much more likely to develop a serious drug eruption than HIV-negative controls. The pathomechanism of this reaction is poorly understood.

Erythema multiforme minor is the most frequently seen of these eruptions. It is more common in children and young adults and can be caused by myriad infections and medications. Exposures to topical antigens such as urushiol in the poison ivy plant have also been reported to cause rashes resembling erythema multiforme minor. The most common cause that has been isolated is HSV. The rash of erythema multiforme minor can be seen in association with a coexisting herpesvirus infection or independent of the viral infection. Most episodes last for 2 to 3 weeks. A subset of patients will have recurrent episodes, often in association with recurrent HSV, but not always. The rash appears acutely as a well-defined macule with a "target" appearance—a red center, a surrounding area of normal-appearing skin, and a rim of erythema that encircles the entire lesion. The peripheral rim is well circumscribed and demarcated from the normal skin. Over a day, the macules may turn into edematous plaques. As time progresses, the center of the lesion becomes purple or dusky red. There may be only one area of involvement or hundreds in severe cases. Erythema multiforme minor affects the palms and soles; the target lesions in these areas can be very prominent and classic in appearance. The mucous membranes of the oral mucosa are involved in 20% of cases of erythema multiforme minor. Edematous pink-red plaques can be seen, as well as the more classic target lesions. If other mucous membranes are involved, the classification of erythema multiforme minor should not be used; the patient more likely has erythema multiforme major. Most cases of erythema multiforme minor self-resolve, but they do have a tendency to recur.

Erythema multiforme major has been considered by many to be the same entity as SJS. This may be true because the pathogenesis and clinical appearance can be similar. However, subtle differences exist and warrant classifying this condition independently. Erythema multiforme major is more likely of the two to be induced by an underlying infection. Both erythema multiforme major and SJS are most often induced by medications. The mucocutaneous surfaces are affected to a significant degree. In severe cases, the mucosal membranes of the respiratory and gastrointestinal tract may also be affected. Erythema multiforme major and SJS typically begin with a nonspecific prodrome of fever and malaise. Fever is the most frequent nonmucocutaneous symptom. The rash begins insidiously as pink macules that quickly develop a dusky purple central region. The typical target-like lesion of erythema multiforme minor is usually absent in SJS but may be seen in erythema multiforme major. Erythema multiforme major is differentiated from erythema multiforme minor in that it affects a larger surface area and affects two mucous membranes. SJS

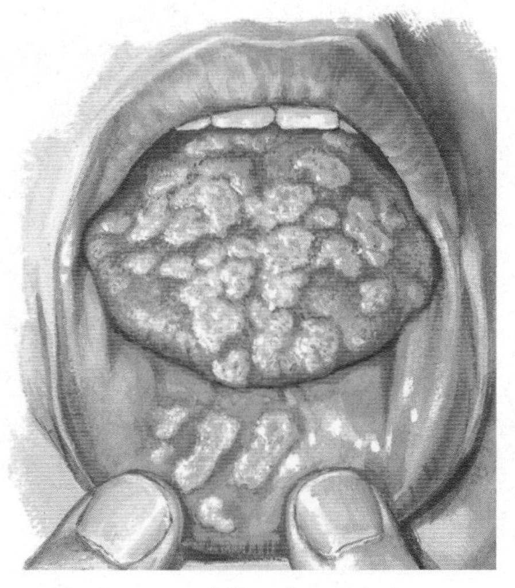
Erythema multiforme exudativum

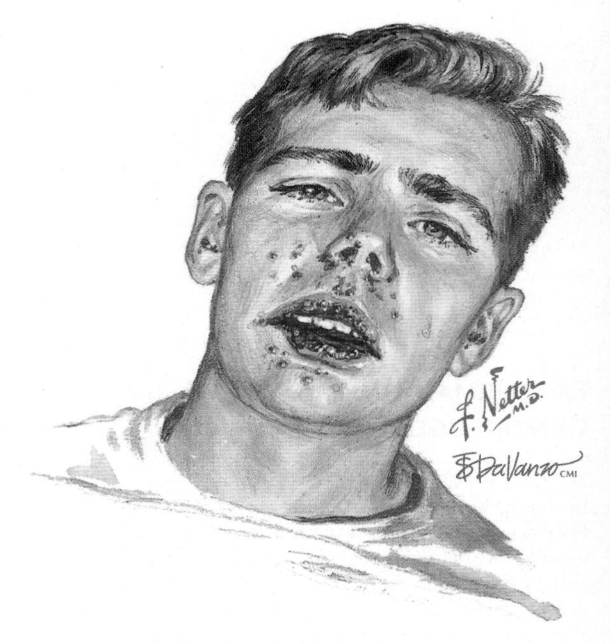

Stevens-Johnson syndrome

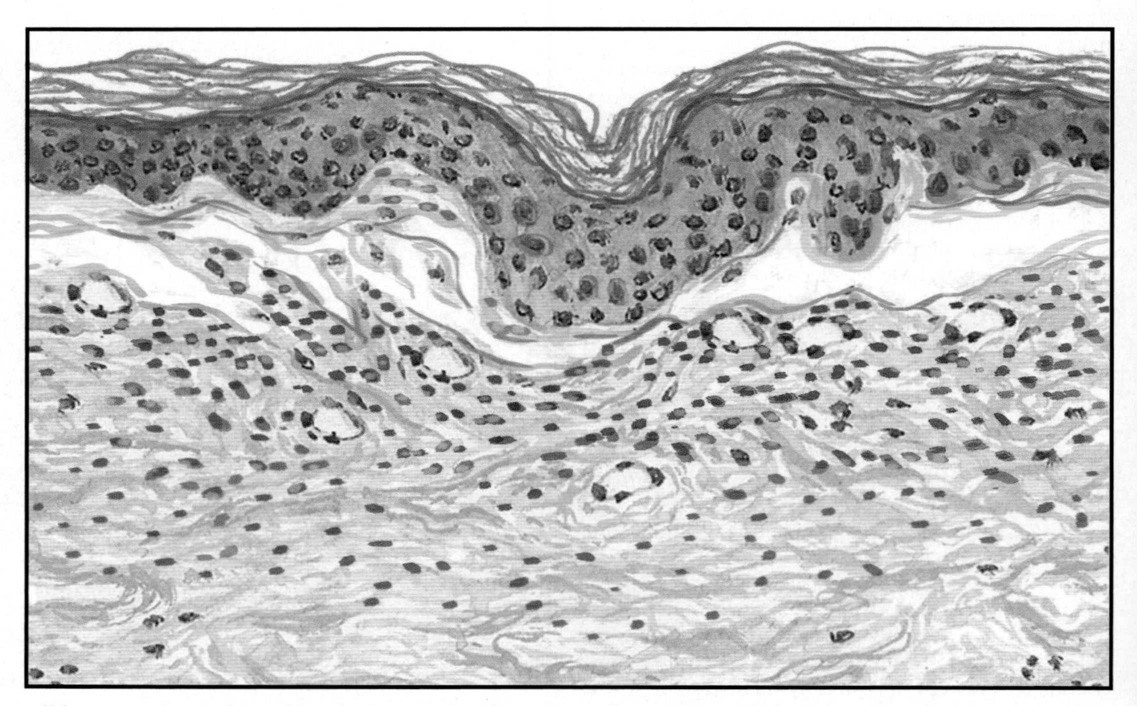
All have similar and overlapping histologic features. A subepidermal blister is forming here due to necrosis of the overlying epidermis. There is a lymphocytic-predominant perivascular infiltrate.

DRUG ERUPTIONS

ERYTHEMA MULTIFORME, STEVENS-JOHNSON SYNDROME, AND TOXIC EPIDERMAL NECROLYSIS (Continued)

is more likely to affect the ocular and urethral mucous membrane.

In SJS the dusky center of the lesion soon begins to blister, first as small vesicles and then coalescing into larger bullae. The extent and body surface area (BSA) of blistering is used to differentiate SJS from toxic epidermal necrolysis. Most consider blistering of 10% of the BSA and involvement of at least two mucosal surfaces to be definitive for SJS. Those cases with 10% to 30% BSA involvement have been termed *SJS–toxic epidermal necrolysis overlap*. Cases with greater than 30% BSA involvement are considered to represent toxic epidermal necrolysis. Light lateral pressure at the edge of a bulla or vesicle is an objective physical test that can be performed at the bedside. Spreading or an increase in size of the blister with pressure indicates separation of the epidermis from the underlying dermis and is termed the *Nikolsky sign*.

Pathogenesis: Erythema multiforme major/SJS is believed to be a hypersensitivity reaction to certain medications or infections. In the case of HSV, HSV DNA has been discovered in the skin lesions of erythema multiforme and induces cell-mediated immunity. For medication-induced cases, the insulting medication is thought to be metabolized into a recognizable antigen or to act as an antigen without metabolic degradation. Antibodies bind to the drug antigen and form antigen-antibody complexes that can deposit in the skin and other regions, causing an inflammatory cascade and the clinical findings.

Histology: The classic histologic picture of erythema multiforme minor and major shows an acute inflammatory infiltrate along the dermal-epidermal junction. The stratum corneum is normal. There is an interface dermatitis with vacuolar degeneration of the basal cell layer. The interface dermatitis leads to necrosis and death of the basilar keratinocytes. If the necrosis spreads and coalesces, small areas of subepidermal blister formation may be seen. Erythema multiforme minor can share some features with fixed drug eruptions. In fixed drug eruptions, melanophages are typically present, whereas this is not the case in erythema multiforme. Biopsy specimens of SJS and toxic epidermal necrolysis show more interface damage and blistering of the skin. The plane of separation is in the subepidermal space.

Treatment: Therapy for erythema multiforme minor and erythema multiforme major is supportive care. The skin lesions typically self-resolve with minimal to no sequelae. Topical corticosteroids may help decrease the time to healing and alleviate symptoms of pruritus. Recurrent episodes of erythema multiforme due to herpesvirus infection can be treated with chronic daily use of an antiviral agent such as acyclovir. This decreases the recurrence of herpes simplex infection and the resulting erythema multiforme reaction. Oral lesions can be treated with topical analgesics; the use of oral steroids is reserved for severe cases.

SJS can be a life-threatening condition and can progress to toxic epidermal necrolysis. For both SJS and toxic epidermal necrolysis, the cause of the reaction should be identified and withdrawn, and infections should be treated appropriately. These patients require aggressive supportive care, including wound care and fluid and electrolyte balancing. Most patients with severe involvement benefit from the experience of a burn unit. SJS and toxic epidermal necrolysis can be treated similarly to burns because the same technical issues are involved. There is no consensus on how to treat these two conditions with medications. The use of oral steroids early in the course of disease may help lessen the overall involvement, but steroids increase the risk of secondary infection and should not be used in patients with infection-induced disease. If used late in the course of disease, they appear not to help and only increase the risk of side effects. IVIG, cyclosporine, and tacrolimus have been used to treat these conditions with varying success. If used early, treatment may modify the disease course; if used late, it is unlikely to be of any help. Plasmapheresis has shown efficacy. The amount of BSA involved with blistering is related to the prognosis. Those with greater BSA blistering tend to fare worse than those with smaller BSA involvement.

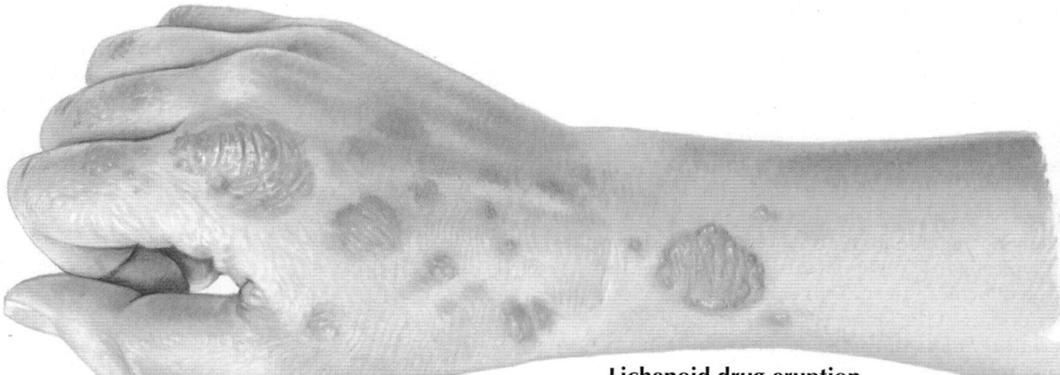

Lichenoid drug eruption. Dusky purple macules and patches.

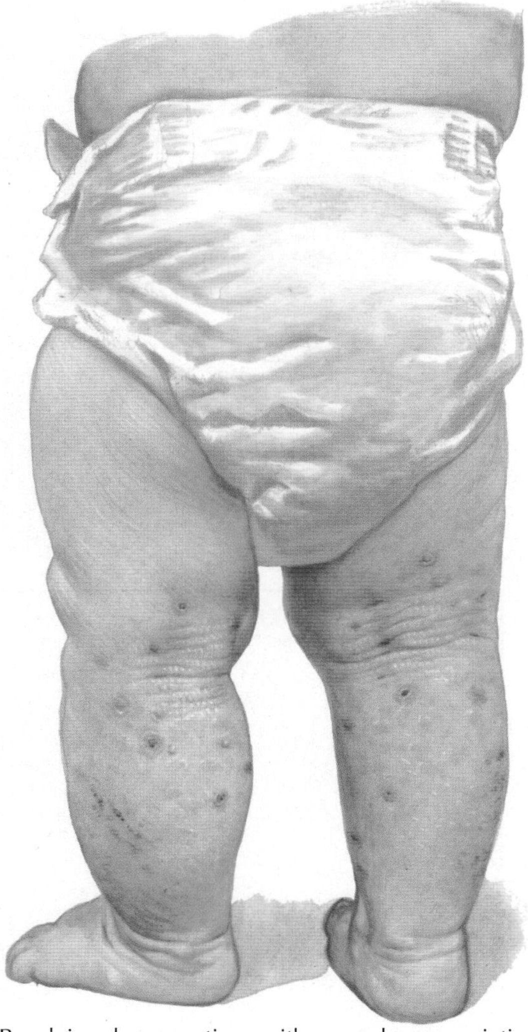

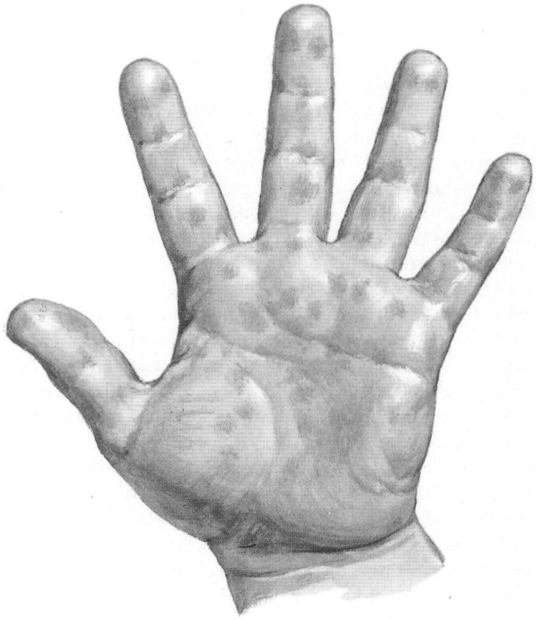

Erythema multiforme frequently affects the palms.

Resolving drug eruptions with secondary excoriations. Drug rashes typically start on the trunk and spread to the extremities.

F. Netter M.D.
C. Machado M.D.

ERYTHEMA NODOSUM

Erythema nodosum, an idiopathic form of panniculitis, can be seen in association with a wide range of inflammatory and infectious diseases. It is, however, most commonly seen during pregnancy or with the use of oral contraceptives. Erythema nodosum is believed to occur as a secondary phenomenon in response to an underlying alteration of normal physiology. The condition typically resolves spontaneously but in some cases can be difficult to treat. Erythema nodosum affects the anterior part of the lower legs almost exclusively.

Clinical Findings: Erythema nodosum is most commonly seen in young adult women. There is no racial predilection. The skin findings in erythema nodosum have an insidious onset. Small, tender regions begin within the dermis and develop into firm, tender dermal nodules, with the anterior lower legs almost always involved. The rash typically affects both lower legs in synchronicity. The lesions can be multifocal or solitary in nature. Most patients have multiple areas of involvement, with varying sizes of the lesions. Involvement of other areas of the body has been reported but is exceedingly uncommon.

The surface of the dermal nodules exhibits a slight red or purplish discoloration to the overlying otherwise normal-appearing epidermis. If ulcerations are present, another diagnosis should be considered, and a biopsy is warranted. Although almost all cases can be diagnosed on clinical grounds; skin biopsies are required for cases that are atypical in location or have unusual features such as ulcerations, surface change, palpable purpura, or other features inconsistent with classic erythema nodosum.

The diagnosis of erythema nodosum should lead to a search for a possible underlying association. One of the most frequent causes is the use of oral contraceptive pills. If the rash is thought to be related to the use of oral contraceptives, they should be discontinued, after which the lesions typically resolve. Pregnancy is another major cause of erythema nodosum. The lesions may be difficult to treat during pregnancy, but they will spontaneously resolve after delivery. Erythema nodosum may also be seen in association with sarcoid. Löfgren syndrome is the combination of fever, erythema nodosum, and bilateral hilar adenopathy that occurs as an acute form of sarcoid. In patients with no known reason for erythema nodosum, a standard chest radiograph should be considered to evaluate for sarcoid or the possibility of an underlying fungal or atypical infection. Valley fever (coccidioidomycosis), which is caused by the fungus *Coccidioides immitis*, has been linked with the development of erythema nodosum. Patients presenting with erythema nodosum who have lived in or traveled to an endemic area should be evaluated for this fungal infection. Streptococcal infection and tuberculosis should also be considered. Erythema nodosum has also been reported to occur in the inflammatory bowel diseases and in Hodgkin lymphoma.

Pathogenesis: The etiology of erythema nodosum is unknown, but it is thought to be a hypersensitivity reaction pattern to multiple unique stimuli. It is theorized that the antigenic stimulus causes the formation of antibody-antigen complexes that localize to the septal region of the adipose tissue.

Histology: Erythema nodosum is a primary septal panniculitis. The inflammation is isolated primarily to the fibrous septa that are present within the subcutaneous tissue. The fibrous septa are responsible for providing a framework for the adipose tissue. No vasculitis is seen, and its presence should trigger reconsideration of the diagnosis. The overlying dermis has a superficial and deep perivascular lymphocytic infiltrate. A characteristic finding is that of Miescher radial granulomas, which represent multiple histiocytes surrounding a central cleft. Multinucleated giant cells are also present within the septal infiltrate.

Treatment: Treatment is primarily symptomatic, and the possibility of an underlying disorder should be pursued. Erythema nodosum induced by medications or pregnancy resolves spontaneously once the medication is withdrawn or after delivery. Cases associated with an underlying infection, malignancy, or inflammatory bowel disease may be longer lasting and may show a waxing and waning course. Topical corticosteroids, compression stockings, elevation, and NSAIDs, such as indomethacin, are first-line therapies. Intralesional steroids can be beneficial in mild cases. Severe cases can be treated with a short course of prednisone. Supersaturated potassium iodide and colchicine have also been reported to be used successfully.

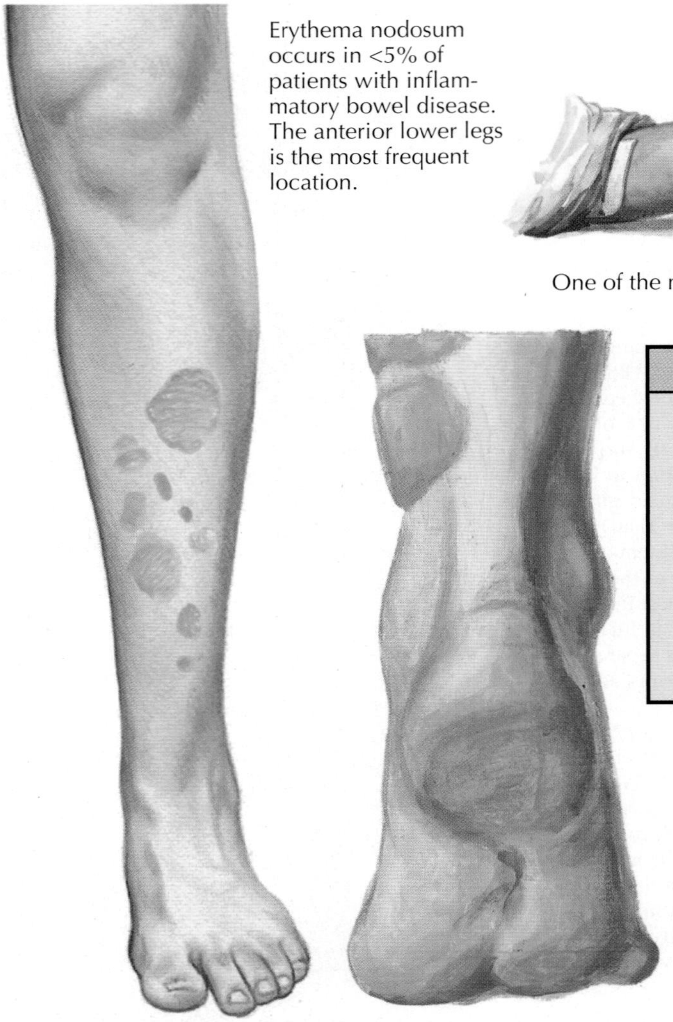

Erythema nodosum occurs in <5% of patients with inflammatory bowel disease. The anterior lower legs is the most frequent location.

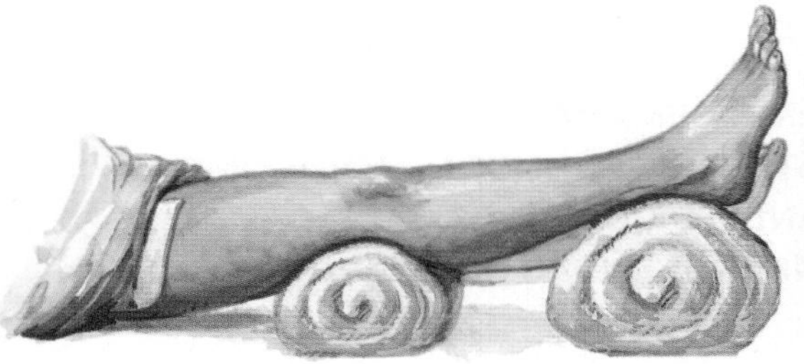

One of the mainstays of therapy is leg elevation.

Main Forms of Panniculitis
Predominantly septal panniculitis
▶Erythema nodosum
Predominantly lobular panniculitis
▶Lipodermatosclerosis
▶α_1-Antitrypsin deficiency panniculitis
▶Erythema induratum
▶Sclerema neonatorum
▶Traumatic panniculitis
▶Pancreatic panniculitis

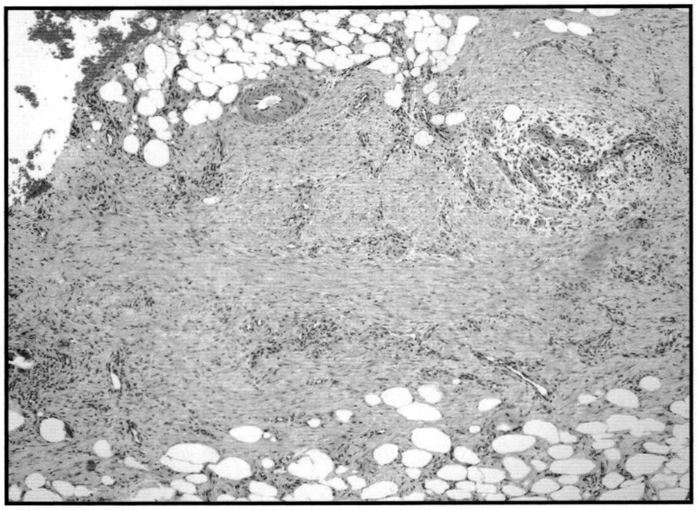

Erythema nodosum is a panniculitis that predominantly affects the septal portions of the adipose tissue. The septal tissue is expanded with a lymphocytic infiltrate.

Fabry Disease

Fabry disease is a rare disease caused by a deficiency in the enzyme α-galactosidase A (ceramide trihexosidase). Fabry disease is also known by its alternative descriptive name, angiokeratoma corporis diffusum. It is inherited in an X-linked recessive pattern and is classified as a lysosomal storage disease. The defect in this enzyme causes a lack of proper metabolism of globotriaosylceramide (ceramide trihexoside) and accumulation of this lipid in tissues throughout the body. Fabry disease affects the skin, kidneys, cardiovascular system, eye, and neurologic system. There is no known cure, but advances in enzyme replacement therapy have shown promising results. Males are more severely affected; females can be affected to varying degrees or can act as carriers. Fabry disease has been estimated to occur in 1 of every 10,000 males with the average age at death being 58 years.

Clinical Findings: The clinical manifestations have a slow onset during childhood; the average age at onset is 5 to 6 years. Due to its X-linked nature, it overwhelmingly affects males. Female heterozygotes can develop milder disease. Acroparesthesias are the initial presenting symptoms in most children. Patients have severe pain in the hands and feet that is episodic in nature and can last from minutes to hours or, in extreme cases, days. The pain is often described as a burning sensation. Episodes of stress can induce the acroparesthesias, which are accompanied by bouts of hypohidrosis or, less commonly, anhidrosis. This inability to sweat properly may lead to heat exhaustion and heat intolerance. Patients also eventually develop varying degrees of hearing loss.

The cutaneous findings consist of numerous angiokeratomas in unusual locations. These fine, red, hyperkeratotic papules occur on the trunk and lower extremities and are almost always located between the umbilicus and the knees. The number of angiokeratomas continues to increase with time, eventually reaching hundreds to thousands. The mucous membranes may also be involved. Presentation of a child or a young adult with multiple angiokeratomas should prompt the clinician to consider the diagnosis of Fabry disease. If the diagnosis of is made, patients should be referred to a specialty center.

The most characteristic ocular finding is that of cornea verticillata. This is a whorl-like corneal opacity that can be observed only by slit-lamp examination. It does not impede vision.

With time, patients begin to develop progressive kidney disease. The earliest sign is often asymptomatic proteinuria. Continued kidney damage eventually leads to chronic renal failure and end-stage renal disease. Maltese cross–shaped deposits are often found in the urine sediment and represent lipid accumulations. Cardiovascular changes can be seen and lead to ischemic heart disease. Stroke and cerebral vascular disease are common and cause a significant degree of mortality.

Diagnosis can be made by evaluating white blood cells for α-galactosidase A activity or for elevated levels of globotriaosylceramide in plasma. Males with classic Fabry disease have less than 1% of proper enzyme activity. DNA gene sequencing can be performed to isolate the exact genetic defect. Genetic testing is the only reliable way to diagnosis females with the disease because female carriers do have some plasma enzyme activity.

Pathogenesis: Fabry disease is caused by accumulation of globotriaosylceramide in various tissues due to improper metabolism caused by a deficiency in the enzyme α-galactosidase A.

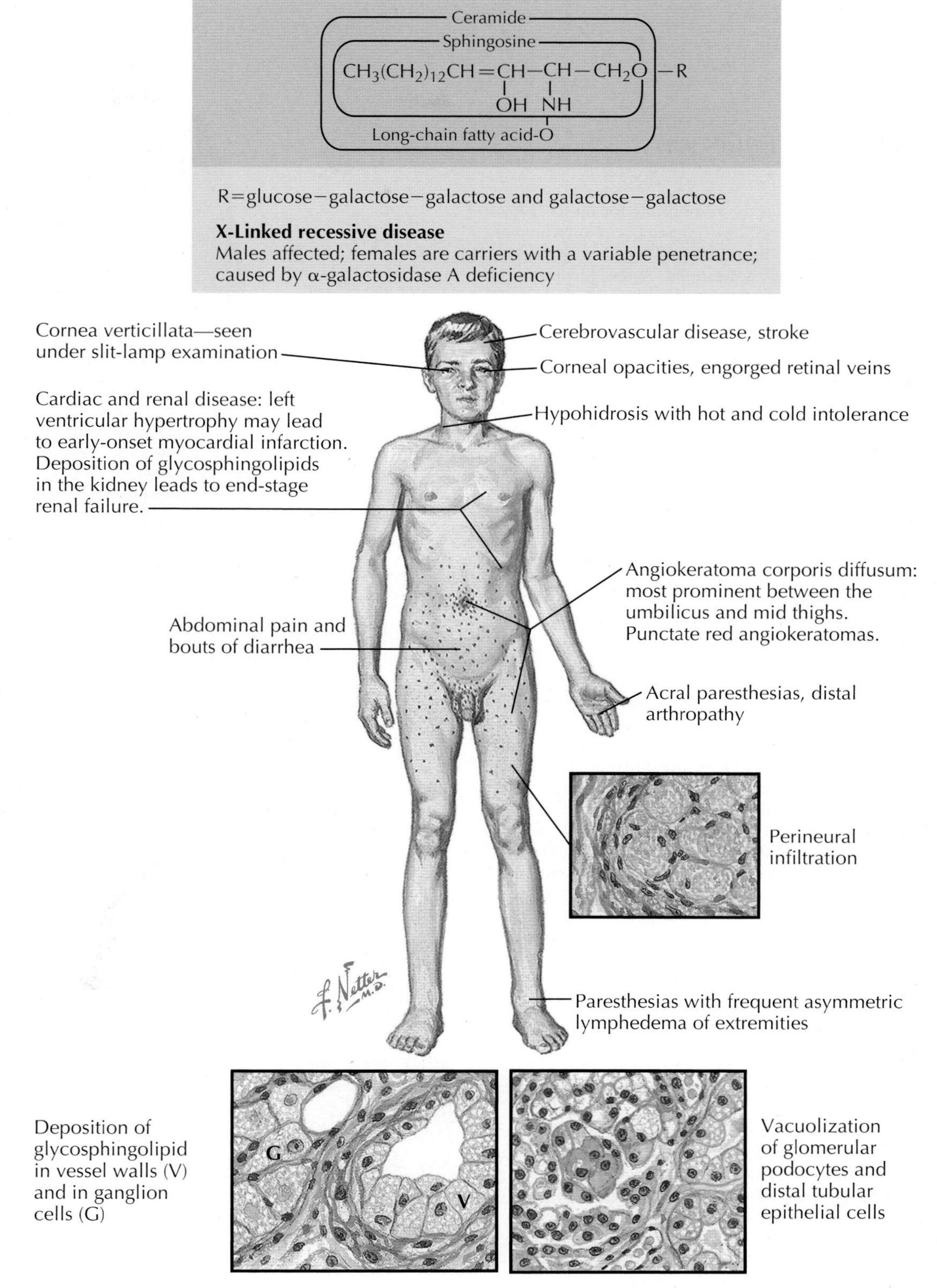

Histology: Skin biopsies are often not helpful in diagnosing Fabry disease. Angiokeratomas are histologically indistinguishable from those seen in other conditions. Electron microscopy can show lysosomal inclusions.

Treatment: Many medications, typically from the antiseizure class, can be used to treat the acroparesthesias. Phenytoin and gabapentin help control the frequency and duration of the episodes. In the past, there were no specific therapies for Fabry disease. End-stage renal disease often required kidney transplantation. Enzyme replacement therapy has been available since 2003 and has begun to have an effect on morbidity in these patients. Chaperone therapy has been used to help the cell transfer α-galactosidase A enzyme into lysosomes. Substrate reduction therapies work by inhibiting globotriaosylceramide production. Gene therapy, including viral vector and gene editing techniques, is being explored.

FIXED DRUG ERUPTION

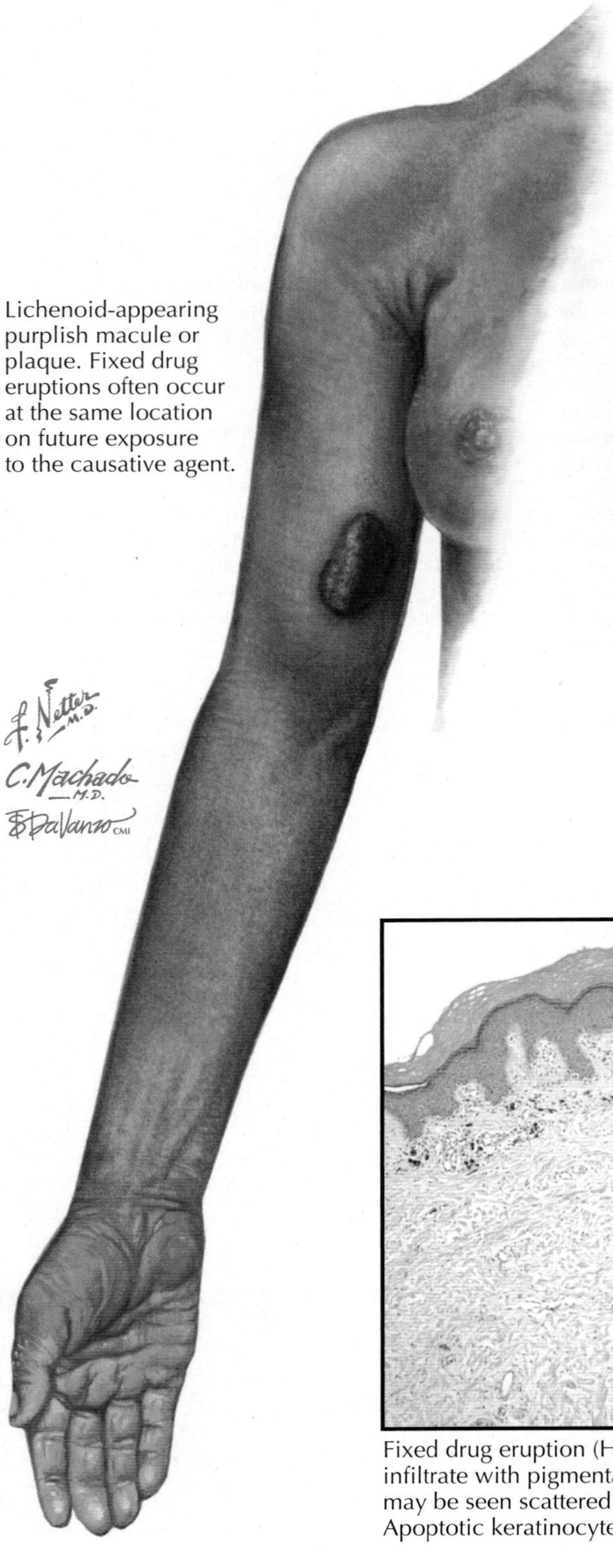

Fixed drug eruptions are responsible for up to 20% of all cutaneous drug rashes. They can occur anywhere on the body and have been reported to occur secondary to a lengthy list of medications. A few medicines in particular have been associated with fixed drug eruptions. One of the most frequent causes in the past was phenolphthalein in over-the-counter laxatives. After the numerous side effects from this medication were revealed, it was withdrawn from the market and is now only of historical significance. Fixed drug eruptions are unique in many ways, both clinically and histologically. The exact pathogenesis is unknown.

Clinical Findings: Clinically, fixed drug eruptions appear as oval to round, dusky red to purple macules with minimal surface change. Some cases have shown bullous-type reactions. The fixed drug eruption is unique in that it recurs in the same location time and time again as the patient is reexposed to the offending agent. Sometimes months may pass between exposures, and yet the reaction recurs in the same location. The glans penis, the oral mucosa, and the hands are the most commonly involved areas, although any area of the skin may be involved. Most individuals have one area of reaction, but some have multiple areas of involvement. It is unusual to have more than five areas involved, but case reports of widespread reactions have been reported. In these cases, the differential diagnosis includes erythema multiforme. Another characteristic feature is the postinflammatory hyperpigmentation that occurs after resolution. This is caused by the considerable amount of melanin pigment incontinence that results from disruption of the dermal-epidermal junction. The hyperpigmentation can take months to years to resolve.

The list of medications that can cause fixed drug eruptions continues to grow. The most frequently reported culprits are the sulfa-based antibiotics, NSAIDs, and tetracycline-based antibiotics. Common over-the-counter medications have also been reported to cause fixed drug eruptions, including acetaminophen and herbal supplements. For this reason, a thorough history that includes both prescription and other medications is required.

A number of rare variants of fixed drug eruptions have been reported and include urticarial eczematous and bullous forms. The majority of fixed drug eruptions are strikingly pigmented, but some rare variants have been shown to be hypopigmented.

Pathogenesis: The etiology is unknown. Research has indicated that $CD8^+$ T cells are the primary cell type within the inflammatory infiltrate. Once activated, these $CD8^+$ T cells produce IFN-γ. This abnormal immune response is responsible for the tissue damage. The precise interaction and mechanism by which certain medications react with the immune system of susceptible individuals to cause the eruptions have not been elucidated.

Histology: Fixed drug eruptions are categorized in the lichenoid pattern of histologic skin disease. These drug reactions show a prominent lichenoid infiltrate with lymphocytes. The infiltrate is associated with very noticeable vacuolar change of the basilar layer of the epidermis and prominent formation of necrotic keratinocytes (Civatte bodies). All cases show melanin incontinence within the dermis, which can be used to differentiate fixed drug eruption from other lichenoid reactions. If present, the bullae form within the subepidermal space in the bullous variant of fixed drug eruption. Rare variants of fixed drug eruption have been described that have included evidence of vasculitis. This form is exceedingly rare.

Treatment: The main goals in therapy are making the correct diagnosis and removing the offending agent. Once done, the lesions heal within weeks to months. Medium-strength to potent topical corticosteroids can be used to help relieve pruritus and potentially speed healing. Fixed drug eruptions often leave an area of postinflammatory hyperpigmentation or hypopigmentation after the initial reaction has resolved. This pigmentary abnormality can last for months to years.

Lichenoid-appearing purplish macule or plaque. Fixed drug eruptions often occur at the same location on future exposure to the causative agent.

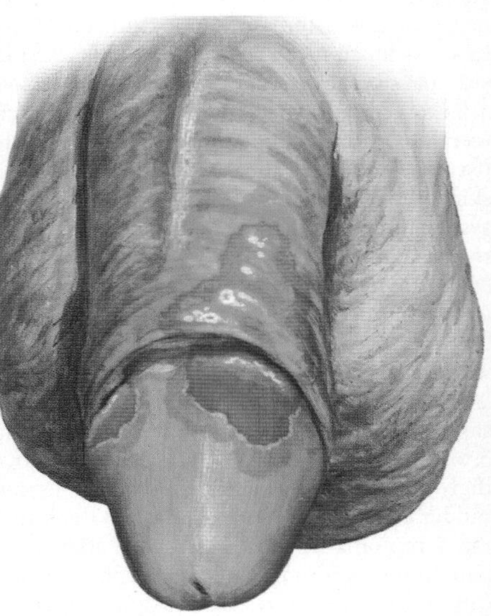

The glans penis is one of the most frequently involved areas in fixed drug eruptions.

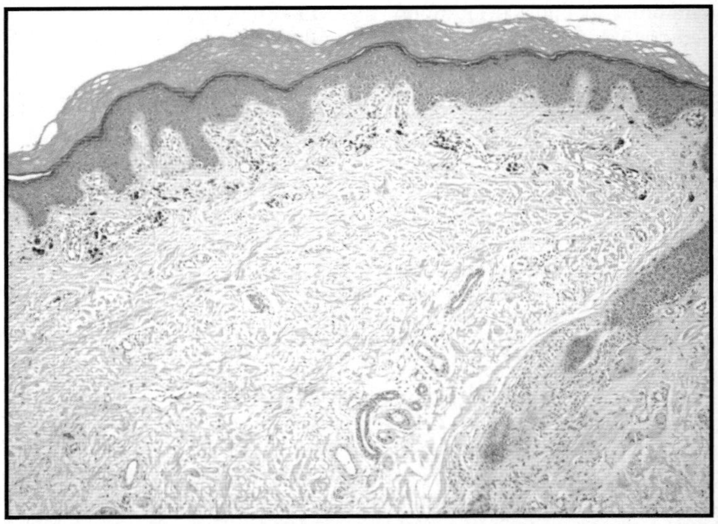

Fixed drug eruption (H&E stain) exhibiting a lymphocytic lichenoid infiltrate with pigmentary incontinence. Some vacuolar alteration may be seen scattered about the epidermal-dermal interface. Apoptotic keratinocytes can be variable in number.

GOUTY ARTHRITIS

Infancy
Inborn metabolic error
but no hyperuricemia or gout

Serum uric acid (mg/100 mL)
10
8
6
4
2
Normal

Puberty
In males, hyperuricemia develops but no clinical signs of gout. In females, hyperuricemia appears later and more rarely.

Adulthood
(30–50 years) Acute gout. Great toe swollen, red, painful.

After repeated attacks
Chronic tophaceous arthritis

Early tophaceous gouty arthritis

Same patient 12 years later, untreated

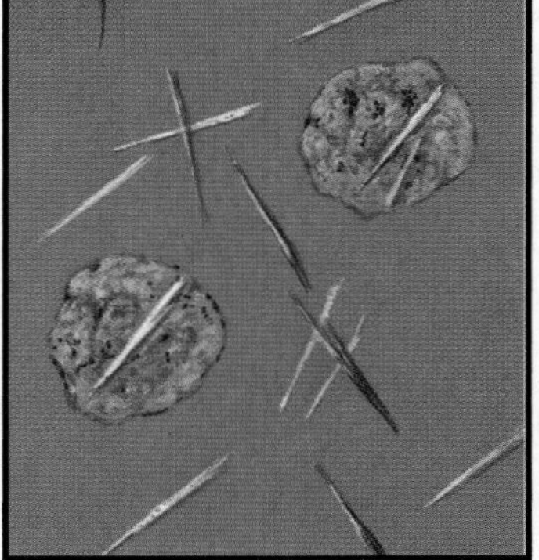
Free and phagocytized monosodium urate crystals in aspirated joint fluid seen on compensated polarized light microscopy

GOUT

Gout is one of the crystal-induced arthropathies caused by precipitation of uric acid crystals in the joint spaces, kidneys, and cutaneous locations. It is divided into acute and chronic phases, which have different presentations and treatments. The human body's immune reaction against the urate crystals causes more damage than the crystals themselves. Gout has been described for centuries and is clinically easily diagnosed. Medications, genetic predisposition, and dietary habits all contribute to cases of gout. Other crystal-induced arthropathies must be considered in the differential diagnosis of gout, the most common being calcium pyrophosphate crystals.

Clinical Findings: Gout is a disease predominantly found in the male population. Its incidence increases with each decade of life. Podagra is the classic presentation of an acute gouty attack. Descriptions of podagra have been published in the medical literature for centuries. It manifests as an acute monoarticular arthritis. The joint most commonly affected is the metatarsophalangeal articulation of the great toe. The clinical signs start as redness overlying the joint, swelling, warmth, and severe pain. Podagra has often been described as one of the most painful experiences a patient can perceive. A clue to the diagnosis is that the pain is often so severe that it appears to be out of proportion to the clinical picture. Patients complain of the slightest movement or touch; they are unable to wear shoes or bear weight on the foot, and they often have trouble with placement of a thin sheet over the affected joint. Acute attacks may be frequent, and the need for therapy is quite apparent. If no treatment is undertaken, an acute case of gout may last 7 days or longer. Any joint in the body can be affected by acute gout, but the great toe is by far the most common. Patients with acute gout have abnormal laboratory test results that can help in the diagnosis. An increased white blood cell count with a left shift is almost always seen. The markers of acute phase reactants are elevated, including the erythrocyte sedimentation rate, ferritin, and C-reactive protein.

The diagnosis can be made at the bedside by joint aspiration and microscopic evaluation. The affected joint is tapped with a fine-gauge needle and aspirated. The aspirate is then evaluated under polarized microscopy. Needle-like, elongated crystals of uric acid are seen freely within the synovial aspirate and also within the leukocytes of patients with gout. Radiographs of the affected joint do not show uric acid crystals and are likely to show only grossly abnormal soft tissue swelling. The serum uric acid level in acute gout can be normal, slightly elevated, or abnormally elevated; therefore this test by itself is unreliable in making the diagnosis.

Chronic gout, which is seen as a sequela of multiple attacks of acute gout, leads to joint destruction and chronic arthritis. Patients with chronic gout may also develop acute episodes of gout. Patients with chronic gout are predisposed to the development of tophaceous gout. This form of gout manifests as skin deposits of urate crystals. It can occur in any location but is most often within the subcutaneous tissue. These tophi appear clinically as subcutaneous nodules, often overlying the extensor joints, particularly the elbows, Achilles tendons, and hands. For some reason, the ear is another area affected by tophi. The nodules of tophi may become thinned and partially translucent. The tophi may show an underlying yellowish appearance beneath the skin, and occasionally the clumping of crystals is appreciated just underneath the skin. With trauma, the nodules occasionally ulcerate, and crystals drain from

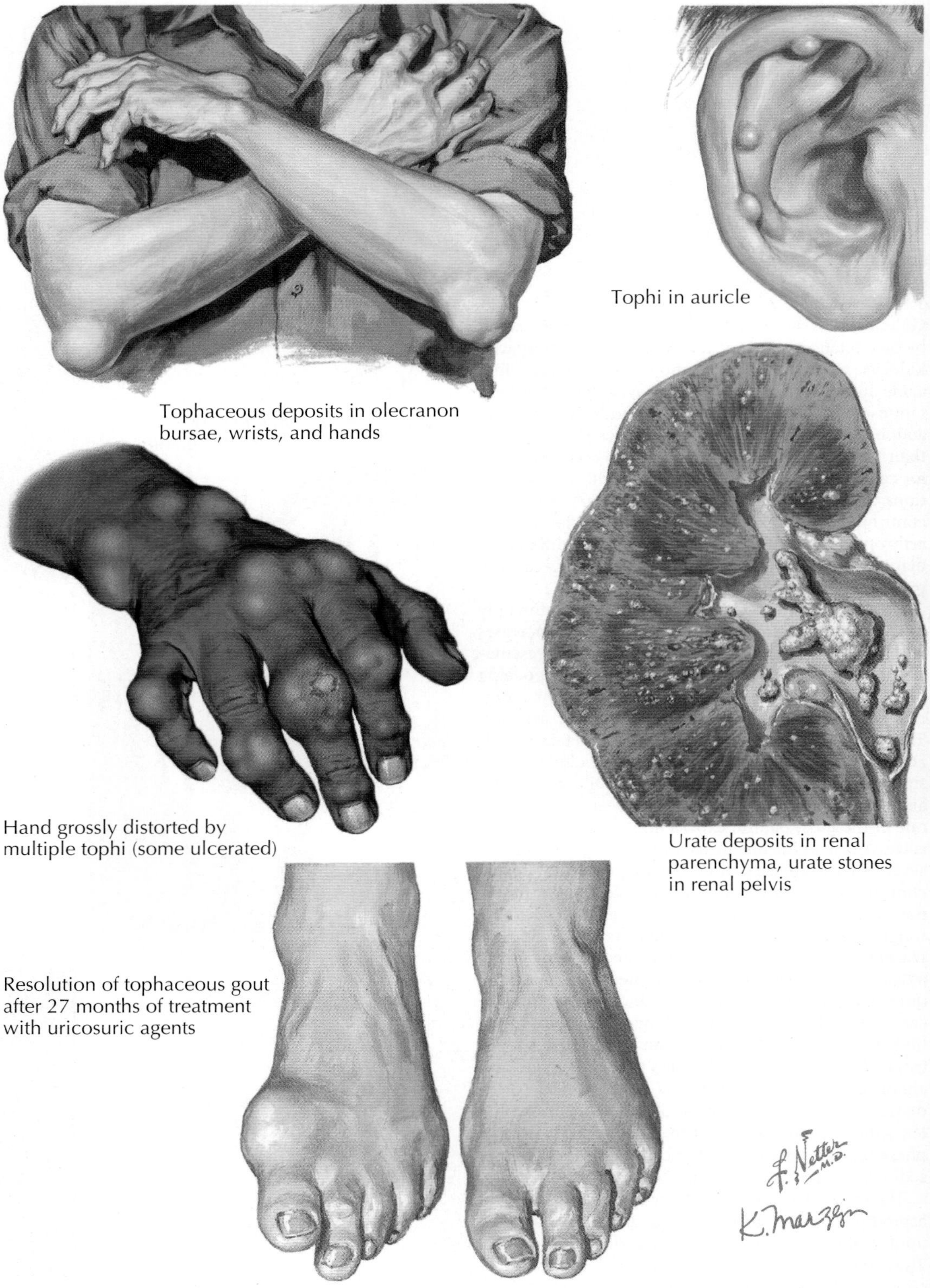

Gout (Continued)

the tophi. Saturnine gout is a specific form of gout that is caused by the consumption of homemade moonshine contaminated with lead.

Pathogenesis: Gout is caused by increased levels of uric acid resulting from a decrease in secretion, an increase in production, or an increase in dietary intake. Underexcretion of uric acid by the kidneys is responsible for most cases of gout. This can result from genetic causes or from use of medications that compete with the transport of uric acid, especially alcohol and the loop diuretics. Uric acid is produced under normal circumstances from the breakdown of purine nucleotides. Patients with Lesch-Nyhan syndrome have a defect in the hypoxanthine-guanine phosphoribosyltransferase enzyme, which is encoded by the gene *HPRT1* and is critical in the purine recycling pathway. This syndrome is seen in children and can lead to severe neurologic disease that is confounded by severe gout. Certain chemotherapies cause severe immediate death of many leukocytes, resulting in the release of a high concentration of uric acid that can overwhelm the body's normal mechanisms of removal, leading to gout. Foods found to have high concentrations of uric acid should be avoided by patients with preexisting gout because they have been shown to exacerbate the disease.

Histology: Biopsies are rarely performed because the clinical scenario is often diagnostic. When tissue of tophi is procured for biopsy, it should be fixed in alcohol because formalin dissolves the uric acid crystals, and they will not be seen on histologic examination. The diagnosis can still be made because the needle-shaped, clefted areas left by the dissolved crystals is characteristic. The crystals can be appreciated on alcohol-fixed tissue and appear needle shaped and birefringent under polarized light. The histologic appearance of gout is much different from that of calcium pyrophosphate, and there is usually no problem differentiating the two conditions. The crystals of pseudogout are rhomboid shaped and weakly birefringent.

Treatment: The therapeutic goal in acute gouty attacks is to control the patient's pain, and NSAIDs have long been the medications of choice. Indomethacin has been widely used for years. Aspirin should never be used in acute gout because it can transiently increase uric acid levels when initiated. Colchicine is another medication used for the treatment of acute gouty attacks. Prednisone can be used to decrease the acute inflammation, pain, and swelling. Medications for the prophylactic treatment of gout are not used in acute episodes because they may make an acute attack worse. They have also been demonstrated to trigger attacks of acute gout on rare occasions.

The most frequently used prophylactic medications to help prevent future acute attacks are allopurinol and probenecid. Allopurinol is used exclusively for patients who overproduce uric acid, and probenecid is used for those whose kidneys underexcrete uric acid. Up to one-third of patients started on allopurinol develop a cutaneous rash. If this happens, prompt discontinuation is wise because allopurinol can lead to a severe drug hypersensitivity syndrome. Allopurinol works by inhibiting the purine breakdown enzyme xanthine oxidase. This ultimately decreases the amount of uric acid produced from the breakdown of purine byproducts. Historically, allopurinol was the first medication devised to inhibit a specific enzyme.

Tophi can be treated with the long-term use of allopurinol or probenecid. Over time, the goal is to mobilize the tissue uric acid and increase its excretion from the body. This can take years. Individual tophi have been surgically removed to help increase range of motion, if located around joints, or to improve cosmesis.

Tophaceous Gout

Tophaceous deposits in olecranon bursae, wrists, and hands

Tophi in auricle

Hand grossly distorted by multiple tophi (some ulcerated)

Urate deposits in renal parenchyma, urate stones in renal pelvis

Resolution of tophaceous gout after 27 months of treatment with uricosuric agents

F. Netter M.D.
K. Marzen

Graft-Versus-Host Disease

With the ever-increasing number of stem cell transplantations and increasing survival rates of patients undergoing these procedures, graft-versus-host disease (GVHD) is becoming more prevalent. Two distinct clinical cutaneous forms exist, acute and chronic, each with its own manifestations and treatment options. Acute GVHD is often manifested by mucocutaneous eruptions that can range from a mild macular rash to life-threatening blistering of the skin. Chronic cutaneous GVHD is entirely different in clinical manifestation than its acute counterpart. The two forms are also seen during specific time frames: acute GVHD is most likely to occur within the first 3 months after transplantation, whereas chronic GVHD occurs later, typically 4 months or longer after transplantation.

GVHD can be seen not only after stem cell transplantation but also in any immunosuppressed patient who has received antigenically and immunologically viable cells from a donor. This may occur during organ transplantation or, rarely, during blood transfusion. The use of leuko-poor blood has helped decrease the chance of GVHD after blood transfusions.

Clinical Findings: Acute GVHD is a common complication after stem cell transplantation. The incidence has been reported to be as high as 90%. The degree of involvement is variable. GVHD affects males and females equally, and there is no racial predilection. Patients who develop acute GVHD typically begin having symptoms soon after their cell counts recover, usually 1 to 2 weeks after transplantation. Skin eruptions that develop within the first week after transplantation are typically not from GVHD. The skin, upper and lower digestive tract, and liver are frequently involved, and these organ systems are evaluated to help make the diagnosis of GVHD. The rash of acute GVHD can range from a fine maculopapular rash to severe blistering of the skin that can resemble toxic epidermal necrolysis and can be life-threatening. It is difficult, if not impossible, to predict the development and course of acute GVHD. These patients take multiple medications, and the differential diagnosis includes a drug rash. Histologic evaluation of a skin biopsy cannot always differentiate the two. The coexistence of mucositis, diarrhea, and elevated liver enzymes makes the diagnosis of acute GVHD more plausible. The constellation of all of these symptoms leads to the diagnosis.

Chronic GVHD has entirely different clinical manifestations. This form of GVHD typically begins 3 to 6 months after transplantation. The skin is most commonly involved. Two distinct forms of chronic cutaneous GVHD occur: lichenoid and sclerodermatous. The lichenoid variant manifests as red papules, patches, and plaques. There is a slight resemblance to lichen planus. The sclerodermatous variant is less common and manifests as thickened, firm skin with poikilodermatous changes. The surface of the skin is shiny, and the loss of adnexal structures is variable. This variant of chronic GVHD can be localized to a small area, or it can be generalized and may include the entire surface area of the skin. The amount of surface area involved is directly related to the morbidity the patient experiences.

Pathogenesis: GVHD is caused by transplanted immune cells that recognize the new host as foreign, leading to inflammatory reactions.

Histology: Histologic evaluation of skin biopsy specimens cannot differentiate acute GVHD from drug exanthems. Acute GVHD has been graded on a histologic scale of 1 to 4. Grade 1 shows basal layer vacuolar and interface changes; grade 2 shows signs of keratinocyte death; grade 3 shows clefting within the subepidermal space; and grade 4 is full bulla formation with epidermal parting.

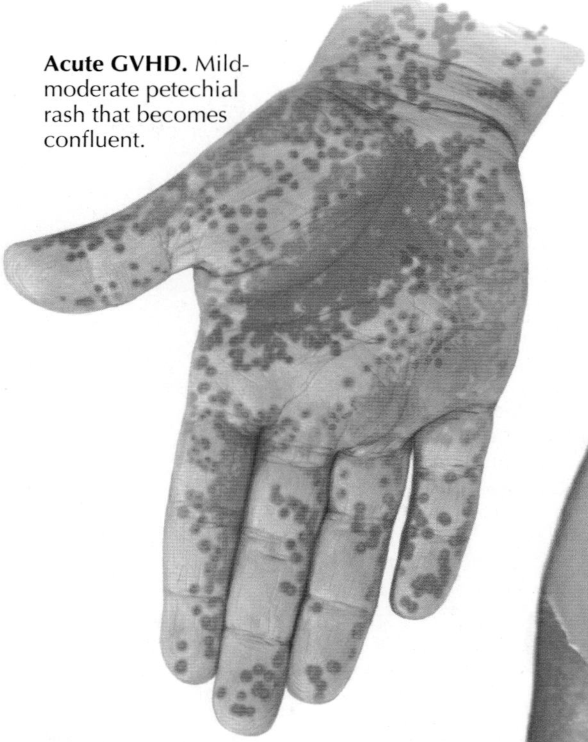

Lichenoid chronic GVHD shows a lichenoid dermatitis with a predominantly lymphocytic infiltrate. The sclerodermatous form of chronic GVHD shows abnormally thick dermal collagen, much like that seen in scleroderma.

Treatment: Prophylactic treatment with cyclosporine or tacrolimus and mycophenolate mofetil has helped reduce acute GVHD. The treatment is based on the clinical symptoms and the type of skin lesions. Corticosteroids are commonly used in both acute and chronic GVHD. The acute form has also been treated with tacrolimus and cyclosporine.

Chronic GVHD is difficult to manage. There is no cure for GVHD, and treatment is directed at stabilizing and improving skin function and increasing the patient's functional capabilities. Phototherapy has been used successfully, as has extracorporeal photopheresis. The protein kinase inhibitors ibrutinib, ruxolitinib, and belumosudil are helpful in treating chronic GVHD.

Acute GVHD. Mild-moderate petechial rash that becomes confluent.

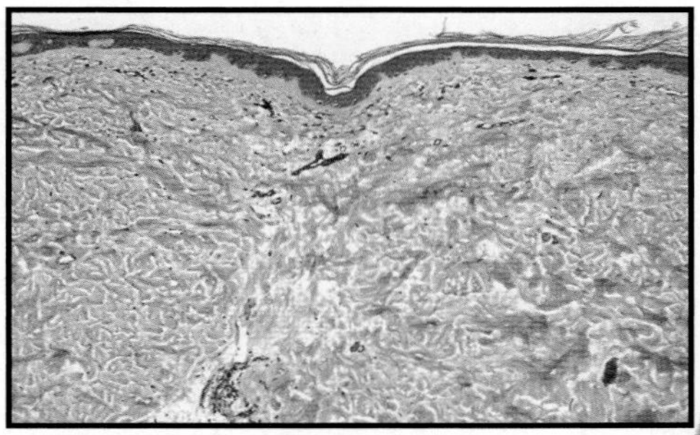

Sclerodermatous GVHD. Unlike acute GVHD, the chronic sclerodermatous form shows thickening of the collagen within the dermis. A thinned atrophic epidermis and a decrease in the number of adnexal structures are also noted.

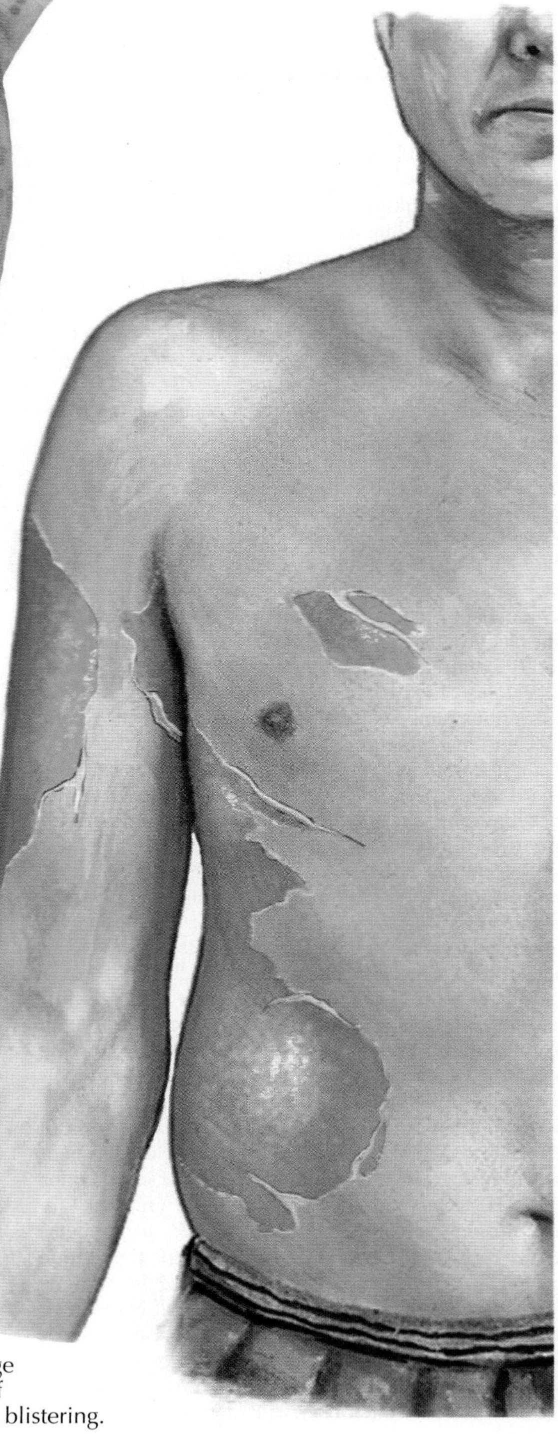

Severe acute GVHD. The skin peels off in large sheets due to necrosis of the skin and subsequent blistering.

C. Machado M.D.
DaVanzo CMI

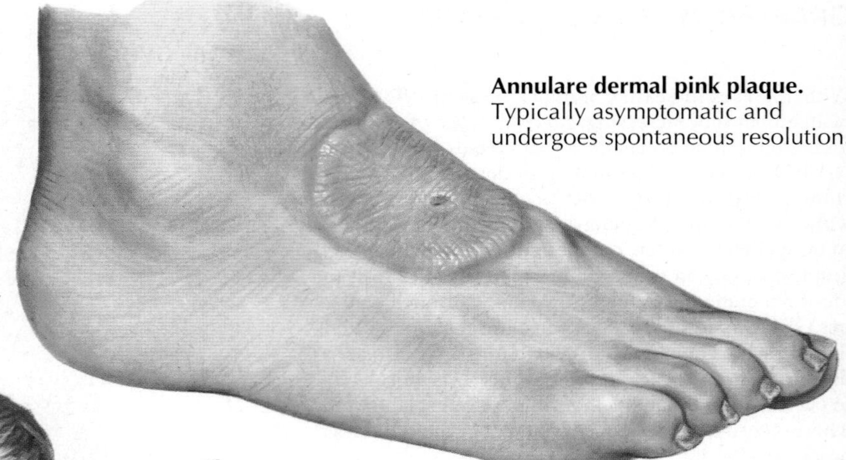

Annulare dermal pink plaque. Typically asymptomatic and undergoes spontaneous resolution.

Generalized granuloma annulare in a child

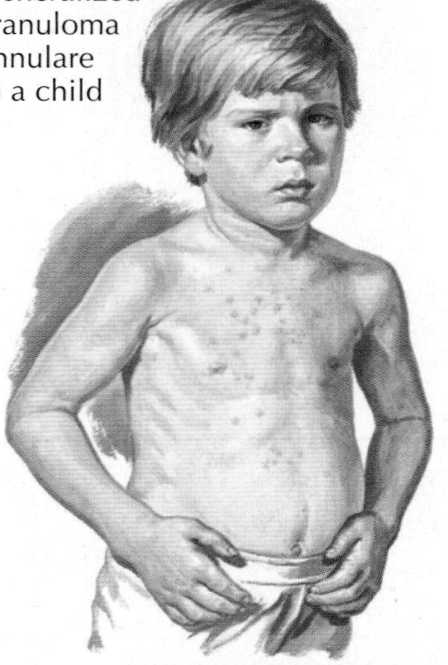

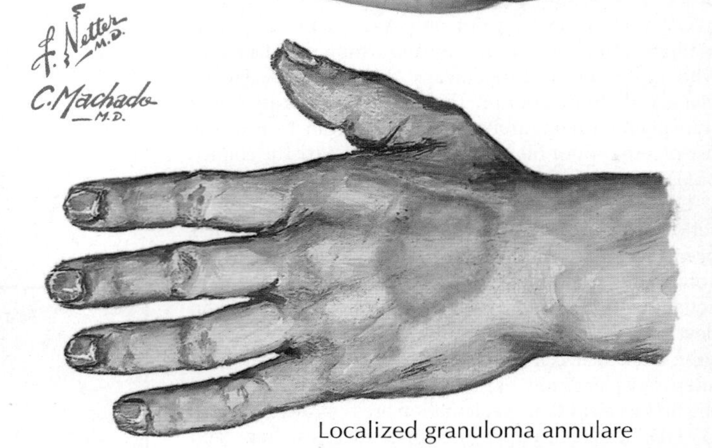

F. Netter M.D.
C. Machado M.D.

Localized granuloma annulare

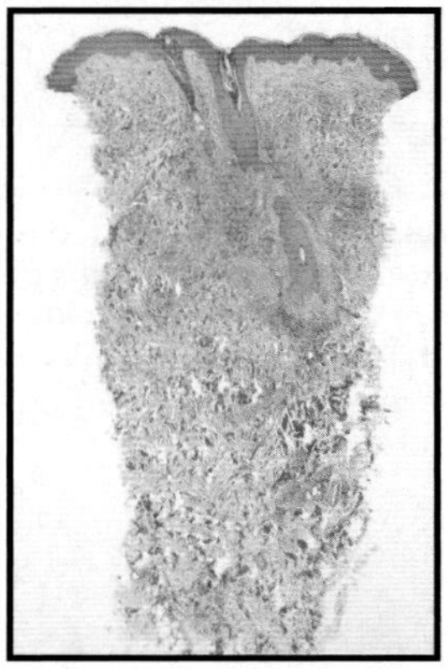

Low power. Granulomatous inflammation throughout the specimen with necrobiotic collagen bundles.

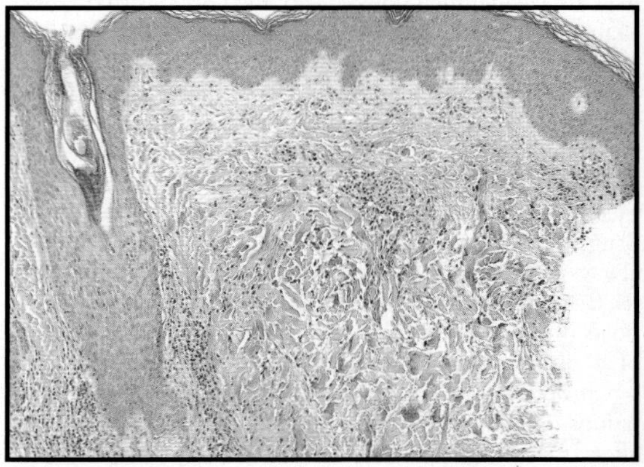

High power. Necrobiotic collagen within the granulomatous region.

GRANULOMA ANNULARE

Granuloma annulare is a commonly encountered rash, with an estimated incidence of 1 in 2500. The etiology of this rash is unknown. There are various clinical presentations, including localized, generalized, subcutaneous, actinic, and perforating forms. The generalized version has been seen in association with diabetes. Individuals with underlying rheumatoid arthritis, lupus and hyperlipidemia may be at higher risk for developing granuloma annulare. Most cases spontaneously resolve. Multiple treatment strategies exist.

Clinical Findings: Granuloma annulare occurs commonly in children but can be seen in any age group. There is no race predilection, but it is three times as common in females as in males. The localized form of granuloma annulare typically starts insidiously as a small, flesh-colored to slightly yellow papule that expands centrifugally. Once the lesion gets to a certain size, its characteristic appearance becomes evident. Fully formed, the area appears as an annular plaque with minimal to no surface change. The plaque appears to have a raised rim around the edge, and the central portion of the lesion is almost normal in appearance. The peripheral rim is slightly yellow in color. The lesions can be entirely flesh colored. Patients experience minimal symptoms. Slight itching may be present. It is not uncommon to have multiple areas of involvement. The dorsal aspects of the feet and hands are common locations for this rash. Some patients relate that their rash improves during the summer months. The lesions can range from small papules a few millimeters in diameter to larger plaques a few centimeters in diameter. If only small papules exist, a biopsy is required for diagnosis. The clinical appearance of the larger plaques is so characteristic that the diagnosis can be made clinically.

The generalized version of granuloma annulare consists of numerous widespread papules and small plaques. In most cases, there are no annulare-appearing plaques; the diagnosis is considered clinically, but a biopsy is required to confirm the diagnosis. This form occurs almost exclusively in adults and may be seen in association with diabetes. Patients with a diagnosis of generalized granuloma annulare should be screened for diabetes. Other variants of granuloma annulare are uncommonly encountered. They include the subcutaneous form, the perforating variant, and the actinic variant. The actinic variant may be considered a unique entity, termed *annular elastolytic giant cell granuloma.* Subcutaneous granuloma annulare manifests as deep-seated nodules within the dermis. A diagnosis is made via biopsy. This variant appears to be more common in children and is frequently located on the lower legs. The perforating variant is the rarest form and is the only variant to exhibit surface change. The areas of involvement show central umbilication that develops small erosions. This is reported to occur most commonly on the dorsal surface of the hands. Involvement of the non–hair-bearing skin of the palms or soles with any variant of granuloma annulare is exceedingly rare.

Pathogenesis: The etiology is unknown. It has been theorized to represent an abnormal immune response to a foreign antigen such as a virus or bacteria. This has not been proven, and many other theories of pathogenesis exist. Both the Th1 and Th2 pathways have been shown to be upregulated in granuloma annulare. Elevated cytokine levels of TNF-α, IFN-γ, IL-12, IL-4, and IL-17 have been demonstrated. Ultimately, the collagen within the lesions is disrupted, and the resulting inflammatory response causes the clinical findings.

Histology: The histologic findings in biopsy specimens of granuloma annulare are very specific. There are areas of necrobiotic collagen with a surrounding granulomatous infiltrate. The collagen is being destroyed centrally. A varying amount of mucin is present. The main histologic differential diagnosis is between granuloma annulare and necrobiosis lipoidica. The inflammation in necrobiosis lipoidica is typically oriented across the entire biopsy specimen in a layered fashion. Histologic variants of granuloma annulare exist, including interstitial granuloma annulare.

Treatment: Localized forms of granuloma annulare that are asymptomatic and not causing any distress to the patient can be left alone. Most cases resolve spontaneously over time with no residual scarring. Topical corticosteroids may be used to decrease the inflammatory response. Intralesional corticosteroids can be used, but the risk of atrophy must be considered. Phototherapy has been used successfully. Psoralen + UVA light (PUVA) therapy has had more success than ultraviolet B (UVB) light therapy, most likely because UVA light penetrates deeper into the dermis than UVB. Phototherapy with UVA_1 appears promising. Successful treatment with systemic agents such as hydroxychloroquine, combination antibiotics, apremilast, and TNF inhibitors has been reported.

Graves Disease and Pretibial Myxedema

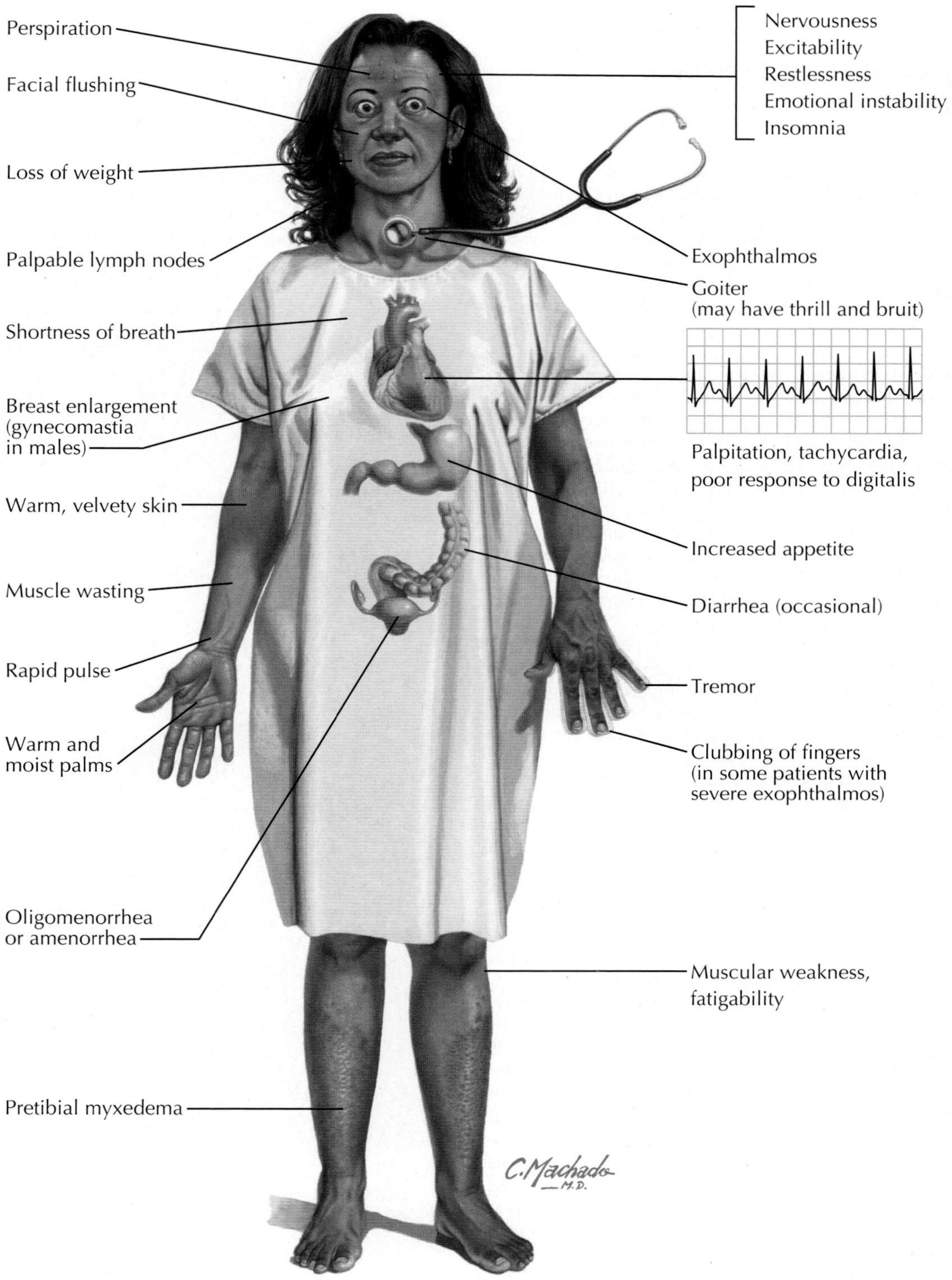

Graves disease is an autoimmune form of hyperthyroidism that is most often seen in the adult population. This autoimmune disease causes the thyroid gland to produce excessive thyroid hormones. These elevated hormone levels result in the clinical manifestations.

Clinical Findings: Graves disease is seen in females more frequently than males, in a ratio of approximately 7:1. Individuals age 30 to 60 years are at highest risk. Most patients have an insidious onset of symptoms. Heat intolerance and nervousness are two of the early and more common findings. Anxiety and emotional difficulties can be life altering. Patients often report difficulty sleeping. Constitutional symptoms can manifest as weight loss, increased appetite, increased sweating, and profound nervousness. Women may experience menstrual irregularities. Cardiac arrhythmias are common as the disease progresses. Hypertension and tachycardia can be two of the earliest cardiovascular signs of the disease. As the disease progresses, exophthalmos becomes prominent, a goiter can be seen or felt, and patients develop pretibial myxedema.

The exophthalmos may lead to intermittent double vision and a feeling of posterior ocular pressure. Photophobia can be a part of the disease, as can frequent tearing and a feeling of "sand" in the eyes that causes pain. Goiter may be noticeable to the patient, and it may be appreciated initially because of difficulty buttoning one's collar. The goiter is diffuse in nature. The thyroid is easily palpable and is firm to the touch. On occasion, the astute clinician can auscultate a bruit over the thyroid gland; this represents the increased blood flow to the growing gland.

Pretibial myxedema is the most widely recognized skin finding in Graves disease. It begins as small, indurated papules that coalesce into plaques on the anterior shin. The plaques indent easily when palpated and clinically act like lymphedema, producing a nonpitting edema. Pretibial myxedema can occur in other areas of the body, but this is a rare finding. The skin is typically warm to the touch and can have a velvety feel. Increased sweating is noticeable most often as warm, moist palms and soles, similar to that observed in patients with hyperhidrosis. Clubbing of the fingers is seen in a small proportion of affected individuals. Facial flushing with an increase in sweating is also seen. Females may develop breast enlargement, and males may develop gynecomastia.

Laboratory testing is needed to help define the condition. Radioactive iodine uptake imaging shows a diffuse, symmetric uptake of iodine in the patient with Graves disease. The pattern of uptake is very different from that seen in patients with a "hot" thyroid nodule, in which the radioactive signal is dramatically increased in the nodule. Thyroid antibody testing is very helpful in differentiating Graves disease from other forms of thyrotoxicosis. Antithyroglobulin, antimicrosomal, antithyroid peroxidase and anti–thyroid-stimulating hormone (TSH) receptor antibodies can be evaluated.

Pathogenesis: Graves disease is an idiopathic autoimmune disease that causes autoantibodies against the TSH receptor. The antibodies act as agonists to the receptor and cause nonstop activation of the TSH receptor on the thyroid. This leads to increased production of thyroid hormones, both triiodothyronine (T_3) and thyroxine (T_4), by the thyroid. The increase in metabolic functioning of the thyroid leads to diffuse enlargement and goiter. The increased production of thyroid hormones and their effects on target tissues lead to the clinical findings. Genetic susceptibility is now well recognized.

Histology: Biopsy specimens of the pretibial skin show substantial volumes of mucin deposits within the middle and lower dermis, between collagen bundles. The mucin is so thick that it causes the dermal collagen bundles to be splayed apart. Overlying hyperkeratosis can be appreciated. Biopsy specimens from clinically unaffected skin may show some of the same histologic findings but on a lesser scale.

Treatment: Treatment of Graves disease is predicated on stopping the excessive thyroid hormone production. Ablation of the thyroid can be achieved with radiation therapy or surgical removal. Medications such as β-blockers are used to lessen the symptoms of the disease until it is under control. Medical management of Graves disease can be achieved with propylthiouracil or methimazole, both of which act to decrease thyroid hormone production. Insulin growth factor receptor (IGF-1R) has been found to be increased in tissue from patients with Graves disease. Teprotumumab, an IGF-1R blocker, is approved to treat exophthalmos and has shown some efficacy in treating pretibial myxedema.

HIDRADENITIS SUPPURATIVA (ACNE INVERSA)

Hidradenitis suppurativa (acne inversa) is a rare chronic, life-altering disease. It can be an isolated clinical finding, or it can be associated with cystic acne, dissecting cellulitis of the scalp, and pilonidal cysts.

Clinical Findings: Hidradenitis suppurativa is most commonly encountered in postpubertal women. The ratio of female-to-male involvement is approximately 3:1. Black individuals are more likely to develop hidradenitis suppurativa, and a genetic predisposition has been determined. This condition preferentially affects areas that are rich in apocrine glands and terminal hairs. The areas most involved are the axillae, groin, and inframammary folds. It is rare in other areas. Hidradenitis suppurativa starts as tiny red papules or nodules that tend to be folliculocentric. The papules are tender and firm to palpation. At this point, the differential diagnosis includes an early folliculitis or furunculosis. As the disease progresses, the hard nodules become fluctuant and spontaneously drain to the surface of the skin. The nodules may coalesce into plaques with varying amounts of scarring. The longer the process has been occurring, the more scarring is prevalent. Eventually, sinus tracts develop that interconnect multiple subcutaneous nodules with multiple cutaneous openings. Clinically, pressing on one of the nodules may produce drainage from a distant sinus tract. The disease is relentless, and new crops of lesions repeatedly develop. Pain is significant and is a main cause of morbidity. Obesity tends to be seen in association with hidradenitis suppurativa. Hidradenitis has been seen in association with Crohn disease, and in the past some believed that hidradenitis suppurativa was a cutaneous form of Crohn disease. Long-standing disease has been associated with the development of squamous cell carcinoma. The tumors tend to be large at diagnosis as the diagnosis is often delayed because the inflammation camouflages the squamous cell carcinoma.

The drainage from the cutaneous nodules often requires extensive bandaging to keep clothing from getting soiled. The drainage has a malodorous, foul smell. The draining sinus tracts and nodules are often colonized with various bacteria, and cultures of the purulent drainage show growth of a number of different organisms, including *Staphylococcus aureus* and streptococcal species. However, this is not primarily an infectious disease, and it is not contagious. The bacteria in these cases are present secondary to the underlying inflammatory condition and the lack of normal cutaneous skin barrier function.

Pathogenesis: Hidradenitis suppurativa is an inflammatory disease with secondary bacterial superinfection and colonization. Routine culturing of the nodules and the drainage is often sterile. Hidradenitis is theorized to be caused by rupture of the mature follicular epithelium along areas of apocrine glands; hence its propensity to occur in areas with high densities of apocrine glands. A hormonal control over the process has been theorized, given that it is more common in postpubertal women and in obese individuals. Once the hair follicle ruptures, an inflammatory cascade is set off and causes the resulting nodules, cysts, fistulas, and scarring. It appears to be a self-perpetuating process. The exact mechanism by which this occurs is unknown.

Histology: Chronic lesions show a dense, mixed inflammatory infiltrate with abscess and sinus tract formation. Varying amounts of fibrosis and scar tissue are present. Apocrine gland inflammation can be appreciated in a fair number of cases. The inflammation extends into the subcutaneous tissue.

Treatment: Therapy is often aimed at reducing inflammation and bacterial superinfection. There is no curative therapy, and many treatments have only anecdotal reports of success. Topical clindamycin and other antibacterial products such as benzyl peroxide are often the first-line agents prescribed for mild disease. Oral antibiotics, typically in the tetracycline class, are often used because they have both antiinflammatory and antibacterial properties. Weight loss must be advocated. Individuals who smoke should be encouraged to cut back and eventually quit. Other agents that have had some success include isotretinoin, acitretin, adalimumab, and infliximab. Intralesional steroids can help calm inflamed papules and nodules. Surgical options include wide local excisions to remove the affected tissue and repair with complex flap closure. Liposuction has also been tried in an attempt to remove the affected apocrine gland hair follicle unit. The only potential for cure is with a surgical approach. This approach seems to work best for axillary disease; groin and inframammary disease almost always recurs after surgery. It is also of the utmost importance to address patients' psychosocial needs because this disease has a devastating toll on patients.

Hidradenitis suppurativa. Abscess, sinus tract formation, and significant scarring lead to exquisitely tender areas of involvement. The axilla, groin, and buttocks are frequently affected.

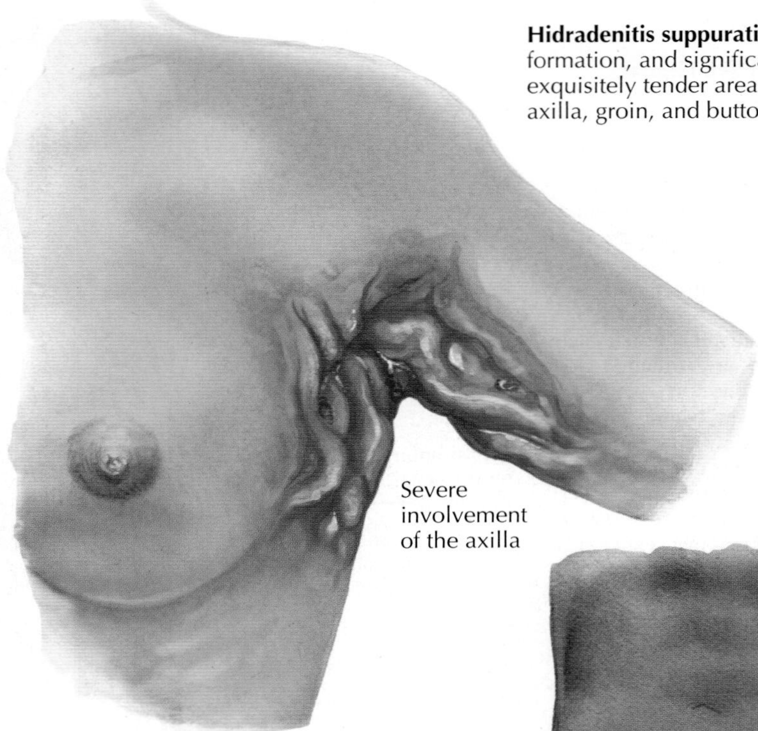

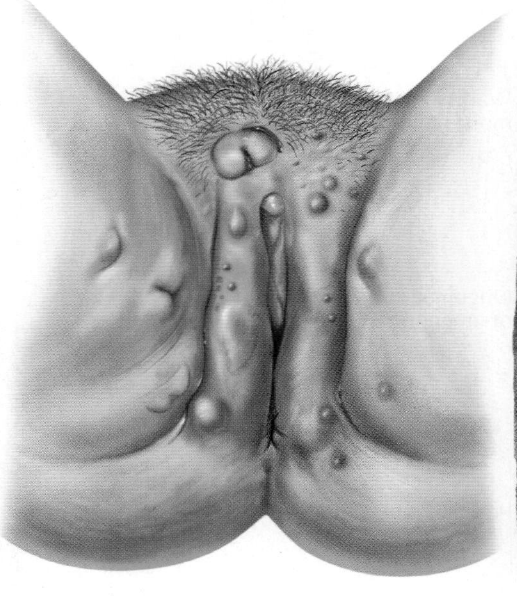

Severe involvement of the axilla

C.Machado M.D.
DaVanzo CMI

Hidradenitis suppurativa (acne inversa) on the groin

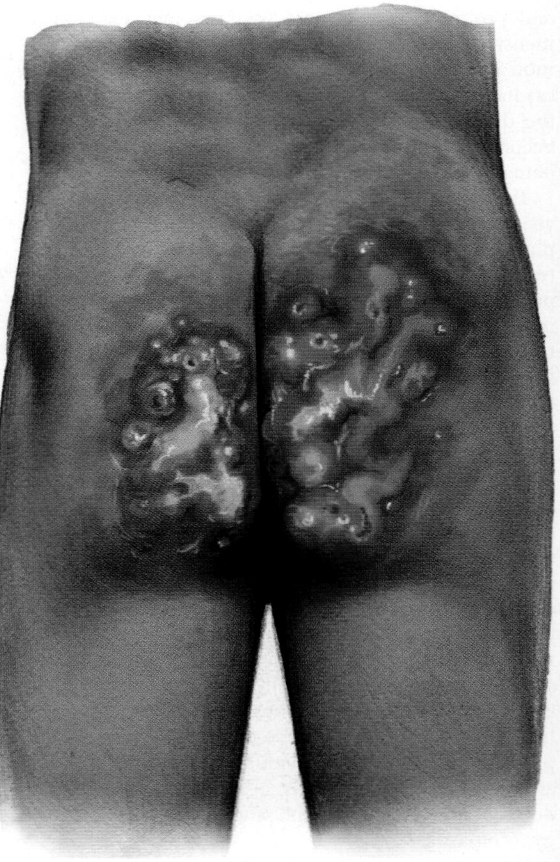

Severe inflammatory hidradenitis suppurativa of the buttocks

Infantile Hemangiomas

Infantile hemangiomas and congenital hemangiomas are two main types of hemangiomas to consider in the infant population. Infantile hemangiomas are the most frequently encountered of the hemangiomas and occur in approximately 4% to 5% of infants. They are most frequently seen in premature infants and infants who weigh less than 1.5 kg. Infantile hemangiomas are more frequently seen in females.

Clinical Findings: Infantile hemangiomas start to appear during the first few weeks of life, whereas congenital hemangiomas are present at birth. There is a predictable natural history for most infantile hemangiomas. The proliferation phase can last an average of 3 to 6 months. After this time, there is a stabilization and then an involution phase. The involution phase often starts when the child is about 1 year of age and can last up to 10 years. During this phase the hemangiomas may develop ulcerations. These can on occasion become secondarily infected and are a source of pain and discomfort. Once resolved, the involved area may show some cutaneous signs such as telangiectasia, atrophy, scarring, and the presence of some fatty fibrosis tissue.

These benign vascular tumors can be classified based on their location within the skin (superficial, deep, or mixed). The more superficially the hemangioma is located, the redder it is in appearance. Superficial infantile hemangiomas will have a bright red and lobulated surface. Deep hemangiomas may not have any surface change and present as nodules within the dermis that are often soft. They often have a bluish hue. Mixed form has areas with both superficial and deep components. Hemangiomas come in all sizes and shapes.

Multiple cutaneous hemangiomas should be evaluated by ultrasound to look for hepatic hemangiomas, which are not infrequently seen in individuals with multiple cutaneous hemangiomas. Large facial hemangiomas should alert the clinician to the possibility that the infant may have PHACE syndrome. This syndrome is composed of **p**osterior fossa malformations, **h**emangioma, **a**rterial defects**, c**oarctation of the aorta, and **e**ye abnormalities. Infants with hemangiomas in the jaw and neck region may also have upper airway involvement, and the airway should be assessed.

Pathogenesis: The etiology of hemangiomas is still not well understood. Many theories have been developed, and each has evidence to support its role. Embolization of placental tissue, maternal hypoxia, the renin-angiotensin system, and a local increase in vasoactive mediators are some of the numerous studied pathogenic mechanisms. More research is necessary to fully document the cause and evolution of hemangiomas.

Histology: Hemangiomas are not routinely biopsied because they are typically diagnosed on appearance and history. Biopsies are usually performed in cases that are not straightforward, and the differential diagnosis includes other forms of vascular anomalies. Infantile hemangiomas in the proliferative phase will show multilobular proliferation of numerous capillaries. The endothelial cells in infantile hemangiomas almost always stain with glucose transporter-1. This stain is rarely positive in other vascular growths, and its presence is a good indicator of infantile hemangiomas. Biopsies during the involution phase show a decrease in the number of capillaries and apoptotic cells, more fibrous fatty tissue, and less mitotic activity.

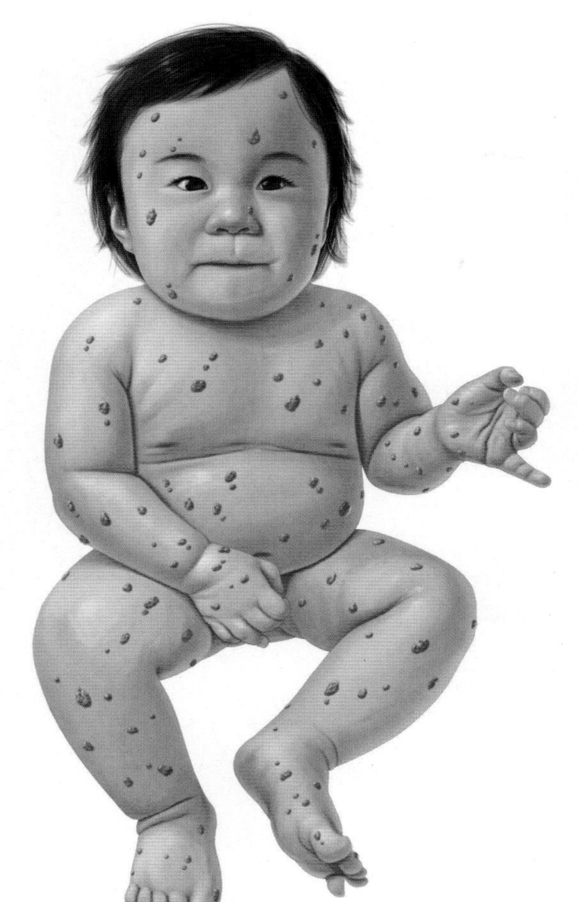

Multiple cutaneous hemangiomas. Infants who develop more than five superficial hemangiomas are given this classification. They are at higher risk for developing hemangiomas of various internal organs.

Paul Kim
C.Machado M.D.

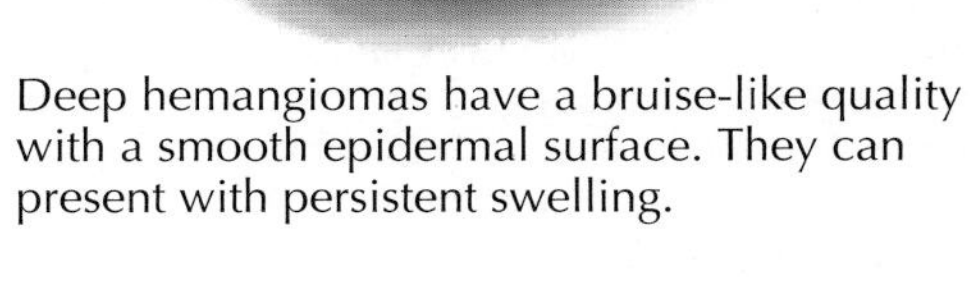

Deep hemangiomas have a bruise-like quality with a smooth epidermal surface. They can present with persistent swelling.

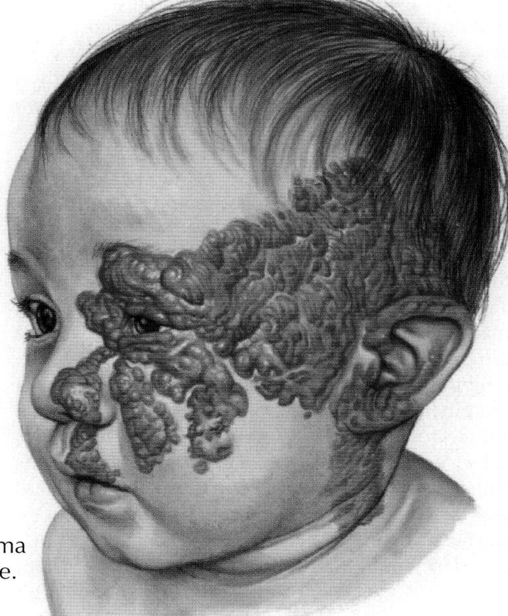

Large segmental cervicofacial hemangioma is one of the features of PHACE syndrome. Superficial hemangiomas are bright red with a textured surface.

Treatment: Many small infantile hemangiomas in noncritical locations often do not require therapy. Infantile hemangiomas that are large or affect critical structures (mouth, airway, eye, anus) are treated with oral propranolol (nonselective β_1- and β_2-blockers) for 6 to 12 months. Care is taken to avoid hypotension and hypoglycemia. This therapy is generally well tolerated. Smaller hemangiomas can be treated with topical timolol. Pulse dye laser is often used during episodes of ulceration. Patients with ulcerated hemangiomas should be monitored for secondary infections, which should be promptly treated with antibiotics. Surgical intervention has become much less frequently performed because of the use of β-blockers. The timing and use of surgery encompass numerous complex factors and require management by surgeons experienced in treating hemangiomas. Surgery can also be used to treat the residual skin changes that may occur after a hemangioma has resolved.

Irritant Contact Dermatitis

Irritant contact dermatitis is one of the most commonly encountered dermatoses in the dermatology clinic. Its true incidence is unknown. Irritant contact dermatitis can be caused by a multitude of factors, and the morphology of its appearance can be varied. One of the most common forms of irritant contact dermatitis is seen on the hands and is caused by occupational exposures to irritant chemicals or excessive handwashing.

Clinical Findings: Irritant contact dermatitis can occur at any age. Some studies show that women are more commonly affected. There is no racial predilection. Many exposures can lead to the development of irritant contact dermatitis. The final clinical manifestations are similar despite the different instigating chemicals. Variations exist in the location of the dermatitis. The hallmark of irritant contact dermatitis is xerosis. Once the skin dries out to a certain point, it becomes inflamed. This leads to the clinical picture of dry pink or red patches. On the hands, painful fissures or splits may occur within the skin lines.

Diaper dermatitis in infants is one specific form of irritant contact dermatitis. The damp diaper rubbing against the child's buttocks and legs can cause skin irritation, red patches, and occasionally erosions. The child can become irritable with pruritus and is at higher risk for secondary bacterial infections.

Many chemicals are direct irritants to the skin, and injuries from these agents are occasionally seen in a dermatologist's office. Exposure of the skin to hydrochloric acid results in skin cell death, necrosis, and inflammation. This, in turn, leads to the development of red patches or plaques with varying amounts of erosion and ulceration. These patients often receive care in an occupational work setting or in the emergency department. The same can be said for exposure of the skin to strong basic chemicals such as sodium hydroxide. Basic chemicals can cause an irritant contact dermatitis that is directly related to the necrotic effect of the chemical on the skin surface.

One of the most common causes of irritant contact dermatitis is frequent handwashing. Soaps remove the sebum that the skin produces as a way of physiologically keeping the skin from drying out. Once the removal of sebum outweighs its production, dryness begins to set in and transepidermal water loss increases. If the skin is not given enough time to repair itself, the epidermis continues to dry out and becomes inflamed. Pink to red patches become evident, and, as the irritation continues, the dryness worsens until fissuring and cracking occur.

Ring dermatitis is another common form of irritant contact dermatitis. Soap residue is believed to build up between the surface of the ring and the skin. This prolonged contact causes an irritant contact dermatitis underlying the ring. It can be misdiagnosed as an allergic contact dermatitis, and on initial presentation these two forms of dermatitis cannot be differentiated. The main differential diagnosis is between an irritant and an allergic contact dermatitis. The two have similar clinical appearances and can be almost impossible to differentiate. Irritant contact dermatitis typically has an acute onset and a decrescendo resolution unless there is repeated exposure to the irritant. Allergic contact dermatitis usually has a crescendo-decrescendo clinical course. These patterns can be helpful in differentiating the two conditions.

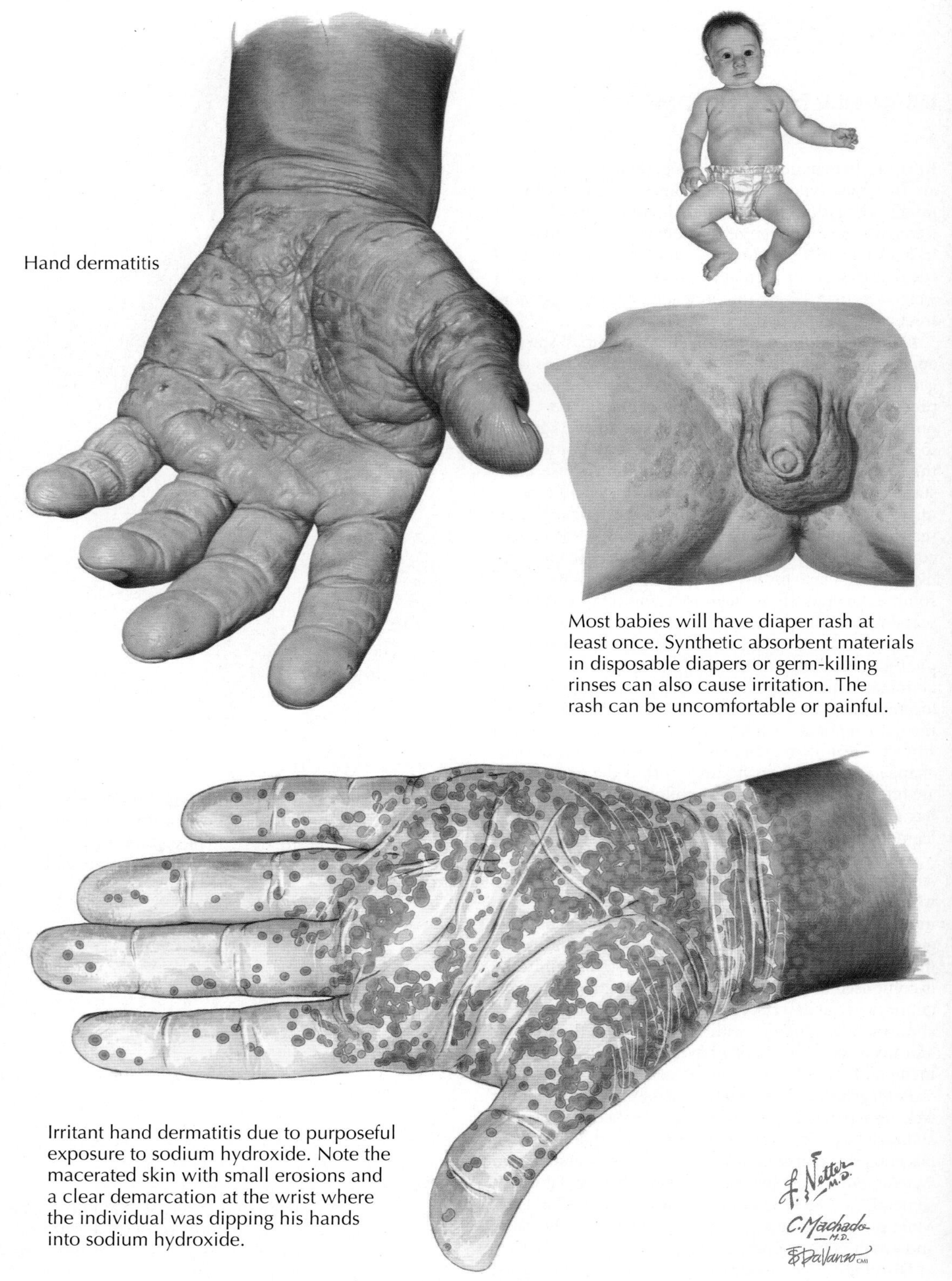

Most babies will have diaper rash at least once. Synthetic absorbent materials in disposable diapers or germ-killing rinses can also cause irritation. The rash can be uncomfortable or painful.

Irritant hand dermatitis due to purposeful exposure to sodium hydroxide. Note the macerated skin with small erosions and a clear demarcation at the wrist where the individual was dipping his hands into sodium hydroxide.

Pathogenesis: Exposure to an irritant chemical, whether an acid or a base, or repeated exposure to soap and water leads to a similar inflammatory cascade. The damaged keratinocytes release myriad inflammatory cytokines. The intensity of the reaction is based on the concentration of the irritant and the exposure time. The recruitment of T cells occurs later in the time course of irritant contact dermatitis compared with allergic contact dermatitis.

Histology: There is a mixed inflammatory infiltrate with a predominance of lymphocytes. Varying degrees of both spongiosis and necrosis of keratinocytes can be seen. In chronic cases, signs of lichenification are noted.

Treatment: The goal of treatment is to eliminate exposure to the irritant. Barrier creams and frequent diaper changes may be all that is needed to resolve irritant contact diaper dermatitis. Hand dermatitis can be treated with a combination of moisturizers, topical corticosteroids, and avoidance of frequent handwashing. If these changes can be accomplished, the prognosis is excellent. Workers with potential occupational exposures to irritant chemicals must be properly trained in handling them and given the correct protective gear to prevent exposure.

Keratosis Pilaris

Keratosis pilaris is an extremely common dermatosis that in mild states can be considered a variant of normal skin. It is usually brought to the clinician's attention as an afterthought, or the clinician observes the condition and tells the patient about it for educational purposes. There are more severe forms of keratosis pilaris in which patients present to the dermatologist for therapy. Many distinct variants of keratosis pilaris exist and are named based on the area of involvement.

Clinical Findings: Keratosis pilaris is found in more than 40% of the adult population and in as many as 80% of children. There is no sex or race predilection. It typically begins soon after a child reaches 5 years of age. Most cases are asymptomatic and are of no concern to the patient or of only cosmetic concern. The upper lateral arms are the most common site of involvement. Small (1–2 mm), pink-to-red follicular hyperkeratotic papules are present to a varying extent. Some are so fine that they are noticeable only on palpation. A small subset of individuals have more extensive disease that can include the upper thighs, shoulders, and cheeks. Widespread cases tend to be more noticeable, and the papules tend to be more inflammatory in nature.

This inflammatory form of keratosis pilaris is also called keratosis pilaris rubra. It is typically manifested by bright red, small, hyperkeratotic papules that may resemble pustules. They can be mistaken for acneiform lesions. A scraping of the inflammatory lesion results in removal of a small keratin plug rather than the contents of an acneiform pustule. The location on the outer arms and upper thighs also helps to differentiate this condition from acne. Both keratosis pilaris and acne are extremely common, and they are often seen together in the same patient.

Ulerythema ophryogenes is a keratosis pilaris variant that manifests in early childhood. The lateral one-third of the eyebrow is affected with minute, red keratotic papules. Hair loss of the lateral eyebrows is common. The rash may affect other parts of the face and may heal with tiny pitted scars. It is almost always seen along with classic keratosis pilaris. Over time, alopecia may develop in the affected regions, especially the lateral eyebrows.

Atrophoderma vermiculata is one of the rare keratosis pilaris variants. It manifests as small, hyperkeratotic plugs on the cheeks that resolve and leave behind small, atrophic scars in a fine, mesh-like pattern.

Erythromelanosis follicularis faciei et colli is similar in nature to atrophoderma vermiculata, but it lacks any evidence of scarring. This condition has been reported to occur most commonly in young men during the second and third decades of life. Postinflammatory hyperpigmentation is another unusual feature not seen with the other variants.

Keratosis follicularis spinulosa decalvans is almost certainly the least common keratosis pilaris variant. It is inherited in a X-linked fashion and thus predominately affects males. It is manifested by areas of skin thickening and follicular plugging along with areas of scarring alopecia. This condition may also affect the eyelashes. Corneal dystrophy and blepharitis can be seen.

Pathogenesis: The exact etiology of keratosis pilaris is unknown. It is believed to be caused by an abnormality in follicular keratinization of the infundibulum, leading to hyperkeratosis.

Histology: Keratosis pilaris is rarely biopsied. A keratin plug is the most prominent feature. The plug is typically 1 to 2 mm in diameter and may lie on top of a meager lymphocytic infiltrate.

Treatment: No therapy is required for most cases. A keratolytic moisturizer or humectant moisturizer works well. These include urea, glycolic acid, lactic acid, and salicylic acid–based moisturizers. After discontinuation, however, the rash of keratosis pilaris returns over a period of a few weeks to months. Many other therapies have been used. Vitamin A derivatives (e.g., tretinoin) are among the more frequently used prescription medications. The cream is applied daily and has been successful in removing the redness and hyperkeratosis.

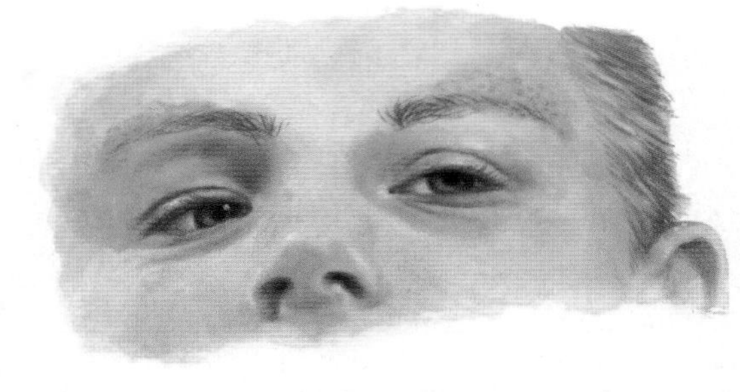

Ulerythema ophryogenes showing loss of the lateral eyebrows

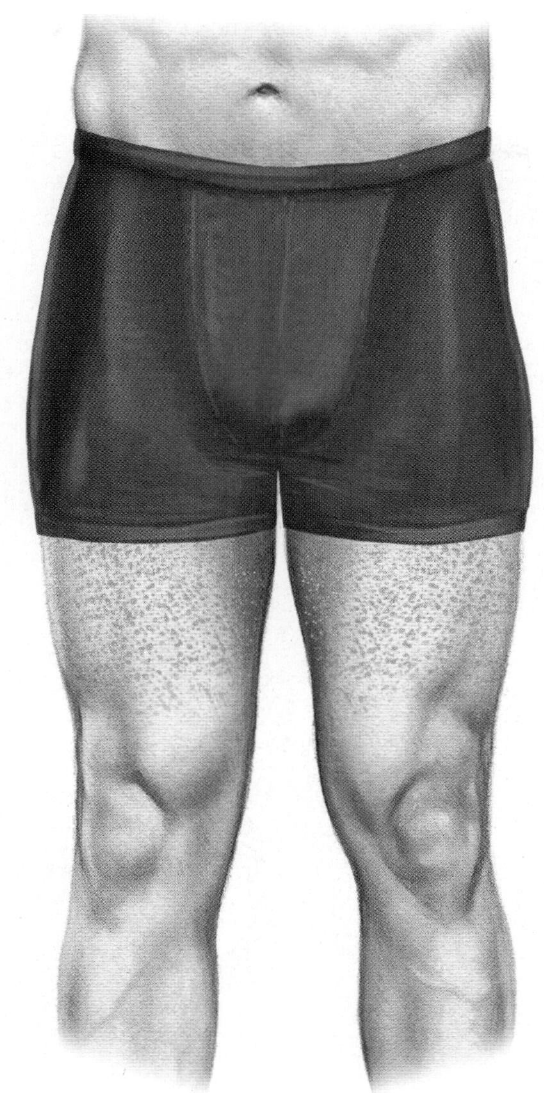

Keratosis pilaris of upper thighs. The upper arms and thighs are two commonly affected areas. Small 1- to 2-mm hyperkeratotic red papules.

C. Machado M.D.
DaVanzo CMI

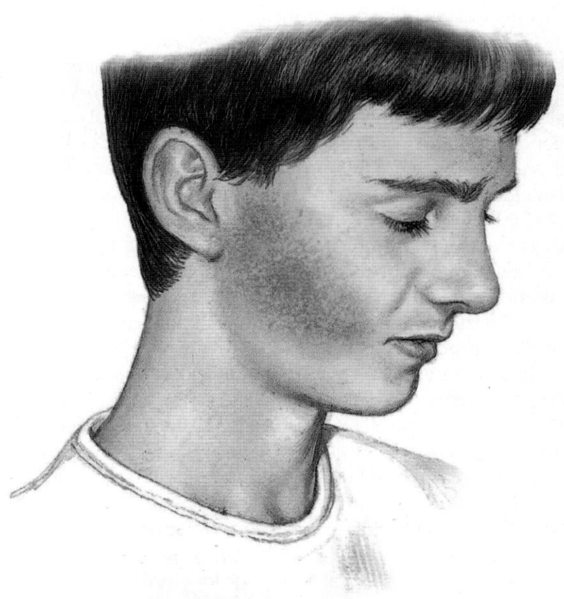

Keratosis pilaris atrophicans faciei. Perifollicular erythema is prominent, as are small regions of atrophic scarring.

Keratosis Pilaris Variants

- ▶ Keratosis pilaris rubra
- ▶ Ulerythema ophryogenes (keratosis pilaris atrophicans faciei)
- ▶ Atrophoderma vermiculata (folliculitis ulerythematosa reticulata)
- ▶ Erythromelanosis follicularis faciei et colli
- ▶ Keratosis follicularis spinulosa decalvans

Langerhans Cell Histiocytosis

Langerhans cell histiocytosis (LCH) is a rare disorder caused by the proliferation of Langerhans cells in various tissues. Historically, the disease was categorized based on the grouping of symptoms and organs affected, with names such as Letterer-Siwe disease and Hand-Schüller-Christian disease. Over 100 histiocytic conditions have been reported. LCH has now been classified with a standardized approach that categorizes LCH into subgroups based on prognosis and extent of involvement. These histiocytoses are a heterogeneous group of diseases that may affect both the skin and various internal organs. The main systemic finding is the accumulation of pathologic Langerhans cells within the affected tissue. The diagnosis is made on clinical, histologic, laboratory, and radiographic findings. The newer classification of LCH is based on the number of organ systems involved. It includes the subtypes of restricted single-system LCH, extensive multisystem LCH, and single-system pulmonary LCH. The extensive multisystem form of LCH can be further divided into cases with and without organ dysfunction. Prognosis and therapy depend on the organ systems involved and the number of systems implicated. Optimal therapy has yet to be determined.

Clinical Findings: LCH is a very rare condition that affects approximately 8 of every 1 million people. There is a 2:1 male-to-female predilection. There is a slight increase in the Hispanic population. Usually, the condition is first noticed in childhood, typically before 3 years of age, but adult-onset disease does occur. LCH isolated to the skin has one of the best prognoses of all of the forms of LCH. Most cases of LCH manifest first in the skin, even before the development of systemic findings; therefore all patients with cutaneous LCH should be routinely screened for systemic diseases.

In infants, the typical presenting skin findings are those of a persistent papulosquamous eruption on the scalp that resembles cradle cap. On closer inspection, small petechiae are observed. These petechiae are very characteristic for LCH and can be easily overlooked. The scalp form is often misdiagnosed as seborrheic dermatitis early in infancy, and frequently it is not until the child is 3 to 6 months old and the rash has persisted that the diagnosis of LCH is entertained. The other common presentation in children is that of persistent diaper dermatitis. The rash has a unique predisposition to affect the groin folds and can be quite inflammatory and resistant to typical therapy for irritant contact dermatitis or diaper dermatitis. The groin rash appears as red to yellowish-orange papules that coalesce into plaques. Ulcerations and erosions are common. Superinfection with bacteria often leads to an odor. These clinical findings typically mimic other common childhood dermatoses. Persistence of the rash or worsening with appropriate therapy for these other dermatoses usually leads the clinician to reevaluate the diagnosis and then perform a skin biopsy to establish the diagnosis. Other skin findings are adenopathy, ear inflammation and drainage from the external ear, and soft tissue swelling. The soft tissue swelling is seen only in patients with underlying bony disorders. Gingival hypertrophy may also be seen, but it is often subtle. Infants may also have premature eruption of their teeth, which is most commonly noticed by the still breastfeeding mother.

Presentation of Langerhans Cell Histiocytosis in Childhood

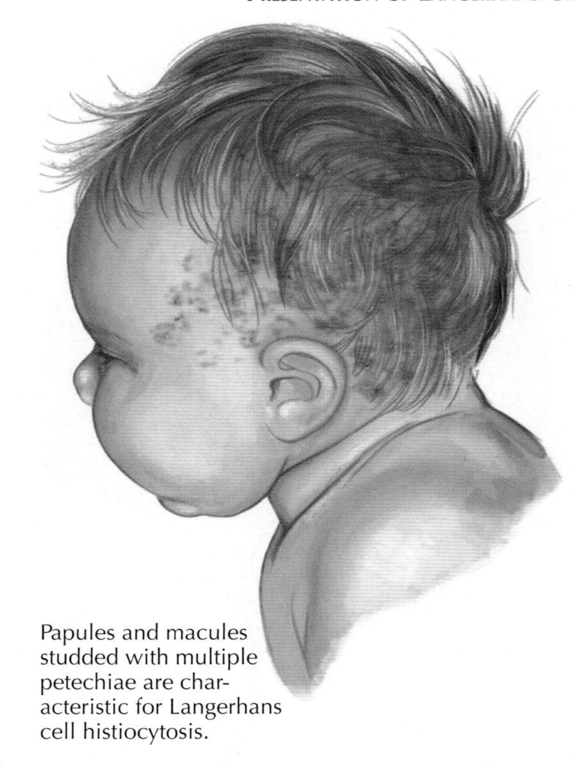

Papules and macules studded with multiple petechiae are characteristic for Langerhans cell histiocytosis.

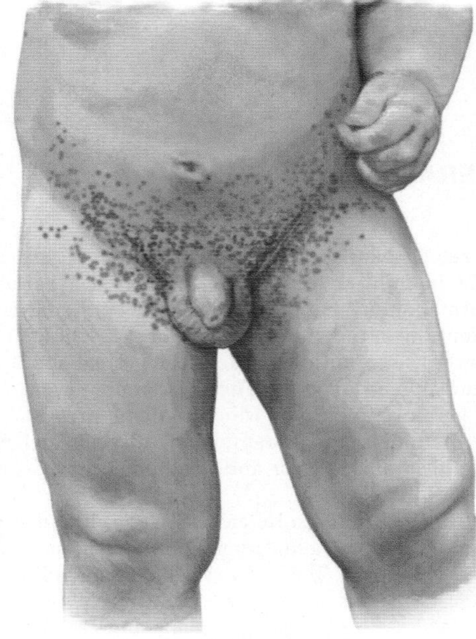

The diaper area is one of the more common areas of involvement with Langerhans cell histiocytosis. This disease should be in the differential diagnosis of diaper rash that does not respond to therapy for dermatitis, especially if petechiae are present.

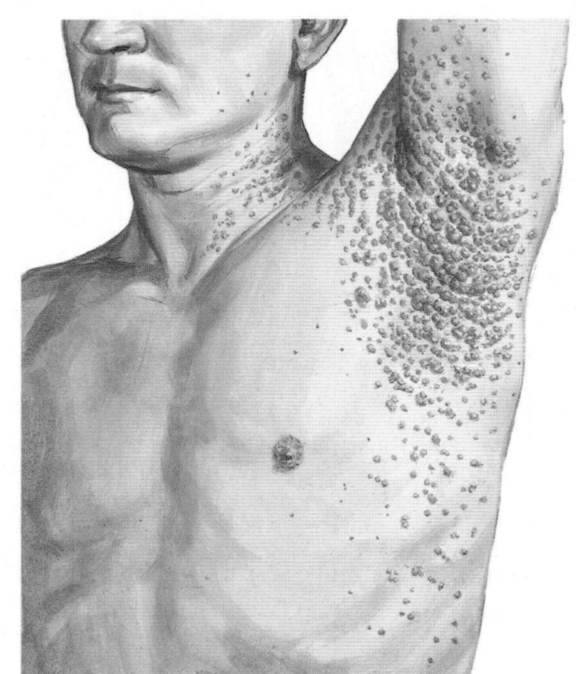

Disseminated Langerhans cell histiocytosis lesions in axilla and on neck and trunk

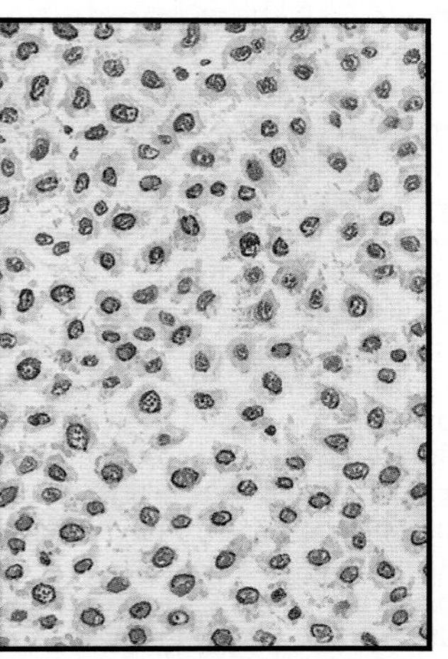

Sheets of Langerhans cell histiocytes with abundant pink cytoplasm and folded nuclei with prominent nuclear grooves

F. Netter M.D.
C. Machado M.D.
DaVanzo CMI

Twenty percent of patients do not exhibit any cutaneous signs of disease and present solely with varying systemic symptoms. The most common extracutaneous form of LCH, formerly designated eosinophilic granuloma, is now called single-system unifocal bone disease. Children present with a painless to slightly tender soft tissue swelling overlying the bony area of involvement, most commonly the calvarium. Palpation of the swelling reveals the fluctuant nature of the soft tissue distention, and in some cases the defect in the underlying bone can be felt. Plain radiographs can help delineate the extent of disease. If one area of bony involvement is found, a skeletal survey should be performed to evaluate for other silent bony lesions, which can occur in up to 15% of cases. The involved bone has a radiolucent appearance that is sharply demarcated from the surrounding bone. Bony involvement has been described to occur in almost every bone in the body. Most cases are inconsequential, but if the involvement affects a critical portion of the spine, the possibility of weakening of the joint and

Langerhans Cell Histiocytosis (Continued)

potential fracture could have life-threatening implications. The term "floating teeth" has been used to describe the finding of radiolucent aspects of the mandible that give the appearance that the teeth are floating without the support of the underlying bone.

LCH can be a life-threatening, progressive disease. The lymphatic system, lungs, hypothalamus, and pituitary are commonly involved. Lymphadenopathy in the region of skin or bony involvement is usually seen. Biopsies of lymph nodes can show involvement with Langerhans cells or dermatopathic changes.

Lung involvement is almost always a component of multisystem disease. Radiographs may be normal or may show cystic spaces or a nonspecific interstitial infiltrate. Pulmonary function testing may reveal a decrease in diffusion capacity and a decrease in forced expiratory volume. Lung abnormalities are frequently seen in adults with LCH.

The pituitary stalk can also be affected in this disease. The eponym *Hans-Schüller-Christian disease* describes patients with LCH who have the constellation of diabetes insipidus, lytic bony lesions, and exophthalmos. The involvement of the pituitary stalk leads to the diabetes insipidus. The lack of antidiuretic hormone causes the excretion of large amounts of dilute urine and increased thirst. The skull is the bony region most commonly involved.

Letterer-Siwe disease is the name given to the constellation of symptoms that include severe skin involvement, hepatosplenomegaly, anemia, and leukopenia. These patients have early onset of disease in infancy and have a poor prognosis because of the aggressiveness and extent of the disease load.

The diagnosis and prognosis of LCH depend on the number of organ systems involved and the extent of disease. Treatment likewise depends on these factors, and a multidisciplinary approach should be taken.

Pathogenesis: The exact etiology is unknown, and there is considerable ongoing research to determine whether this is a clonal malignant process or a reactive process. The Langerhans cells present within the areas of involvement have a different morphology from their normal counterparts. The affected Langerhans cells are round, without dendritic processes, and have been found to express different cell surface markers. The clonal Langerhans cells are $CD1a^+/CD207^+$ cells and have continuous activation of the MAPK pathway. *BRAF* and *MAP2K1* gene mutations have been found in LCH, but no single gene defect has been described as pathogenic.

Histology: Histologic findings from the skin and other involved tissues are only slightly different. The main pathology is found within the sheets of abnormal-appearing Langerhans cells. On microscopic evaluation, the cells have kidney bean–shaped nucleus and show varying amounts of epidermotropism. Immunohistochemical staining shows CD1a, S100, and CD207 positivity. On electron microscopy, the characteristic tennis racket–shaped Birbeck granules are seen.

Treatment: Therapy is determined by the extent and location of disease state. Mild, localized cutaneous single-system disease may be observed and watched carefully for the development of systemic involvement. Supportive care is given with topical antiinflammatory agents and antiinfectives to help treat and prevent possible infections, especially infections of the intertriginous region in infants. A small percentage of patients experience spontaneous remission. Single bony lesions may also remit spontaneously.

Bony lesions have been treated with resection of the involved tissue, curettage of the region, and systemic steroid therapy. Steroid use has been associated with recurrences after the drug is stopped.

Multisystem disease is treated in myriad ways depending on the burden of disease, the systemic involvement, and the patient's symptoms. The disease can be difficult to treat, and systemic chemotherapies are the mainstay of treatment. Vinblastine- or etoposide-based regimens are most commonly used as first-line therapy. MAPK pathway inhibitors and BRAF inhibitors are being studied. Some refractory disease has been treated with ablative chemotherapy and subsequent stem cell transplantation.

Eosinophilic Granuloma

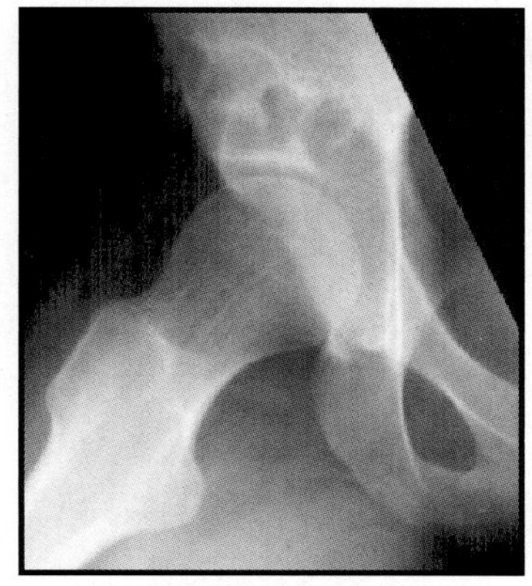

Radiograph shows loculated, bubble-like, radiolucent lesion in supraacetabular region of right ilium.

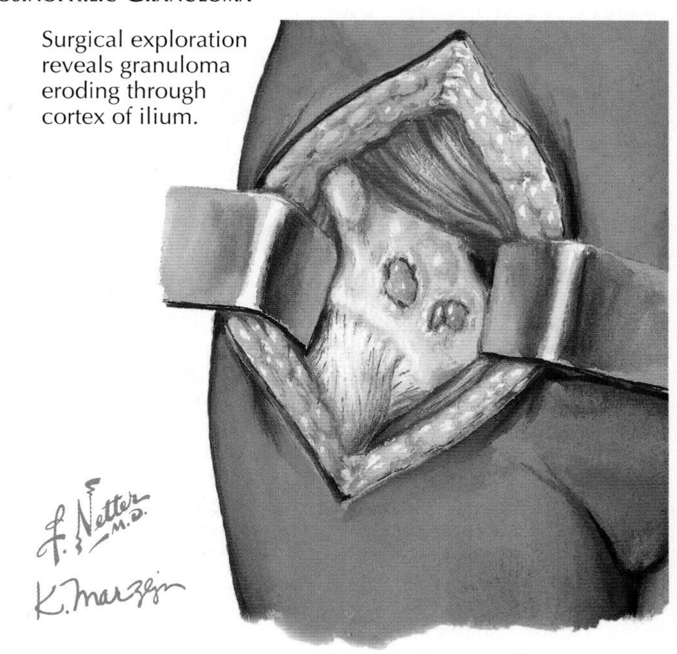

Surgical exploration reveals granuloma eroding through cortex of ilium.

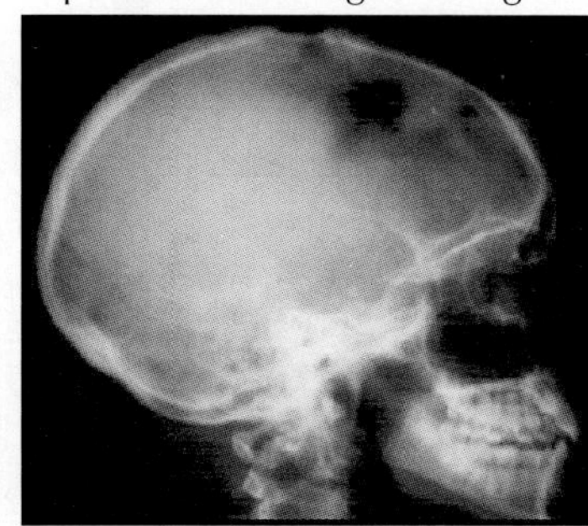

Variegated defects in flat bones of skull

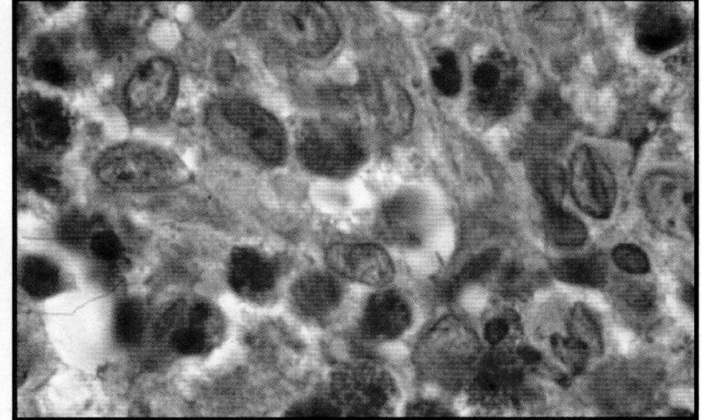

Section reveals pale-staining, foamy histiocytes interspersed with bilobed eosinophils (H&E stain).

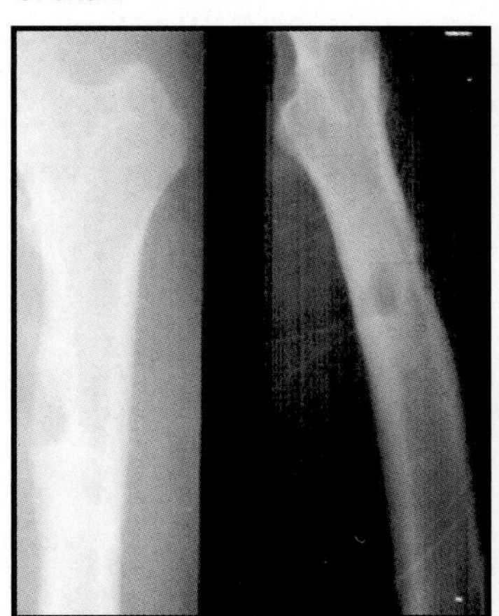

Anteroposterior and lateral views show typical marginated, radiolucent lesions in femoral shaft.

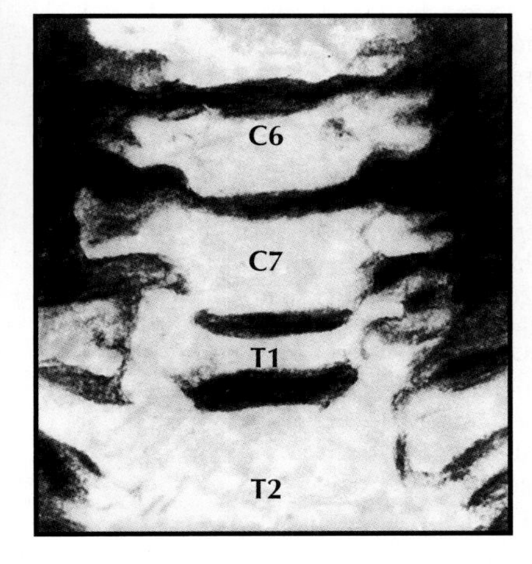

Marked narrowing of first thoracic vertebra that led to spinal cord injury in 13-year-old boy. Vertebra plana in young patients strongly suggests eosinophilic granuloma.

LEUKOCYTOCLASTIC VASCULITIS

Many forms of vasculitis can affect the skin, the most common being leukocytoclastic vasculitis. Other forms of vasculitis known to affect the skin as well as other organ systems include Churg-Strauss vasculitis, Henoch-Schönlein purpura, granulomatosis with polyangiitis, polyarteritis nodosa, and urticarial vasculitis. Leukocytoclastic vasculitis is by far the most frequently encountered of the cutaneous vasculitides. The causes and pathomechanisms vary, and diagnosis and treatment depend on the results of the clinical and histologic evaluations.

Clinical Findings: Leukocytoclastic vasculitis has no racial or sex predilection and is most commonly seen in the adult population. Leukocytoclastic vasculitis most commonly affects the lower extremities or dependent areas of the body. For example, this form of vasculitis is most commonly seen on the legs of ambulatory patients and on the back and buttocks of bedridden patients. The clinical hallmark of vasculitis is the presence of palpable purpura. The rash may start as small, pink, violaceous macules that rapidly develop into red or purple palpable papules; hence the term *palpable purpura*. Most of the lesions of palpable purpura are uniform in size, but they can range from minute to 1 cm or more in diameter. Patients are most likely to report mild itching, pain, or no symptoms at all, and the rash is what brings them to see the clinician. Mild constitutional symptoms are often present, with mild fever, fatigue, and malaise regularly reported. Skin-specific symptoms can range from mild pruritus to pain and tenderness on palpation.

The etiology of cutaneous leukocytoclastic vasculitis is heterogeneous. Many cases are idiopathic in nature, with the most common causes being infections and medications. Leukocytoclastic vasculitis can also be a sign of an underlying malignancy. Almost every possible infection (bacterial, viral, parasitic, and fungal) has been reported as an initiating factor for leukocytoclastic vasculitis. Medications are a common culprit and can easily be overlooked if a thorough history is not obtained. If the offending infection is treated properly or the offending medication is removed, the vasculitis resolves in approximately 1 month. The symptoms also cease, often faster than the rash resolves. Postinflammatory hyperpigmentation with some hemosiderin deposition often is a residual finding after the lesions have cleared. This resolves slowly over 6 to 12 months. When diagnosed, individuals should have their kidney function assessed (blood urea nitrogen and creatinine ratio and urinalysis) because the kidney is the most frequently affected internal organ.

Pathogenesis: Leukocytoclastic vasculitis is a type III hypersensitivity reaction. Soluble antigens are believed to become complexed with antibodies. As these antigen-antibody complexes enlarge, they get trapped in the tiny vasculature of the dependent regions of the body. There, they can initiate the complement cascade and cause endothelial cell wall death, recruitment of neutrophils, and continued blood vessel destruction, leading to the typical cutaneous findings.

Histology: The pathology is centered on the blood venules in the dermis. A prominent neutrophilic infiltrate is present. Degeneration of the neutrophils is always seen, with nuclear dust; this is termed *leukocytoclasis*. Fibrinoid necrosis of the vessel walls is easily seen. Extravasated red blood cells are seen in the vicinity of the vasculitis. Thrombosis of affected vessel walls is a secondary finding and is not the primary pathology.

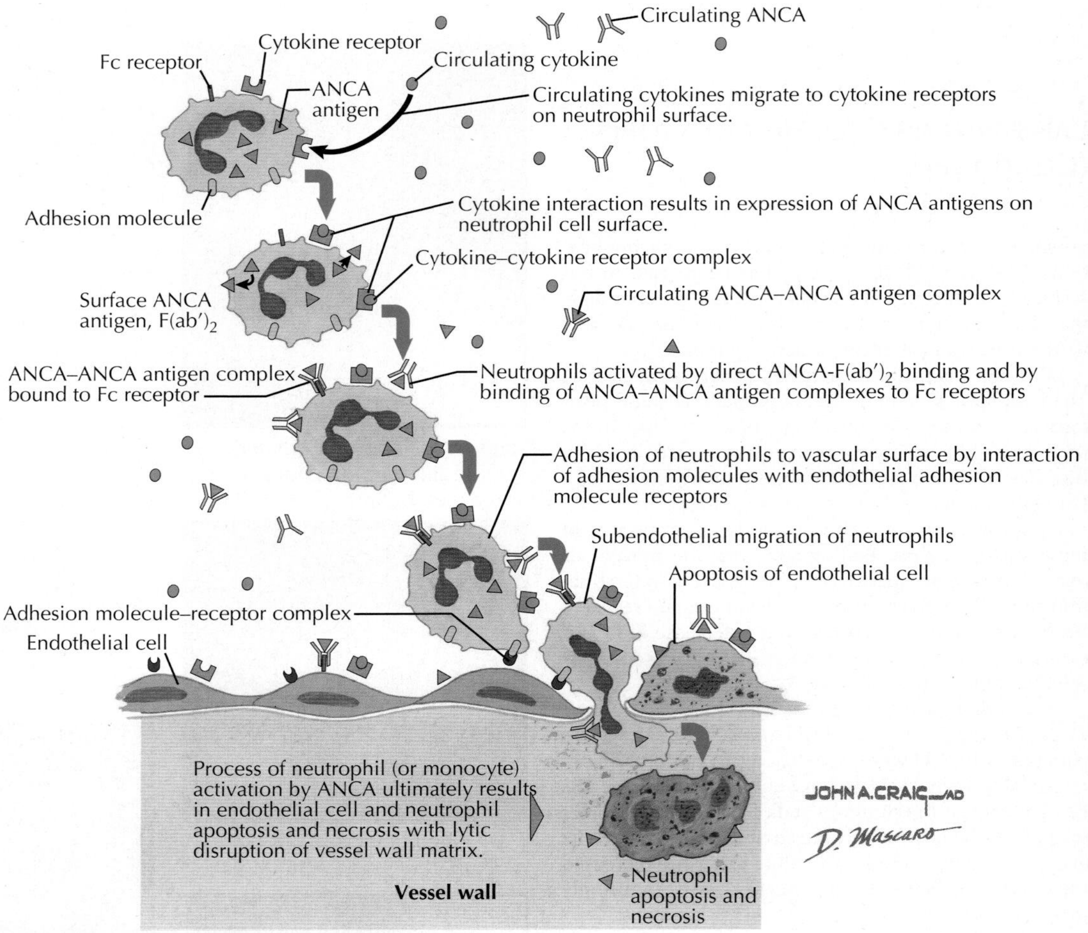

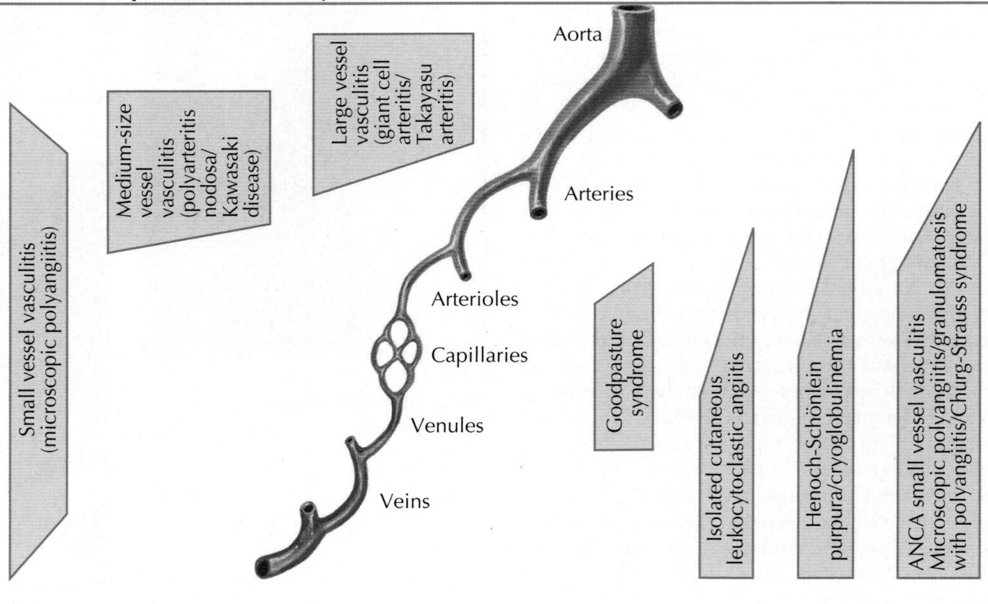

Treatment: Therapy is based on the cause of the leukocytoclastic vasculitis. Offending medications should be withdrawn and replaced with substitutes of a different class. Infections must be thoroughly treated. The use of topical high-potency corticosteroids is helpful in some cases, and oral steroids may be used in medication-induced leukocytoclastic vasculitis. In cases of infection-induced vasculitis, prednisone should be reserved until after the infection has been properly treated. Idiopathic vasculitis is treated with oral steroids, and often a search for an infection or other cause is undertaken. A thorough history and physical examination are needed, as well as some screening laboratory tests. Random laboratory testing usually is not helpful unless the history or review of symptoms points in a particular direction. If patients experience more than simply very mild systemic symptoms, an evaluation should be done to rule out the more serious forms of vasculitis.

Lichen Planus

Lichen planus is a common inflammatory skin disease. It is unique in that it can affect the skin, the mucous membranes, the nails, and the epithelium of the hair follicles. Lichen planus most commonly affects the skin, but the other areas can be involved either solely or in conjunction with one another. Lichen planus that involves the skin tends to spontaneously remit within 1 to 2 years after onset, whereas the oral version is almost always chronic.

Clinical Findings: Lichen planus can affect people at any age, but it is much more common in adulthood. It has no sex or racial predilection. The rash is classically described as flat-topped, polygonal, pruritic, purple papules. Frequently, a whitish, lacy scale, referred to as *Wickham striae*, overlies the papules. Lichen planus is unusual in that the pruritus causes most patients to rub the area rather than scratch. Lichen planus exhibits the Koebner phenomenon, and often areas of linear arrangement are seen secondary to trauma or rubbing. This is helpful when clinically examining a patient because scratch marks and excoriations are rarely seen, whereas lichenification from repeated rubbing of the lesions is frequently seen. The rash tends to be more prominent on flexural surfaces, especially of the wrists. The glans penis is another distinctive location in which lichen planus commonly occurs.

Many clinical variations of lichen planus have been described. An afflicted individual may have more than one morphology. Hypertrophic lichen planus has the appearance of thickened, scaly plaques with a rough or verrucal surface. Areas on the periphery may appear more classic in nature. This variant can be difficult to diagnosis clinically, and often a biopsy is required. It also can be difficult to treat effectively, and it runs a chronic course. Rarely, hypertrophic lichen planus has been reported to transform into malignant squamous cell carcinoma. Bullous lichen planus is an extremely uncommon variant that usually occurs on the lower extremities. The vesicle or bulla typically forms within the center of the lichen planus lesion.

Lichen planopilaris is the term given to describe lichen planus affecting the terminal hair follicles. This is most common on the scalp and leads to a scarring alopecia. The typical findings are small, erythematous patches surrounding each hair follicle. As the disease progresses, loss of hair follicles is observed, signifying that scarring is taking place. The central crown is the area most often affected. It is uncommon for the entire scalp to be affected. Once scarring has occurred, the hair loss is permanent. Lichen planopilaris runs a chronic waxing and waning clinical course.

Lichen planus may affect the mucous membranes of the oral cavity, the genital region, and the conjunctiva. These areas appear as glistening patches with lacy, white reticulations on the surface. Mucous membrane lichen planus has a higher tendency to ulcerate than the cutaneous form does. There have been reports of malignant transformation to squamous cell carcinoma. For this reason, long-term follow-up is required. Lichen planus may also affect the nail matrix and nail bed, leading to dystrophy and nail abnormalities. The most frequently seen nail abnormality is longitudinal ridging, but the most characteristic nail finding is pterygium formation.

Generalized lichen planus

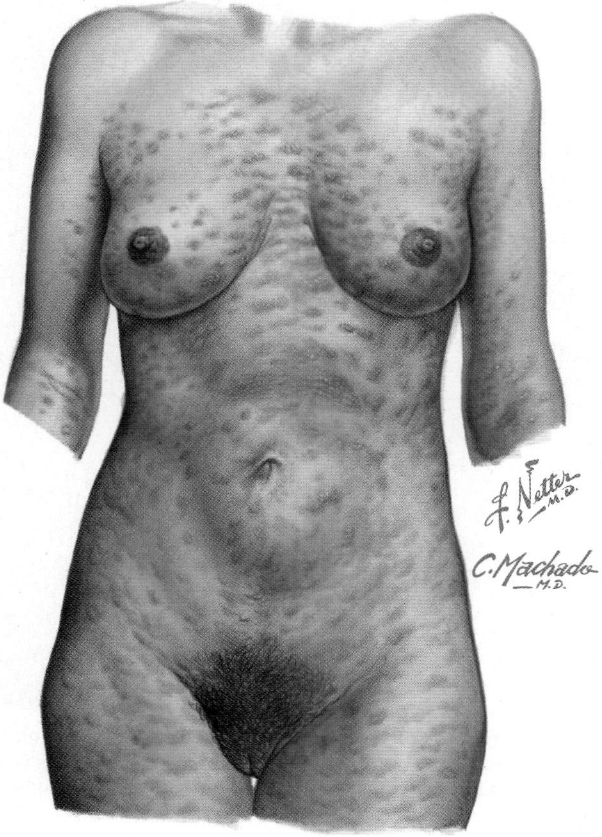

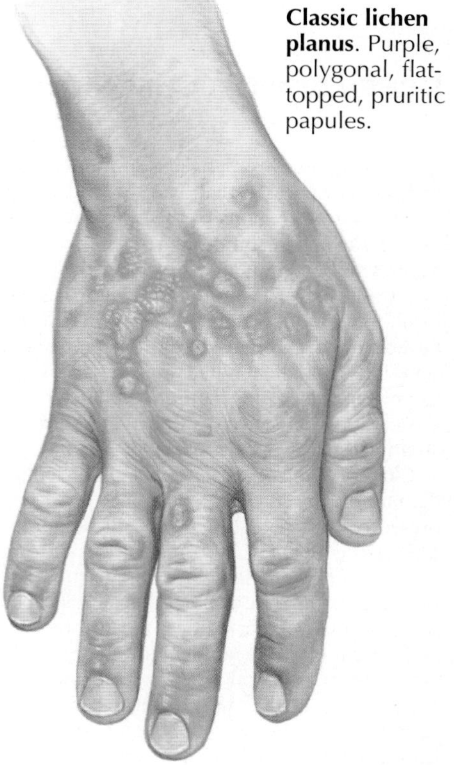

Classic lichen planus. Purple, polygonal, flat-topped, pruritic papules.

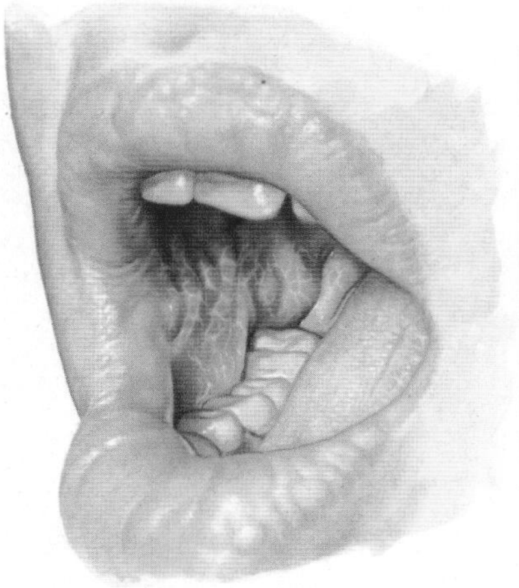

Oral lichen planus

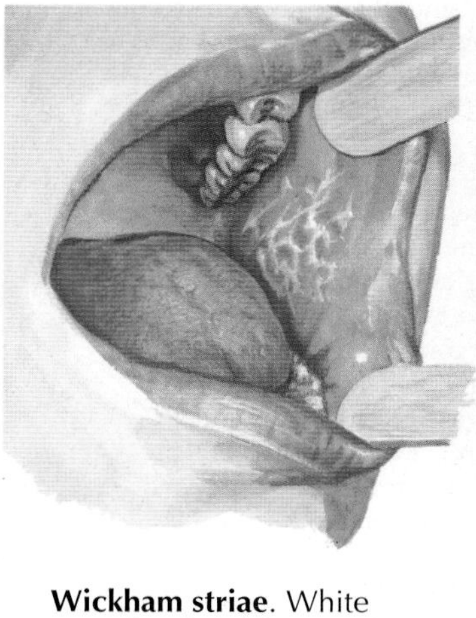

Wickham striae. White reticulated patches on the buccal mucosa.

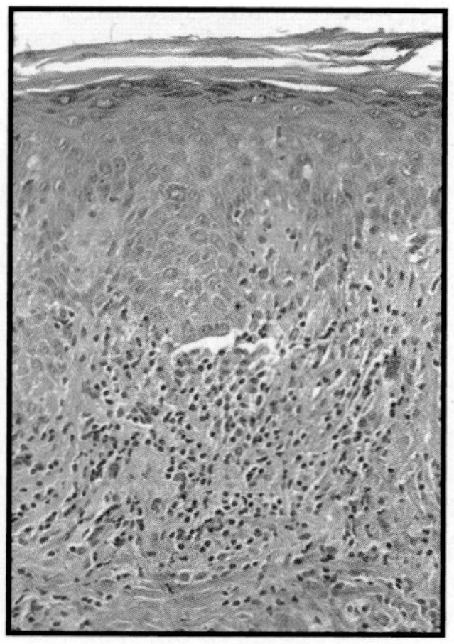

Histology of lichen planus. Lichenoid lymphocytic infiltrate with "saw-toothing" of the rete ridges, decreased granular cell layer, and a Max Joseph space at the dermal-epidermal junction.

Pathogenesis: Lichen planus appears to be mediated by an abnormal T-cell immune response. The T-cells act locally on the keratinocytes to induce the clinical findings. It is a mixed $CD4^+$ and $CD\ 8^+$ T-cell inflammatory infiltrate. Genetic predisposition has been described with association with various HLA markers. The exact pathomechanism has yet to be described.

Histology: The lesions show characteristic findings that include a dense lichenoid lymphocytic infiltrate along the dermal-epidermal border. Necrotic keratinocytes are frequently encountered within the hyperplastic epidermis and have been named Civatte bodies. Hypergranulosis is a prominent feature, as is the "saw-tooth" pattern of epidermal hyperplasia. The presence of eosinophils should lead the clinician to consider the diagnosis of a lichen planus–like drug eruption or lichenoid contact dermatitis.

Treatment: Isolated lesions can be treated with topical corticosteroids or immunomodulators. Up to two-thirds of skin lesions resolve spontaneously. Patients with widespread disease present a therapeutic challenge. Ultraviolet phototherapy, oral corticosteroids, and oral retinoids such as acitretin and isotretinoin have been used. Mucosal disease tends to be chronic and can be resistant to treatment. Many systemic agents have been used to treat persistent disease.

LICHEN SIMPLEX CHRONICUS

Lichen simplex chronicus is a commonly encountered chronic dermatosis that can be initiated by many events. Certain regions of the body are more prone to developing lichen simplex chronicus, such as the lower leg and ankle region and the posterior scalp, but it can occur anywhere. The initiating factor can be any skin insult that induces itching. The itch-scratch cycle is never broken, and the skin in the region being manipulated takes on a lichenified appearance. This is believed to be a localized skin condition that has no systemic associations or causes. Many therapies have been attempted with varying rates of success.

Clinical Findings: There is a slight female preponderance and no racial predilection. Most patients who present with lichen simplex chronicus do not relate an underlying insult that initiated the chronic itching. Some report a previous bug bite, trauma, or initiating rash such as allergic contact dermatitis caused by poison ivy. Involvement is localized to one region of the body, most often the ankle. Other commonly involved areas are the occipital scalp and the anogenital region. Patients report that they have a constant itching or burning sensation, and they respond to it by chronically rubbing or itching the area. Initially, a fine red patch with some excoriations is present. As the condition becomes chronic, the rash takes on the clinical appearance of lichen simplex chronicus. The skin becomes thickened and lichenified. There is an accentuation of the normal skin lines, and the region of involvement shows varying degrees of hyperpigmentation. Small excoriations and even small ulcerations may occur if the pruritus is severe and the patient cannot control the itching.

The cycle of pruritus and itching is perpetuated and can last for years to decades if untreated. Patients often relate that stressful events can initiate a flare of preexisting lichen simplex chronicus. They also regularly state that the itching is worse during the evening hours just before sleep. It is theorized that the cortex is not as busy processing information at that time, and areas of the brain that are responsible for itching become activated or disinhibited from cortical control. Even with treatment, some cases last for years. Patients typically become frustrated with therapy and are willing to pursue the help of other clinicians or ancillary medical caregivers, such as acupuncturists. A fully developed area of lichen simplex chronicus is a well-defined lichenified plaque with excoriations and blood-tinged crust.

Pathogenesis: The exact pathomechanism of development is unknown. Initiating events have been investigated, including insect bite reactions, underlying atopic diathesis, anxiety, stressful events, and other psychiatric conditions. Many patients have none of these factors, yet the clinical and pathologic picture is identical.

Histology: The epidermis is acanthotic with elongation of the rete ridges. A varying amount of parakeratosis is present, with excoriations and superficial ulcerations observed in some cases. The collagen bundles within the papillary dermis show a vertical arrangement, parallel to the rete ridges. The rete ridges are irregular in elongation, unlike the regular pattern seen in psoriasis. A varying degree of epidermal spongiosis is seen but no epidermotropism. The inflammatory infiltrate is composed primarily of lymphocytes.

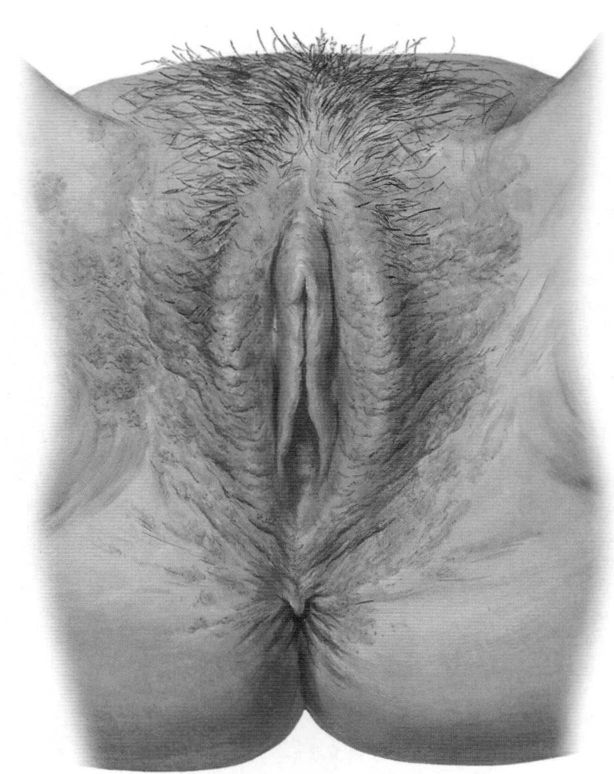

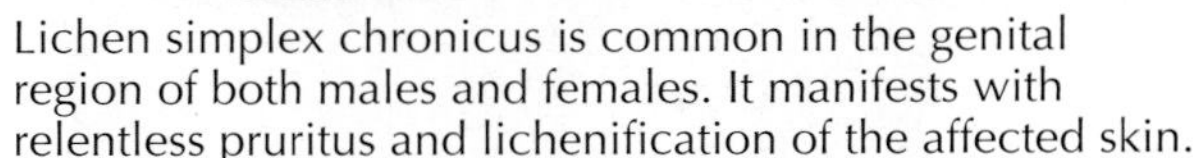

Lichen simplex chronicus is common in the genital region of both males and females. It manifests with relentless pruritus and lichenification of the affected skin.

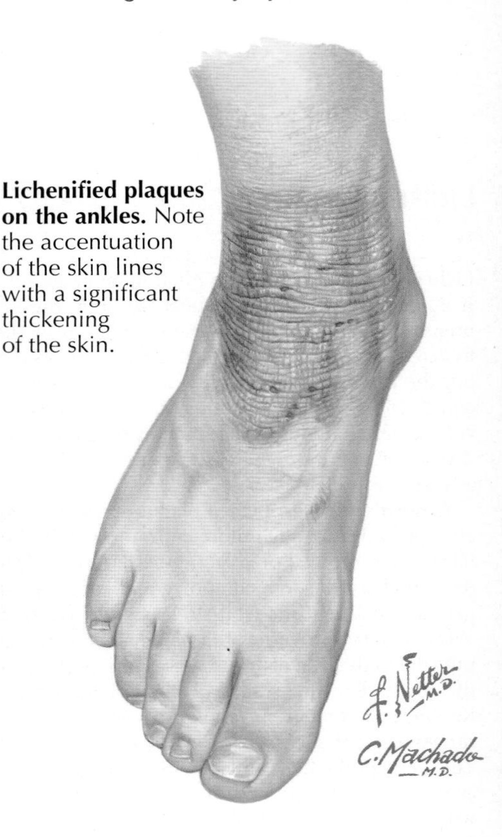

Lichenified plaques on the ankles. Note the accentuation of the skin lines with a significant thickening of the skin.

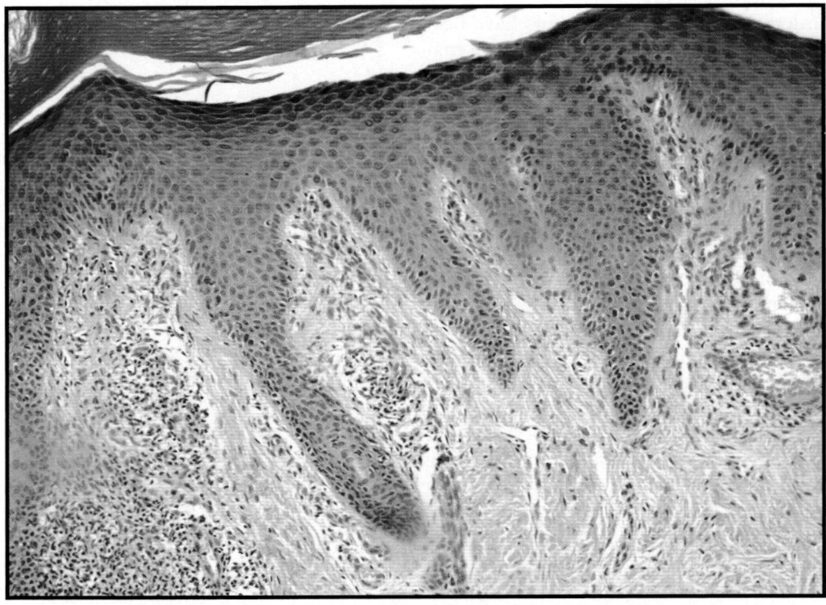

Acanthosis with elongation of the rete ridges. Patchy hyperkeratosis and parakeratosis. Vertically arranged collagen is present within the dermal papilla.

Treatment: Therapy is often directed at breaking the itch-scratch cycle. This is attempted with a combination of topical high-potency corticosteroids and oral antihistamines or gabapentin. The sedating antihistamines work better than the newer, nonsedating ones. Topical steroids may be used under occlusion for better penetration of the lichenified region. Intralesional injection with triamcinolone may be attempted. Capsaicin, which is derived from capsicum peppers, may be used. This agent works by depleting the superficial nerve endings of substance P, the neurotransmitter required for the itching sensation. Patients should be advised to trim their fingernails to help prevent trauma when they scratch. Behavioral modification may be attempted, but it is best accomplished by a professional psychiatrist or psychologist. Precipitating causes such as stress should be addressed. Patients often have remissions with frequent relapses.

Lower Extremity Vascular Insufficiency

Vascular insufficiency of the lower extremity is a common finding in the older population. Factors that increase the risk of vascular disease include diabetes, obesity, smoking, hypertension, and hypercholesterolemia. Both the venous and the arterial systems may be affected, and the signs and symptoms are unique to each. The combination of venous and arterial insufficiency is commonly seen in older patients with diabetes, especially those who smoke. Abnormalities of the lymphatic system may cause findings similar to those of venous insufficiency. Risk factors for lymphatic disease include prior surgeries (e.g., inguinal lymph node dissection), radiotherapy, and idiopathic lymphedema.

Clinical Findings: Venous insufficiency is a common disease that has no racial or ethnic predilection. It has been reported to be slightly more common in women. Venous insufficiency eventually leads to venous stasis and ulcerations. It has been estimated to be the cause of more than 50% of lower extremity ulcerations, with arterial insufficiency being the next most common cause, and neuropathic causes and lymphedema accounting for the remainder.

The first signs of venous insufficiency may be the development of varicose veins or smaller dilated reticular veins. As time progresses, venous stasis changes are seen, including dry, pink to red, eczematous patches with varying amounts of peripheral pitting edema. Red blood cells are extravasated into the dermis where, over time, they break down and form hemosiderin deposits, which appear as brown to reddish macules and patches. Continued venous hypertension, stasis, and swelling may eventually lead to a venous stasis ulcer. These ulcers are most commonly present on the medial malleolus region of the ankle but can occur almost anywhere on the lower extremity. They are usually nontender, but some can be exquisitely painful.

Arterial insufficiency is most often caused by atherosclerosis of the larger arteries of the lower extremity. Patients often have coexisting risk factors, including older age, hypertension, smoking, diabetes, and hypercholesterolemia. Arterial ulcers are slightly more common in men, and there is no racial predilection. The clinical presenting signs are often dependent rubor, claudication, and rest pain. Physical examination confirms the absence of peripheral pulses in the dorsal pedal and posterior tibial arteries. At this point, the patient is at high risk for arterial ulcerations and subsequent gangrene. Surgical intervention is the only viable means of treatment.

Pathogenesis: Venous drainage of the lower extremity is accomplished via the superficial and deep systems of veins that are connected through horizontally arranged communicating vessels. These veins contain one-way bicuspid valves that prevent backflow and work with the action of muscle contraction to force the venous flow in a superior direction, eventually to empty into the inferior vena cava. The flow of venous blood toward the vena cava is the primary responsibility of the leg muscles, especially the calf muscle. Patients with sedentary lifestyles are at higher risk for venous insufficiency. During ambulation, the venous pressure normally decreases as the blood flow is increased toward the vena cava. If an abnormality exists and this does not occur, venous hypertension ensues. Congenital absence of the venous valves, incompetent valves, and a history of deep venous thrombosis are just three of the potential reasons for venous insufficiency. Once venous hypertension occurs, the patient is at risk for development of venous stasis and venous ulcerations.

Arterial insufficiency is caused by a slow narrowing of the arteries due to cholesterol plaque. This narrowing restricts the amount of blood flow to the tissue. Once the flow is decreased to less than the requirement needed for muscle and normal physiologic functioning, symptoms arise.

Histology: Biopsies should not be performed in cases of arterial insufficiency because they lead to ulcerations, infections, and, most likely, emergent surgery. Histologic evaluation of venous ulcerations shows a nonspecific ulcer, edema, proliferation of superficial dermal vessels, and extravasated red blood cells with a varying amount of hemosiderin deposition.

Treatment: Venous insufficiency is treated with a combination of compression and leg elevation. Losing weight and increasing the activity level may also help. Removal of incompetent veins may help. Arterial insufficiency is best treated surgically with stent placement or arterial bypass of the narrowed artery. The treatment for the patient's underlying hypertension, hypercholesterolemia, and diabetes should be maximized. Individuals must quit smoking. Pentoxifylline has also been used, with variable success, in early disease.

Vascular Insufficiency in Diabetes

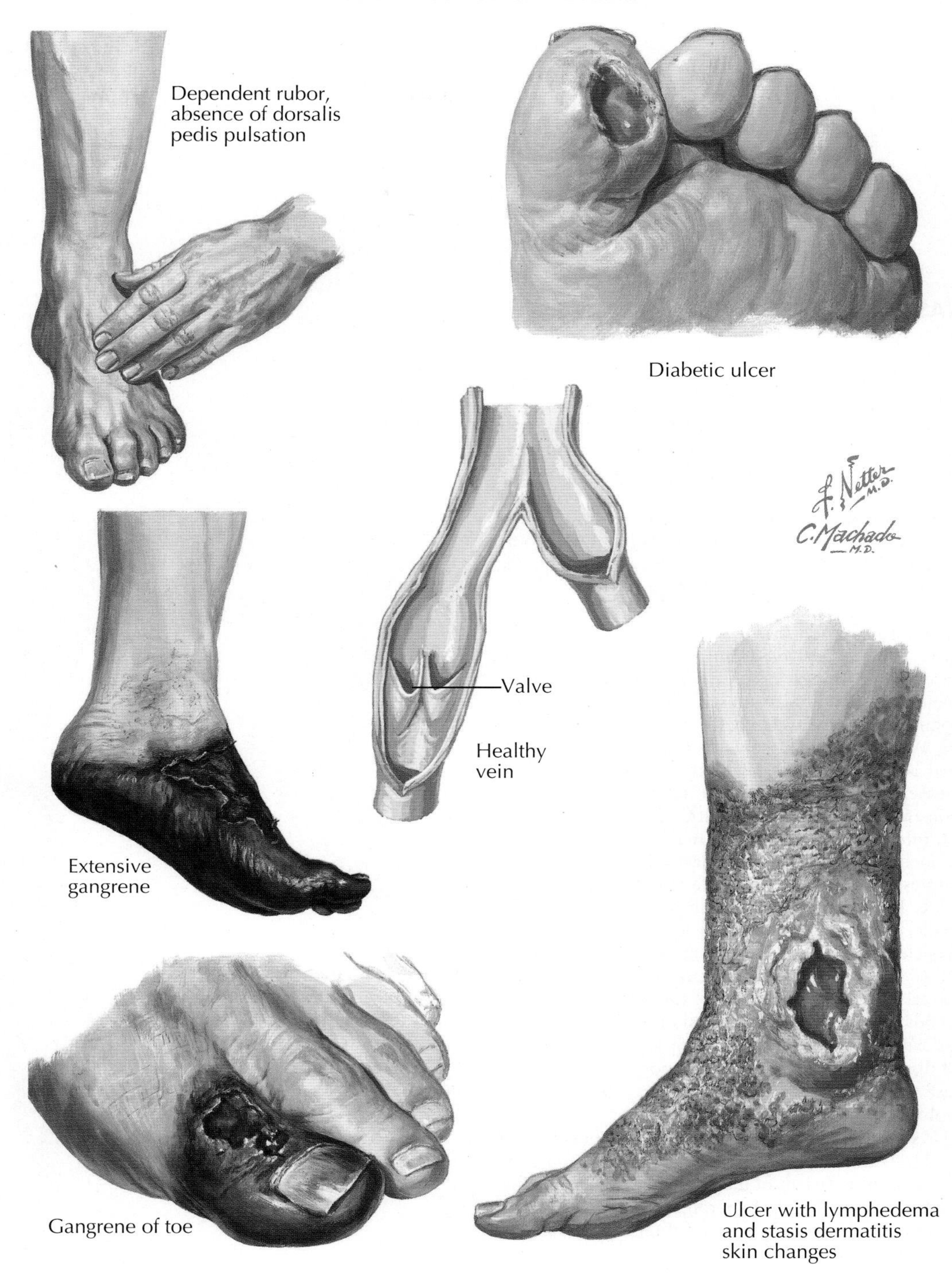

Mast Cell Disease

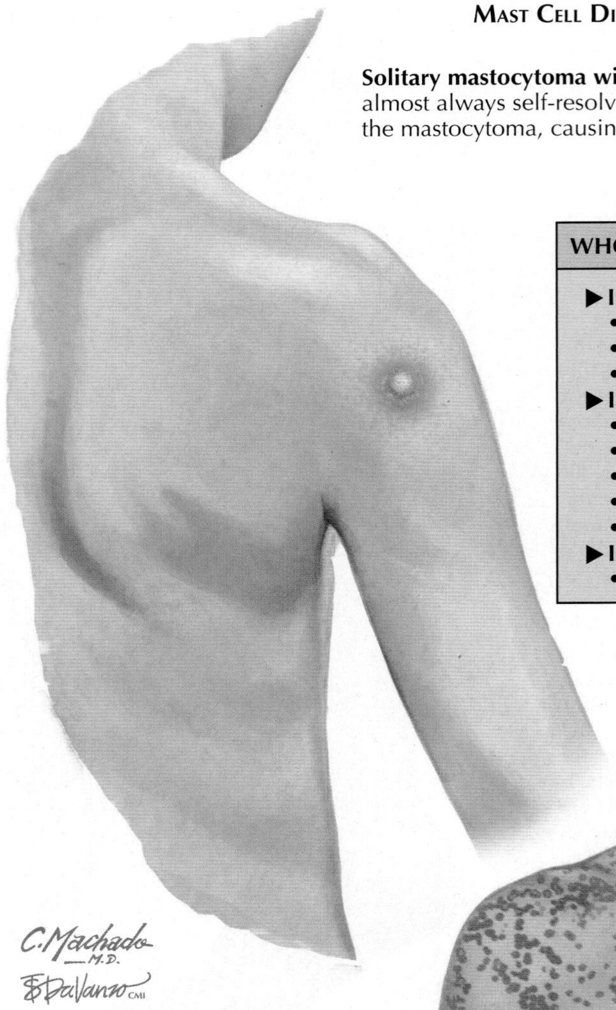

Solitary mastocytoma with Darier's sign. Solitary mastocytomas almost always self-resolve. Darier's sign is elicited by rubbing the mastocytoma, causing urtication.

WHO 2016 Classification of Mastocytosis
▶ **I Cutaneous mastocytosis**
• Urticaria pigmentosa/maculopapular
• Diffuse cutaneous
• Mastocytoma
▶ **II Systemic mastocytosis**
• Indolent
• Smoldering
• Aggressive
• Associated with hematologic malignancy
• Mast cell leukemia
▶ **III Sarcoma**
• Mast cell sarcoma

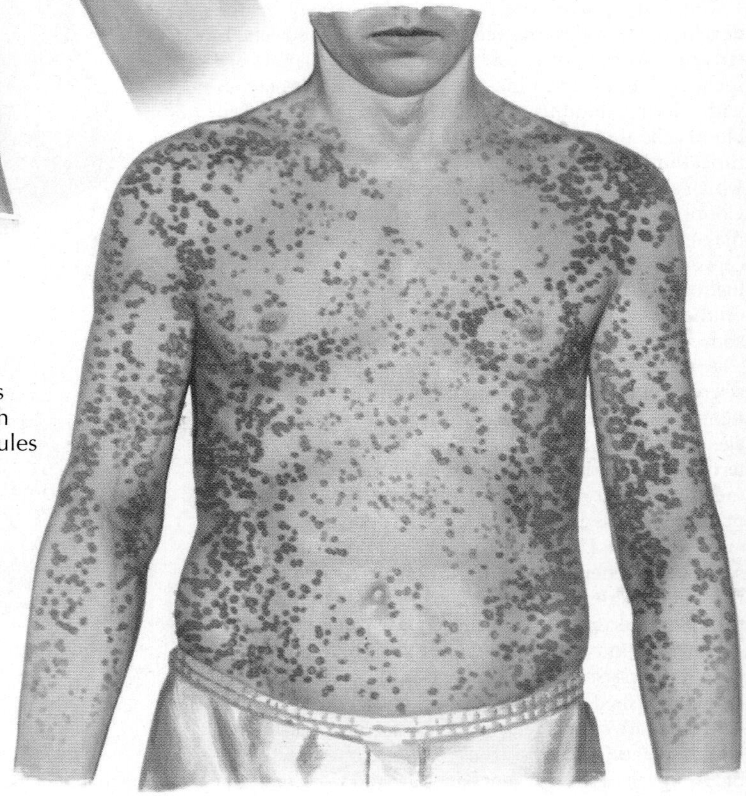

C. Machado M.D.
DaVanzo CMI

Urticaria pigmentosa. This is the most common form of cutaneous mastocytosis. It can manifest with reddish-brown macules and papules and in severe cases with vesicles and bullae.

MAST CELL DISEASE

Mast cell disease is an uncommon condition that has several clinical variants and subtypes. It can be seen as a solitary finding, as in the solitary mastocytoma, or it can result in widespread cutaneous disease, as in urticaria pigmentosa. Most mast cell disease is caused by an abnormality in the *c-kit* gene *(KIT)*. There are many other forms of mast cell disease, most in the benign category; some affect the skin predominantly, and others are more systemic in nature. One systemic type is the rare mast cell leukemia. Other systemic forms have been reported, such as mast cell sarcoma, and carry a poor prognosis. It is important to recall that mast cells are derived from the bone marrow and share certain things in common with other hematopoietic cells. Cutaneous mast cell disease has a better prognosis than the systemic forms of mast cell disease. The World Health Organization (WHO) has developed a simplified classification system for mast cell disease broken down into two main categories, cutaneous and systemic, with a third category of sarcoma.

Clinical Findings: Solitary mastocytoma is one of the most common of all the mast cell disease types. It manifests in early childhood, often in the first few years of life. It appears as a yellowish to brownish macule, papule, or plaque. On rare occasions, a lesion develops a vesicle or bulla. Most lesions are asymptomatic until rubbed or scratched. When this takes place, a localized urticarial reaction occurs above the mastocytoma and extends into the surrounding skin. This sign, called Darier's sign, can be used in any of the cutaneous mast cell diseases to help make the diagnosis. These solitary mast cell collections almost always spontaneously resolve with no sequelae.

Urticaria pigmentosa is a more diffuse affliction of the skin with mast cells; it has been reported to be the most common variant of mast cell disease. From a few to hundreds of slightly hyperpigmented macules and plaques occur across the surface of the skin. Some develop into vesicles and bullae. This most commonly occurs in early childhood but has also been reported to occur in adulthood. Most children are diagnosed on the basis of the clinical presentation and demonstration of a positive Darier's sign. The condition typically runs a benign course in children, and most cases spontaneously remit over a few years and then disappear at about the time of puberty. Adult-onset urticaria pigmentosa is a more chronic disease that rarely remits. Special care should be taken to continually screen adult patients for the development of systemic mast cell involvement.

Telangiectasia macularis eruptiva perstans is a less commonly seen variant of mast cell disease. It occurs almost exclusively in the adult population. Patients often present with widespread telangiectases in unusual locations such as the back, chest, and abdomen. There can be a background erythema, and Darier's sign may or may not be present. The most common symptom is pruritus. The appearance can be bothersome for some. It is most often limited to the skin, but the clinician should evaluate for systemic involvement. The WHO removed this a separate variant in the 2016 classification.

Measurement of the serum tryptase level is the most accurate means of screening for systemic involvement with mastocytosis. Levels in the normal range indicate cutaneous disease only; levels greater than 20 ng/mL are indicative of systemic involvement, and further systemic workup is warranted. Urine histamine and histamine metabolites can also be assessed but seem to be less sensitive and less specific than the serum tryptase level. If systemic involvement is considered, further testing with a bone marrow biopsy may be indicated. Molecular genetic testing can be performed on the bone marrow sample to assess for *KIT* mutation.

Mast Cell Disease (Continued)

Mast Cell Degranulation Blockers

Mast cell degranulation effects

A. Antigen reacts with antibody (IgE) on membrane of mast cells, which respond by secreting pharmacologic mediators.

Vagus nerve

Mast cell degranulation blockers

Histamine

SRS-A (slow-reacting substance of anaphylaxis)

ECF-A (eosinophil chemotactic factor of anaphylaxis)

Prostaglandins

? Serotonin

? Kinins

Mucous gland hypersecretion

Smooth muscle contraction

Increased capillary permeability and inflammatory reaction

Eosinophil attraction

B. End-organ (airway) response compounded by nonspecific reactions (ciliostasis, particle retention, and cell injury)

F. Netter M.D.

J. Perkins MS, MFA

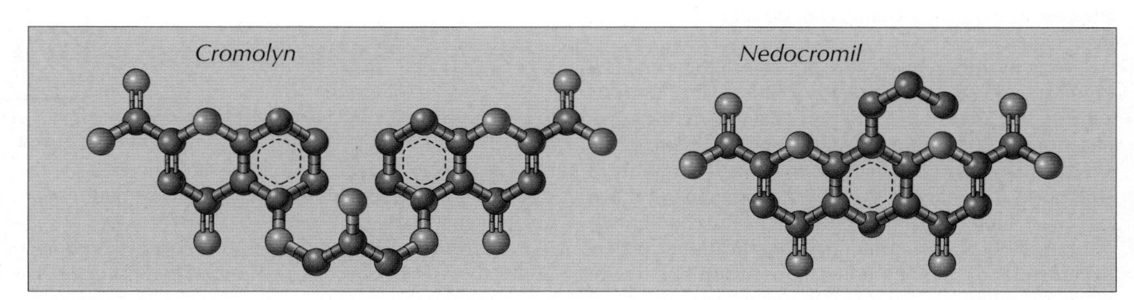

Pathogenesis: Mast cell disease is caused by a mutation in *KIT*. *KIT* is a protooncogene that encodes a protein called stem cell factor receptor (SCFR). SCFR is a transmembrane tyrosine kinase protein. This receptor is prominent in two skin cell types, mast cells and melanocytes. It is also present on a host of other primitive hematologic cell types. Stem cell factor is also known by various other names, including KIT ligand, CD117, steel factor, and mast cell growth factor. It is the molecule that binds to the transmembrane SCFR and acts to promote the reproduction of mast cells. The activating mutation of SCFR seen in mast cell disease causes an upregulation of signaling via this pathway and an uncontrolled proliferation of mast cells. The continuous activation of the stem cell factor allows for prolonged survival of mast cells, which also contributes to their increased number. Numerous mutations of *KIT* have been described, and it is believed that the different mutations play a role in the varied clinical expression of the disease. The most common mutation is a D816V mutation caused by replacement of the normal aspartic acid at the 816 position with a valine amino acid.

Darier's sign is caused by direct release of histamine and other inflammatory mediators from the excessive collection of mast cells within the affected skin. On direct stimulation such as scratching or rubbing, the mast cells automatically release the contents of their granules. These granules contain histamine and other vasoactive substances that cause edema, redness, and pruritus.

Histology: The histologic features depend on the form of mast cell disease. Most skin biopsy specimens show an excessive number of mast cells, typically surrounding the cutaneous vasculature. These mast cells are best appreciated with special staining techniques. The Leder (chloracetate esterase) stain, Giemsa stain, and toluidine blue stain are the most commonly used special stains to help highlight the cutaneous mast cells. CD117 immunostaining also stains mast cells.

Treatment: Cutaneous mast cell disease in children is often self-limited and resolves spontaneously with time. Therapy with antihistamines may help decrease the pruritus and provide symptomatic relief until the condition resolves on its own. The most important aspect for children with cutaneous mast cell disease, especially urticaria pigmentosa, is to avoid agents or physical insults that may cause massive degranulation of mast cells. These triggers include medications such as anesthetics, narcotics, polymyxin B, and many others. Physical triggers include extremes of temperature, vigorous exercise, repeated rubbing of the involved skin, and many other stimuli that differ from individual to individual.

Antihistamines are the mainstay of therapy. The leukotriene inhibitors are also used as adjunctive therapy to the antihistamines. Cromolyn is a mast cell stabilizer that is not absorbed through the gastrointestinal tract. Its use is limited to treatment of coexisting diarrhea caused by mast cell disease of the gut. Telangiectasia macularis eruptiva perstans has been treated with the 585-nm pulsed dye laser to decrease the redness and telangiectasias for cosmetic purposes.

Depending on the symptoms and the body systems involved, systemic chemotherapy may be warranted to decrease the mast cell load. These agents rarely put patients into long-term remission, and the response is transient. Some success has been achieved in treating systemic disease with the tyrosine kinase inhibitors such as imatinib. Resistance to imatinib therapy is believed to be due to various mutations in c-kit. Newer therapies that target multiple tyrosine kinases are being developed, such as midostaurin. These newer medications are able to inhibit c-kit's resistance to imatinib. Stem cell transplantation has a potential for cure.

MORPHEA

En coup de sabre. Rare form of localized morphea on the forehead and face. May be associated with Parry-Romberg syndrome.

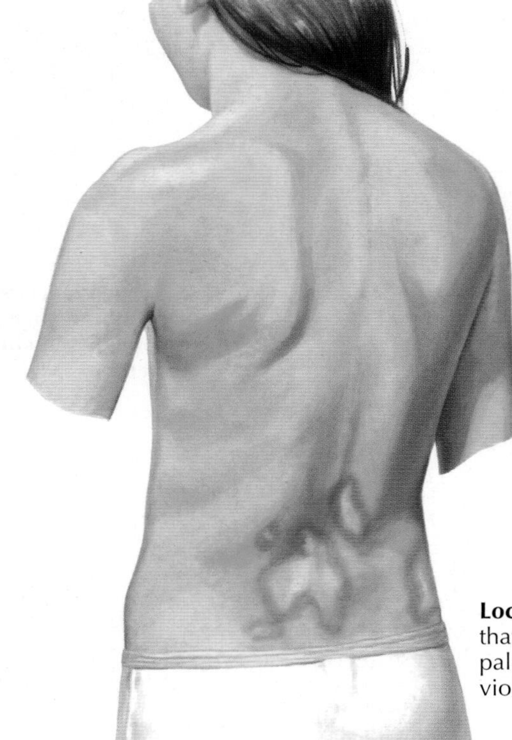

Localized morphea. Atrophic plaques that are firm and nonflexible on palpation. Often surrounded by a violaceous or erythematous rim.

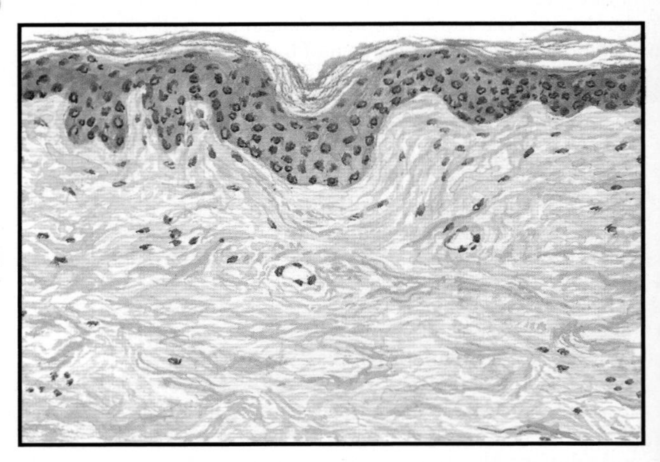

Progressive systemic sclerosis (scleroderma). Typical skin changes in scleroderma: extensive collagen deposition and epidermal atrophy.

Morphea is an idiopathic inflammatory dermatosis of the skin and subcutaneous tissue. The most common form is solitary, but many clinical variants have been described, including linear, guttate, and generalized forms. A small subset of patients (<1%) progress to progressive systemic sclerosis. Many patients do not seek medical advice because the onset is insidious or the area of involvement is so small that it is hardly noticeable or bothersome.

Clinical Findings: Morphea can be seen in any race and at any age, but it is typically seen in young White females. The ratio of females to males has been estimated at 2:1. Morphea begins as a small erythematous macule. The lesion expands outward with a violaceous to red border. As it expands, the central portion becomes slightly hypopigmented and indurated in nature. The trunk is the most commonly involved region of the body. Most areas of involvement are asymptomatic to slightly pruritic. If the involved area crosses over a joint, there may be some loss of motion of the affected joint and pain with flexion and extension. The main differential diagnosis is between morphea and lichen sclerosis et atrophicus. Lichen sclerosis et atrophicus is typically more strikingly white in coloration and is less indurated.

Many variants of morphea have been described. Guttate morphea manifests with tiny, teardrop-shaped hypopigmented macules with slight induration scattered about the trunk or extremities. The induration of guttate morphea is not nearly as prominent as that of localized morphea and may not be appreciable. These guttate lesions may be impossible to distinguish clinically from lichen sclerosis et atrophicus, and a biopsy is the only way to differentiate the two. Biopsies are not always conclusive, and the term *morphea–lichen sclerosis overlap* has been used to describe lesions with features of both conditions. Generalized morphea is a rare variant with extensive involvement of the cutaneous surface. By definition, generalized morphea does not have systemic involvement, differentiating it from progressive systemic sclerosis. However, patients with generalized morphea may develop atrophy of the adipose and muscle tissues underlying the areas of involvement.

Linear morphea, also called linear scleroderma, is a unique cutaneous variant that is well described and has a distinctive appearance and potential underlying complications. It is commonly found along the length of the affected extremity. This form occurs most commonly in childhood. The affected skin may become bound down and cause limb length discrepancies as the child grows. Joint mobility is also a potential complication. Cortical hyperostosis of the long bones underneath the area of linear morphea has been well reported and is termed melorheostosis. Subtypes of linear morphea have been given the names en coup de sabre and Parry-Romberg syndrome.

En coup de sabre is a specific type of morphea that occurs along the forehead as well as partially onto the cheek and into the scalp. It appears as a depressed linear furrow from the scalp vertically down the forehead. The appearance can be subtle or extremely noticeable and can cause significant cosmetic problems. Parry-Romberg syndrome is linear morphea that occurs vertically across the face, causing hemifacial atrophy. The underlying adipose tissue, muscle, and bone are involved, with significant disfigurement. Patients may have neurologic involvement leading to seizures.

Pathogenesis: The pathogenesis of morphea is poorly understood. It is believed to be caused by immune system dysregulation of Th1, Th2, and Th17 cytokines. $CD4^+$ T cells have been shown to increase IL-4 production, which in turn causes an increase in transforming growth factor-β (TGF-β). TGF-β has been shown to induce collagen production. This sets off the cutaneous reaction in which an excessive amount of collagen is produced locally by fibroblasts. Potential factors that may initiate the reaction are endothelial damage, radiation damage, certain *Borrelia burgdorferi* infections, and fibroblast abnormalities. These ultimately lead to increased collagen, fibronectin, and elastin production and deposition. *Borrelia*-induced morphea has yet to be described in the United States; it has been reported in Europe and Asia.

Histology: A punch biopsy specimen of morphea appears as a well-formed cylinder. The dermis is expanded with excessive amounts of collagen. A slight inflammatory infiltrate is often seen along the dermal-subcutaneous border. Plasma cells are common.

Treatment: Therapy for localized morphea is not needed but can be attempted with topical corticosteroids, calcipotriene, and phototherapy. Linear morphea should be treated because it has significant functional and cosmetic implications. Immunosuppressive agents such as methotrexate and prednisone have been the most thoroughly studied therapeutic agents. Newer agents that target cytokines, toll-like receptors, peroxisome proliferator-activated receptors, chemokines, and dendritic cells are being studied.

MYXEDEMA

Myxedema is seen in patients with untreated severe hypothyroidism. This condition results from a total lack of thyroid hormone secretion and resultant deposition of mucopolysaccharides into the skin and other organs. Many skin and systemic findings are present in severe hypothyroidism. This is a condition seen predominately in adults. The infantile form, called *cretinism*, is still found in parts of the world that do not routinely test newborn infants. If left untreated, intellectual disability and various neurologic deficits can occur. Myxedema is a rarely seen disease with a high mortality rate.

Clinical Findings: Patients usually develop severe hypothyroidism slowly. It can be caused by autoimmune thyroiditis, a thyroid tumor, a pituitary tumor or infarction, or hypothalamic disease. It can also be seen after treatment of hyperthyroidism with improper replacement of thyroid hormone. The onset of symptoms begins as mild, nondescript findings and advances to severe clinical disease as the lack of thyroid hormone worsens. Patients have many constitutional symptoms and always report fatigue, cold intolerance, and a generalized malaise. Constipation and weight gain are almost universal. Some patients develop a pericardial effusion and bradycardia. Neurologic reflexes are blunted, and patients report slow mental reflexes.

The skin findings are specific to myxedema and can help make the diagnosis. Patients develop diffuse, nonscarring alopecia. The hair is often dry and breaks easily. The lateral half of the eyebrows is shed. Fingernails become brittle and lift off the nail bed. The facial features appear lethargic. Periorbital edema is prominent. Dry skin is severe and can mimic ichthyosis vulgaris. The skin on the lips is thickened, as is the tongue. The tongue may enlarge to the point that the impression of the teeth is seen on its lateral edges. If the infiltrate of mucopolysaccharides is extreme, the scalp can become thickened and furrowed, taking on the appearance of cutis verticis gyrata. The skin may acquire a subtle yellow hue because of carotenemia; this is most likely to be observed on the glabrous skin.

Laboratory findings are diagnostic and necessary. Nonspecific mild anemia is seen, consistent with anemia of chronic disease. Hypercholesterolemia and hyponatremia are two of the nonspecific findings. Electrocardiography shows bradycardia and a prolonged PR interval. The results of various thyroid hormone tests are characteristic. An elevated level of TSH is confirmatory for a diagnosis of primary hypothyroidism. T_4 levels are low and can be measured in various ways.

It is critical to differentiate adult generalized myxedema, as seen in hypothyroidism, from pretibial myxedema. Pretibial myxedema is a marker for hyperthyroidism, not hypothyroidism.

Pathogenesis: Thyroid hormone is required for multiple metabolic pathways to work properly, including the breakdown of glycosaminoglycans. When there is a decrease or a total lack of thyroid hormone, glycosaminoglycans cannot be properly metabolized, and they accumulate in the subcutaneous tissue, most prominently in the tissue of the face and scalp. This leads to the characteristic skin findings in myxedema.

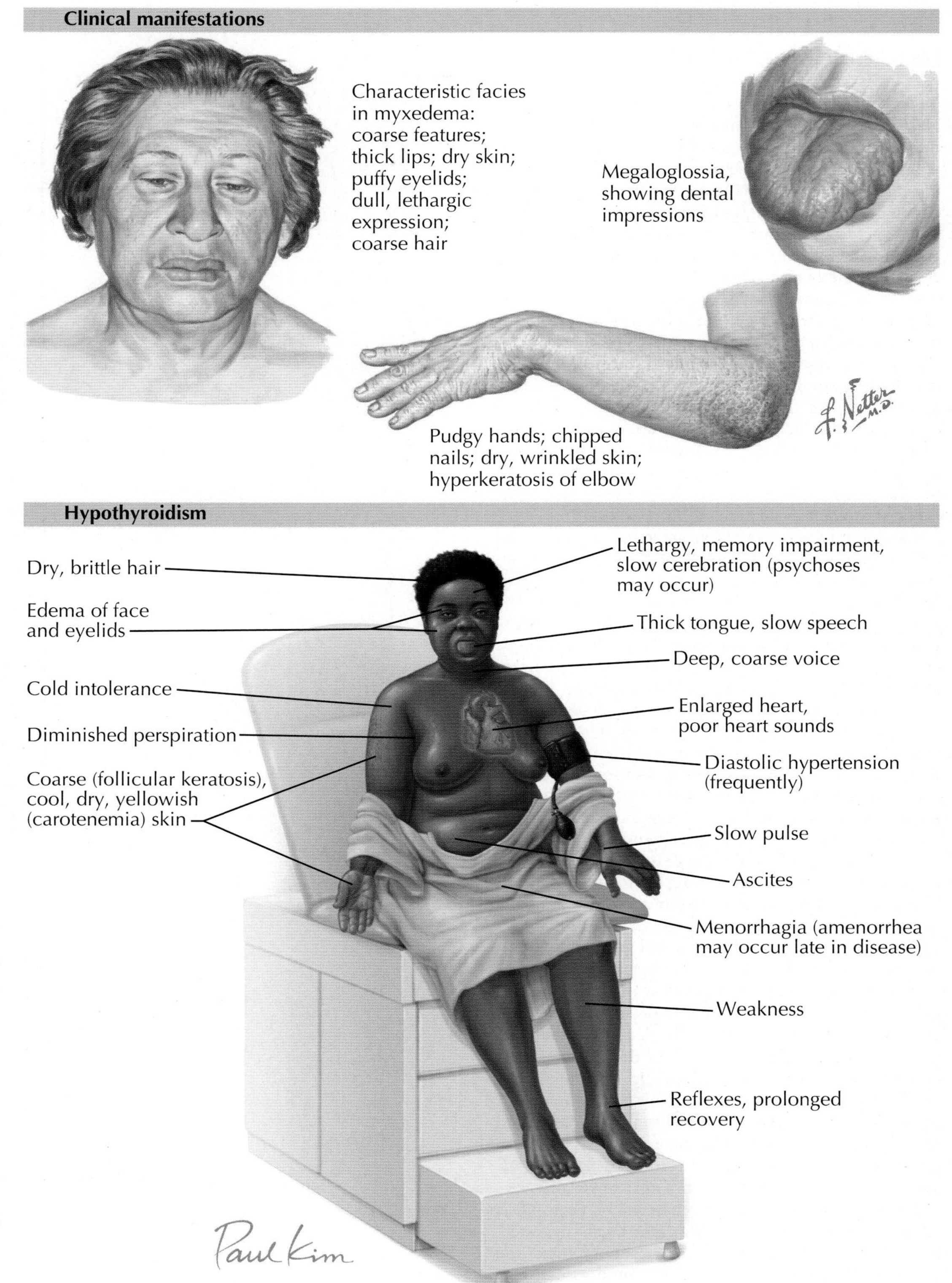

Histology: Biopsy specimens of involved skin show mild deposition of mucin between collagen bundles within the dermis. Hyaluronic acid makes up the majority of the mucin deposits. The alopecia is nonscarring.

Treatment: Prompt recognition and diagnosis of myxedema is required. It is a fatal condition if left untreated, and myxedema coma is precipitated by a total lack of thyroid hormone. Thyroid replacement with levothyroxine (synthetic T_4) is required. Supportive care is necessary until the patient can be adequately stabilized. To determine the cause of hypothyroidism, it is necessary to probe for underlying thyroid cancer, pituitary dysfunction, or other hypothalamic disease. Prompt recognition of the skin manifestations and referral to an endocrinologist can be lifesaving. Once proper thyroid replacement has been achieved, the skin and hair findings slowly resolve over time.

NECROBIOSIS LIPOIDICA

Necrobiosis lipoidica is frequently encountered in the dermatology clinic. It is regularly seen in association with diabetes; in these cases it is referred to as *necrobiosis lipoidica diabeticorum*. However, not all cases are seen in conjunction with diabetes mellitus, and the name *necrobiosis lipoidica* is a more inclusive designation. Patients who present with necrobiosis lipoidica should be evaluated for underlying diabetes and screened periodically over their lifetime because 60% to 80% will have or develop some form of glucose intolerance. Necrobiosis lipoidica has been reported to appear anywhere on the skin, but it is most frequently encountered on the anterior lower extremities. It has a characteristic clinical appearance, and the diagnosis can often be made on clinical grounds alone, without the use of a skin biopsy. The histologic findings are diagnostic for necrobiosis lipoidica. A punch or excisional biopsy is the best method for diagnosis because a shave biopsy does not allow proper histologic evaluation of this condition.

Clinical Findings: There appears to be no sex or racial predilection, and the disease is most commonly diagnosed in early adulthood. In most instances, necrobiosis lipoidica occurs on the anterior lower extremities. The rash typically begins as a tiny red papule that slowly expands outward and leaves behind a depressed, atrophic center with a slightly elevated rim. The borders are very distinct. They are slightly elevated and have an inflammatory red appearance. The lesions are well demarcated from the surrounding normal-appearing skin. The individual plaques show variability in size from a few millimeters to 5 to 6 cm in diameter, and in some rare cases the entire aspect of the anterior lower legs is affected. The plaques have a characteristic orange-brown coloration and significant atrophy. The underlying dermis appears to be thinned dramatically; the dermal and subcutaneous veins can easily be seen and appear to be popping out of the skin. When palpated, the center of the lesions feel as if there is no dermal tissue present at all. The difference between palpation of the normal surrounding skin and palpation of affected skin is striking.

A small percentage of patients with necrobiosis lipoidica experience ulcerations that can be slow and difficult to heal. They are typically caused by traumatic injury to the involved area. Rarely, transformation of chronic ulcerative necrobiosis lipoidica into squamous cell carcinoma has been reported. This transformation is more likely to be a result of the chronic ulceration and inflammation than the underlying necrobiosis lipoidica. Other associations seen with necrobiosis lipoidica include thyroid disease and inflammatory bowel disease.

Pathogenesis: The pathomechanism of necrobiosis lipoidica is unknown. Theories have been suggested, but no good scientific evidence has pinpointed the cause. Collagen degradation and immune complex deposition in abnormal vasculature, possibly due to diabetic changes, are the main pathogenic theories.

Histology: The histology of necrobiosis lipoidica is characteristic. A punch or excisional biopsy is needed to ensure a full-thickness specimen. There is a "cake layering" appearance to the dermis, with necrobiotic collagen bundles within palisaded granulomas alternating with areas of histiocytes and multinucleated giant cells of both the foreign body and the Langhans type. The differential diagnosis histologically is between granuloma annulare and necrobiosis lipoidica. In necrobiosis lipoidica, the inflammatory infiltrate contains less mucin and more plasma cells. The inflammation in necrobiosis lipoidica also tends to extend into the subcutaneous adipose tissue.

Treatment: Treatment is typically initiated with the use of high-potency topical steroids. It may seem counterintuitive to treat an atrophic condition with topical corticosteroid creams, which can cause atrophy. In cases of necrobiosis lipoidica, however, the high-potency steroid agents do not lead to an increase in the atrophy. The steroid agents act to decrease and stop the inflammatory infiltrate from occurring and perpetuating itself. Intralesional injections of triamcinolone have also been successful. Many other agents have been anecdotally reported to be successful in treating this condition (TNF-α inhibitors, UV light, calcineurin inhibitors), although they have not been tried in standardized, placebo-controlled studies. Gaining control of the underlying diabetes does not seem to play a role in the outcome of the skin disease. Ulcerations should be treated with aggressive wound care, and compression garments should be worn if edema or venous insufficiency is present. Ulcers may take months to heal. Once the inflammation has been stopped, most people have residual atrophy that may be permanent or may improve slightly with time.

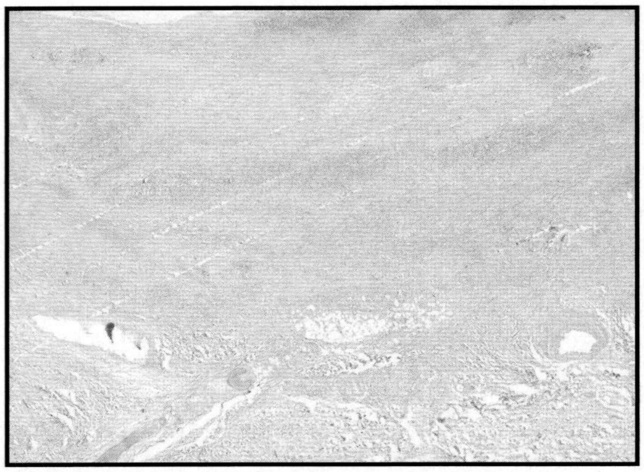

Medium power. A mixed granulomatous infiltrate is present throughout the dermis, and there is a "cake layering" effect.

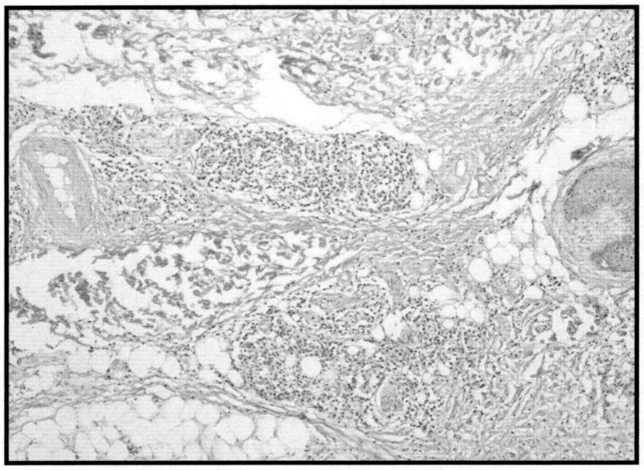

High power. Close-up view of a layer of necrobiotic collagen between two layers of diffuse granulomatous inflammation.

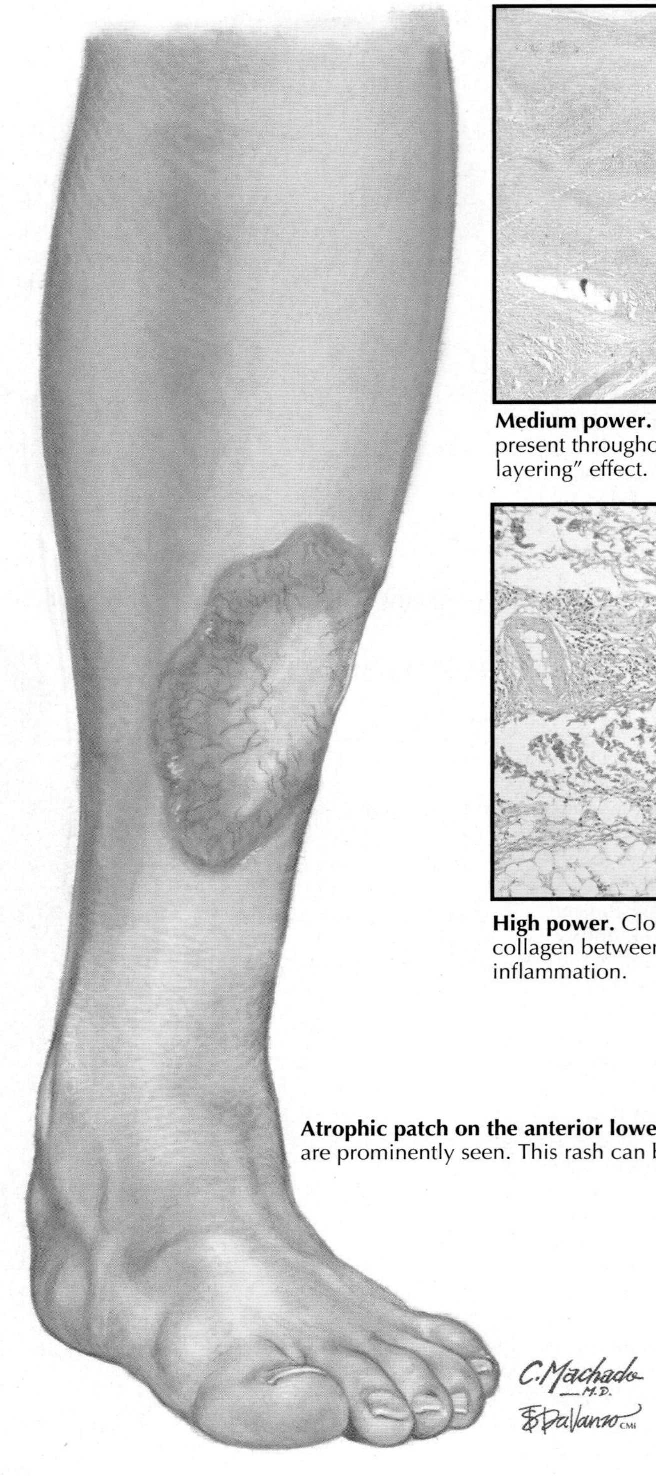

Atrophic patch on the anterior lower leg. Dermal blood vessels are prominently seen. This rash can be associated with diabetes.

Necrobiotic Xanthogranuloma

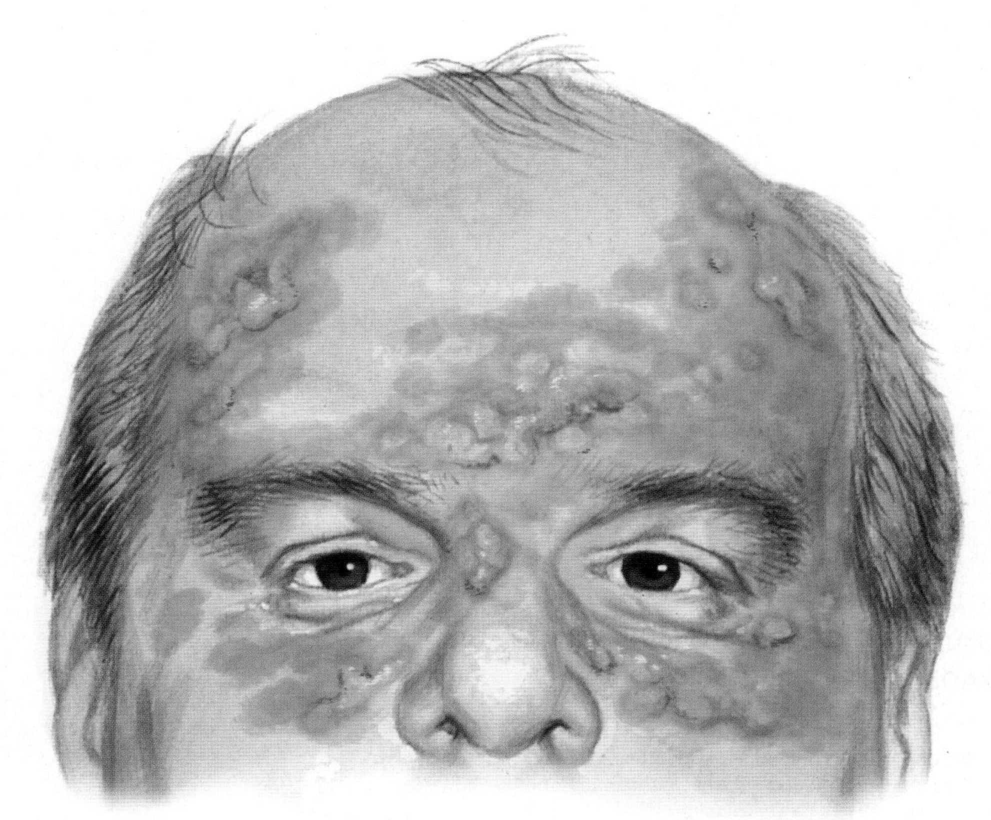

Patches and plaques on the face. Necrobiotic xanthogranuloma is most frequently encountered in a periocular location.

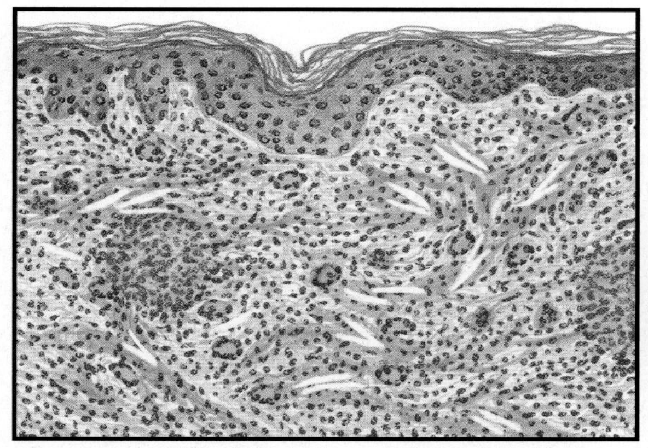

Low power. Diffuse dermal granulomatous infiltrate with giant cells.

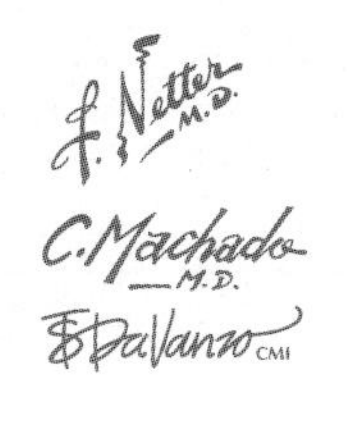

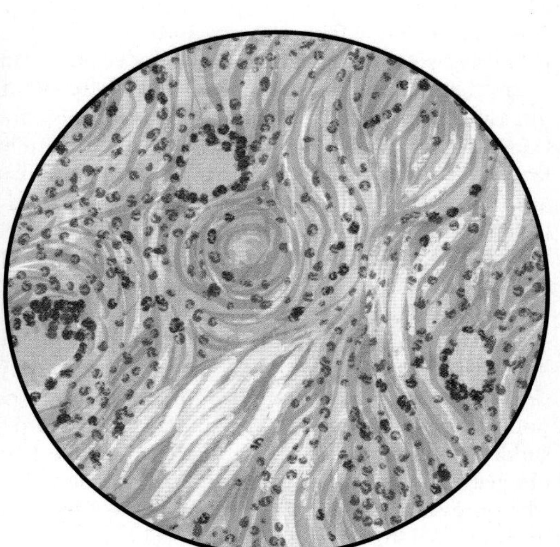

High power. The giant cells can be best appreciated on higher power microscopy. The giant cells are predominantly the Touton type.

Necrobiotic xanthogranuloma is a rare skin condition that is frequently associated with an underlying monoclonal gammopathy. It was first described in the early 1980s and is considered a non–Langerhans cell histiocytosis. Since then, many cases have been reported that have confirmed this to be a distinct, albeit unusual and infrequently encountered, skin condition. The pathologic findings of necrobiotic xanthogranuloma are distinctive and are required to make the diagnosis. Patients with this diagnosis need to be monitored routinely to screen for the development of monoclonal gammopathy and the possibility of multiple myeloma.

Clinical Findings: So few cases of necrobiotic xanthogranuloma have been reported that no firm conclusion can be made on the epidemiology of the disease. However, it is a disease of older adulthood, with almost all cases occurring after the age of 50 years. No race or sex predilection has been noted. The lesions have been reported to occur anywhere on the human body, but they are found most often on the forehead, cheeks, and temporal regions around the eyes. The periorbital region is almost always affected. Necrobiotic xanthogranulomas are typically yellowish to red papules and plaques. There may be intervening atrophy between the areas of involvement. The leading edge of the plaques may have a red or violaceous hue. Occasionally, nodules form. Secondary ulceration is frequently reported, as are telangiectases and dilated dermal vessels, which are most prominent in the regions of atrophy. The ulcerations take an extended period to resolve. Most patients are distraught by the appearance of the rash and report a mild pruritus, although many have no symptoms. The clinical differential diagnosis includes forms of planar xanthomas. A skin biopsy helps differentiate these conditions. This disease progresses over time and typically does not spontaneously remit.

Patients almost always report dry eyes or have objective findings of proptosis. In rare cases, necrobiotic xanthogranuloma affects the lacrimal gland and retrobulbar fat tissue.

Necrobiotic xanthogranuloma is associated with an immunoglobulin G-κ monoclonal gammopathy in most cases. The presence of a gammopathy requires a bone marrow biopsy to help evaluate for multiple myeloma. A small percentage of patients with this gammopathy have or will develop multiple myeloma. Other frequently abnormal laboratory tests in necrobiotic xanthogranuloma include an elevated erythrocyte sedimentation rate, a decreased level of complement C4, and leukopenia. Many other abnormalities have been described, providing more evidence that this is a systemic disease and not an isolated skin disease. Lesions of necrobiotic xanthogranuloma have also been described to occur in the upper respiratory system and in the heart.

Pathogenesis: The pathogenesis has been theorized to be an antibody response to a self-antigen, most likely a form of lipid. The presence of vast amounts of paraprotein may also play a role in the pathogenesis of the rash. The exact etiology is unknown.

Histology: The biopsy findings of necrobiotic xanthogranuloma are unique and characteristic. A punch biopsy or excisional biopsy should be performed to allow adequate evaluation. On first glance, the entire dermis is filled with inflammatory cells. The inflammation is granulomatous and present in the dermis and subcutaneous fat. A unique and characteristic finding, when seen, is that of cholesterol-filled, needle-shaped clefts within the granulomatous infiltrate. Giant cells, both the foreign body type and the Touton type, are commonly seen. The granulomatous infiltrate surrounds and envelops necrobiotic collagen tissue. There is usually an underlying, predominantly lobular panniculitis without vasculitis.

Treatment: Therapy is difficult. No randomized prospective studies have been performed on this rare condition, so only anecdotal therapies have been reported. Topical and oral steroids have been somewhat successful. IVIG has shown promise and has a better side effect profile than the chemotherapeutic agents. Chemotherapeutic agents have been used with variable success, including the alkylating agents. Results have been varied, with some patients experiencing long-term remission. IVIG and steroids currently are first-line treatments. Patients should be screened for gammopathy and for the development of multiple myeloma. The presence of myeloma portends a worse prognosis.

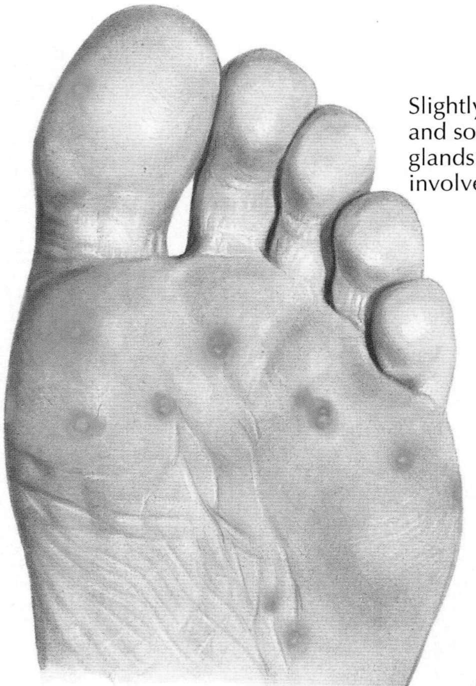

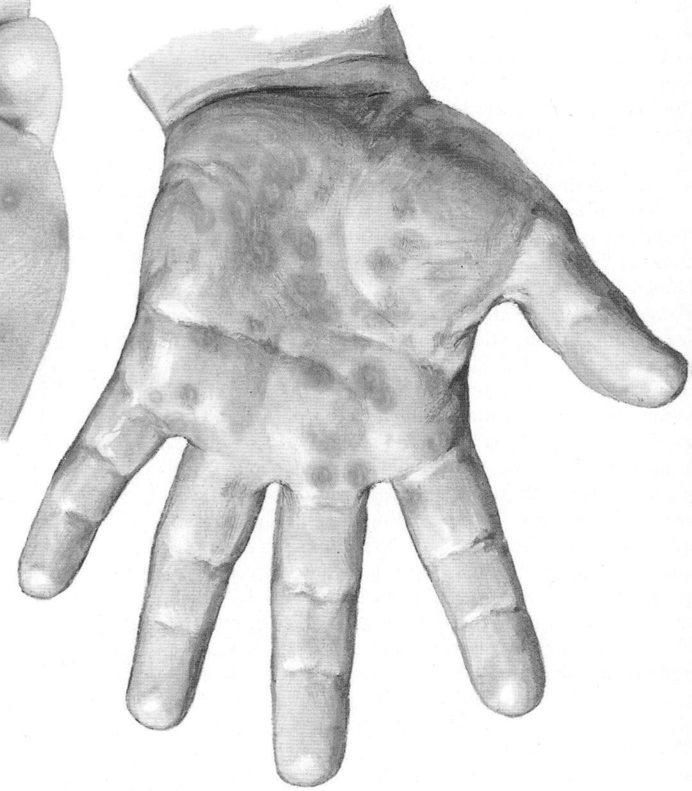

Slightly tender, pink-red macules and papules on the palms and soles caused by inflammation of the eccrine sweat glands. Palms and soles are the most frequent site of involvement, likely due to the high density of eccrine glands.

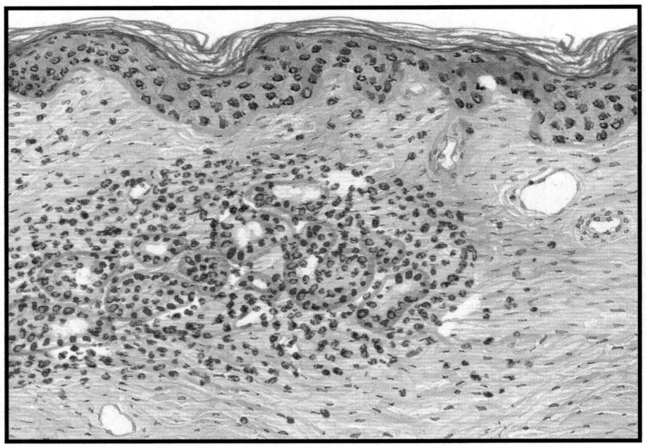

Low power. A neutrophilic infiltrate surrounds the dermal eccrine glands.

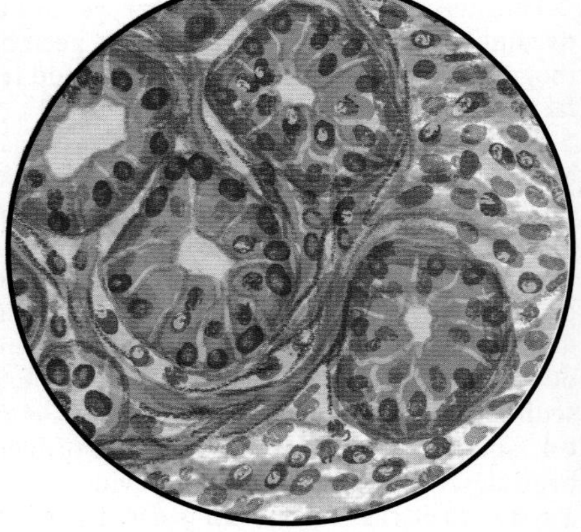

High power. Neutrophils infiltrating the eccrine ductal apparatus.

Neutrophilic Eccrine Hidradenitis

Neutrophilic eccrine hidradenitis is also known by other names, such as *palmoplantar eccrine hidradenitis* and *idiopathic recurrent plantar hidradenitis*. These names imply that it is seen only on the palms and soles. Neutrophilic eccrine hidradenitis is a more accepted term because it includes all cases independent of location. This peculiar and uncommon rash can be seen anywhere on the body that eccrine glands are present. The palms and soles have a higher density of eccrine glands than other regions, which may be one reason why the disease is seen more frequently in this site. This condition has been frequently described in patients with leukemia who are undergoing chemotherapy, particularly acute myelogenous leukemia. It has been reported to occur in other clinical settings, including HIV infection, bacterial infections, and other malignancies, with the use of medications other than chemotherapeutics, as well as in patients with no other associations.

Clinical Findings: Clinically, neutrophilic eccrine hidradenitis manifests in myriad ways. It usually occurs in association with an underlying predisposing condition such as those listed previously. Patients develop the sudden onset of tender red to purple papules and nodules with minimal to no ulceration. The papules blanch when pressed. The palms and soles are most frequently involved, but this condition can occur anywhere on the body. The papules often merge into larger plaques. The lesions may be asymptomatic, slightly tender, painful, or pruritic. Fever can be present. The differential diagnosis includes hot foot syndrome, which is caused by pseudomonal bacterial infections. This condition typically affects the foot, and it can be associated with folliculitis, such as hot tub folliculitis. Patients usually have a benign medical history and have had recent exposure to a hot tub or swimming pool.

Pathogenesis: Chemotherapy-induced neutrophilic eccrine hidradenitis is believed to occur secondary to accumulation of the chemotherapeutic agent within the eccrine glands to a level that is toxic to the secretory cells of the gland, resulting in cell necrosis. The neutrophilic inflammation is poorly understood. Only theories exist on the pathogenesis of non–chemotherapy-induced neutrophilic eccrine hidradenitis; the true pathogenesis is unknown.

Histology: The histologic evaluation requires a punch biopsy or excisional biopsy to evaluate the eccrine glands. A shave biopsy is usually inadequate. There is a striking amount of neutrophilic inflammation in and around the eccrine apparatus. The eccrine glands show varying degrees of necrosis. No vasculitis is present.

Treatment: Treatment is supportive. Underlying infections must be treated adequately. The main goals are pain control and prevention of secondary infection. If the patient's neutrophilic eccrine hidradenitis is caused by a chemotherapeutic agent, a change in the chemotherapy regimen can be considered. If the patient's regimen cannot be changed, topical corticosteroids and nonsteroidal antiinflammatory agents may be used. If this is unsuccessful, dapsone and colchicine may be considered because of their antineutrophilic effects. Oral steroids have been used with variable success. No placebo-controlled studies have been performed for this condition.

METABOLIC PATHWAYS AND CUTANEOUS FINDINGS OF OCHRONOSIS

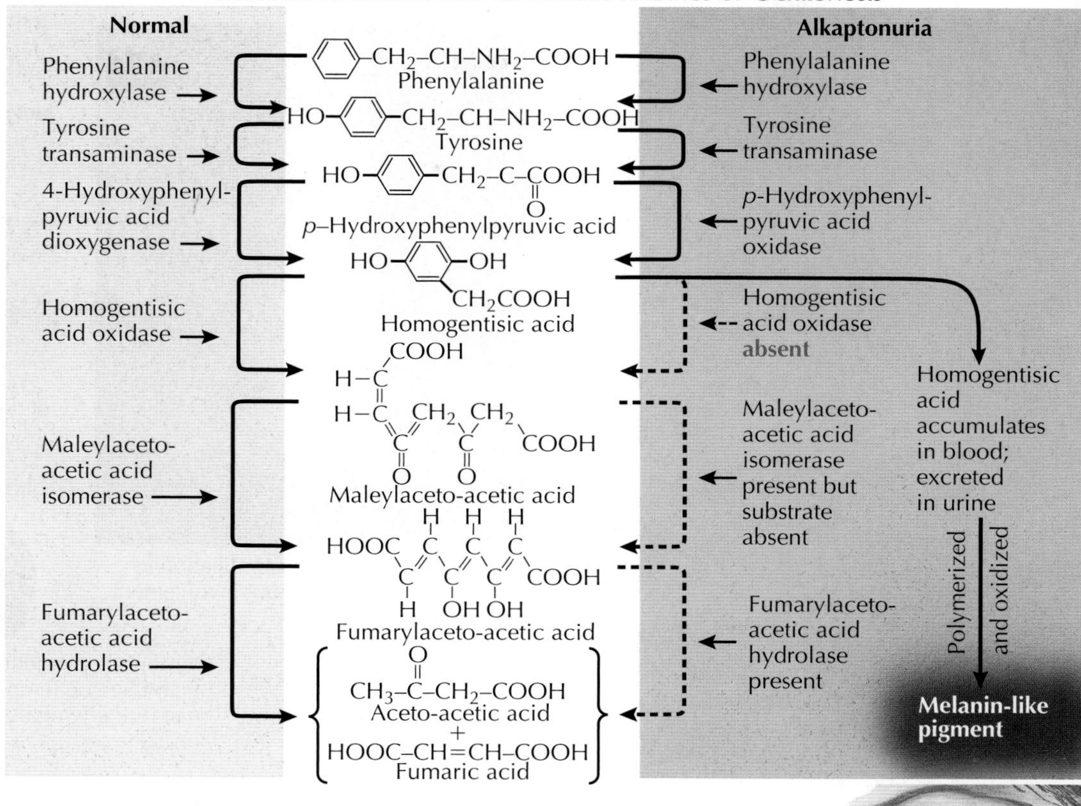

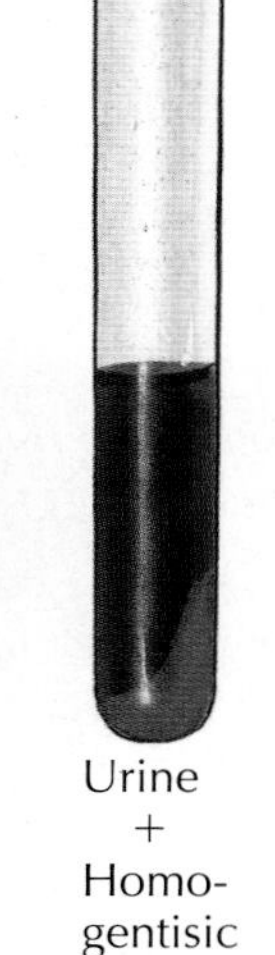

Pigmentation of cartilage of ear and of cerumen

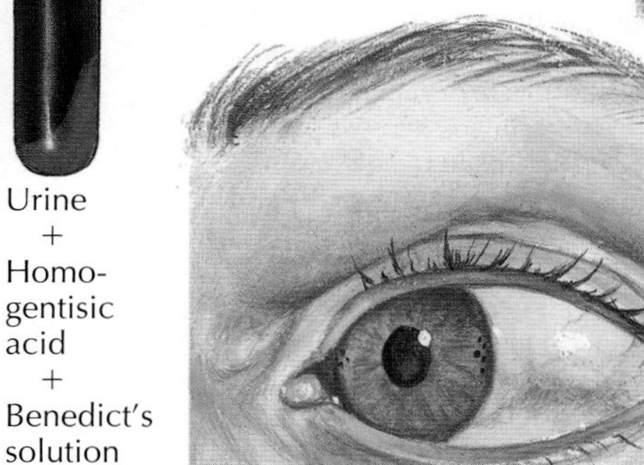

Pigmentation of sclera and pigment spots at margin of cornea

OCHRONOSIS

Ochronosis is the name given to the blue-black pigmentary clinical findings of alkaptonuria. Alkaptonuria is caused by an inborn error of metabolism resulting from a defect or deficiency of the enzyme homogentisic dioxygenase. A complete lack of the enzyme in the kidneys and liver is responsible for the buildup of the homogentisic acid. Alkaptonuria is transmitted in an autosomal recessive manner. Homogentisic acid oxidase is responsible for the metabolism of homogentisic acid, which is a breakdown product of the amino acids phenylalanine and tyrosine. This enzyme metabolizes homogentisic acid into maleylacetoacetic acid, which is eventually converted to fumaric acid and acetoacetic acid. When the homogentisic acid oxidase enzyme is deficient, as in alkaptonuria, homogentisic acid accumulates in the blood and is excreted in the urine. The disease has a slow, insidious onset, and patients often initially present in young adulthood.

Clinical Findings: The first clinical sign is that of dark urine found in an affected baby's diaper, which often causes concerned parents to seek medical advice. If left to stand for a few hours, the urine turns dark black because of the oxidative effects of the atmosphere. The urine can be alkalinized with a strong basic solution such as sodium hydroxide; addition of the basic solution to a sample of urine promptly turns it dark black. Benedict's reagent can also be used to test the urine of patients with alkaptonuria; when it is added, the supernatant turns dark black, which is diagnostic of alkaptonuria. Males and females have the same incidence of disease, but, for an as-yet unknown reason, males tend to have a more severe clinical course. Life span is normal.

As the homogentisic acid accumulates in these patients, it begins depositing in skin and cartilage tissue, for which it has an affinity, becoming visibly noticeable around the fourth decade of life. The sclera is one of the first areas to be noticeably involved. A subtle brown discoloration begins to form on the lateral aspect of the sclera and continues to darken over the lifetime of the patient. The ear cartilage becomes dark brown to almost bluish because of the accumulation of the homogentisic acid. The cerumen is dark black, and evaluation of the ear may also show a darkening of the tympanic membrane and the stapes, incus, and malleus bones of the inner ear. The patient may experience tinnitus.

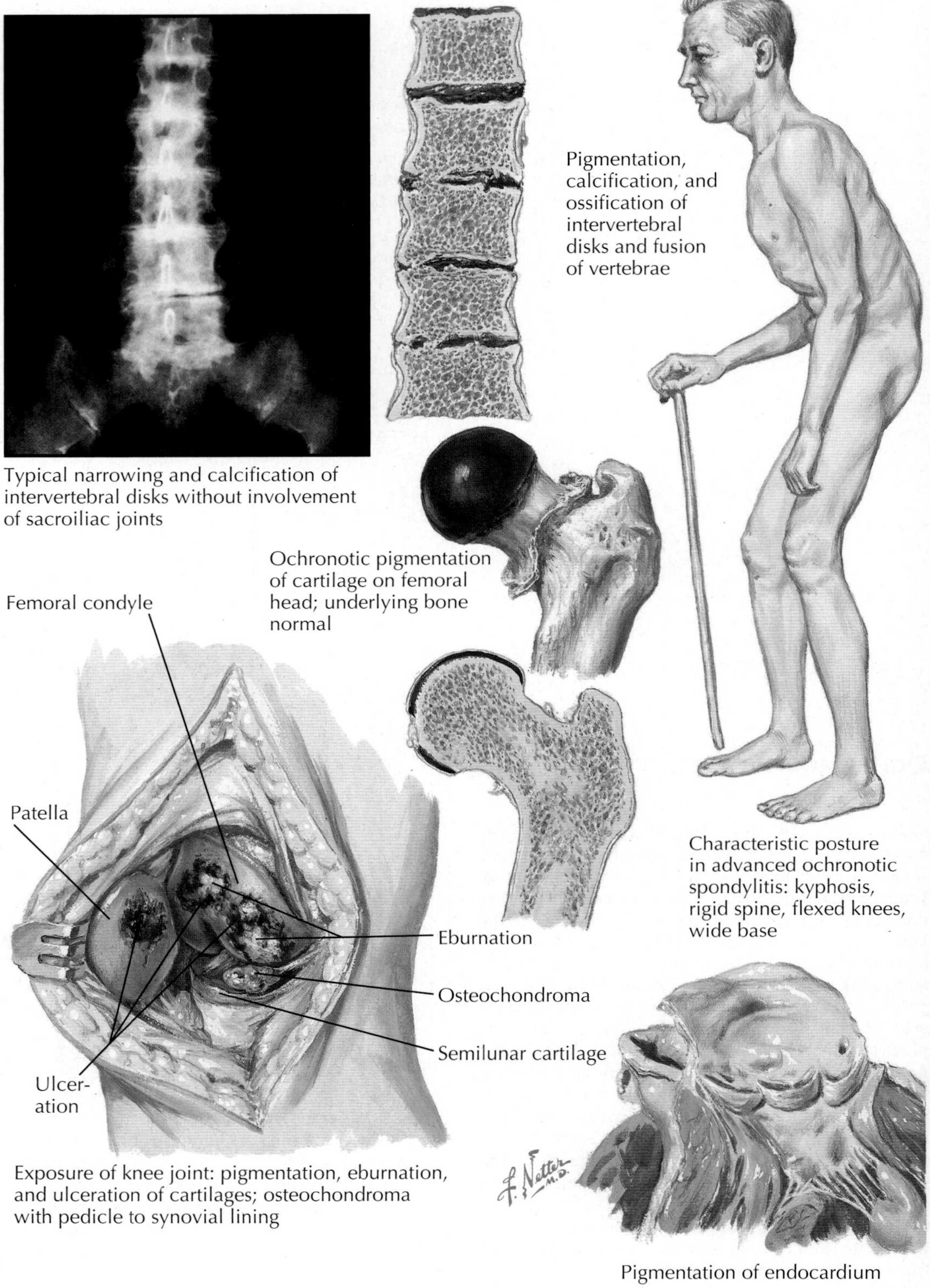

Ochronosis (Continued)

With time, the skin in various regions begins to become hyperpigmented. This first occurs in areas with a high concentration of sweat glands. The axillae and the groin are noticeably affected. The excessive homogentisic acid is secreted in the sweat, and the pigment discolors the surrounding skin. The cheeks are also prominently affected.

The most disabling aspect of this disease is the deposition of homogentisic acid in the fibrocartilage and hyaline cartilage. This leads to severe degenerative joint disease at an early age. Severe arthritis is most prominent in the spine and the large joints of the extremities. The pigment alters the cartilage and makes it brittle and friable. The cartilage begins to fragment and disintegrate and can become embedded in the synovial tissue, causing synovial polyps. The intervertebral disks become severely pigmented and begin to calcify because of the massive destruction of the cartilage. The disks are destroyed, causing a severe reduction in the patient's height, as well as chronic pain and rigidity of the spine. Eventually, the heart, prostate, aorta, and kidneys all show evidence of ochronosis.

Pathogenesis: Ochronosis is the result of an autosomal recessive inherited disorder that causes the affected patient to be deficient in the enzyme homogentisic dioxygenase. Over time, this deficiency leads to the accumulation of homogentisic acid in various tissues throughout the body and the subsequent clinical manifestations.

Histology: The findings on skin biopsy are pathognomonic for ochronosis. Large ochre bodies are found within the dermis. These are obvious on low-power microscopy and can be used to confirm the diagnosis.

Systemic Findings of Ochronosis

Typical narrowing and calcification of intervertebral disks without involvement of sacroiliac joints

Pigmentation, calcification, and ossification of intervertebral disks and fusion of vertebrae

Ochronotic pigmentation of cartilage on femoral head; underlying bone normal

Characteristic posture in advanced ochronotic spondylitis: kyphosis, rigid spine, flexed knees, wide base

Femoral condyle

Patella

Eburnation

Osteochondroma

Semilunar cartilage

Ulceration

Exposure of knee joint: pigmentation, eburnation, and ulceration of cartilages; osteochondroma with pedicle to synovial lining

Pigmentation of endocardium

Treatment: No known cure is available. Physical therapy and joint replacement increase flexibility and range of motion and help decrease morbidity. Pain control is critically important. Some researchers advocate a diet low in phenylalanine and tyrosine, although the success of this approach is anecdotal at best. Researchers around the globe are currently studying nitisinone, an inhibitor of the enzyme 4-hydroxyphenylpyruvic acid dioxygenase. It acts by decreasing the production of homogentisic acid, thereby reducing homogentisic acid deposition in tissue. This, in turn, should theoretically help decrease joint destruction and morbidity in these patients. Nitisinone is a medication used currently to treat tyrosinemia. Chaperone and enzyme replacement therapy are also being studied.

ORAL MANIFESTATIONS IN BLOOD DYSCRASIAS

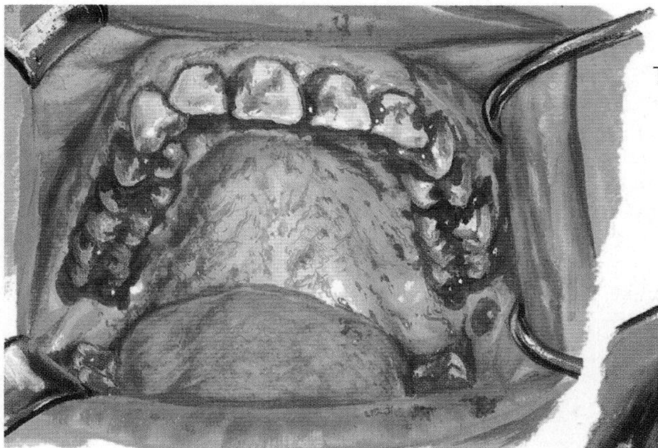

Many systemic hematologic diseases have cutaneous findings as well as oral mucosal findings that are unique and can be the presenting clinical sign of the underlying disease. Awareness of the oral manifestations of these disorders is of paramount importance. Oral manifestations of blood dyscrasias can be seen in agranulocytosis, pernicious anemia, leukemia, polycythemia vera, and thrombotic thrombocytopenic purpura (TTP).

Clinical Findings: Agranulocytosis has been shown to produce oral ulcerations and erosions. Several different causes of agranulocytosis may result in these clinical findings. Medication-induced agranulocytosis is the most frequent cause of a decreased absolute neutrophil count of less than 500/µL. Numerous medications can cause this reaction, including dapsone, methotrexate, and a host of chemotherapeutic agents. A rare autosomal recessively inherited disease called *infantile genetic agranulocytosis* (severe congenital neutropenia), or Kostmann disease, has been described. These patients present in the first months of life with recurrent oral ulcerations, multiple bacterial infections, and severely depressed absolute neutrophil counts. Death is the norm by 1 year of age unless the disease is correctly diagnosed and treated. Successful therapy is achieved with G-CSF or, in more advanced cases, with stem cell transplantation. Even with successful G-CSF treatment, patients still develop oral ulcerations and severe periodontal disease. This is caused by the lack of an antimicrobial peptide, which allows certain bacteria to proliferate unabated. The species most frequently found is *Actinobacillus actinomycetes comitans*. These individuals have a defect in the *HAX1* or *ELA2* genes.

Pernicious anemia is caused by a deficiency of vitamin B_{12}. This deficiency is most commonly seen in individuals with an inability to absorb vitamin B_{12} or in strict vegetarians. Pernicious anemia can manifest with a macrocytic anemia and neurologic complications. Hunter glossitis is a form of atrophic glossitis that affects the tongue, leading to atrophy of the tongue filiform and fungiform papillae. The tongue takes on a beefy red appearance with a smooth surface. Varying degrees of glossodynia and a decreased ability to taste are associated symptoms.

Gingival infiltration with leukemic cells may be the presenting sign of acute leukemia, and gingival bleeding is the most frequent oral manifestation of leukemia. Oral ulcerations are commonly associated with the gingival leukemic hypertrophy. The periodontal tissue appears red and swollen, with varying grades of gingivitis. The gums may grossly enlarge to cover the majority of the teeth. This form of leukemic infiltration is seen almost exclusively in acute myelomonocytic leukemia (M4) and acute monocytic leukemia (M5). It is estimated to occur in two-thirds of patients with M5 disease and in 20% of those with M4 disease. Other forms of leukemia have been implicated in causing gingival enlargement to a much lesser degree.

Polycythemia vera (previously termed *polycythemia rubra vera*) is caused by excessive production of red blood cells, which results in abnormally high hemoglobin and hematocrit values. The majority of cases are complicated by thrombosis. Most of these patients have a mutation in the *JAK2* gene, which encodes a Janus family tyrosine kinase protein. The ability to test for these mutations has made diagnosis much easier. Oral manifestations are limited to the tongue and gingival mucosa. The tongue may become slightly enlarged, smooth, and hyperemic. Bleeding from the gingival mucosa can also be seen. The disease is manifested by many other systemic signs and symptoms.

TTP is a rare, life-threatening disease that can develop rapidly. It is manifested by the formation of microthrombi throughout the small vasculature. This causes multisystem organ failure and rapid death if not promptly treated. Most cases have been found to be caused by a hereditary defect in the *ADAMTS13* gene or by decreased platelet levels induced by medications or autoimmunity. *ADAMTS13* encodes a plasma metalloprotease, which is important in regulating von Willebrand factor function. Oral manifestations of the disease include widespread petechiae and ecchymosis of the tongue, gingival, labial, and buccal mucosa. Petechial hemorrhages of the gums may appear later in the course of the disease.

Thrombocytopenic purpura, diffuse bleeding

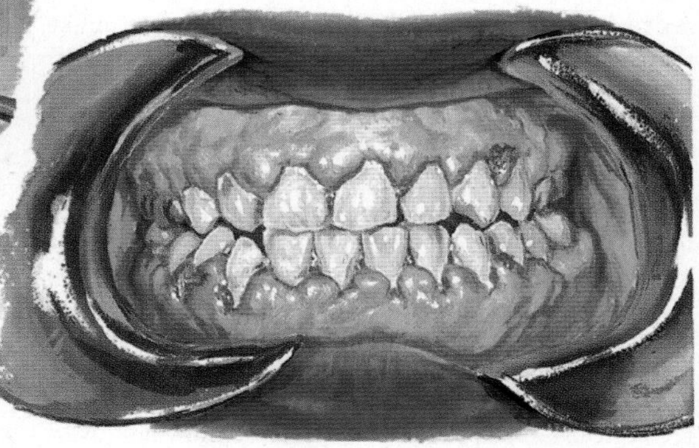

Leukemia (chronic), gingival infiltration

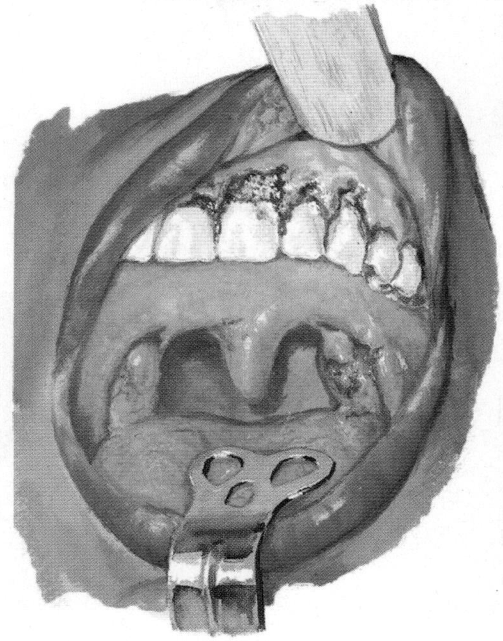

Agranulocytosis, multiple oral ulcers

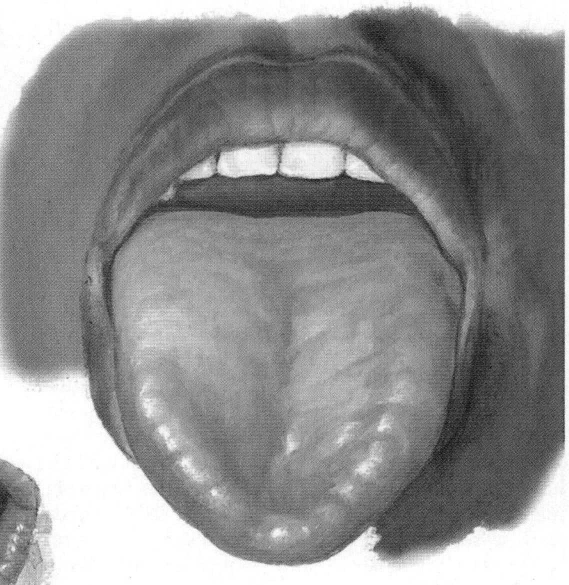

Pernicious anemia, smooth red tongue

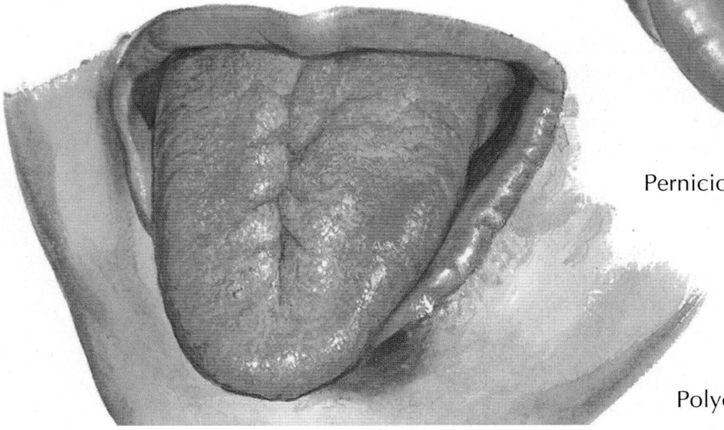

Polycythemia vera, beefy red tongue

PHYTOPHOTODERMATITIS

Phytophotodermatitis is a specific form of phototoxic or photoirritant contact dermatitis. The offending agent is a plant species from certain families. This form of dermatitis has an insidious onset and is typically preceded by little to no inflammation, which can make diagnosis difficult. Recognition of the key clinical features and the species of plant involved helps make the diagnosis.

Clinical Findings: Phytophotodermatitis is caused by certain species of plants that come into contact with the skin. Lone contact with skin is not enough to cause the inflammatory reaction and subsequent postinflammatory hyperpigmentation; after exposure to the plant material, there is a time frame during which the exposed area must be introduced to UV radiation. The plant oils and resins in combination with the correct UV source lead to the characteristic rash. The areas of involvement are typically asymptomatic and do not show any overt inflammatory features. They appear as hyperpigmented, irregularly shaped macules on the skin.

The most typical clinical scenario encountered is one in which the patient comes into contact with a plant that contains a psoralen compound. The most frequently reported cause is the juice of a lime *(Citrus aurantifolia).* This plant is categorized within the Rutaceae family. The Rutaceae family is a widespread family of plants that cause these types of reactions, with the lime being by far the most common offender.

Patients often describe the use of a lime in a mixed drink while vacationing on the beach. The lime juice contacts the skin, and when the skin is exposed to a specific threshold of UV light, the reaction develops. Most often, patients do not report the presence of any acute symptoms. If the reaction is severe, burning occurs acutely and the diagnosis is relatively straightforward. However, most reactions are subtle and do not appear for a few days to weeks. Patients typically return home from vacation and notice a subtle hyperpigmentation around the mouth or scattered on the body where they have splashed or consciously applied the juice from a lime during sunbathing. The hyperpigmentation may last for months to years. On rare occasions, a severe acute reaction occurs with edematous red papules that coalesce into plaques with or without vesicle formation.

The families of plants capable of initiating this type of reaction all contain the chemical psoralen. Psoralen is a potent photosensitizer that is used clinically. Once purified, it can be given orally in the form of PUVA therapy or painted on for topical PUVA therapy. It is especially helpful for treating refractory hand and foot dermatoses.

Pathogenesis: Almost all the plants responsible for phytophotodermatitis come from four specific families: Umbelliferae, Rutaceae, Moraceae, and Leguminosae. These plants contain potent photosensitizers in varying concentrations. The chemicals responsible for photosensitization are the furocoumarins; more specifically, the psoralens. Psoralens are by far the most important of the photosensitizer chemicals. On contact, psoralen penetrates the skin. Subsequent exposure to UVA light in the spectrum of 320 to 400 nm causes pyrimidine dimers to form within the DNA strands exposed to the psoralen, which interrupt DNA synthesis. For solitary acute exposures, the human body is able to repair these DNA errors. Patients who have undergone multiple PUVA treatments are at an increased risk for developing skin cancers because of the chronic nature of the DNA damage that PUVA causes.

Histology: The pathologic features depend on the timing of the biopsy. An acutely inflamed lesion shows a superficial perivascular lymphocytic infiltrate and dermal edema with apoptotic keratinocytes within the epidermis. Late lesions show melanophages within the dermis.

Treatment: Acute areas of involvement can be treated with cool compresses, analgesics, and topical corticosteroid creams. The main issue in management is dealing with the prolonged postinflammatory hyperpigmentation. No therapy has been shown to be helpful, but almost all reactions resolve slowly over time. Care should be taken not to perform a treatment that may lead to a worse cosmetic outcome. Avoidance is the best strategy to prevent this form of dermatitis.

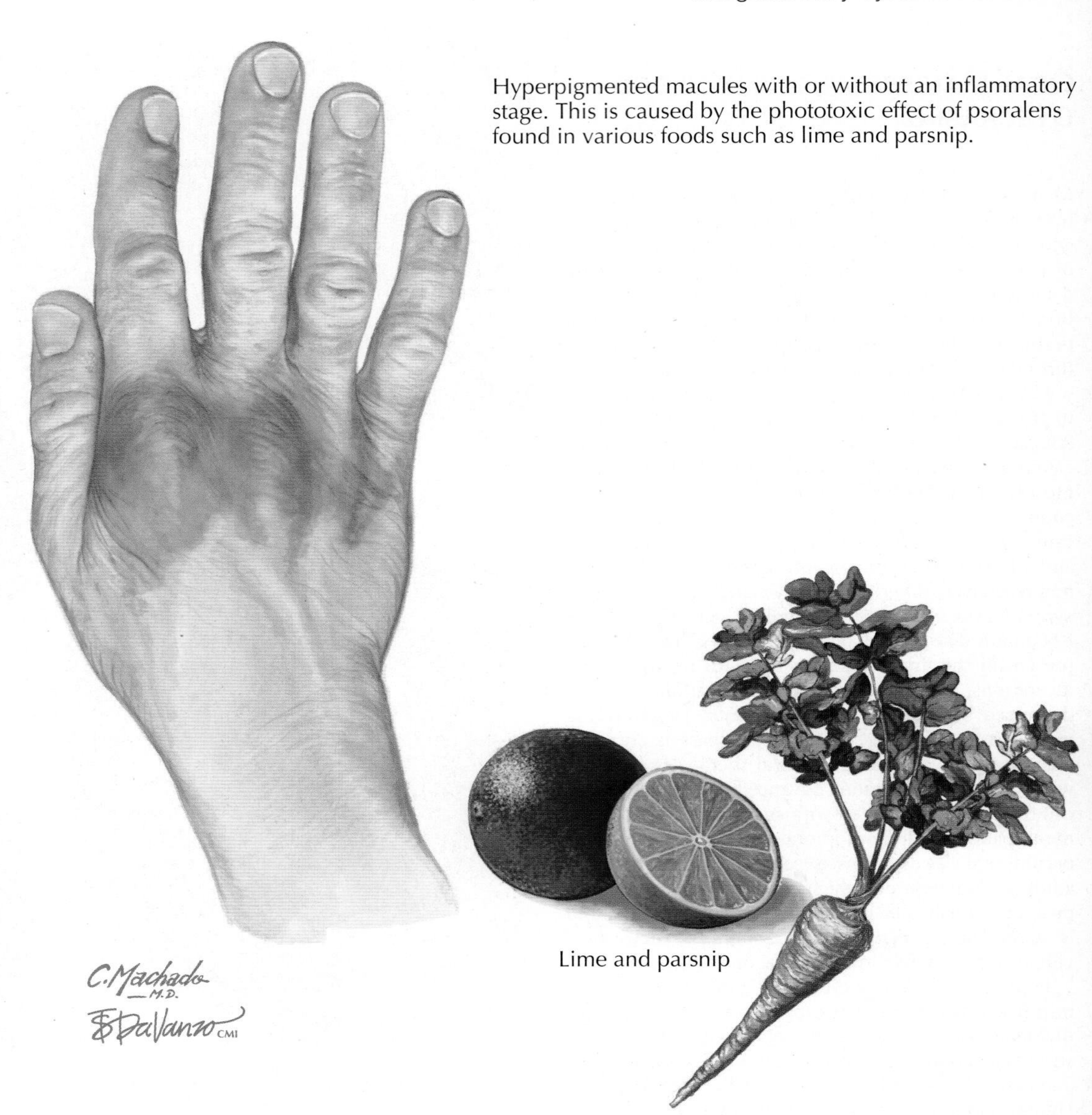

Hyperpigmented macules with or without an inflammatory stage. This is caused by the phototoxic effect of psoralens found in various foods such as lime and parsnip.

The lime is the most frequent cause of this reaction. Bartenders and beach vacationers who drink beverages with a slice of lime are commonly afflicted.

Families of Plants Known to Cause Phytophotodermatitis and Some Representative Species	
Umbelliferae	**Rutaceae**
▶ Dill–*Anethum graveolens*	▶ Rue–*Cneoridium dumosum*
▶ Parsley–*Petroselinum crispum*	▶ Lemon–*Citrus limon*
▶ Parsnip–*Heracleum sphondylium*	▶ Lime–*Citrus aurantifolia*
▶ Giant hogweed–*Heracleum mantegazzianum*	▶ Orange–*Citrus sinensis*
Moraceae	**Leguminosae**
▶ Fig–*Ficus carica*	▶ Scurf pea–*Psoralea corylifolia*

Pigmented Purpura

The pigmented purpuras are a group of idiopathic rashes that can occur at any age. They are grouped together because of their similar clinical and histologic presentations. They are believed to be caused not by vasculitis, but by inflammation of the small cutaneous capillaries, which produces capillaritis. The rash is typically of no clinical significance to the patient, but it can cause significant cosmetic concern, and the purpuras must be differentiated from other conditions that can cause similar rashes. The five rashes that make up the pigmented purpuric family are Schamberg disease, eczematous pigmented purpura of Doucas and Kapetanakis, pigmented purpura of Gougerot and Blum, lichen aureus, and Majocchi disease (annular telangiectatic pigmented purpura). Many medications have been shown to cause pigmented purpura–like eruptions.

Clinical Findings: These entities are grouped together for many reasons. They are believed by some to be slightly different manifestations of the same disease state, and the histopathology of all of the variants is strikingly similar. Pigmented purpuric dermatoses are benign and are not associated with any underlying abnormality. They can occur at any age. They are almost entirely asymptomatic in nature. The true incidence of these conditions is unknown because they are often not reported, but they are believed to occur very commonly.

Schamberg disease is the most frequently encountered pigmented purpuric eruption. It almost universally begins on the lower extremities. It manifests as tiny (1-mm) cayenne pepper–like petechial macules of the skin. Over time, a brownish-red hyperpigmented background forms secondary to the extravasation of red blood cells and their subsequent breakdown within the skin, which releases hemosiderin. The lesions are nonblanching and nonpalpable. The rash may spread proximally up the lower extremity but rarely affects other areas of the body. Most patients are referred to the dermatologist to rule out vasculitis, which is easily done by not finding any evidence of palpable purpura. The rash is almost always entirely asymptomatic, and patients frequently complain only of the appearance. If widespread petechia are seen, a platelet count should be performed to look for thrombocytopenia. If the platelet count is normal, a skin biopsy of the upper extremity or truncal area of involvement should be performed to evaluate for the very rare form of pigmented purpuric mycosis fungoides.

Eczematoid pigmented purpura of Doucas and Kapetanakis is a rare variant that manifests with petechiae and hyperpigmentation but is also associated with an overlying eczematous eruption. This form is typically pruritic and can show secondary excoriations.

Pigmented purpura of Gougerot and Blum is also known as lichenoid pigmented purpura. Small, light pink to purple papules form on the lower extremities. They can initially be mistaken for lichen planus. Biopsies of these papules show a lichenoid infiltrate. This pigmented purpura can be distinguished from Schamberg disease in that the skin findings are palpable. There is no true palpable purpura.

Lichen aureus can be seen at any age and manifests with the presence of multiple tiny, golden-colored macules that coalesce into a large macule or patch. Lichen aureus can occur anywhere on the body and is solitary in nature.

The involved regions in Majocchi disease show annular patches with petechiae and hyperpigmentation from hemosiderin deposition. This is a rare form of pigmented purpura that typically starts on the legs and spreads slowly over time.

Lichen aureus. Golden-colored macules and patches are characteristic of lichen aureus. This is one of the variants of pigmented purpura.

Schamberg disease. Cayenne pepper–like petechiae. This asymptomatic idiopathic rash is almost exclusively seen on the lower legs.

C. Machado M.D.
DaVanzo CMI

Extravasated erythrocytes and a lymphocytic vasculitis are the key histologic features.

Pathogenesis: The pigmented purpuric dermatoses are believed to be caused by capillaritis. The exact etiology is unknown. Venous hypertension in association with capillary fragility appears to be important in the development of pigmented purpura.

Histology: The histologic findings are similar across all variants. Dilated blood vessels are seen with extravasation of red blood cells found prominently in the dermis. The extravasation is seen in the vicinity of the capillaritis. The infiltrate is predominantly lymphocytic and perivascular in location. The presence of hemosiderin is easily seen in chronic lesions and is subtle in early lesions.

Treatment: There is no agreed-upon standard therapy, and withholding therapy is a frequently used option. Anecdotally, topical corticosteroids may be tried for a few weeks. Oral vitamin C and bioflavonoids have been reported to be successful, again mostly in anecdotal reports. Drug-induced cases improve after discontinuation of the offending agent.

PITYRIASIS ROSEA

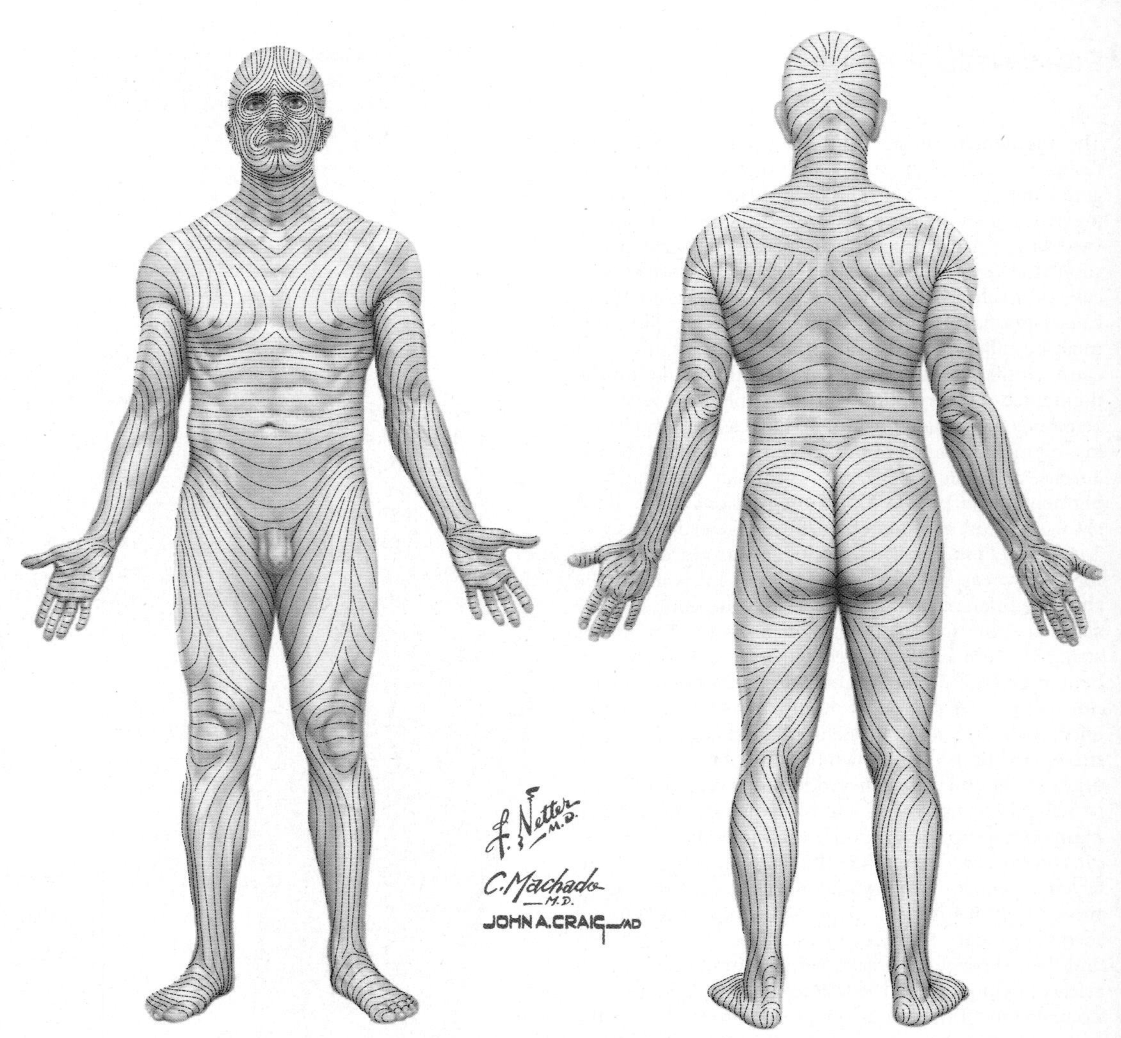

The rash of pityriasis rosea follows the skin tension lines (Langer's lines).

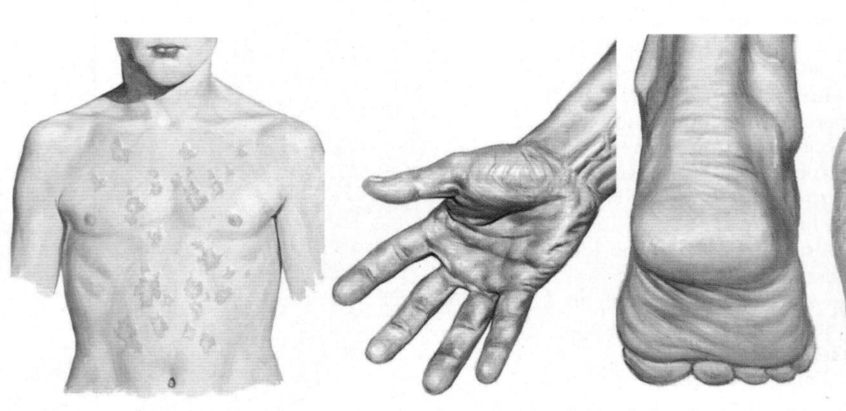

Generalized thin oval patches are distributed on the trunk following the skin tension lines.

The palms and soles are typically unaffected in pityriasis rosea. If they are affected, a rapid plasma reagin blood test must be obtained to rule out secondary syphilis.

Secondary syphilis affecting the sole

Pityriasis rosea is a common idiopathic rash with a characteristic onset and distribution. It is a self-limited rash that spontaneously resolves within a few months. A few distinct clinical variants have been described. The main goal in management is to differentiate pityriasis rosea from other rashes that can have a similar clinical picture.

Clinical Findings: Pityriasis rosea is a common rash of young adults and children. It has no racial or sex predilection. It is most often seen during the spring and fall months. Clustering of cases has been reported. A small but significant subset of patients have had a preceding upper respiratory tract infection. This has led some to search for a viral cause of the rash, although none has been found. The rash of pityriasis rosea often has a varying morphology, but it most commonly begins with a herald patch. The herald patch, or mother patch, is the first noticeable skin lesion. It typically precedes the entire outbreak of pityriasis rosea by a few days. The herald patch is a 2- to 4-cm pink-red patch with fine adherent scale that commonly occurs on the trunk. After a few days, smaller, oval-shaped patches 0.5 to 1 cm in diameter begin appearing on the trunk and extremities. The rash follows the skin tension lines and has a peculiar "fir tree" pattern, which mimics the down-sloping branches of a fir tree. The rash typically spares the face and glabrous skin.

Patients may report mild to moderate pruritus, but most are asymptomatic. The main differential diagnosis includes guttate psoriasis and, in cases that affect the palms and soles, secondary syphilis. Pityriasis rosea is a self-limited, spontaneously resolving rash. It typically does not last longer than 2 to 3 months. Guttate psoriasis usually begins after a streptococcal infection and does not exhibit a herald patch. The teardrop-shaped patches of guttate psoriasis also do not follow the skin tension lines, a fact that can be used to differentiate the two. Tinea corporis is almost always in the differential diagnosis of any rash that has a patch-type morphology and fine surface scale. Tinea corporis can be easily diagnosed with a microscopic KOH evaluation of a small scraping of the skin. Widespread tinea is almost always associated with onychomycosis, and it is more commonly seen in patients who are taking chronic immunosuppressive agents or using topical steroids. That history can be used to help differentiate the two conditions. The rash of secondary syphilis is the great mimicker. Any patient who has pityriasis rosea that affects the palms and/or soles should be tested for syphilis.

A few unique variants of pityriasis rosea exist. One is papular pityriasis rosea. This form more commonly affects school-aged children with Fitzpatrick type IV, V, or VI skin. This version tends to be a bit more widespread and more pruritic. Instead of small, oval-shaped patches, this variant consists of small (0.5-cm) papules that have a minuscule amount of surface scale. It runs the same benign course, with self-resolution after a few weeks to months. On healing, postinflammatory hyperpigmentation or hypopigmentation may result and may persist for several months.

Pathogenesis: Many attempts to isolate a viral or a bacterial element in patients with pityriasis rosea have been met with frustration. To date, no infectious cause has been determined. The true nature and cause of pityriasis rosea remain elusive.

Histology: A superficial and deep lymphocytic and histiocytic infiltrate is seen surrounding the vessels of the dermis. Varying amounts of extravasated red blood cells are appreciated within the upper dermis. The stratum corneum demonstrates differing degrees of acanthosis and parakeratosis.

Treatment: No therapy is needed. Most cases are asymptomatic and mild. Pruritus can be treated with oral antihistamines and adjunctive topical steroids. The use of oral erythromycin, twice a day for 2 weeks, was shown in some to decrease the duration of the rash. In certain cases, UV light therapy is very helpful in treating the rash and pruritus. If there is any consideration for syphilis in the history or the physical examination, serologic blood tests should be performed.

Pityriasis Rubra Pilaris

Pityriasis rubra pilaris (PRP) is an idiopathic rash that has many cutaneous manifestations. It is an uncommon entity that often manifests with near-erythroderma. There are several clinical variations of the condition, and it has a characteristic histologic pattern, although this pattern is not always seen on microscopic examination.

Clinical Findings: PRP has a unique bimodal age of distribution, with an early onset of disease in the first 5 years of life and adult onset in the sixth decade. There is no sex or racial predilection. PRP tends to run a chronic course. It starts insidiously with small follicular, keratotic, pink to red papules. In the classic form the rash starts on the trunk and spreads in both the caudal and cephalic directions. These papules have been described as "nutmeg grater" papules. The papules coalesce into larger patches and plaques. Eventually, large surface areas are involved, with a near-erythroderma. Characteristic islands of sparing occur within the erythrodermic background. These islands of completely normal skin are usually small, a few centimeters in diameter, but can be much larger. The islands typically have an angulated shape and are rarely perfectly round or oval. The palms and soles become thickened and yellowish-orange in color. This is a highly characteristic feature of PRP referred to as "carnauba wax–like" palms and soles. Fissuring is very common within the keratoderma and can be a source of pain and a site for secondary infection.

PRP has historically been separated into five subtypes: classic adult, classic juvenile, atypical adult, atypical juvenile, and a circumscribed or localized form. The classic adult and classic juvenile forms are the most common variants encountered. They typically run a chronic clinical course, with most cases spontaneously resolving a few years after onset. The circumscribed form presents with scattered, well-demarcated plaques with follicular prominence. Atypical variants do not show the characteristic cephalocaudal advancement. Paraneoplastic variants of PRP have been described. Onset of the malignancy precedes the rash of PRP, and patients seem to improve with treatment of the underlying tumor. This is a very rare clinical scenario. Patients with HIV infection seem to be at a higher risk for developing PRP.

The differential diagnosis of classic forms of PRP includes psoriasis, drug rash, and cutaneous T-cell lymphoma. Skin biopsy and clinical pathologic correlation help the clinician make a firm diagnosis.

Pathogenesis: The etiology is undetermined. Initial theories on the formation of PRP had centered on abnormal metabolism of vitamin A or an abnormal immune response to a foreign antigen. These theories have not been thoroughly proven and are unlikely to be the sole initiating factor. The report of a familial form of PRP has shed some light on the etiology. The familial form has shown an increased nuclear factor–kappa B signaling, which is known to increase inflammation. Individuals with HIV have a higher risk of developing PRP, and treating HIV-associated PRP with antiretrovirals has been successful. This has led researchers to look at potential viral initiating factors.

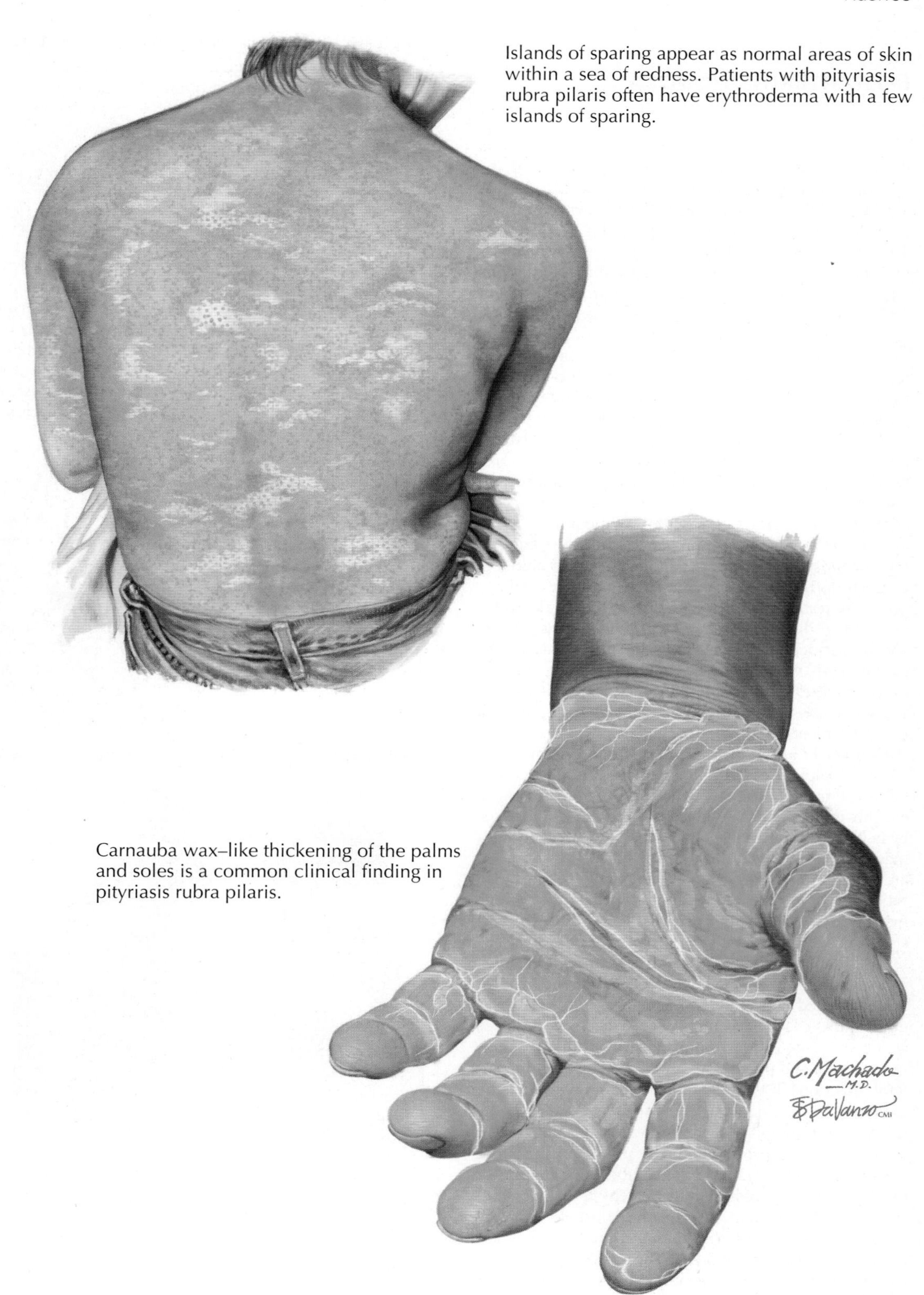

Islands of sparing appear as normal areas of skin within a sea of redness. Patients with pityriasis rubra pilaris often have erythroderma with a few islands of sparing.

Carnauba wax–like thickening of the palms and soles is a common clinical finding in pityriasis rubra pilaris.

Histology: The pathognomonic histologic finding in PRP is the appearance of alternating layers of parakeratosis and orthokeratosis, in both vertical and horizontal directions, lending the appearance of a chess board. This pattern is not always present, and sometimes it can be seen only with close inspection.

Treatment: Therapy for PRP is difficult. Many agents have been used with varying degrees of success. Topical corticosteroid wet wraps, oral retinoids, and UV therapy have long been used as first-line agents. The retinoids are considered first-line therapy, and both isotretinoin and acitretin have been used. Topical calcineurin inhibitors and calcipotriene have shown some efficacy. Immunosuppressants have been used, including methotrexate, azathioprine, and cyclosporine. Anti–tumor necrosis factor inhibitors as well as anti-IL-12 and IL-23 inhibitors appear to be efficacious in some cases.

POLYARTERITIS NODOSA

Polyarteritis nodosa is a rare chronic form of vasculitis of the medium to small arteries with potential for significant cutaneous and systemic manifestations. It is a rare condition, with an estimated incidence of 5 per 1 million persons. There is no race or sex predilection. The symptoms depend on the organ system involved and the extent of vasculitis. The clinical manifestations and organ systems involved vary dramatically from person to person, leading to a heterogenous disease state. Uniquely and for unknown reasons, the respiratory system is spared. Polyarteritis nodosa has been found in some cases to be a chronic, non–life-threatening disease that affects only the skin. More often, it is a multisystem disease, with the skin being affected along with other organ systems. Many other organ systems may be involved, and the skin features may be the presenting sign of the disease. Excisional skin biopsies of cutaneous lesions of polyarteritis nodosa show the characteristic necrotizing vasculitis of medium to small arteries within the deep reticular dermis. The cutaneous diagnosis of polyarteritis nodosa should alert the clinician to the possibility of systemic disease, and appropriate testing should be undertaken to evaluate for widespread disease. Most cases of polyarteritis nodosa are idiopathic, but this condition can be seen in association with viral infections, malignancy, or autoimmune disease. Coinfection with the hepatitis B virus is the most classic and most frequent association with polyarteritis nodosa.

Clinical Findings: The primary cutaneous manifestation is palpable purpura. Cutaneous findings tend to be spread over wide areas of the body and are not found entirely in dependent regions, as is the case with leukocytoclastic vasculitis. Deeper, tender dermal nodules may form. These nodules usually follow the course of an underlying artery. The patient may develop livedo reticularis of the extremities, and secondary ulcerations may form as the vasculitis progresses and causes necrosis of the overlying skin. Diagnosis of the type of vasculitis is difficult to make from clinical examination alone. Tissue sampling is needed to determine the type of vessel affected by the inflammatory vasculitis. There is no diagnostic lab test available. Polyarteritis nodosa has also been shown to have nonspecific findings, such as red macules and papules, that mimic drug eruptions or viral infections. If the only organ system involved is the integumentary system, the prognosis is good, and the disease typically follows a chronic, treatable course.

Once the diagnosis of cutaneous polyarteritis nodosa has been made, a systemic evaluation must be undertaken to pursue potential life-threatening involvement. If other organ systems are involved, the patient will need to undergo systemic therapy, and a multidisciplinary approach is required. The sensory nerves are almost always affected by mononeuritis multiplex. This leads to peripheral neuropathy, which is cited as the most common extracutaneous finding in polyarteritis nodosa. The kidneys, heart, and gastrointestinal tract are also routinely affected, which can lead to life-threatening complications. Renal artery aneurysms can form along the branches of the renal artery and can become thrombosed. This leads to wedge-shaped infarcts in the kidney with varying amounts of kidney function loss. Gastrointestinal arterial infarcts can also cause bowel ischemia and symptoms of an acute abdomen. The central nervous system (CNS) and the musculoskeletal system are also frequently affected.

Polyarteritis nodosa with characteristic multisystem involvement

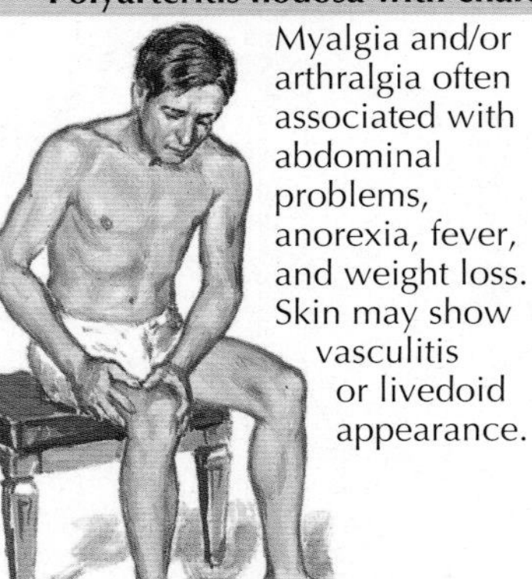

Myalgia and/or arthralgia often associated with abdominal problems, anorexia, fever, and weight loss. Skin may show vasculitis or livedoid appearance.

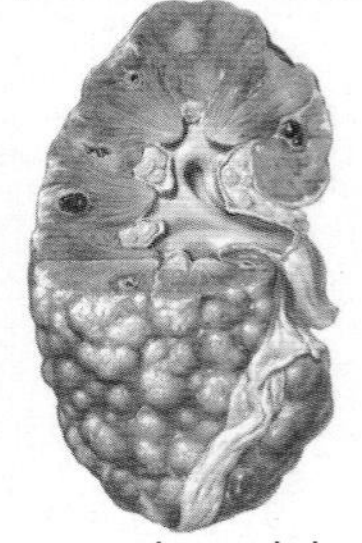

Coarsely nodular, irregularly scarred kidney. Cut section reveals organizing infarcts and thrombosed aneurysms in corticomedullary region.

Hypertension common

Angiogram showing microaneurysm of small mesenteric artery

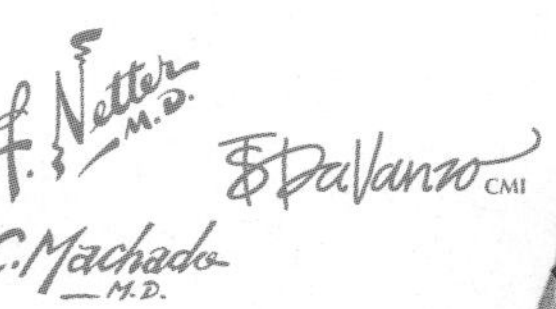

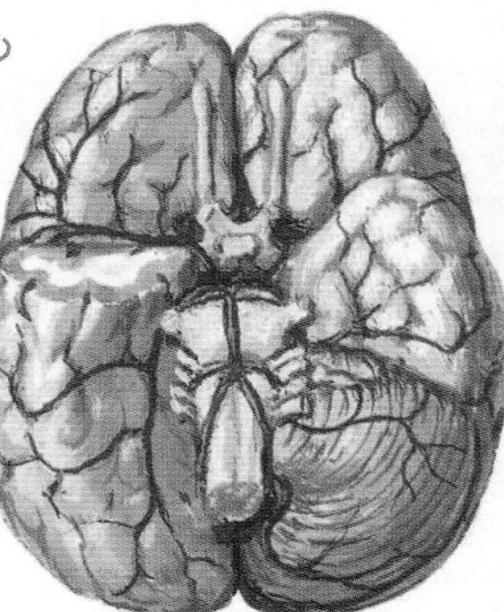

CNS involvement may cause headache, ocular disorders, convulsions, aphasia, hemiplegia, and cerebellar signs.

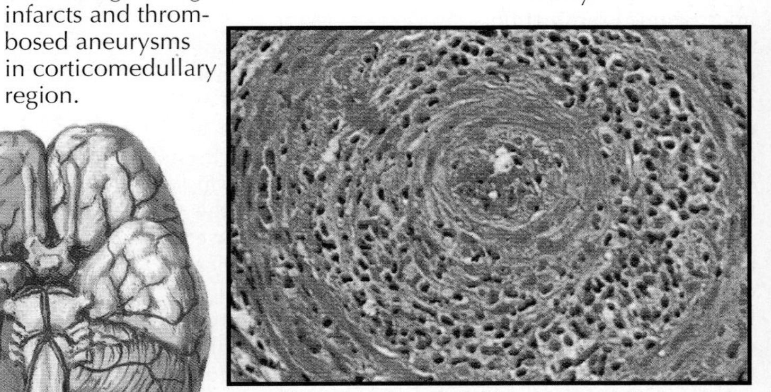

Inflammatory cell infiltration and fibrinoid necrosis of walls of small arteries lead to infarction in various organs or tissues.

Mononeuritis multiplex with polyarteritis nodosa

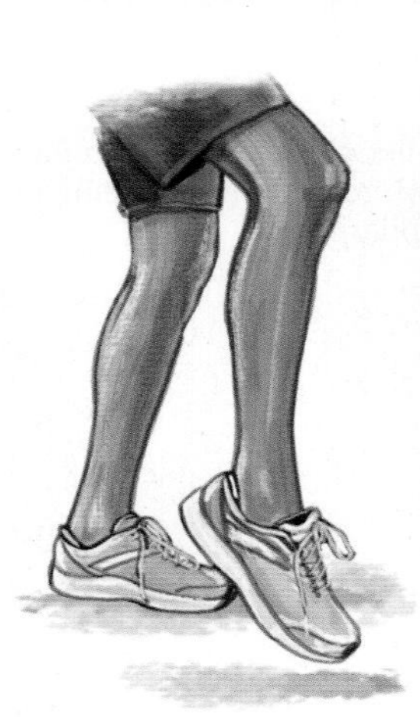

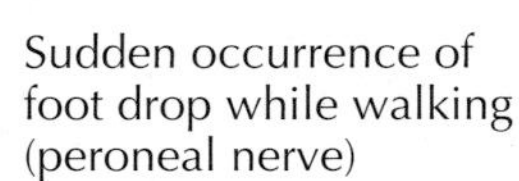

Sudden occurrence of foot drop while walking (peroneal nerve)

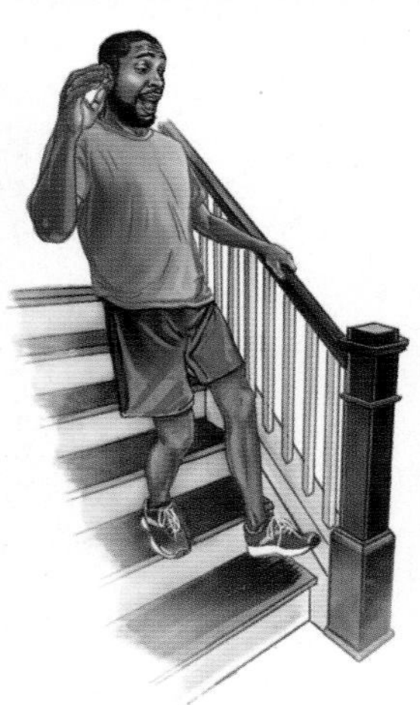

Sudden buckling of knee while going downstairs (femoral nerve)

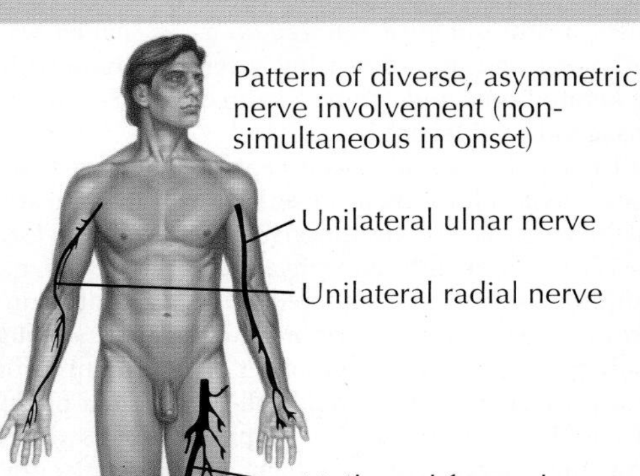

Pathogenesis: The pathomechanisms that incite polyarteritis nodosa are poorly understood. Hepatitis-induced polyarteritis is believed to be partially caused by viral disruption of arterial endothelial cells as a result of circulating antigen-antibody complexes.

Histology: Necrotizing vasculitis of medium and small arteries in the deep reticular dermis is the hallmark of polyarteritis nodosa. The inflammatory infiltrate is predominantly made up of neutrophils with an admixture of other leukocytes. Fibrinoid necrosis is prominent, and intraluminal clotting is often seen. Depending on the type of skin lesion biopsied, varying amounts of skin necrosis are seen. This is most commonly observed in areas of infarcted skin and ulceration.

Treatment: The first-line therapy is with oral corticosteroids. The use of steroid-sparing agents early in the course of the disease may help decrease steroid-induced side effects. Methotrexate, mycophenolate mofetil, and azathioprine are the main steroid-sparing agents. Cyclophosphamide is the major steroid-sparing agent used for severe cases. Therapy for polyarteritis nodosa induced by hepatitis B virus infection is targeted at the replicating viral particles.

Pruritic Urticarial Papules and Plaques of Pregnancy

Pruritic urticarial papules and plaques of pregnancy (PUPPP), also known as *polymorphous eruption of pregnancy*, is the most common dermatosis associated with pregnancy. The name describes the variable appearance of the rash. Idiopathic in nature, it is seen most commonly during an expectant mother's first pregnancy. It has been shown to have no bearing on pregnancy outcome or on the fetus or newborn. It is diagnosed on clinical grounds and rarely biopsied. There are no associated laboratory abnormalities. The classic history and variable morphology of the rash are characteristic.

Clinical Findings: PUPPP occurs during the late third trimester of pregnancy or soon after delivery. The rash almost always begins within the striae distensae of the abdomen. Small urticarial papules and plaques begin to form within the striae. They are extremely pruritic and cause significant discomfort. As the name implies, the rash can have a polymorphous nature. Papules, plaques, macules, and even small vesicles have been described. The rash may spread from the abdomen to other regions of the body. PUPPP has been described to occur more commonly during a patient's first pregnancy with a male fetus. The reasons for this are unknown. The rash spontaneously remits after delivery, in most cases within 2 to 4 weeks. Patients with onset after delivery typically have a shorter course, with 1 week of severe itching followed by remission soon afterward. PUPPP typically does not recur in subsequent pregnancies. PUPPP also does not flare when birth control medications are started after pregnancy, as seen in herpes gestationis.

The main differential diagnosis is between PUPPP and prurigo gestationis. Prurigo gestationis has no primary lesions and manifests as diffuse itching with excoriations. Liver function enzymes may be elevated in this condition. Prurigo gestationis is associated with an increased risk for prematurity. Scabies infection can also be highly pruritic and can be considered in the differential diagnosis. Scabies is easily diagnosed with a scraping and microscopic evaluation of a burrow. Scabies can have its onset at any time during a pregnancy, and urticarial papules and plaques within striae are not typically seen. If seen, they are not as numerous or uniform in appearance as PUPPP lesions. Herpes gestationis, also known as *pemphigoid gestationis* or bullous pemphigoid of pregnancy, is the most severe of all the pregnancy-associated rashes. It can begin as urticarial red plaques on the abdomen and then spread to other regions. Compared with PUPPP, it tends to occur earlier in pregnancy. The biggest differentiating point is that the rash of herpes gestationis will begin to blister; small vesicles form and quickly coalesce into larger bullae. Bullae are never seen in PUPPP. Herpes gestationis is caused by maternal antibody formation against hemidesmosomal antigens. Titer levels can be measured, and the most commonly found antibody is against the 180-kd bullous pemphigoid antigen (BP180). There is a risk of prematurity and low birth weight with this rash. Oral corticosteroids are often needed to keep herpes gestationis under control. The rash remits after delivery but tends to recur during subsequent pregnancies, and it can flare when an affected patient starts taking birth control medications.

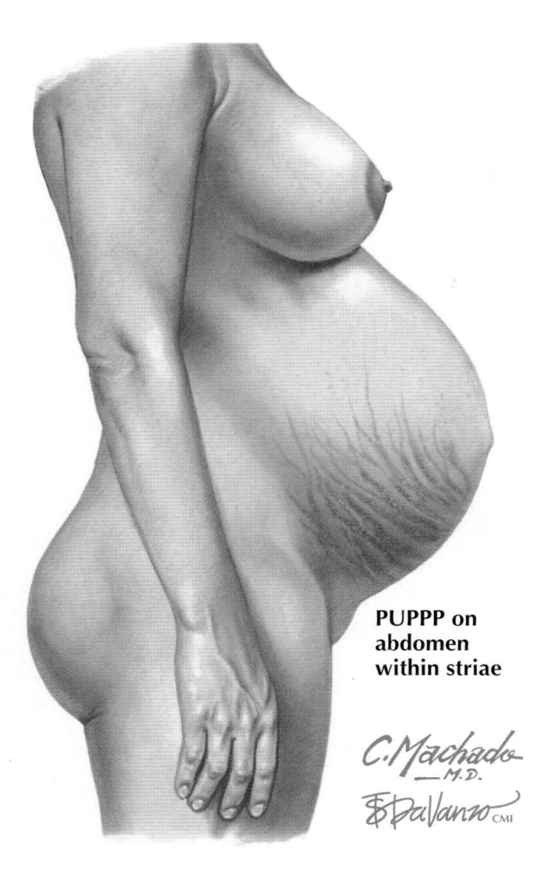

PUPPP on abdomen within striae

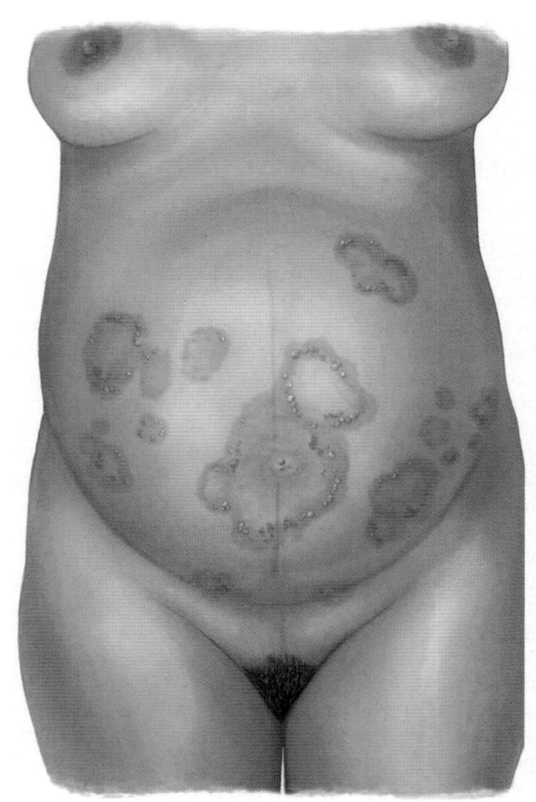

Herpes gestationis. Also known as bullous pemphigoid of pregnancy. Pruritic bullae develop on a background of erythematous or urticarial-appearing skin.

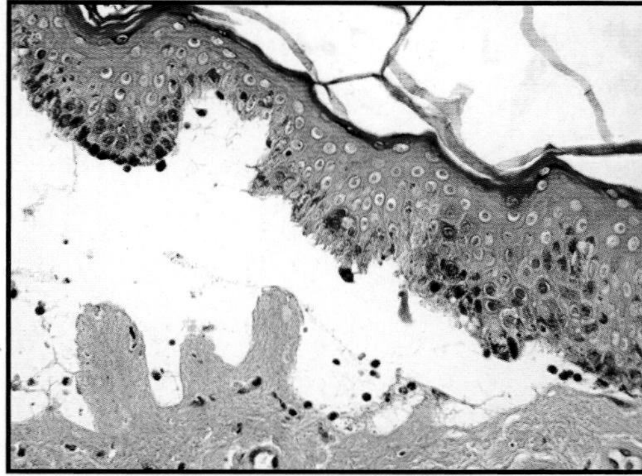

Herpes gestationis (pemphigoid gestationis) (H&E stain). Prominent subepidermal bulla formation is seen along the specimen. Separation is caused by antibodies against the BP180 protein, which leads to bulla formation.

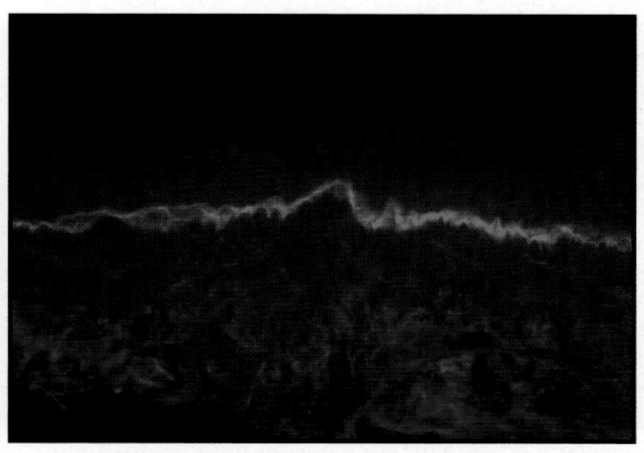

Immunofluorescence. Immunofluorescence studies show linear staining of C3 along the basement membrane zone in herpes gestationis.

Pathogenesis: The etiology is unknown. PUPPP is most commonly seen in first pregnancies and possibly is more common in multiple-birth pregnancies. The exact roles played by skin distention, hormonal changes, and interactions with the immune system in the pathogenesis of PUPPP are being studied.

Histology: Histologic findings of PUPPP biopsy specimens are nonspecific; there is a superficial and deep perivascular lymphocytic infiltrate. Occasional eosinophils are seen, with some dermal edema.

Treatment: The main treatment for PUPPP is supportive care and suppression of the itching symptoms. There are no ill effects on the fetus, and expectant mothers can be given topical medium- or high-potency corticosteroids to help decrease the itching. Occasionally, antihistamines such as diphenhydramine are also needed to control the itching.

PSEUDOXANTHOMA ELASTICUM

Pseudoxanthoma elasticum is a rare genetic disorder with both cutaneous and systemic findings. It is inherited in an autosomal recessive manner. This disease is caused by a defect in an ATP-binding protein found in many tissues, including the skin, eye, gastrointestinal tract, and cardiovascular system. The cutaneous findings often precede the appearance of the systemic findings. Recognition of the cutaneous findings can help lessen the risk of systemic complications. A multidisciplinary approach to the care of these patients is required. The skin findings have no bearing on mortality.

Clinical Findings: Pseudoxanthoma elasticum manifests in late childhood or early adulthood, and there is no race or sex predilection. The cutaneous findings are almost always the first sign of the disease. The skin on the neck is most commonly affected early and most severely. There is a "plucked chicken skin" appearance to the skin. Small yellow papules are studded within the involved region and over time coalesce into larger, symmetric plaques. The intervening skin has a dull appearance with a fine pebbly texture. The neck is by far the area most noticeably affected, but other regions may become involved, including the intertriginous areas. A rare generalized cutaneous form has been reported. The mucous membranes may also become involved, with tiny yellow papules. As time progresses, the skin may become loose, appearing to hang from the body, which can be a significant cosmetic concern to the patient. The areas of cutaneous involvement are essentially asymptomatic. On occasion, mild pruritus is reported. A nonspecific skin finding seen with increased frequency in pseudoxanthoma elasticum is elastosis perforans serpiginosa. This perforating disorder has been described to occur in many different clinical settings and is caused by the transepidermal elimination of damaged elastic tissue. The reason this occurs in pseudoxanthoma elasticum is unknown.

It is important to diagnosis this disease at a young age so that some of the severe systemic complications can be prevented. The globe is affected in pseudoxanthoma elasticum. The first sign is a yellowish discoloration of the retina. Later in life, cracks or ruptures in Bruch's membrane can be seen on funduscopic examination; these are termed *angioid streaks*. Angioid streaks have a later age at onset than the cutaneous findings do. Abnormalities of the elastic fibers in Bruch's membrane are responsible for their formation. Angioid streaks can be seen in many disorders of connective tissue and are not specific for pseudoxanthoma elasticum. Retinal hemorrhage and resultant visual field loss are the most severe ophthalmologic complications.

Cardiovascular and gastrointestinal manifestations arise because of the abnormal calcification of elastic tissue within blood vessel walls. Gastrointestinal hemorrhage may occur and may be life-threatening. Angina and hypertension may occur from involvement of the coronary and renal arteries, respectively.

Pathogenesis: Pseudoxanthoma elasticum is inherited in an autosomal recessive fashion and is caused by a defect in the *ABCC6* gene. This gene is responsible for encoding the multidrug resistance–associated protein 6, which is also known as ATP-binding cassette transporter 6. This protein is found within the liver and kidneys and is expressed at low levels in the tissues affected by this disease. It has been proposed that the defect causes a metabolic abnormality, possibly resulting in a buildup of a metabolite that damages the elastic fibers in the affected tissue.

Histology: Findings on skin biopsies are very characteristic and show abnormal fractured, calcified elastic tissue within the dermis. The findings can be accentuated with special staining methods to highlight the calcified elastic fibers. However, the diagnosis can be made easily on routine hematoxylin and eosin staining.

Treatment: Therapy is directed at preventive care. Routine cardiovascular and ophthalmologic examinations can help keep hypertension and early signs of retinal disease in check. Retinal hemorrhages must be treated acutely by an ophthalmologist. Routine examinations for blood in the stool and routine gastrointestinal examinations are warranted to screen for gastrointestinal bleeding, which is the main cause of morbidity and mortality in these patients. Patients should be encouraged to stay within a healthy weight range and not to smoke. Most patients live a normal life span.

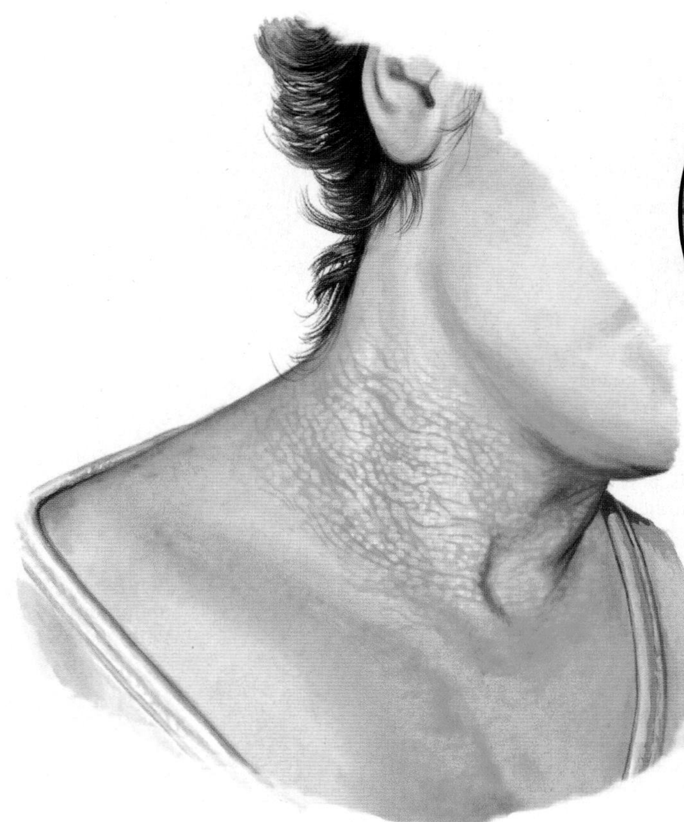

The neck is often the first area of skin involvement. Often clinically noted to have the appearance of "plucked chicken skin".

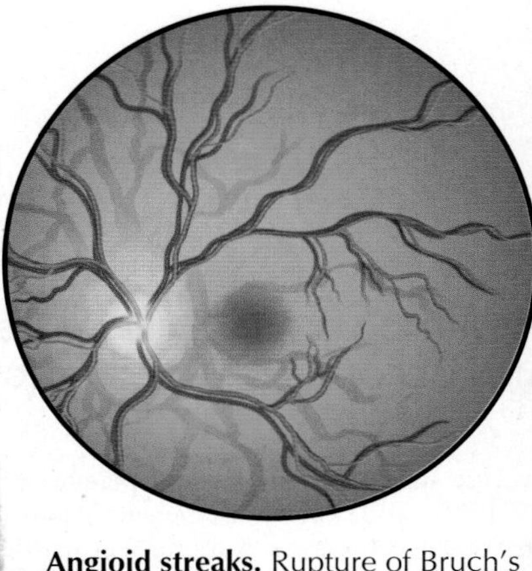

Angioid streaks. Rupture of Bruch's membrane, likely due to abnormal calcification of the membrane, can be seen in pseudoxanthoma elasticum on slit-lamp examination.

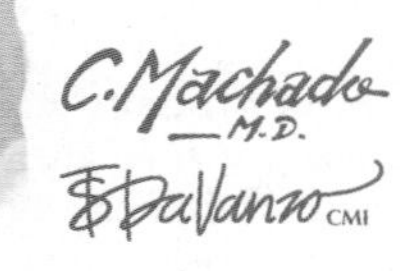

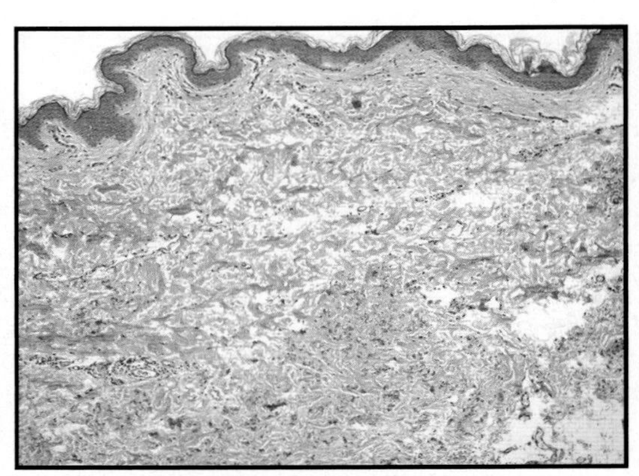

Low power (H&E). Fragmented and calcified elastic fibers appear as basophilic clumps within the middle to lower dermis. This is highly characteristic for pseudoxanthoma elasticum.

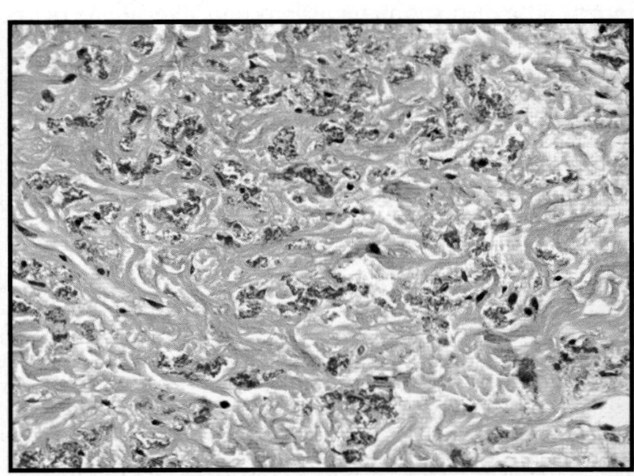

High power (H&E). Basophilic clumping of calcified elastic fibers that have become fragmented is well appreciated in this high-power view. The abnormality in the elastic fibers leads to the various clinical manifestations of the disease.

PSORIASIS

Psoriasis is an autoimmune disease that affects 1% to 2% of the U.S. population. There is a large regional variation in the incidence of psoriasis. Scandinavian countries have a much higher incidence than the rest of the world, and the Native American population has one of the lowest rates of psoriasis. Much has been learned about the pathogenesis of psoriasis, and dramatic advances in therapy have helped many patients. Psoriasis is grouped with the other papulosquamous skin diseases because of its ability to form patches and plaques. It can cause joint disease as well as skin disease. The total effect that psoriasis has on patients cannot be judged solely on the basis of skin involvement because the disease has been shown to have profound psychological and social effects as well. There is no known cure for psoriasis, but research is moving forward, and new therapies are actively being developed.

Clinical Findings: Psoriasis is a papulosquamous skin disease that can affect people at any age of life. There is no sex predilection. Approximately 40% of affected individuals have a family history of psoriasis. Most patients with early age at onset tend to have a more severe course of disease. Psoriasis often starts with silvery, ostraceous, scaly patches and plaques with a predilection for the knees, elbows, and scalp. The term *ostraceous scale* refers to the oyster shell–like appearance of the hyperkeratotic scale that is oriented in a concave manner. The term *rupioid scale* is used to describe the psoriatic plaques that appear to mimic the cone shape of limpet shells. A characteristic clinical finding is that of Woronoff's ring, the peripheral rim of blanching seen around the early psoriatic plaques. Woronoff's ring is specific to psoriasis and most likely is caused by localized vasoconstriction surrounding the area of the lesion, which has an increased blood flow. Auspitz's sign is another characteristic clinical sign used to differentiate psoriasis from other rashes. It refers to the pinpoint bleeding that occurs after the upper scale has been physically removed from a psoriatic plaque. There is a striking symmetry to the rash. Psoriasis can have various skin morphologies, and there are several well-recognized clinical variants with distinctive clinical findings.

Psoriasis vulgaris is the most common form of psoriasis encountered. It manifests with symmetrically located, silvery, scaly patches and plaques on the scalp, knees, elbows, and lower back. Patients can have a small amount of body surface area involvement, or they can have widespread disease approaching near-erythroderma. The face is usually spared from patches and plaques of psoriasis. Patients with a higher body surface area of involvement tend to have a higher risk for development of psoriatic arthritis and psoriatic nail disease. All patients with psoriasis exhibit the Koebner phenomenon. Koebnerization of psoriasis occurs when a previously normal area of skin is traumatized and psoriatic plaques develop within the traumatized skin.

HISTOPATHOLOGIC FEATURES AND TYPICAL DISTRIBUTION OF PSORIASIS

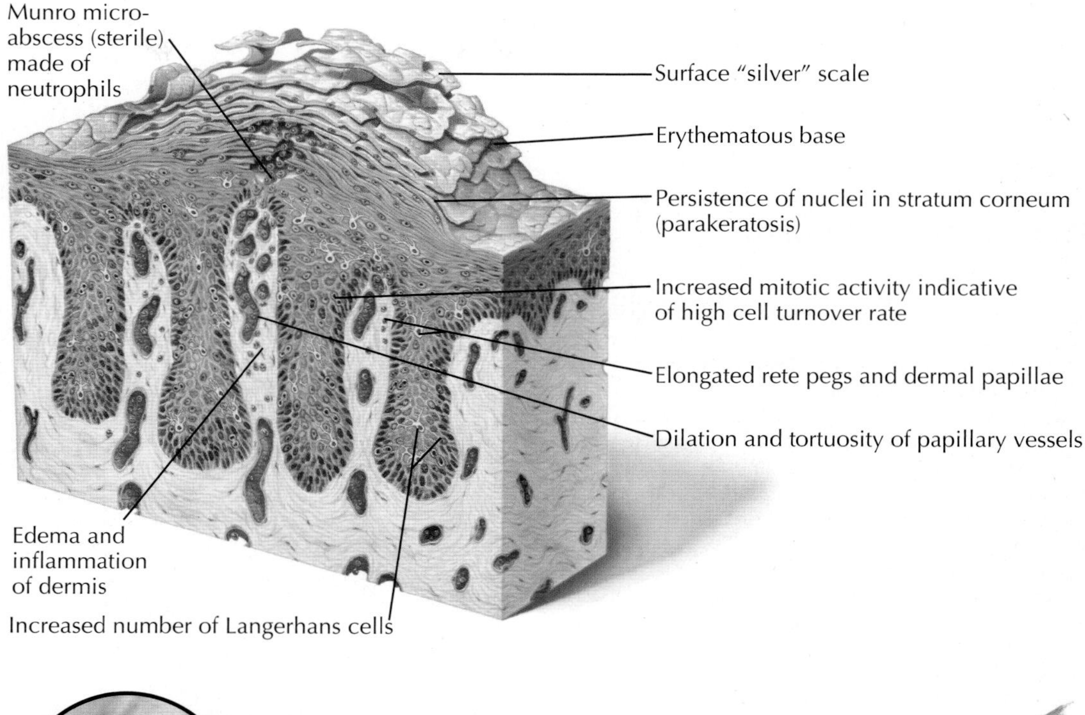

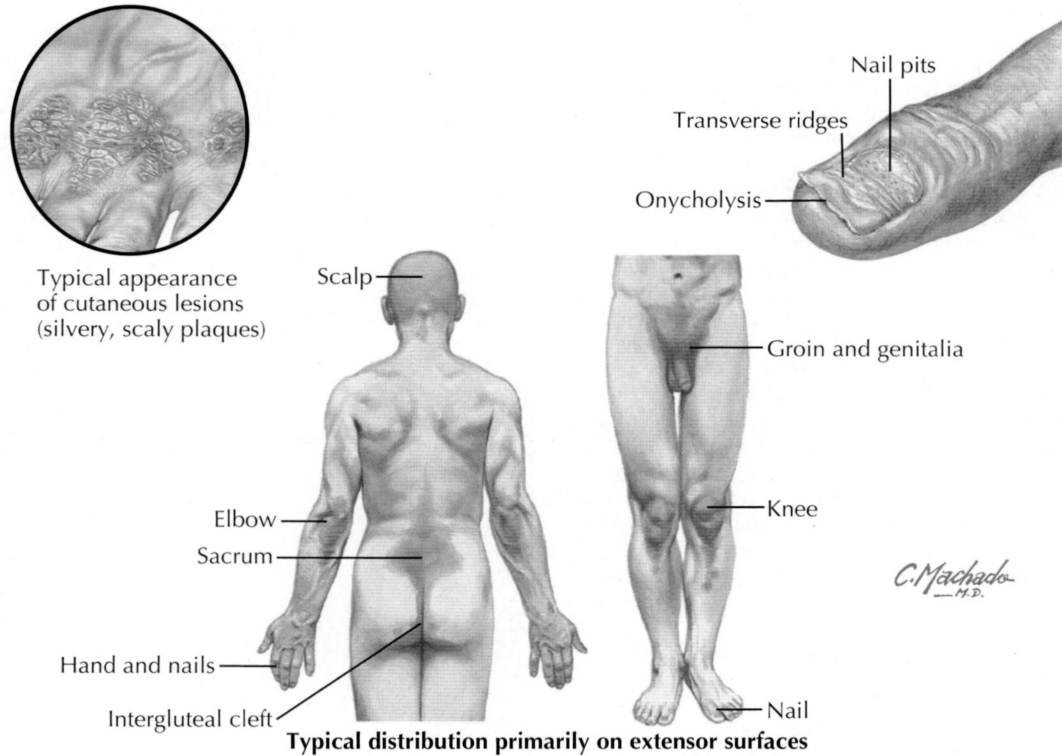

Typical distribution primarily on extensor surfaces

Inverse psoriasis is a well-recognized clinical variant that manifests in intertriginous areas of the groin, gluteal cleft, axillae, and umbilicus. The patches tend not to be as thick as in the other forms, and the scale is fine. This is because of their location in occluded areas, which have an increased amount of moisture that helps to keep the scale to a minimum. The patches can be bright red and are often misdiagnosed as a cutaneous *Candida* infection. Inverse psoriasis is also symmetric in nature and can present therapeutic challenges.

Guttate psoriasis is a variant of psoriasis that can occur after an infection, most notably a streptococcal bacterial infection. The guttate lesions develop soon after or during the infection and appear as tiny teardrop-shaped patches with fine adherent scale. The word *guttate* means "droplet," and the lesions of guttate psoriasis appear as tiny droplets of psoriatic patches found generalized over the skin, as if areas of psoriasis had developed within sprinkled water droplets. Children with guttate psoriasis may have only one isolated

Inverse Psoriasis and Psoriasis in the Genital Area

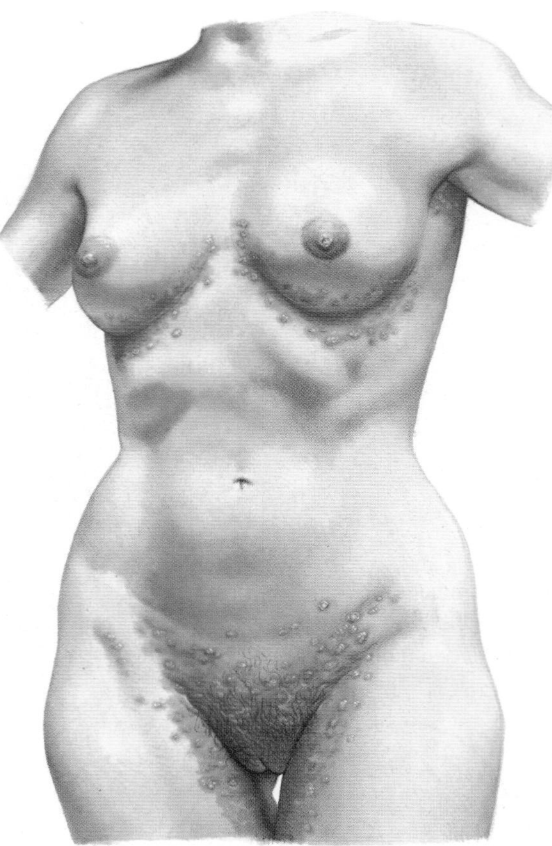

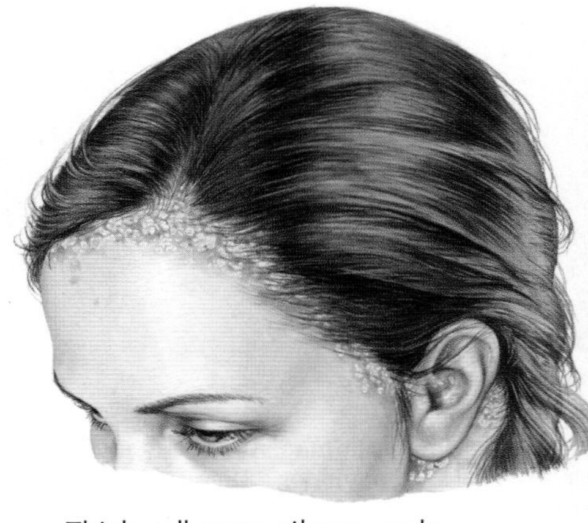

Thick, adherent, silvery, scaly patches and plaques on scalp

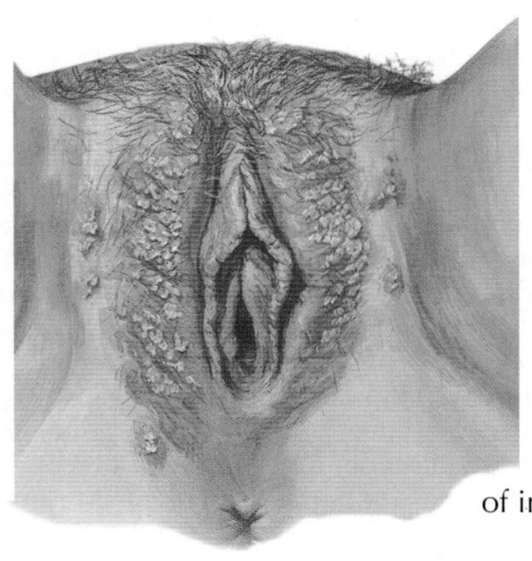

Typical appearance of intertriginous lesion

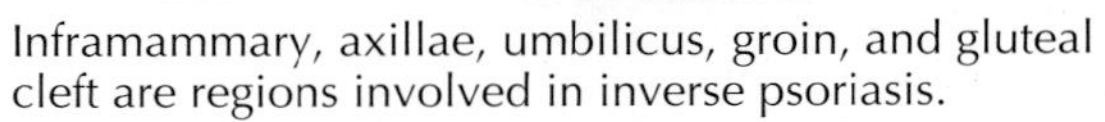

Inframammary, axillae, umbilicus, groin, and gluteal cleft are regions involved in inverse psoriasis.

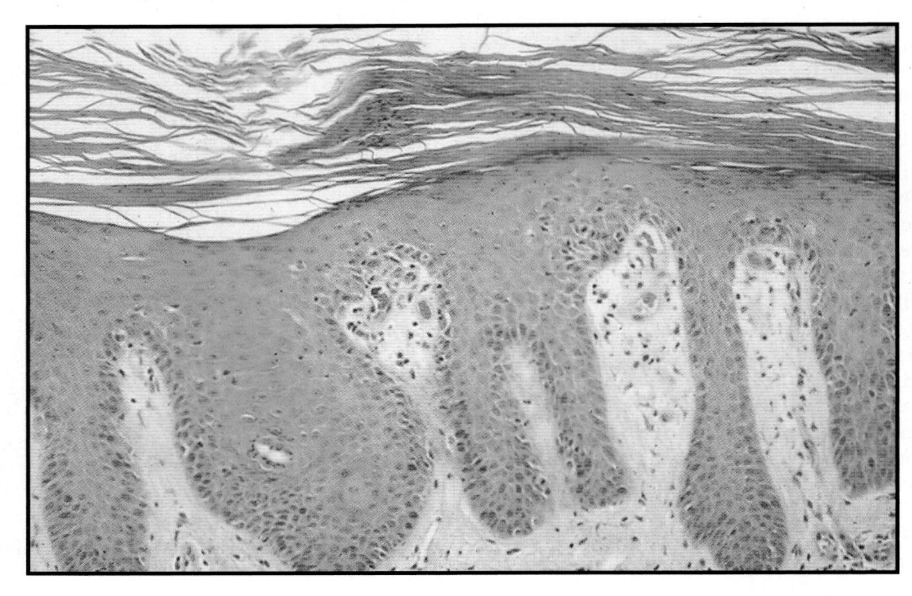

Regularly spaced and shaped acanthosis of the epidermis, with telangiectatic vessels in the papillary dermis

F. Netter M.D.
C. Machado M.D.

Psoriasis (Continued)

episode after a streptococcal infection and no evidence of psoriasis thereafter. Adults with guttate psoriasis, on the other hand, almost always develop psoriasis vulgaris at some later point.

Scalp psoriasis is a unique variant that occurs only on the scalp. Patients report thick, scaly patches that itch and can cause a dramatic amount of seborrhea. Most patients who present with localized scalp psoriasis eventually develop areas of psoriasis elsewhere on their bodies.

Pustular psoriasis is a rare and distinctive form. It can occur in patients with a preexisting history of psoriasis, or it can be the initial presenting morphology. The diagnosis is straightforward in a patient with a long-standing history of psoriasis who develops a pustular flare. The most common reason for this is the rapid withdrawal of systemic corticosteroids, such as when a patient with psoriasis is prescribed methylprednisolone for an unrelated condition (e.g., allergic contact dermatitis due to poison ivy). The rapid decrease in the dose of the corticosteroid can induce a pustular flare. The patches of psoriasis develop pinpoint (1–2 mm) pustules that can coalesce into superficial pools of pus. These patients are often ill appearing and can have associated hypocalcemia. Patients presenting with pustular psoriasis without a preexisting history of psoriasis pose a difficult diagnostic problem at first. The differential diagnosis is among psoriasis, a pustular drug eruption, and Sneddon-Wilkinson disease. A skin biopsy and clinical follow-up eventually make the diagnosis clear.

Nail psoriasis is most often associated with severe psoriasis vulgaris and psoriatic arthritis. It can occasionally be a solitary finding. Oil spots, onycholysis, nail pitting, and variable amounts of nail thickening can be present. Nail disease is refractory to most topical therapies, and systemic therapy is often required to get a good clinical response. Nail psoriasis is a marker for psoriatic arthritis, and patients with nail psoriasis are at a higher risk for development of psoriatic arthritis.

Palmar and plantar psoriasis is another of the less commonly seen clinical variants. It can manifest on the palms and soles as red, scaly patches and plaques or as patches studded with a variable number of small pustules. This variant of psoriasis is more commonly found in females, and smoking has been shown to make the clinical course worse.

Psoriatic erythroderma is a rare variant seen as a sequela of steroid withdrawal or of other, undefined triggers. It manifests with near-total redness of the skin. The redness is caused by massive vasodilation of the cutaneous vasculature, which can lead to high-output cardiac failure. These patients often require inpatient treatment.

Psoriatic arthritis can manifest in association with psoriatic skin disease or as arthritis with nail findings. Patients typically present with an asymmetric oligoarticular arthritis, symmetric polyarticular arthritis, distal interphalangeal–predominant disease, spinal spondylitis, or arthritis mutilans. Arthritis mutilans is the rarest form of psoriatic arthritis, but it is life-altering and can lead to a devastating loss of function. Psoriatic arthritis is considered a seronegative form of inflammatory arthritis.

Pathogenesis: Psoriasis is an autoimmune disease caused by an abnormality within the T cells of the immune system. There is a genetic susceptibility, and the HLA Cw6 locus is the most commonly found (but not the only) susceptibility factor in patients who develop psoriasis. The success of therapy with cyclosporine, a medication that dramatically decreases T-cell function, was one of the first clues to the pathogenesis of psoriasis. Patients with psoriasis given this medicine almost always have rapid clinical improvement.

T-cell lymphocytes and dermal dendritic cells are the most likely precursor cells to be the cause of pso-

Psoriatic Arthritis

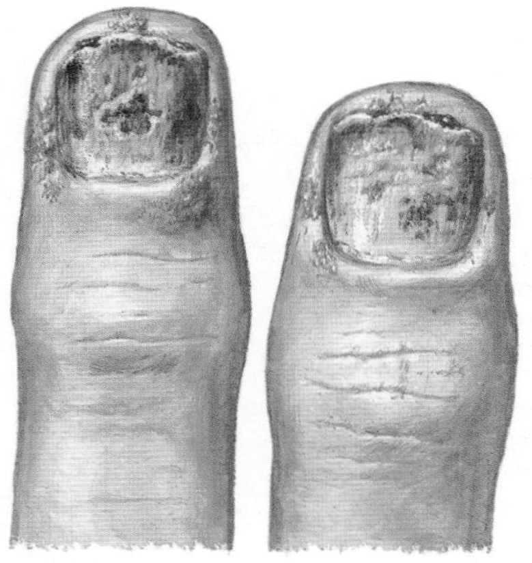

Pitting, discoloration, and erosion of fingernails with fusiform swelling of distal interphalangeal joints

Psoriatic patches on dorsum of hand with swelling and distortion of many interphalangeal joints and shortening of fingers due to loss of bone mass

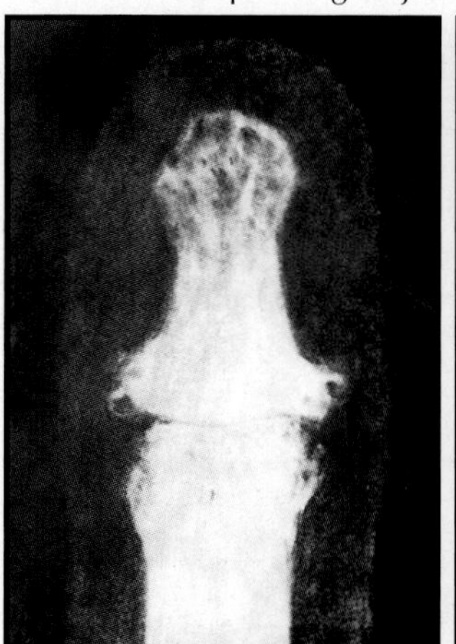

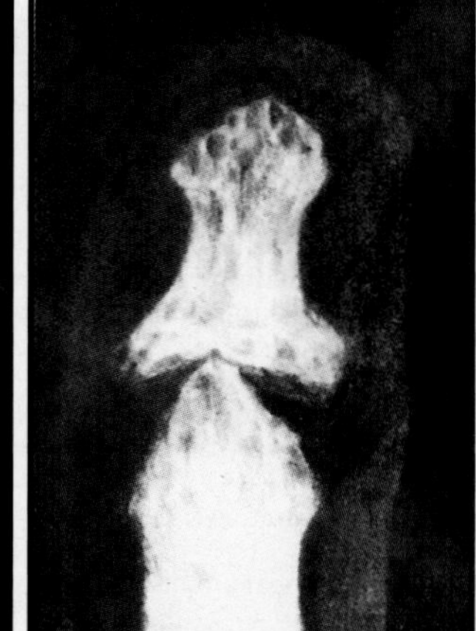

Radiographic changes in distal interphalangeal joint. *Left,* In early stages, bone erosions are seen at joint margins. *Right,* In late stages, further loss of bone mass produces "pencil point in cup" appearance.

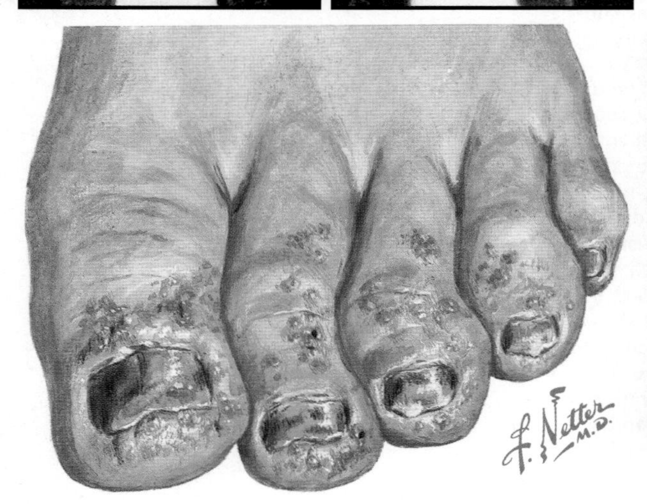

Toes with sausage-like swelling, skin lesions, and nail changes

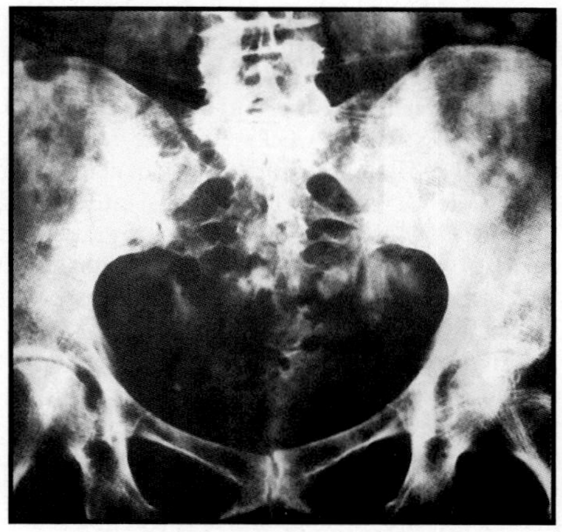

Radiograph of sacroiliac joints shows thin cartilage with irregular surface and condensation of adjacent bone in sacrum and ilia.

Psoriasis (Continued)

riasis; they are both found in increased numbers in psoriatic plaques. $CD8^+$ T cells are the predominant lymphocyte found within the epidermis; they contain the cutaneous lymphocyte antigen (CLA) on their cell surface. CLA is important because it directs these cells into the skin. There is a proliferation of Th1, Th17, and Th22 cells in psoriatic plaques. Each of these cells can secrete unique cytokines such as TNF-α, IL-17, and IL-22. These abnormal cytokine levels have become the target of many therapies. Many subsets of dermal dendritic cells have been found within psoriatic plaques. Dendritic cells have been shown to be potent stimulators of T cells and are believed to be required to propagate the inflammatory reaction. These two cell types interact and change the local cytokine profile into one that is proinflammatory and provides a milieu required for the development of the clinical findings of psoriasis. What is still unknown is the initial stimulus that sets off this cascade of events and how it is propagated and perpetuated.

Histology: Histologic examination of biopsy specimens of psoriasis vulgaris show regular psoriasiform hyperplasia of the epidermis. Multiple normal-appearing mitotic figures are seen within keratinocytes. Neutrophils are prominent within the stratum corneum and within the lumen of the papillary dermal blood vessels. Mounds of parakeratosis are seen in the stratum corneum and contain many neutrophils. The papillary dermis shows a proliferation of ectatic capillary vessels with a perivascular infiltrate made up of lymphocytes, Langerhans cells, and histiocytes. Collections of neutrophils within the stratum corneum are called Munro microabscesses. Kogoj microabscesses are similar collections of neutrophils within the stratum spinosum. There is a decrease in the thickness of the granular cell layer. With time, some of the tips of the rete ridges coalesce and form thickened ends.

Pustular psoriasis shows varying amounts of intraepidermal pustules; acanthosis and psoriasiform hyperplasia are not prominent. Again, there are multiple dilated capillary blood vessels in the papillary dermis.

Treatment: There is no cure for psoriasis. Treatment should be based on the amount and location of the psoriatic plaques and consideration of the psychological well-being of the affected individual. Small areas in discrete locations can be treated with topical corticosteroids, anthralin, tar compounds, or vitamin D or A analogs or left alone without therapy. UV therapy with natural sunlight, narrow-band UVB, or PUVA has been used with great success. Often, combinations of therapies are implemented.

As the body surface area of involvement increases or the psychological well-being of the individual is affected such that systemic therapy is warranted, many agents are available to treat the psoriasis. Phototherapy with narrow-band UVB or PUVA has been used for decades with excellent results. In the long term, these therapies increase the patient's risk of developing skin cancers, and lifelong dermatologic follow-up is required.

Oral systemic agents are also used for moderate to severe psoriasis. Methotrexate taken on a weekly basis has been used for years. Oral cyclosporine has been used with great success for erythrodermic and pustular psoriasis. Its use is limited to 6 to 12 months because of nephrotoxicity. Many biologic agents have become available over the past 2 decades. These medications are given by subcutaneous, intramuscular, or IV injection. They include the TNF-α inhibitors, the IL-17 and IL-12/IL-23 inhibitors, and the solitary IL-23 inhibitors. All of these agents have had excellent response rates. They are all considered to be immunosuppressive, and patients taking these medications need close clinical follow-up because they are at increased risk for infections and possibly systemic cancers, such as lymphoma, after years of use. Acitretin, apremilast, and JAK inhibitors are oral medications that in a subset of patients can have excellent results.

RADIATION DERMATITIS

With the ever-increasing use of adjunctive radiotherapy for a plethora of indications in the treatment of cancer, radiation dermatitis has been increasing in incidence. There are acute and chronic forms of radiation dermatitis, and their development is based on the total dose of radiation received. The skin is particularly sensitive to radiation damage, and it responds to the radiation in various ways. In the 1950s, the use of radiation to treat common skin conditions such as acne, tinea, and many common dermatoses was widespread. It was not until a better understanding of the long-term effects of radiation was achieved that this practice was discontinued. Localized or widespread radiotherapy is still used for some skin conditions, but it is most commonly reserved to treat malignancies such as tumor-stage mycosis fungoides or as an adjunctive therapy for melanoma, squamous cell carcinoma, Merkel cell carcinoma, or, uncommonly, unresectable basal cell carcinoma. External-beam radiotherapy can cause other complications depending on where it is administered. Irradiation of the head and neck region, for example, often produces xerostomia and mucositis. Dysphagia is also a possibility. If care is not taken to protect the globe, vision alteration or blindness may occur.

The method by which the radiation dose is given (fractionated, hyperfractionated, or accelerated hyperfractionated) is less critical in the development of radiation dermatitis than the total dose or the coexisting use of chemotherapy. Chemotherapy in combination with radiotherapy dramatically increases the chance of radiation dermatitis. Individuals with an underlying connective tissue disease are at highest risk of developing radiation dermatitis.

Clinical Findings: Radiation dermatitis can be divided into an acute form and a chronic form. The acute form begins within weeks after the radiation therapy has started. There is a graded scale of acuity from grade I to grade IV. Almost all patients undergoing radiotherapy develop some symptoms of grade I radiation dermatitis. Grade I is defined as a slight erythema of the skin overlying the radiation site associated with xerosis of the skin. Grade II manifests with more inflammatory red patches and edema. Grade III shows evidence of bright erythema, edema, and desquamation of the epidermis. Grade IV manifests as full-thickness skin necrosis, erythema, and ulcerations. This is the least common form of acute radiation dermatitis but the most severe, and it requires immediate management.

Chronic radiation dermatitis is commonly seen many months to years after exposure to radiation. Poikilodermatous skin changes are most prominent, and there is a thickening and hardness to the exposed skin. Poikiloderma manifests as telangiectasias, atrophy, and hyperpigmentation and hypopigmentation. Hair loss is common, as is the loss of all appendageal structures such as eccrine glands and apocrine glands. The hair loss is permanent.

Treatment: Therapy for acute radiation dermatitis is grade dependent. There is no acceptable or reliable prophylactic method to prevent radiation dermatitis. Grade I acute dermatitis is treated with moisturizers, and the use of a low-potency cortisone cream can be considered. Grade II or III acute dermatitis should be treated with moisturizing creams such as zinc oxide paste. Strict sun protection is required. Medium-potency corticosteroids may be used, and care should be taken to avoid superinfection. If a cutaneous infection is suspected, culture and use of appropriate antibiotics is required. Grade IV dermatitis requires treatment by a team of wound care specialists adept at treating burns.

Chronic radiation dermatitis itself does not require therapy unless the patient experiences severe tightness or hardness of the skin. In anecdotal reports, pentoxifylline has been successful in softening the areas of chronic radiation dermatitis. Hyperbaric oxygen has been used with varying results. Topical moisturizers may help with the dryness. Pulsed dye laser can be used to treat telangiectasias. The most critical aspect is routine inspection of the area of chronic radiation dermatitis for the development of skin cancers, most commonly basal cell carcinoma and squamous cell carcinoma.

EFFECTS OF RADIATION ON HUMANS

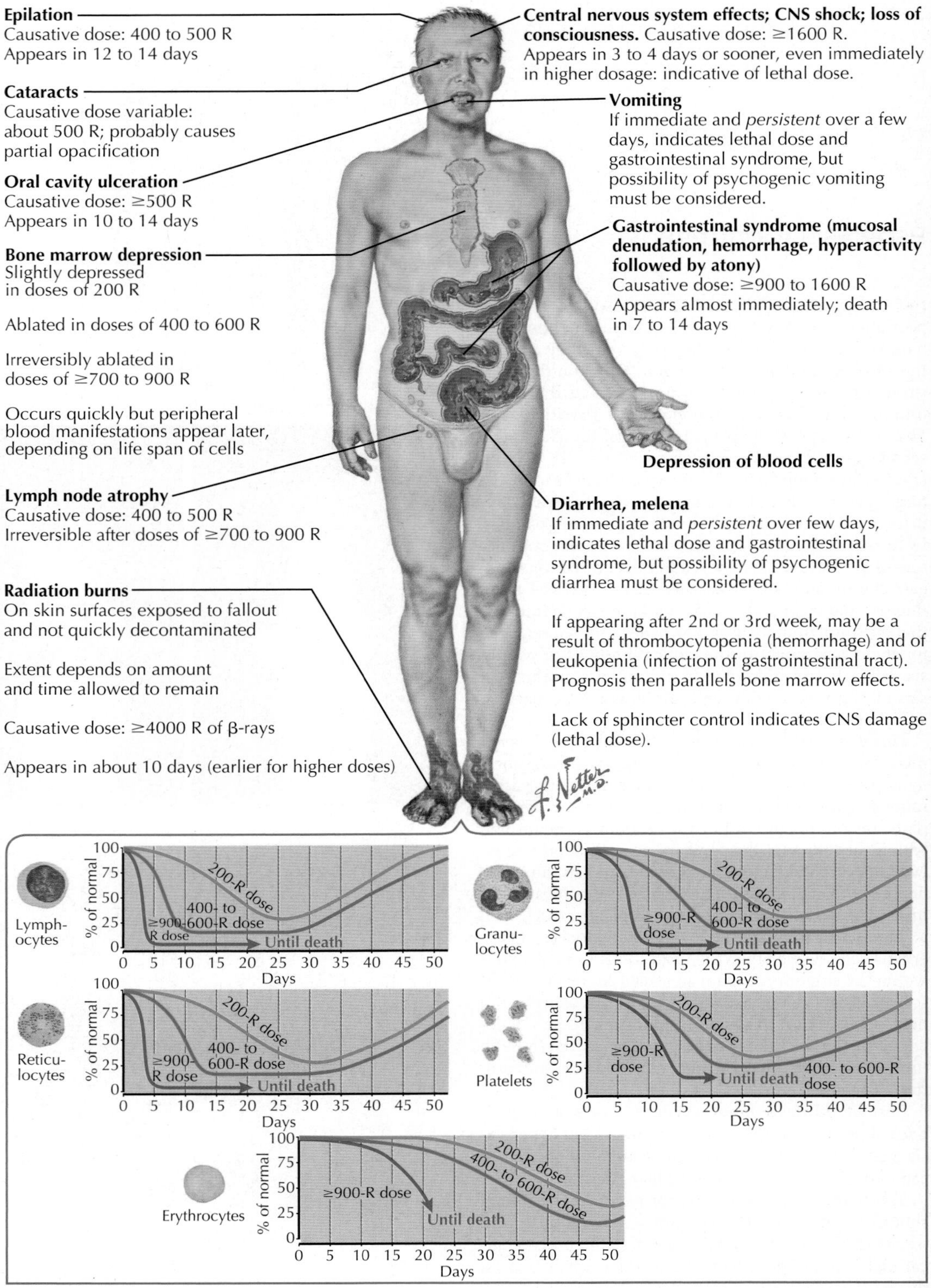

Epilation
Causative dose: 400 to 500 R
Appears in 12 to 14 days

Cataracts
Causative dose variable: about 500 R; probably causes partial opacification

Oral cavity ulceration
Causative dose: ≥500 R
Appears in 10 to 14 days

Bone marrow depression
Slightly depressed in doses of 200 R
Ablated in doses of 400 to 600 R
Irreversibly ablated in doses of ≥700 to 900 R
Occurs quickly but peripheral blood manifestations appear later, depending on life span of cells

Lymph node atrophy
Causative dose: 400 to 500 R
Irreversible after doses of ≥700 to 900 R

Radiation burns
On skin surfaces exposed to fallout and not quickly decontaminated
Extent depends on amount and time allowed to remain
Causative dose: ≥4000 R of β-rays
Appears in about 10 days (earlier for higher doses)

Central nervous system effects; CNS shock; loss of consciousness. Causative dose: ≥1600 R. Appears in 3 to 4 days or sooner, even immediately in higher dosage: indicative of lethal dose.

Vomiting
If immediate and *persistent* over a few days, indicates lethal dose and gastrointestinal syndrome, but possibility of psychogenic vomiting must be considered.

Gastrointestinal syndrome (mucosal denudation, hemorrhage, hyperactivity followed by atony)
Causative dose: ≥900 to 1600 R
Appears almost immediately; death in 7 to 14 days

Depression of blood cells

Diarrhea, melena
If immediate and *persistent* over few days, indicates lethal dose and gastrointestinal syndrome, but possibility of psychogenic diarrhea must be considered.
If appearing after 2nd or 3rd week, may be a result of thrombocytopenia (hemorrhage) and of leukopenia (infection of gastrointestinal tract). Prognosis then parallels bone marrow effects.
Lack of sphincter control indicates CNS damage (lethal dose).

F. Netter M.D.

Lymphocytes — % of normal vs. Days (0–50): 200-R dose; 400- to 600-R dose; ≥900-R dose; Until death
Granulocytes — % of normal vs. Days (0–50): 200-R dose; 400- to 600-R dose; ≥900-R dose; Until death
Reticulocytes — % of normal vs. Days (0–50): 200-R dose; 400- to 600-R dose; ≥900-R dose; Until death
Platelets — % of normal vs. Days (0–50): 200-R dose; 400- to 600-R dose; ≥900-R dose; Until death
Erythrocytes — % of normal vs. Days (0–50): 200-R dose; 400- to 600-R dose; ≥900-R dose; Until death

REACTIVE ARTHRITIS

Reactive arthritis comprises a unique constellation of clinical findings. The syndrome is believed to be precipitated by an infectious agent, often shigella or chlamydia. The hallmark of the disease is an inflammatory arthritis.

Clinical Findings: Reactive arthritis usually affects men in the third to fifth decades of life. The most frequent skin findings are balanitis circinata and keratoderma blennorrhagica. Balanitis circinata manifests as small psoriasiform, pink-to-red patches on the glans penis. It can appear identical to psoriasis. Keratoderma blennorrhagicum is less common than balanitis circinata. It occurs on the soles and palms, with the soles predominating. Small papulosquamous papules, patches, and plaques occur on the glabrous skin. Small, juicy papules and pustules can be scattered throughout the involved skin; the clinical appearance can mimic psoriasis. Some scholars think that reactive arthritis and psoriasis are one in the same, but other clinical findings of reactive arthritis make them worthy of differentiation.

The unique clinical hallmarks that separate reactive arthritis from psoriasis are the triad of urethritis, conjunctivitis, and arthritis. Urethritis typically is the initial clinical finding. It often begins a few days to 1 week after an infection. The infective agent that most commonly precipitates this syndrome is *Chlamydia trachomatis*. Gastrointestinal bacterial infections have also been shown to initiate the reaction, including infections with *Shigella flexneri*, *Salmonella* species, *Yersinia enterocolitica*, and *Campylobacter jejuni*. Dysuria, urinary frequency, and pyuria can be the presenting findings. Women with severe urethritis can develop cervicitis, cystitis, and pyelonephritis. Men are prone to development of cystitis and prostatitis. A few days to weeks later, the patient develops conjunctivitis and arthritis. The conjunctiva is red and injected with a weeping exudate. Iritis and uveitis are rare manifestations but can occur.

Reactive arthritis is considered a seronegative form of arthritis. It is typically polyarticular and affects the large joints such as the knees and hips. The joints become swollen, red, and tender. Movement can be restricted because of pain. Most cases spontaneously resolve, but a subset of patients develop chronic progressive destructive arthritis.

Some patients develop nondescript small, discrete oral ulcers that can appear the same as aphthous ulcers. They can be nontender, and this feature can be helpful in differentiating them from other forms of oral ulcers. These ulcers spontaneously resolve in most cases. Laboratory testing shows seronegativity. Testing for both rheumatoid factor and ANAs is negative. The sedimentation rate is often extremely elevated. Patients frequently carry the HLA-B27 marker, which has been found to occur with a higher than expected frequency in patients with ankylosing spondylitis and reactive arthritis. However, most patients who test positive for the HLA-B27 marker never develop either of these conditions. There is no blood test that can make the diagnosis of reactive arthritis. Radiographs can be helpful in assessing joint inflammation and joint destruction. The diagnosis of reactive arthritis is made on clinical grounds. Most patients do not exhibit all the findings mentioned, and the diagnosis is based on the number of clinical findings and the length of time the patient has had them. The American College of Rheumatology has published criteria to help make the diagnosis.

Pathogenesis: The leading theory is that an infection in a susceptible individual sets off this immunologic reaction. HLA-B27 seems to be a marker that is frequently positive in patients with reactive arthritis, but only a small subset of HLA-B27–positive patients develop the disease. The exact pathomechanism is unknown. A bacterial antigen may cause epitope spreading and initiate the autoimmune reaction.

Histology: The pathologic findings are nondiagnostic and appear identical to those of psoriasis. Psoriasiform hyperplasia of the epidermis is prominent, along with neutrophils. Increased numbers of blood vessels are seen in the dermis.

Treatment: Any underlying infection must be sought and appropriately treated with the correct antibiotic therapy. Nonsteroidal antiinflammatory drugs are used to treat the arthritis. An ophthalmologist should be consulted to evaluate the globe. Corticosteroid eyedrops are frequently used. Topical steroids can be used to treat the skin manifestations. Many patients experience a spontaneous remission in a few months. Chronic cases are most frequently treated with either sulfasalazine or methotrexate.

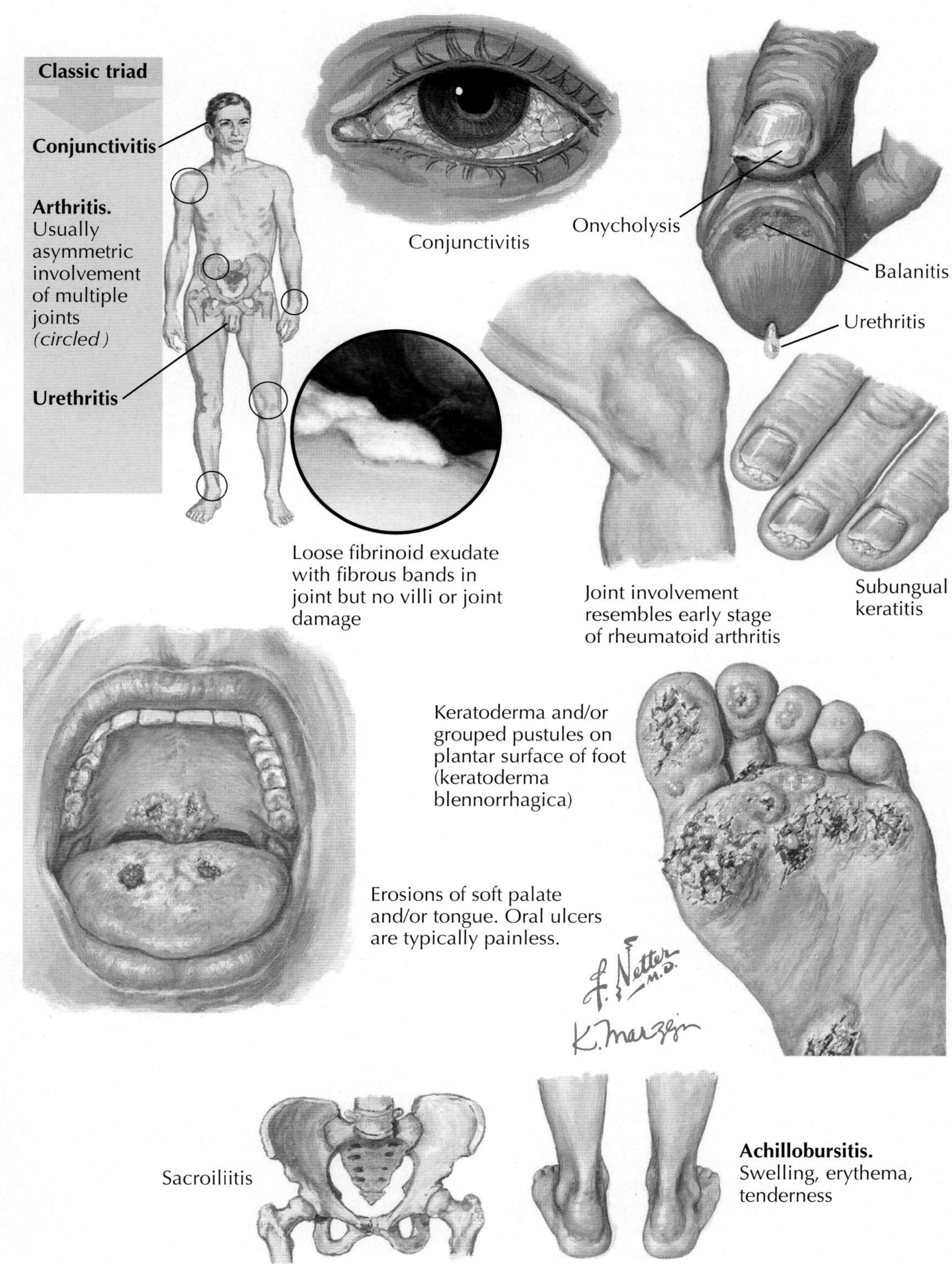

Rosacea

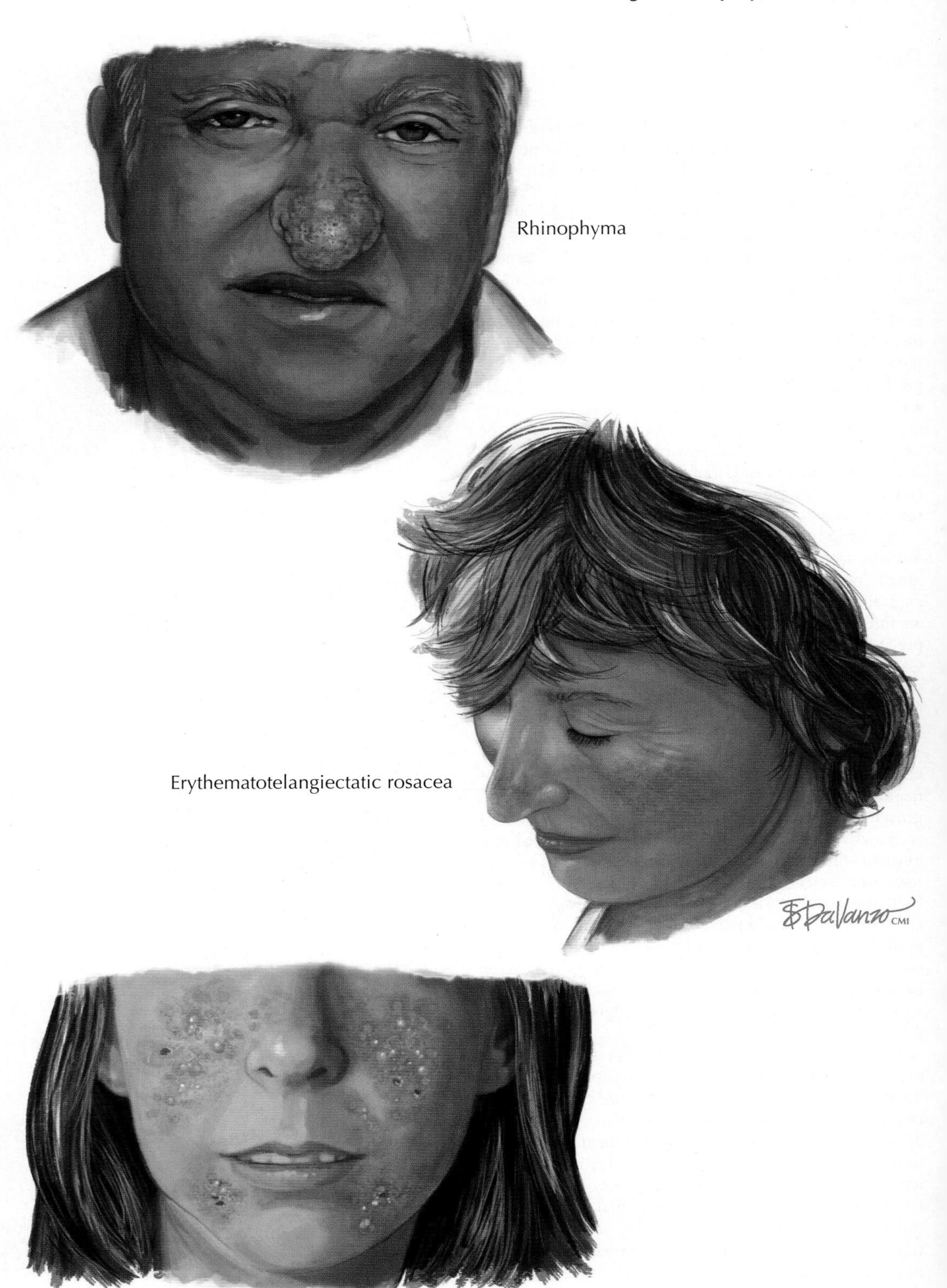

Rhinophyma

Erythematotelangiectatic rosacea

Rosacea fulminans

Rosacea is an extremely common chronic dermatosis. This inflammatory dermatosis is associated with many triggers or initiating factors that can cause a flare of the underlying inflammatory response. There are various subtypes, including erythematotelangiectatic; papular pustular, ocular, and phymatous varieties; and rosacea fulminans. The erythematotelangiectatic form is the most common subtype. Rosacea fulminans is the least common but by far the most severe form.

Clinical Findings: Rosacea is most often seen in White individuals, especially those of northern European heritage, but can occur in any race. There is a slight overall female predominance. The phymatous form occurs almost exclusively in men. The peak age at onset has been estimated to be in the third to fourth decades of life. Most patients start with a subtle redness to their cheeks and nose. The forehead and ears are less commonly affected. Most patients notice a trigger or inciting factor that makes their skin flush. Triggers include alcohol, spicy foods, hot liquids (e.g., coffee, tea), and exposure to extremes of temperature. Patients can have any, all, or none of the typical triggers. On exposure to a trigger, patients often experience a warmth to the skin and flushing of the areas involved by rosacea.

The diagnosis is typically straightforward and is made on clinical grounds; however, the differential diagnosis in some cases can include other causes of flushing and lupus erythematosus. The butterfly rash of lupus erythematosus can look very similar, and occasionally a skin biopsy is required to help differentiate the two. This is unusual because the systemic manifestations of lupus are not seen in rosacea. This scenario is most common when a patient with known lupus erythematous presents with a facial rash and the underlying lupus must be differentiated from coexisting rosacea as the cause.

Other common forms of rosacea are the papular pustular and ocular forms. Patients with the papular pustular form typically start off with the erythematotelangiectatic form and progress to this subtype over time. Not every case of erythematotelangiectatic rosacea progresses, however. Patients begin to develop crops of inflammatory papules and pustules, predominantly on the nose and cheeks. The forehead and chin can also be involved. The appearance can be hard to differentiate from acne, but these patients typically have triggers, some flushing, and a later age at onset. The back and chest are not involved by rosacea. Patients with ocular rosacea present with conjunctivitis and blepharitis. These are manifested clinically by redness of the conjunctiva and a feeling of "sand" in the eye. It can be a solitary finding, but it is more commonly seen in conjunction with skin disease.

Phymatous rosacea is caused by massive overgrowth of sebaceous glands with edema and enlargement of the structures affected. This is most common on the nose of men, in which cases it is called *rhinophyma*. The appearance of the nose can become distorted, leading to a red, edematous, bulbous deformity with accentuated follicular openings.

Rosacea fulminans is a rare variant that can have an acute onset of severe papules, pustules, nodules, and cyst formation.

Pathogenesis: The etiology of rosacea is unknown. Subtypes are most likely a heterogeneous group of similar-appearing disease states.

Histology: The findings on skin biopsy in rosacea depend on the form that is biopsied. The erythematotelangiectatic form typically shows a few dilated blood vessels and dermatoheliosis. A sparse, superficial lymphocytic infiltrate may surround adnexal structures. Papular rosacea shows perifollicular abscesses. An interesting finding with unknown relevance is that of multiple *Demodex* mites within the hair follicle passage. A granulomatous form of rosacea can be seen histologically.

Treatment: Sun protection and sunscreen use are important for all patients with rosacea, especially the erythematotelangiectatic form. The use of topical and oral antibiotics (e.g., topical metronidazole, sulfacetamide, oral tetracyclines) has long been the mainstay of therapy. Topical azelaic acid has also been helpful. α_2-Adrenergic agonists act as vasoconstrictors and can be used topically to decrease erythema. Avoidance of triggers is helpful in some individuals. The 585-nm pulsed dye laser has provided excellent results in treating the underlying redness from telangiectatic blood vessels. Isotretinoin has been used in severe cases, including rosacea fulminans. Rhinophyma is typically treated with a surgical approach to debulk the extra tissue and reshape the nose.

CUTANEOUS MANIFESTATIONS OF SARCOID

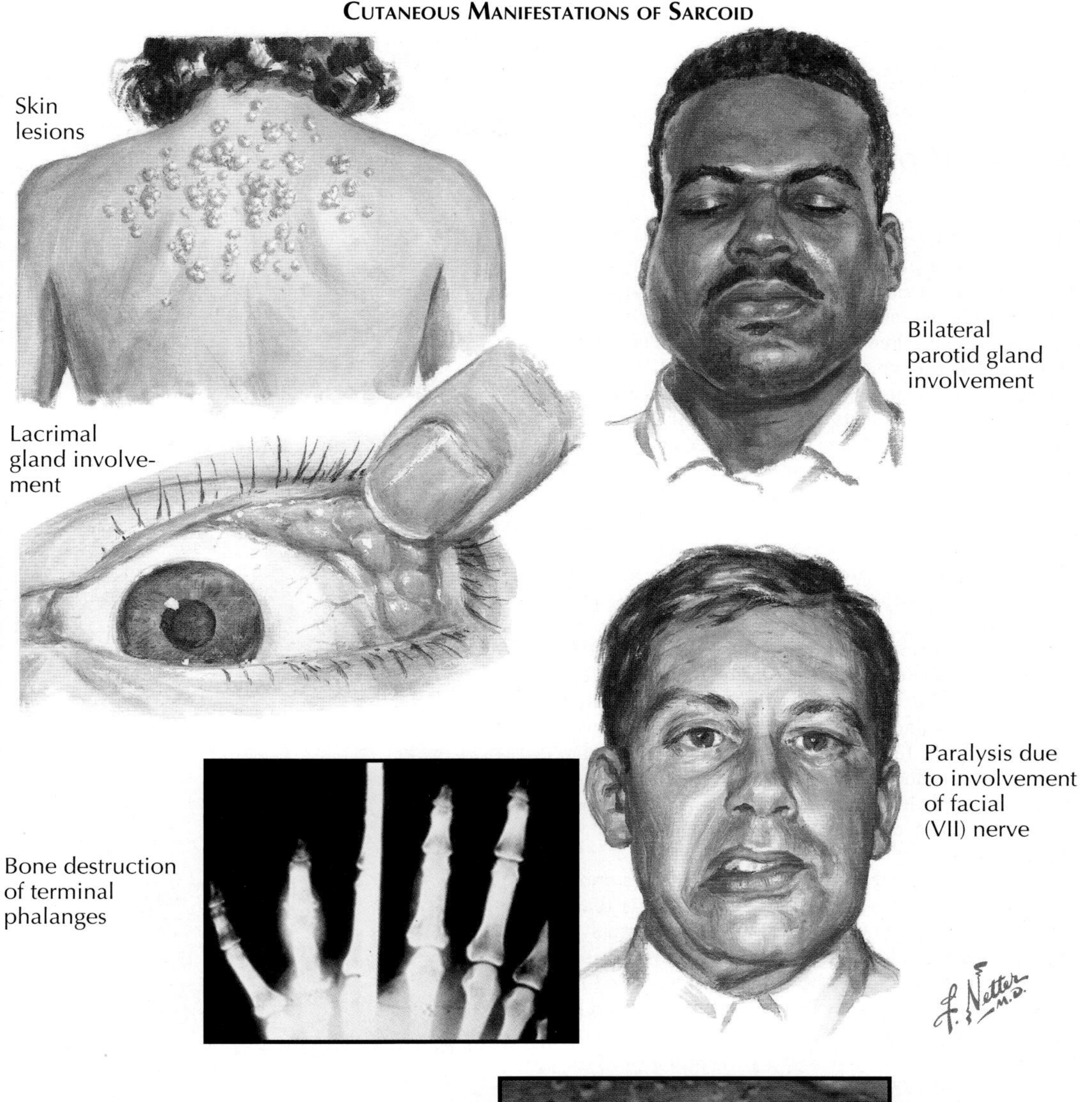

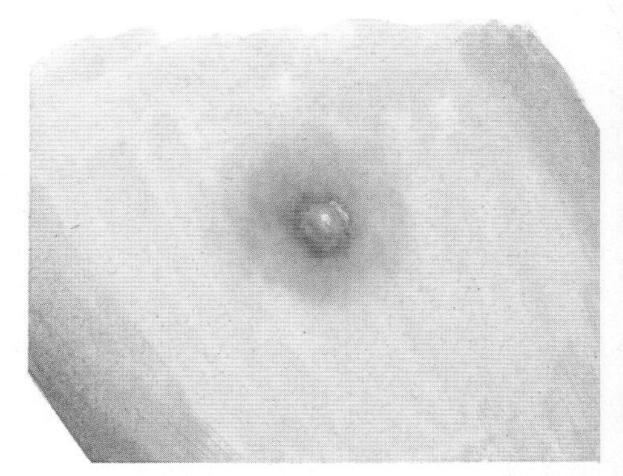

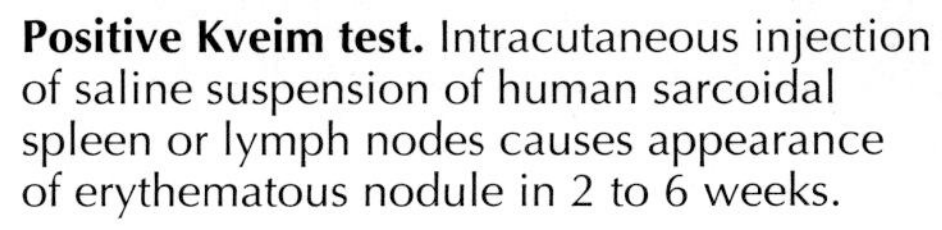

Positive Kveim test. Intracutaneous injection of saline suspension of human sarcoidal spleen or lymph nodes causes appearance of erythematous nodule in 2 to 6 weeks.

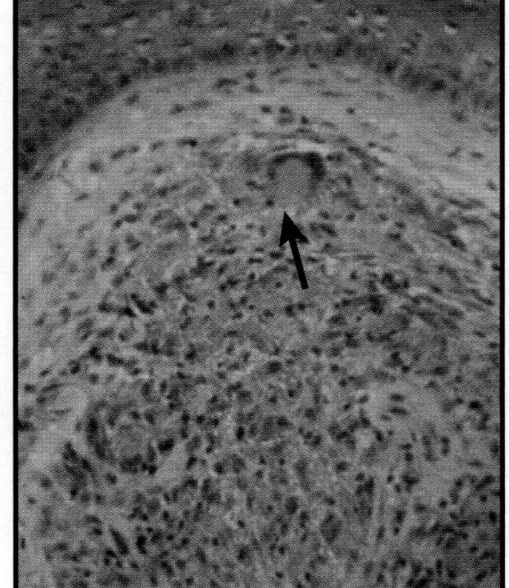

Biopsy of nodule. Typical sarcoidal granuloma (dense infiltration with macrophages, epithelioid cells, and occasional multinucleated giant cells [*arrow*]).

SARCOID

Sarcoid, or sarcoidosis, is a relatively common condition that can affect numerous organ systems. There is a wide spectrum of disease activity, from localized skin disease to widespread involvement of the integumentary, pulmonary, cardiac, renal, gastrointestinal, ophthalmic, endocrine, neurologic, and lymphatic systems. However, most cases are mild in nature and can be controlled with proper care. Although an infectious etiology has often been theorized, no conclusive evidence has been established. This idiopathic condition can produce multiple skin findings. When found, the skin findings should initiate a systemic workup to evaluate for underlying organ involvement.

Clinical Findings: Sarcoidosis can occur in any ethnic population, but it is seen at a higher rate in Black individuals. It also has a higher incidence in women. Onset usually is before age 40 years. Up to 90% of patients with sarcoid have a benign clinical course with no increased mortality rate. Sarcoidosis has been reported to occur in a familial form, which has led researchers to look for specific genetic defects that could explain the disease. However, sarcoid remains an idiopathic multisystem disease. There are many distinct clinical expressions of the disease that are common enough that they have been named, including Löfgren syndrome, lupus pernio, Darier-Roussy sarcoid, Heerfordt syndrome, and Mikulicz syndrome.

Sarcoid can affect the skin in a multitude of ways. There are both specific and nonspecific skin findings. The most common nonspecific skin finding is erythema nodosum, which affects the lower anterior extremities. It manifests as tender subcutaneous nodules or plaques. Examination of biopsy specimens shows a nonspecific form of septal panniculitis. The etiology of erythema nodosum in patients with sarcoid is poorly understood.

The lesions of sarcoid that occur within the integumentary system are quite varied. The most common specific skin lesion is a slightly brownish to red-brown papule, plaque, or nodule with varying amounts of hyperpigmentation. Sarcoid is a mimicker of many other conditions, especially in its skin lesions. Macular lesions, ulcerations, subcutaneous nodules, annular plaques, ichthyosiform erythroderma, and alopecia have all been described as potential presentations of sarcoid.

The extracutaneous organ system most commonly involved is the pulmonary system. There is a relatively straightforward classification that describes the stages of pulmonary sarcoid based on radiographic findings. The higher the radiographic stage, the more severe the disease. Isolated bilateral hilar adenopathy is the most common pulmonary finding and is the basis for stage I radiographic disease. These patients are most commonly asymptomatic, and the adenopathy is found on routine radiographic testing. Any findings of pulmonary sarcoid should prompt referral to a pulmonologist for pulmonary function testing.

Löfgren syndrome is defined by the acute onset of erythema nodosum, almost exclusively in young adult women; it is seen in association with fever, bilateral hilar adenopathy, and uveitis. Other, nonspecific constitutional signs are often present. The erythrocyte sedimentation rate is uniformly elevated. This syndrome is most commonly seen in young White women and typically resolves spontaneously within 2 to 3 years.

Lupus pernio is the name given to the clinical findings of specific cutaneous sarcoid involvement of the nose and the rest of the face. This form of sarcoid is quite resistant to therapy, runs a more prolonged course, and is often difficult to treat. The skin findings are typically shiny brown-red plaques, papules, and nodules overlying the nose and other regions of the face. The involvement can become so severe as to cause disfigurement of the nose. Lupus pernio has no relation to the autoimmune disease lupus. Lupus pernio can be very difficult to treat, and systemic immune suppression is often required.

Subcutaneous sarcoidosis, also called *Darier-Roussy sarcoid*, is an uncommon condition that manifests as

SARCOID (Continued)

subcutaneous plaques or nodules of varying size. This is a rare finding in patients with sarcoid. It manifests as slightly tender dermal plaques or nodules with an overlying hyperpigmentation or normal-appearing skin. A biopsy specimen taken from one of the subcutaneous nodules shows the typical findings of sarcoid.

Heerfordt syndrome is an extremely rare version of sarcoidosis that manifests more commonly in young adult men than in women. It is manifested by fever, parotid gland hypertrophy, and lacrimal gland enlargement in association with facial nerve palsy and uveitis. Neurologic involvement with sarcoidosis may cause papilledema and cerebrospinal fluid pleocytosis, indicating an inflammatory reaction pattern. Meningism can occur with headache, spinal stiffness, and photophobia.

Mikulicz syndrome is not specific to sarcoid. It is manifested by bilateral enlargement of various glands, including the parotid, submandibular, and lacrimal glands. The tonsillar tissue may also be involved. Fever is common, as is the subsequent development of dry eyes and mouth due to the widespread, often painless, inflammation of the affected glands. It has been seen with uveitis and is considered by some as a variant of Sjögren syndrome.

Diagnostic testing to confirm sarcoid includes, most importantly, a tissue biopsy. Tissue sampling is diagnostic and should initiate a search for other organ system involvement. Laboratory testing may show elevated levels of serum calcium and angiotensin-converting enzyme. Chest radiographs can identify a spectrum of disease that is staged by certain criteria. Patients uniquely show a decreased ability to mount a delayed-type hypersensitivity reaction. This may be manifested by an inability to react to intradermally placed antigens such as tuberculin or *Candida* and is termed *anergy*. In the past, patients with sarcoid were frequently found to have a positive Kveim test. This test is no longer clinically performed because of the danger of transmitting a bloodborne pathogen. The test was performed by interdermal placement of a small amount of a suspension of human spleen and lymph node that had been affected by sarcoid, similar to the placement of a purified protein derivative test for tuberculosis. This test was found to be positive in more than 85% of patients with sarcoid.

Mortality is uncommon but may occur secondary to severe cardiac, renal, or pulmonary involvement.

Pathogenesis: The exact etiology of sarcoidosis is unknown. For years, scientists have been looking at the potential causative link between sarcoid and an infectious agent, usually an atypical mycobacterial agent. However, no conclusive evidence has been reported to indicate that sarcoid is caused by an infectious disease. It has been theorized that sarcoid occurs in a genetically susceptible individual who has had an environmental exposure (infectious agent or chemical exposure). The exposure allows for the sarcoidal inflammation to occur in those susceptible individuals.

Histology: The classic finding of multiple, noncaseating epithelioid granulomas with a sparse surrounding inflammatory infiltrate is the hallmark of sarcoidosis. The granulomatous findings are consistent across all of the various tissues affected by sarcoid. Many nonspecific histologic findings can also be seen, but not on a consistent basis; these include Schaumann bodies and asteroid bodies.

Treatment: The treatment for sarcoid has been consistent over time and includes nonspecific immunosuppression, most commonly with oral corticosteroids such as prednisone. Isolated cutaneous findings may be treated with topical corticosteroids or intralesional steroid injections. Methotrexate is a steroid-sparing agent that is used for difficult-to-control disease and for lupus pernio. The anti–tumor necrosis factor medications infliximab and adalimumab have been used with some success. The use of hydroxychloroquine has also been advocated for treatment of cutaneous sarcoid. Azathioprine, mycophenolate mofetil, IVIG, JAK inhibitors, and rituximab have all been used with varying success in more severe cases.

SYSTEMIC MANIFESTATIONS OF SARCOID

Relative frequency of organ involvement in sarcoidosis

Brain + (15%)
Eyes ++ (20%)
Nasal and pharyngeal mucosa, tonsils + (10%)
Salivary glands + (1%)
Lymph nodes ++++ (80%)
Lungs ++++ (80%)
Heart ++ (20%)
Liver ++++ (70%)
Spleen ++++ (70%)
Skin ++ (30%)
Bones ++ (30%)

Perivascular infiltration, chiefly of histiocytes in cardiac interstitium

Granuloma with giant cell in heart wall

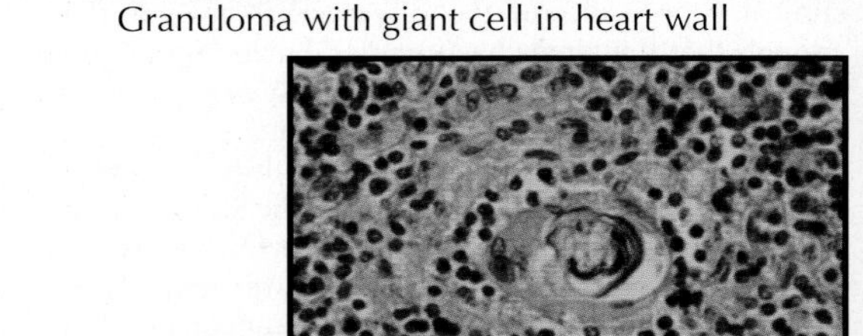
Schaumann body (concentrically laminated, calcified body) in a mediastinal lymph node giant cell

Sectioned lung in advanced sarcoidosis. Fibrosis in central zone with bullae near surface of upper lobe, one of which contains an aspergilloma.

Typical epithelioid cell granulomas with occasional giant cells

SCLERODERMA (SYSTEMIC SCLEROSIS)

Typical skin changes in scleroderma: extensive collagen deposition and some epidermal atrophy

Characteristics. Thickening, tightening, and rigidity of facial skin, with small, constricted mouth and narrow lips, in atrophic phase of scleroderma.

Sclerodactyly. Fingers partially fixed in semiflexed position; terminal phalanges atrophied; fingertips pointed and ulcerated

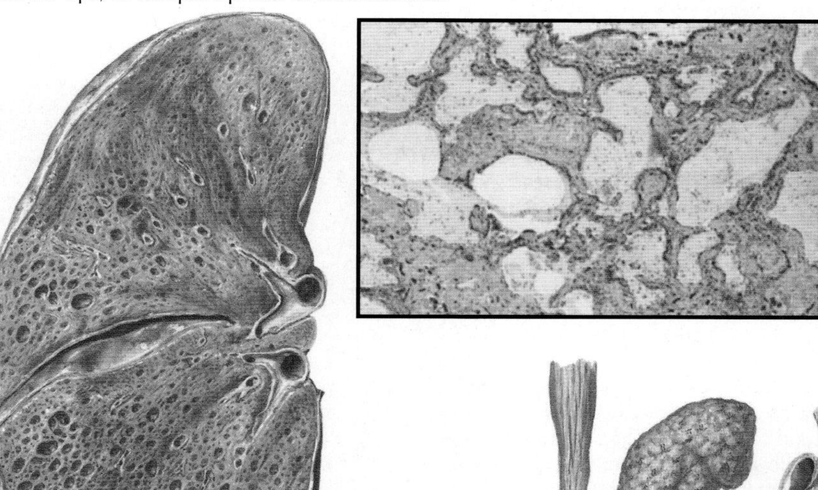

Microscopic section of lung. Fibrosis with formation of microcysts, many of which represent dilated bronchioles.

Grossly sectioned lung. Extensive fibrosis and multitudinous small cysts. Visceral pleura thickened but not adherent to chest wall.

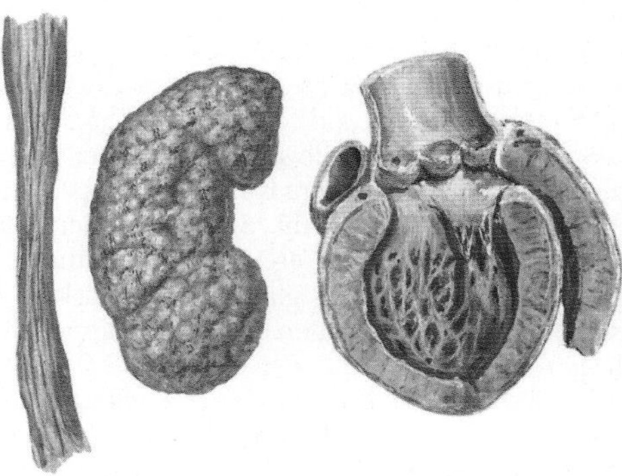

Esophagus, kidneys, heart, skin, and other organs, as well as joints, may also be affected.

Scleroderma, or systemic sclerosis, is a rare idiopathic, life-threatening connective tissue disease that involves many organ systems. There is often an insidious onset of diffuse skin thickening, sclerodactyly, Raynaud phenomenon, capillary nailfold loops, and tightening of the skin around the orifice of the mouth. This is a progressive disease with significant morbidity and mortality from organ fibrosis and vascular dysfunction. Autoantibody production is a hallmark, and various antibody profiles can be seen.

Clinical Findings: Systemic sclerosis is an unrelenting connective tissue disease that predominantly affects young adult women. There is no racial predilection. It occurs across all ethnic backgrounds. Skin findings are variable from patient to patient, but all have a persistent and relentless sclerosis of the skin. It begins insidiously; the skin slowly begins to thicken and harden, causing the underlying dermis to become firm to palpation. The progressive sclerosis causes digital tip ulceration as the peripheral distal blood vessels begin to thrombose. The hair shafts in the affected skin disappear at a slow and steady, almost unnoticeable rate. This is caused by crowding out of the hair follicles by the excessive production of dermal collagen.

As the dermal sclerosis progresses, skin tightness is noticed, and the patient may become aware of difficulty with movement of the fingers. The tightness around the mouth is manifested by an increase in the furrowing circumventing the oral orifice and inability to open the mouth as wide as was once possible. Patients may lose the ability to make facial expressions as the skin tightens and hardens in place. Patients may be left in an expressionless state.

The skin overlying the sclerosis develops hyperpigmentation and hypopigmentation; this has been given the name "salt-and-pepper discoloration." The skin develops a shiny, smooth appearance. The capillary loops around the nailfolds become enlarged and engorged and are visible without magnification. These dilated capillary loops occur in up to three quarters of all patients with progressive systemic sclerosis.

Sclerodactyly is the term given to the progressive thickness and associated tightness of the digits. It is caused by the overabundance of collagen production within the dermis.

Systemic sclerosis is a multisystem disorder that not only affects the skin but also causes significant, life-threatening damage to internal organs. The esophagus is affected early, and patients report dysphagia and an inability to swallow food easily. Aspiration of food and liquids is common and often leads to aspiration pneumonia. Pulmonary fibrosis is a leading cause of morbidity and mortality. Patients report shortness of breath and a cough. Pulmonary hypertension is almost universally seen. Conduction defects can develop in the cardiovascular system, and thickening of the myocardial wall may cause a constrictive cardiomyopathy. The kidneys are also involved, and a subset of patients develop renal failure and hypertension.

There are two main subsets of disease: diffuse cutaneous systemic sclerosis and limited systemic sclerosis. The limited version is typically seen distal to the elbows and knees, and the diffuse version is much more widespread.

Pathogenesis: The initiating factor causing the fibroblast to make ever-increasing amounts of collagen in an unregulated manner is unknown. Many possible targets are being explored as potential causes of progressive systemic sclerosis, including fibroblasts, endothelial cells, various environmental antigens, and internal defects within T cells. Numerous autoantibodies are present.

Histology: The histologic findings in the skin are characteristic. Punch biopsy specimens are very square on gross evaluation because of the increased amount of dermal collagen. Microscopic evaluation shows an increased amount of collagen that replaces everything, including the adnexal structures and subcutaneous fat. The extensive collagen is so vast that it can appear as an amorphous eosinophilic mass with nothing between the collagen bundles. A sparse inflammatory infiltrate is present at the interface of the collagen and underlying remaining tissue. Plasma cells may be prominent.

Treatment: Treatment for this skin disease is difficult. Pruritus can be controlled with antihistamines and topical corticosteroids. UV phototherapy has been used. The deeper-penetrating UVA rays work best and are often administered in the form of PUVA therapy. Systemic corticosteroids, methotrexate, cyclophosphamide, JAK inhibitors, prostacyclin, rituximab, mycophenolic mofetil, IVIG, infliximab, and many others have been used to treat scleroderma. Systemic sclerosis requires a multidisciplinary approach to achieve the best therapeutic results.

SEBORRHEIC DERMATITIS

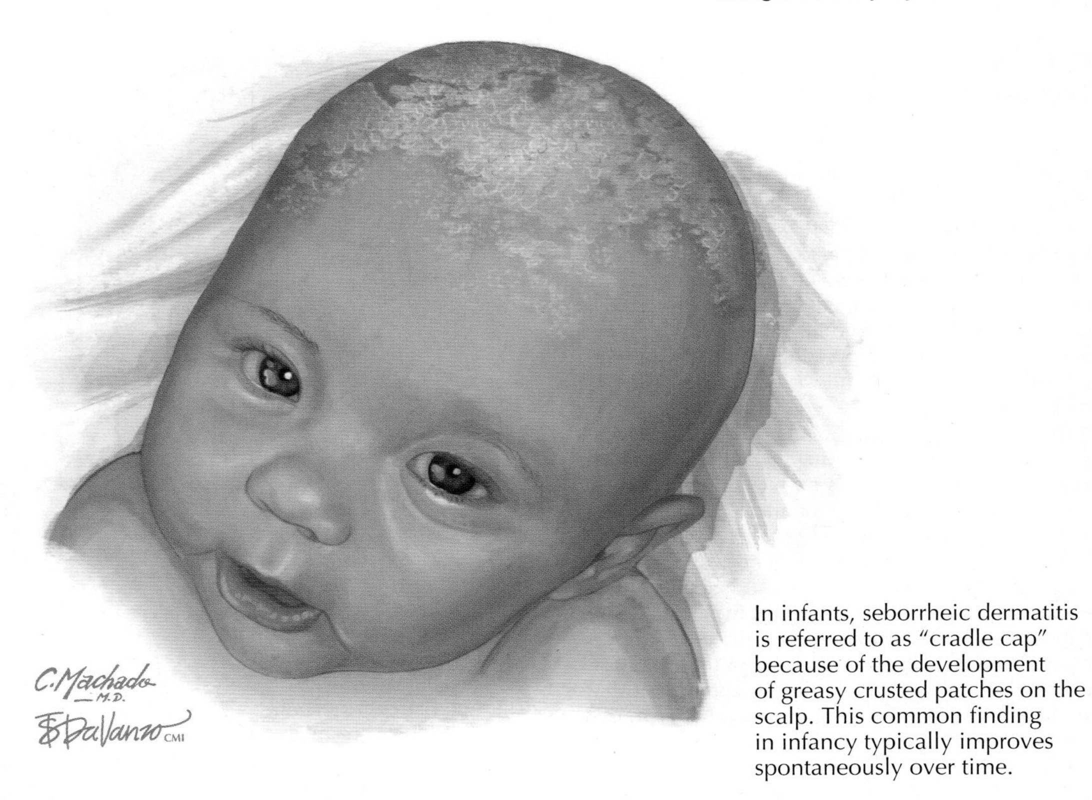

In infants, seborrheic dermatitis is referred to as "cradle cap" because of the development of greasy crusted patches on the scalp. This common finding in infancy typically improves spontaneously over time.

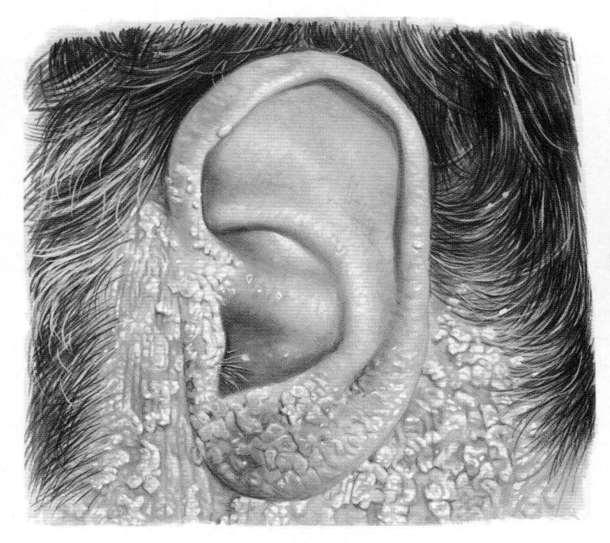

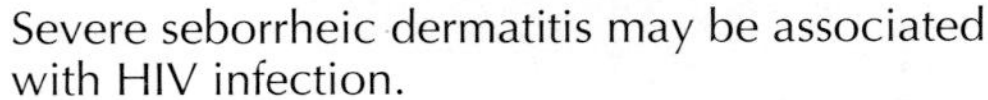

Severe seborrheic dermatitis may be associated with HIV infection.

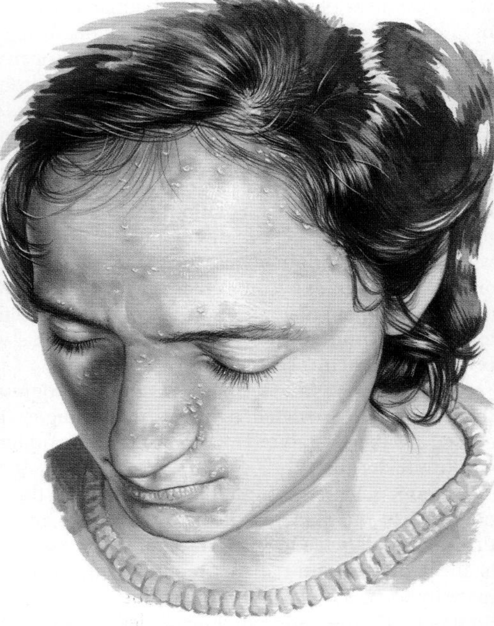

Seborrheic dermatitis in adults frequently manifests with greasy yellow, scaly patches in the scalp, ears, and eyebrows and along the nasolabial fold.

Seborrheic dermatitis is a commonly encountered rash with a bimodal age distribution. There is an infantile and an adult form. The two forms do not resemble each other clinically and are distinct in appearance. The infantile form has also been named "cradle cap" because of its prominent location on the scalp. The adult form has been found in association with many underlying conditions, although it is most commonly seen as an isolated skin finding.

Clinical Findings: The infantile form of seborrheic dermatitis manifests in the first weeks of life and lasts a few months at most. It affects males and females equally, and there is no racial predilection. The typical location of involvement is the scalp. Most cases are mild and do not cause the parents to seek the advice of a medical professional. These mild cases manifest with a fine scale that may be slightly greasy or adherent. The child is unaware of the dermatosis, and it resolves spontaneously. Rarely, an infant develops greasy yellow, scaly patches and even plaques across the entire scalp (cradle cap). The dermatitis may become more inflamed, and weeping from the patches or plaques may ensue. The infant may try to scratch at the areas, indicating that pruritus is present. In these severe cases, weeping patches and plaques may also be seen in the groin and axillary folds. Only in the most exceptional of cases does the rash disseminate, but it has the ability to affect any region of the body. It can be misdiagnosed as tinea capitis.

The adult version is chronic in nature and affects a higher percentage of people than does the infantile form. Because of its chronicity, patients often seek medical advice. There is also quite a bit of clinical variability in adult seborrheic dermatitis. The face is the most involved site, with a predilection for the nasolabial fold, eyebrows, ears, and scalp. Most cases are mild and consist of greasy yellow to slightly red, scaly patches. The scalp involvement is similar in appearance. Patients often report dandruff. Seborrheic dermatitis has a propensity to affect the areas of the skin that have a high density of sebaceous glands. On occasion, patients also have involvement on areas of the upper chest and back.

Many conditions have been associated with the adult form of seborrheic dermatitis, including Parkinson disease and other chronic neurologic disorders. Adult onset of severe seborrheic dermatitis has been reported to occur with a higher incidence in patients with underlying HIV infection. HIV-associated seborrheic dermatitis tends to be widespread, with severe facial involvement. Patients who present with sudden-onset severe seborrheic dermatitis should be assessed for HIV risk factors.

Pathogenesis: The exact pathogenesis is unknown. Seborrheic dermatitis is believed to be caused by an interaction of various components of the skin, including the production of sebum, with the normal skin immune system response to the fungus *Malassezia furfur*. How these factors play in the formation of seborrheic dermatitis is not completely understood.

Histology: Seborrheic dermatitis is almost never biopsied to confirm the diagnosis. Classic biopsy specimens show parakeratosis overlying a slightly spongiotic epidermis with a mild lymphocytic perivascular infiltrate in the dermis. Spores of fungus can be seen lying on the surface of the epidermis.

Treatment: Most cases of infantile seborrheic dermatitis can be ignored or treated with daily baths and a bland emollient. More involved cases can be treated with more frequent shampooing of the scalp and the use of a mild topical corticosteroid. The use of ketoconazole cream has also been advocated in some cases.

Because of its chronic nature, adult seborrheic dermatitis is treated with topical ketoconazole as a first-line therapy. Other azole antifungal agents are just as effective. The addition of a weak topical corticosteroid used intermittently can also lead to excellent results. The scalp is most commonly treated with a ketoconazole-based shampoo or a tar- or selenium-based shampoo. Severe cases may respond to courses of oral antifungals. There is no cure for seborrheic dermatitis, but most therapeutic regimens, if adhered to, lead to an excellent clinical response.

Skin Manifestations of Inflammatory Bowel Disease

Crohn disease and ulcerative colitis are common autoimmune gastrointestinal disorders with many cutaneous findings. Most patients do not have the cutaneous findings, but a small proportion of the population with inflammatory bowel disease develop one of the cutaneous manifestations, which include pyoderma gangrenosum, aphthous ulcerations, oral candidiasis, erythema nodosum, and metastatic Crohn disease. Ocular manifestations include iritis and conjunctivitis. Arthritis, although not a skin manifestation, can produce red, tender swelling around an afflicted joint space.

Clinical Findings: Ulcerative colitis and Crohn disease are more commonly seen in Whites. Crohn disease is slightly more common in women, and ulcerative colitis affects men and women equally. Up to 20% of individuals with inflammatory bowel disease have a family history of the condition. Ulcerative colitis affects the large intestine, whereas Crohn disease has been shown to affect any part of the gastrointestinal tract.

Skin manifestations occur in 5% to 10% of those affected by inflammatory bowel disease. The most common skin finding is erythema nodosum. Erythema nodosum manifests as tender dermal nodules predominantly on the anterior lower legs. They typically are symmetric in location. There are many associations with erythema nodosum in addition to inflammatory bowel disease, including pregnancy, use of birth control medications, sarcoidosis, deep fungal infections such as coccidiomycosis, and an idiopathic form. The etiology and pathogenesis are unknown. Erythema nodosum can occur in areas other than the pretibial region, but this is uncommon.

Pyoderma gangrenosum is one of the most severe skin manifestations of inflammatory bowel disease. It can manifest as a small, red papule or pustule that can rapidly expand to form a large ulceration with a violaceous undermined rim. The ulcer may form in a cribriform pattern. The skin involved develops small cribriform ulcerations centrally that expand outward and coalesce into one large ulcer. These ulcers are extremely tender and cause significant morbidity. Pyoderma gangrenosum can also be seen as an idiopathic finding or in association with an underlying malignancy, typically in the lymphoproliferative group. It has been estimated that approximately 1% of patients with inflammatory bowel disease develop pyoderma gangrenosum. Pyoderma gangrenosum has a propensity to develop in a peristomal location after surgical placement of an ostomy. Pyoderma in this location compromises the ostomy seal and can lead to infection

Aphthous ulcers can occur anywhere within the oral mucosa. They are shallow ulcerations with a white fibrinous base. They are quite tender and can cause patients to avoid eating because of the severe discomfort. Oral candidiasis is typically an iatrogenic manifestation of inflammatory bowel disease. Most patients are prescribed systemic steroids to treat their underlying disease, which predisposes them to the development of *Candida* infections, both oral and vaginal.

Arthritis is seen in approximately 10% of patients with inflammatory bowel disease and is considered to be in the seronegative classification of inflammatory arthropathies.

Metastatic Crohn disease is a unique manifestation. It represents the spread of the granulomatous disease onto the skin. It most commonly occurs in areas with close approximation to the gastrointestinal tract, such as the perianal and perioral regions. It manifests as tender, draining papules and nodules. A peculiar variant has been described to occur along the inguinal creases. It appears as fissures or ulcerations that can penetrate deeply into the dermis and even the subcutaneous fat tissue. It has been described as slit-like or knife-like linear ulcerations. Isolated genital swelling is another unusual presentation of metastatic Crohn disease. Metastatic Crohn disease has been described in many other cutaneous locations. This form of cutaneous disease can be difficult to treat.

Other rare skin findings seen in association with inflammatory bowel disease are skin fistulas, vasculitis including polyarteritis nodosa, urticaria, Sweet syndrome, epidermolysis bullosa acquisita, and psoriasis.

Pathogenesis: The pathogenesis of these cutaneous manifestations of inflammatory bowel disease is unknown. They are theorized to be caused by an autoimmune mechanism of defective cell-mediated immunity.

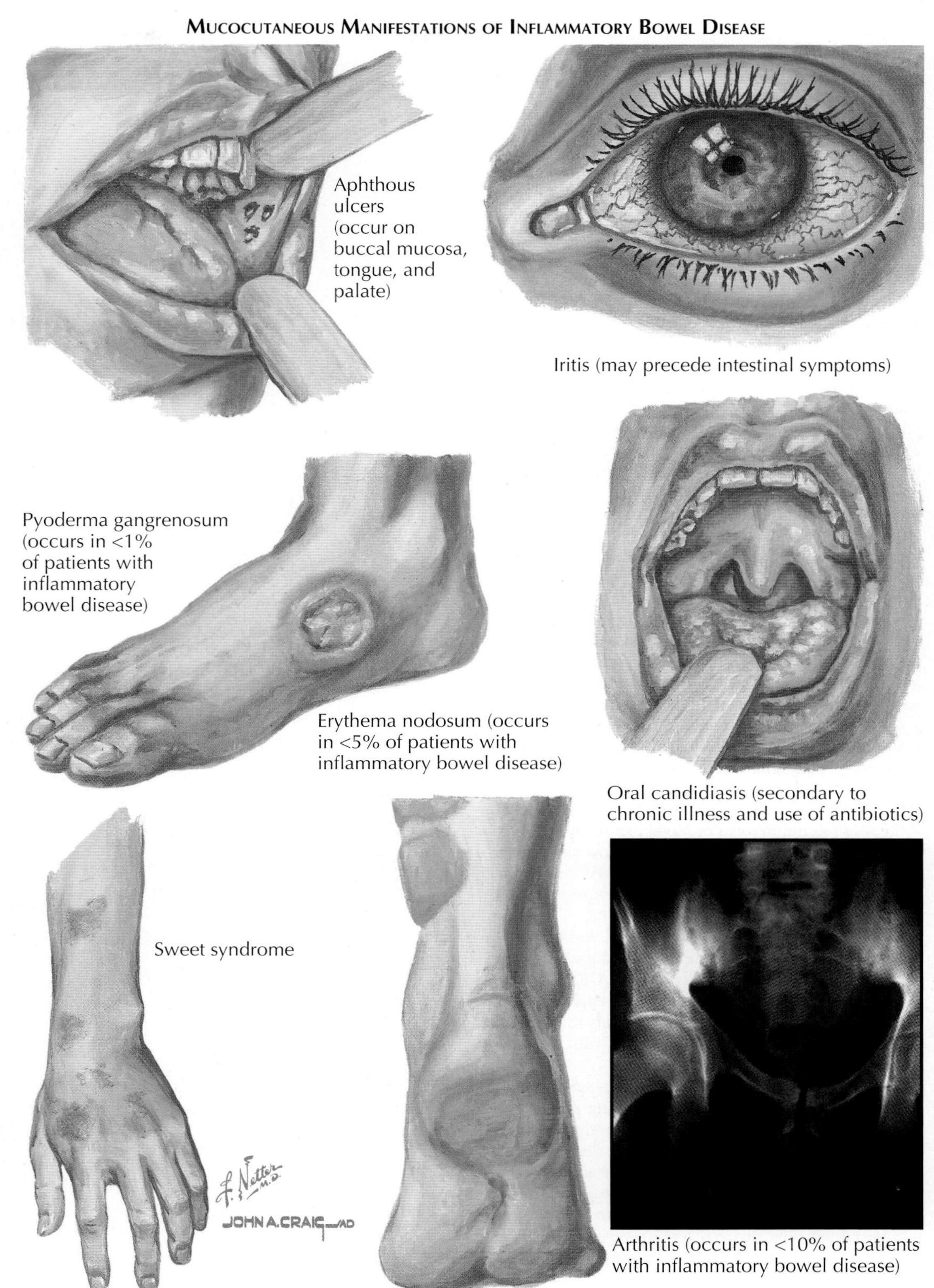

Skin Manifestations of Inflammatory Bowel Disease (Continued)

Cutaneous Manifestations of Inflammatory Bowel Disease

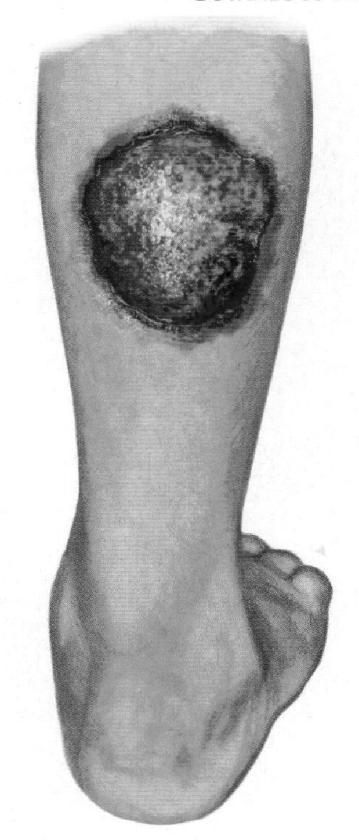

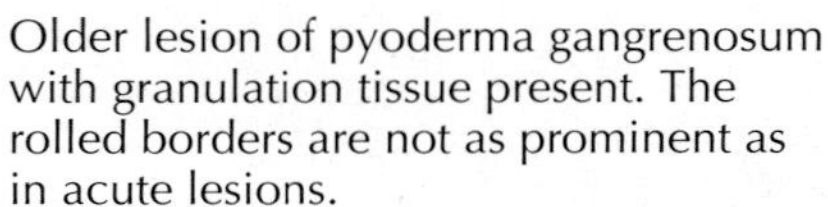

Older lesion of pyoderma gangrenosum with granulation tissue present. The rolled borders are not as prominent as in acute lesions.

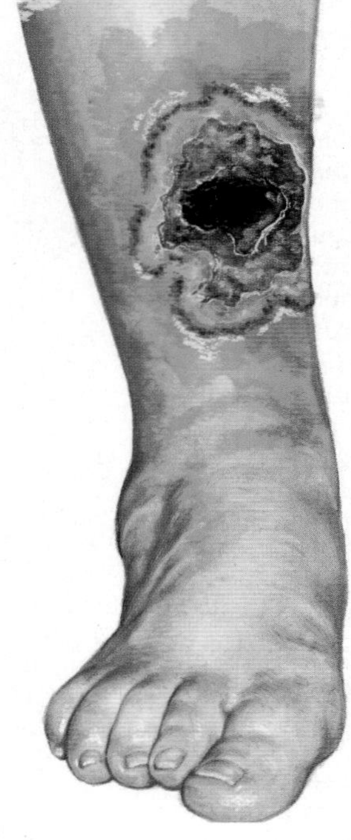

Cribriform ulceration with a purple surrounding border is characteristic of pyoderma gangrenosum.

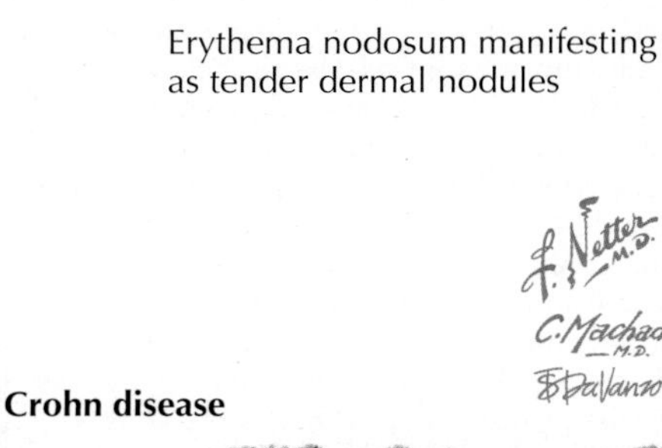

Erythema nodosum manifesting as tender dermal nodules

Crohn disease

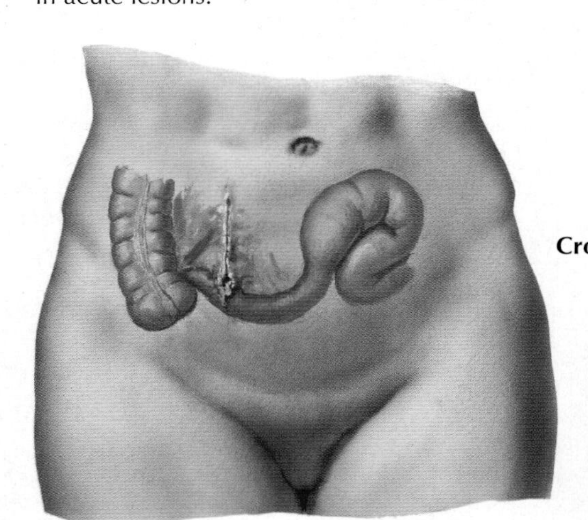

External fistula (via appendectomy incision)

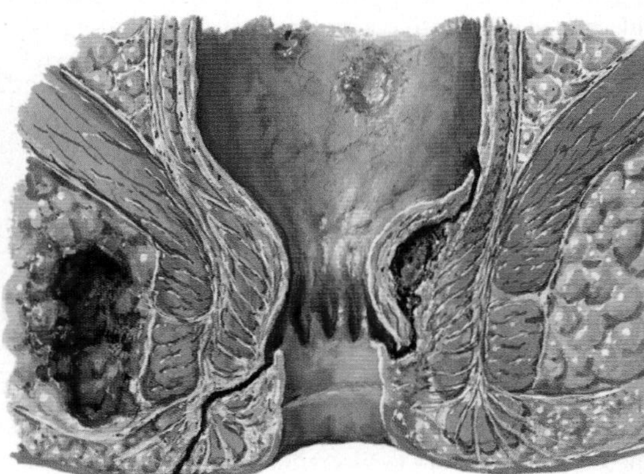

Perianal fistulae and/or abscesses

Metastatic Crohn disease is believed to be caused when the inflammatory bowel disease recognizes the skin as gut tissue and develops the same granulomatous process within the cutaneous structures.

Histology: Pyoderma gangrenosum shows nonspecific ulceration when biopsied. The findings are nondiagnostic, and the diagnosis is one of exclusion. The presence of multiple neutrophils should trigger an investigation for cutaneous infection, and appropriate tissue cultures should be performed and found negative before a diagnosis of pyoderma gangrenosum is made. The appearance of pyoderma gangrenosum histologically is highly dependent on the time and type of lesion biopsied. Early lesions show a follicle-centered neutrophilic infiltrate with a dermal abscess. As the lesions progress, ulceration is seen with a predominant neutrophilic infiltrate. The ulcers are often very deep and enter the subcutaneous tissue. Changes of vasculitis can often be seen, but they are believed to be caused by the overlying ulceration; the vasculitis is not thought to be the predominant pathologic process.

Biopsy specimens of erythema nodosum show a septal panniculitis. The fibrous septa are inflamed with a mixed inflammatory infiltrate with heavy lymphocyte predominance. Giant cells are frequently seen within the widened septal tissue. A unique finding is that of Miescher radial granuloma formation, in which multiple histiocytes are arranged flanking a small area. They are organized circumferentially around a central slit-like space. The reason for this finding is unknown. Erythema nodosum is the most common form of septal panniculitis.

Aphthous ulcerations, if biopsied, show small ulcerations or erosions of the mucosa. The predominant cell type found within the infiltrate is the neutrophil. These findings are nonspecific.

Oral candidiasis should be diagnosed without a skin biopsy. A scraping of the white oral plaques shows an easily removed, whitish, sticky tissue. A KOH microscopic examination shows candidal elements. Histologic examination of a biopsy specimen reveals the candidal organisms on the surface of the mucosa, with an underlying mixed inflammatory infiltrate.

Metastatic Crohn disease is a unique phenomenon. It is histologically described as noncaseating granulomas. These granulomas are identical to the bowel granulomas. The skin granulomas are centered in the dermis but can be seen around blood vessels and into the adipose tissue.

Treatment: Therapy is aimed at controlling the underlying bowel disease. If it is well controlled, the skin manifestations typically resolve. Conversely, if the bowel disease is poorly controlled, the skin disease will be poorly controlled as well. Skin manifestations can be used as a sign of active bowel disease. If a patient who has been in a long remission suddenly develops pyoderma gangrenosum, it is highly plausible that the bowel disease has become active once more. Ulcerative colitis can be cured by colectomy. Crohn disease cannot be cured by colectomy because it affects the entire gastrointestinal tract, and surgery is typically done to treat complications that arise from the disease. Oral or IV immunosuppressive medications are used to treat both these conditions. Oral prednisone, sulfasalazine, azathioprine, methotrexate, mycophenolate mofetil, JAK inhibitors, and IV infliximab have shown excellent results in patients with these chronic diseases. Numerous biologic medications have been developed to treat inflammatory bowel disease, including anti-integrin agents, IL-13/IL-23 inhibitors, and TNF-α inhibitors. They also have the added benefit of helping the skin disease. Cyclosporine and prednisone have shown excellent results in treating pyoderma gangrenosum. Intralesional triamcinolone can be attempted on small, early lesions of pyoderma gangrenosum.

Oral aphthous ulcers can be treated with topically applied steroid gels or ointments compounded in dental paste formula to increase adherence to the mucosa. Topical anesthetics are commonly used.

Erythema nodosum can be treated with compression stockings, topical potent steroids, and oral steroids in severe cases. Intralesional injection of triamcinolone is also effective. Metastatic Crohn disease is difficult to treat and requires systemic immunosuppressive agents such as azathioprine, prednisone, or infliximab. It is best treated by a multidisciplinary approach.

Stasis Dermatitis

Stasis dermatitis is a common chronic dermatosis seen almost exclusively on the lower extremities. The inflammation can lead to long-lasting discoloration, ulceration, and infection. Underlying systemic disease such as congestive heart failure and renal insufficiency can predispose to stasis dermatitis. Any condition that results in chronic edema of the lower extremities has the potential to induce stasis dermatitis.

Clinical Findings: Stasis dermatitis is a chronic inflammatory skin disease that indicates underlying insufficiency of the venous return system. It is most commonly seen in the older population, and there is no sex or racial predilection. Most often, congestive heart failure is the associated disease causing the edema. Many other conditions of venous insufficiency can also be causative, including varicose veins and postsurgical complications, such as after saphenous vein harvest for coronary artery bypass surgery or an inguinal lymph node dissection.

Stasis dermatitis is a skin manifestation of a wide range of underlying venous diseases. The lower extremities account for more than 99% of cases of stasis dermatitis, and the diagnosis in other areas of the body should be questioned. The legs tend to have a range of edema, from the very mild amount that accumulates at the end of a long day of standing to severe chronic edema that is always present. Red-brown eczematous patches, some with a light-yellow discoloration, typically begin around the medial malleolus. As the condition progresses, the patches begin to spread and can encompass the entire lower extremity, although much more commonly they are found at knee level or just below knee level. There can be complete confluence of the dermatitis around the affected limb, or it can affect only part of the leg. The skin becomes hyperpigmented and thickened.

The rash is almost always symmetric, and it is not uncommonly misdiagnosed as bilateral lower extremity cellulitis. The rash is typically pruritic, and the itching can be so severe as to cause excoriations and small ulcerations. Depending on the severity, weeping vesicular patches and plaques can form. A rare bulla can also be seen in some cases, and bullous pemphigoid must be included in the differential diagnosis. Varicose veins are often present on examination, or there may be a history of bypass surgery. If left untreated, venous stasis can lead to venous ulcerations, which have been described as slightly painful ulcerations on the lateral malleolus. The ulcerations can occur anywhere on the leg and in some cases are very tender. Peripheral pulses are intact, and this physical examination finding helps rule out arterial insufficiency. If the ulcerations and edema are not controlled, the ulcerations will continue to expand and can become secondarily infected; if they become deep enough, they can lead to underlying osteomyelitis or cellulitis. These neglected cases can end in loss of the affected portion of the limb if medical therapies do not successfully clear the infection and ulcerations.

Pathogenesis: Increased pressure within the venous system of the lower extremity causes extravasation of serum and blood into the surrounding dermis and subcutaneous tissue. As the edema in the lower extremity worsens, the skin begins to develop signs of chronic inflammation mediated by the abnormal location of fluid.

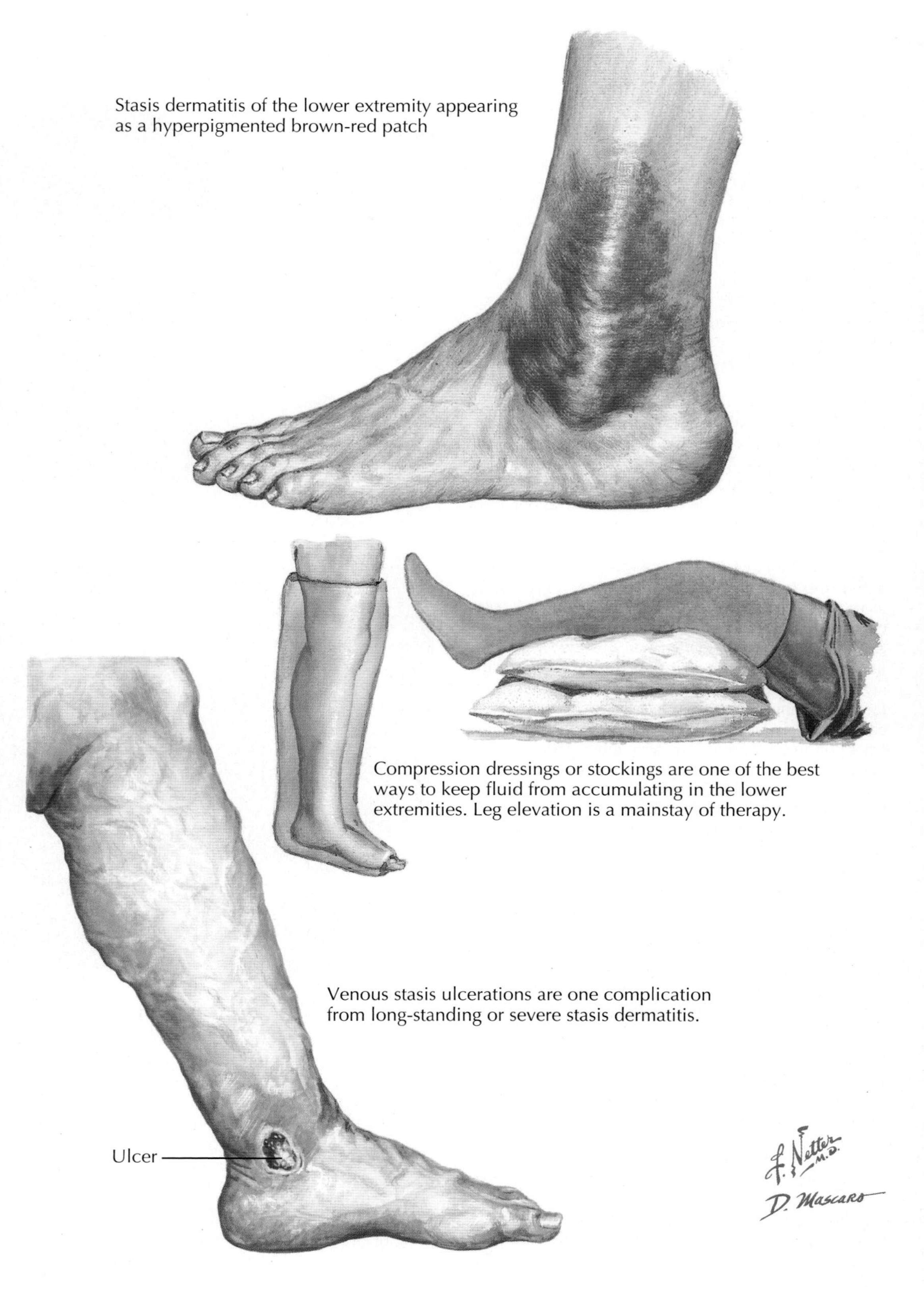

Histology: Biopsies are not routinely performed in stasis dermatitis, and the diagnosis is almost always made clinically. In those cases that are biopsied, histologic examination shows an increase in small vessels, extravasation of red blood cells, and hemosiderin deposition within the dermis. The epidermis shows varying degrees of spongiotic dermatitis.

Treatment: The rash can be treated symptomatically with topical corticosteroids and emollients. The main goal of therapy is to restore the proper venous flow. Depending on the underlying reason for the stasis dermatitis, this may or may not be possible. If it is not possible, the mainstay of therapy is the use of compression stockings or wraps. However, the compliance rate is low because of difficulty putting them on and discomfort. Patients who use compression gear and topical corticosteroids typically have a good prognosis. Cases caused by incompetent veins often improve when the varicosity is removed.

URTICARIA

Urticaria is a commonly encountered skin condition with a multitude of causes. There are primary and secondary forms of urticaria. Most secondary causes are acute in nature and can be explained by an underlying disease state, medication, or food. Urticaria can be a manifestation of many disease states, such as Muckle-Wells syndrome. Urticaria can also be a secondary sequela of an underlying malignancy, acute or chronic infection, genetic disease, or rheumatologic disease. It can also be seen as an acute reaction in a patient with anaphylaxis.

Primary urticaria can be divided into subsets of disease. The most common type is chronic idiopathic urticaria. Other forms of primary urticaria include the physical urticarias. There are many forms of physical urticaria, and provocative testing can determine the type. There is no known cure for urticaria, but most cases of primary urticaria spontaneously resolve within 2 to 3 years.

Clinical Findings: Primary idiopathic urticaria is one of the most frequently encountered forms of urticaria. It is more frequently seen in adult females. It is seen equally across all races. If no underlying cause is found and the urticaria lasts longer than 6 weeks, it is designated *chronic idiopathic urticaria.* This form of urticaria comes and goes at will with no provocative or remitting factors. Lesions appear as evanescent, pink to red, edematous plaques called hives. They can occur anywhere on the body and can cause much distress to the patient because of their appearance and because they induce severe pruritus. Patients are particularly distressed when the hives affect the face and eyelids, causing periorbital and periocular swelling. Patients with chronic urticaria usually undergo a battery of laboratory and allergy tests. A complete blood count, metabolic panel, chest radiograph, and measurements of thyroid-stimulating hormone and antithyroid antibodies should be performed, as well as testing for various infectious diseases if the medical history warrants. Testing for hepatitis B, hepatitis C, and HIV infection can be done in the appropriate clinical setting. Patients with a travel history often undergo stool examinations for ova and parasites. A full physical examination is warranted, together with age-appropriate cancer screening. Most patients with chronic urticaria have no appreciable cause for their hives and are diagnosed as having chronic idiopathic urticaria.

Physical urticarias are a group of conditions that cause hives; they represent a unique form of chronic idiopathic urticaria in that there is a precipitating factor. There are many types of physical urticaria, including aquagenic and cholinergic forms as well as cold-, pressure-, solar-, and vibratory-induced urticaria. These forms are diagnosed based on the results of provocative testing. The clinical history often leads to diagnosis and the appropriate testing regimen. As an example, a patient may develop hives only under tight-fitting socks. This is typical for pressure-induced urticaria. If the patient develops hives on appropriate provocative testing, the diagnosis is made.

Pathogenesis: The pathogenesis of urticaria is poorly understood. Mast cells play a critical role. A stimulus causes mast cells to release histamine, which acts on the local vasculature to increase vascular permeability. The increased permeability causes localized swelling. Some forms of urticaria, such as those seen in anaphylaxis, are caused by a type I hypersensitivity reaction. Other forms of secondary urticaria may be caused by specific IgE antibodies that interact with mast cells.

Many medications have been shown to cause mast cell degranulation without an IgE-mediated pathway. The most common of these are opiates and anesthetic agents. Biochemical transmitters other than histamine also play a role in urticaria; they include the leukotrienes, serotonin, and various kinins.

Histology: The histologic findings in urticaria are bland. The specimen typically shows a superficial perivascular lymphocytic infiltrate with some dermal edema. The epidermis is normal. In fact, the skin can be entirely normal appearing.

Treatment: Treatment of chronic idiopathic urticaria is based on symptom relief. Antihistamines are the first-line therapy and can be used in combination. The lack of response can be frustrating for both patient and physician. Omalizumab, an anti-IgE medication, has good efficacy in treating chronic idiopathic urticaria that does not respond to antihistamine therapy. Physical urticarias are treated in the same manner, with emphasis on avoidance. Patients who can avoid exposure to the physical stimulus responsible for the urticaria have been shown to have better clinical outcomes.

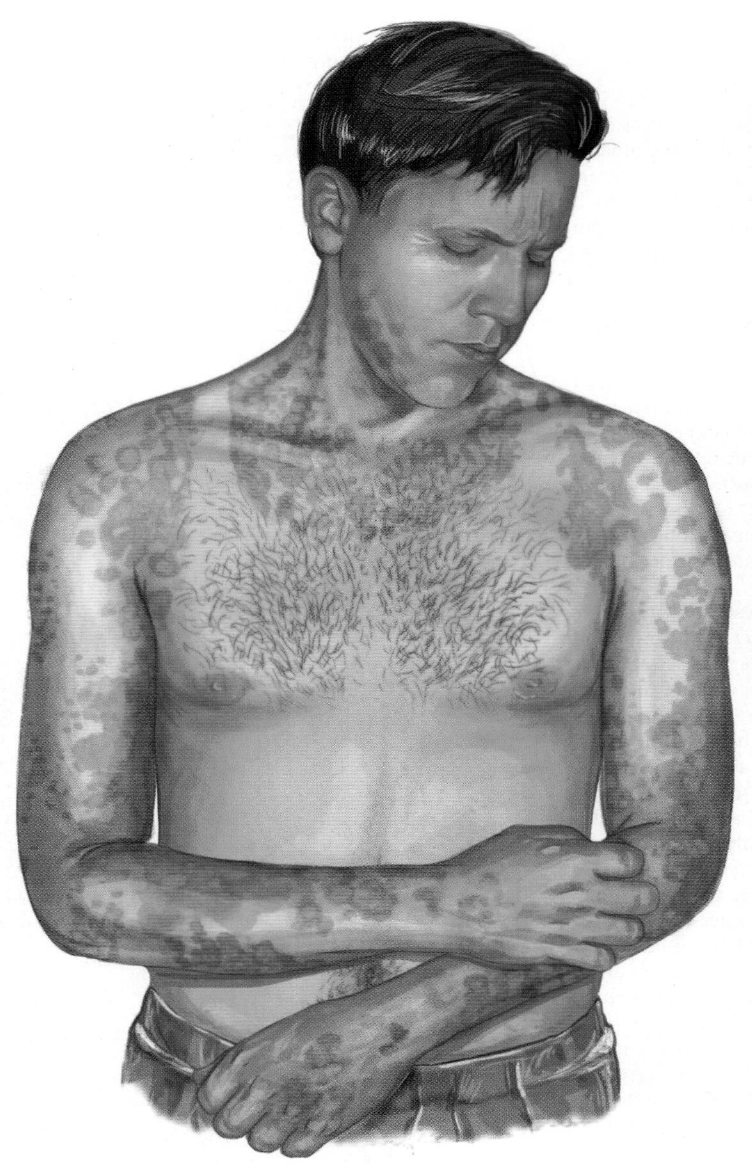

Solar Urticaria: Note the areas affected are only those exposed to the sun in this sleeveless shirt–wearing man.

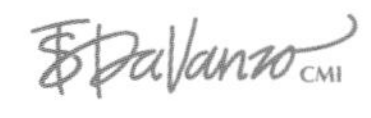

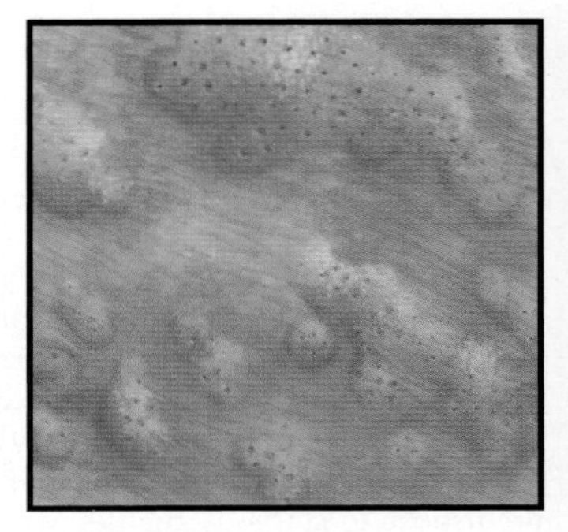

Urticaria: Pink edematous plaques with follicular accentuation caused by the dermal edema.

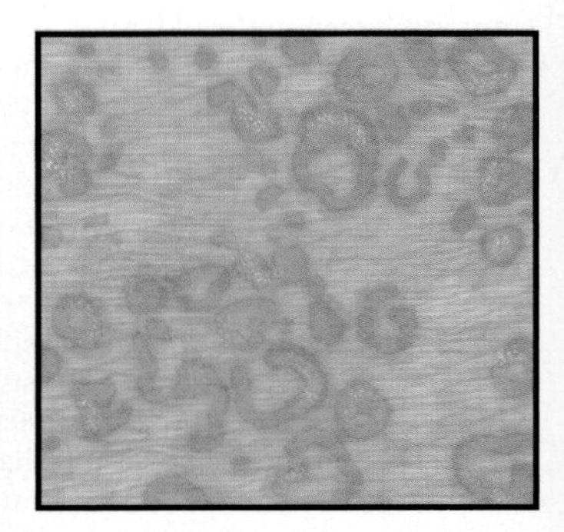

Annular and serpiginous urticaria: This is a less commonly seen variant of urticaria.

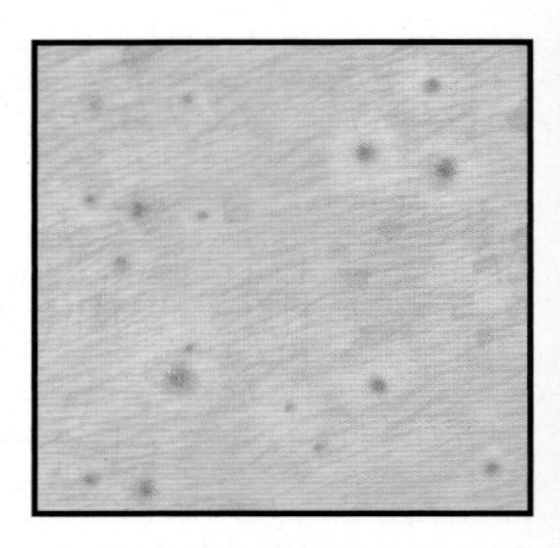

Cholinergic urticaria: This form of urticaria can be induced by increasing the body temperature through exercise or submersion in a warm bath.

VITILIGO

Vitiligo is a common acquired skin disease with multiple clinical variants. Vitiligo occurs because of loss of function or complete loss of melanocytes within the epidermis and follicular epithelium. There are many theories as to its development, but it is believed to be an autoimmune skin disease. Vitiligo may be seen in association with other autoimmune conditions. Patients afflicted with vitiligo are often psychologically affected by the disease.

Clinical Findings: Approximately 1% of the population is affected by vitiligo. It has been reported to occur at any age, but it is most common in the teenage years and the early twenties. There is no sex or racial predilection. A small percentage of cases are familial in nature. The exact inheritance pattern and the reason for this configuration are unknown. Many clinical variants of vitiligo exist. All forms have varying degrees of involvement of the skin. When melanin is no longer produced, patients are left with depigmented macules. These macules appear as stark white areas of skin, which can be a few millimeters to many centimeters in diameter. The areas of involvement have a well-defined border region. Hair within the areas of depigmented skin may also be depigmented. With time, the loss of pigment in the hair becomes more prominent. Hair depigmentation within the regions of vitiligo is not universal, and normal-appearing pigmented hair may grow within such an area. Most commonly, no inflammation is seen, and the areas are completely asymptomatic in nature.

Patients with Fitzpatrick type I skin are less obviously affected than those with Fitzpatrick type VI skin. The areas of vitiligo will not tan after sun exposure. Sun exposure typically makes the difference between affected and nonaffected skin more noticeable, as it increases melanin production in the unaffected skin, resulting in a darkening or tanning of the skin around the vitiliginous region. The areas of vitiligo are prone to easy burning and must be protected.

Various clinical variants or classifications of vitiligo exist, including localized, generalized, linear, trichrome, and blaschkoid variants. The generalized form can cause near-universal involvement of the skin, with only a few tiny islands of normal-appearing skin remaining within the areas of vitiliginous skin. Linear areas of involvement are rare and typically affect a limb. Blaschkoid vitiligo follows the embryologic Blaschko lines.

Pathogenesis: The exact cause of vitiligo has yet to be determined. The leading theory on its development is the autoimmune theory. An unknown trigger causes the immune system to begin destroying melanocytes. The immune system recognizes melanocytes as somehow abnormal and causes their destruction. This is mediated through cytotoxic $CD8^+$ T-cell production of IFN-γ. The autoimmune theory also may explain why vitiligo is seen clustered with diabetes, thyroid disease, and other autoimmune conditions.

Histology: There is no inflammation, and hematoxylin and eosin staining of the biopsy specimen may appear normal unless compared with a biopsy specimen from unaffected skin. When this is done, the lack of melanin production and melanocytes is appreciated. Special staining to accentuate melanocytes can make this difference much more visible.

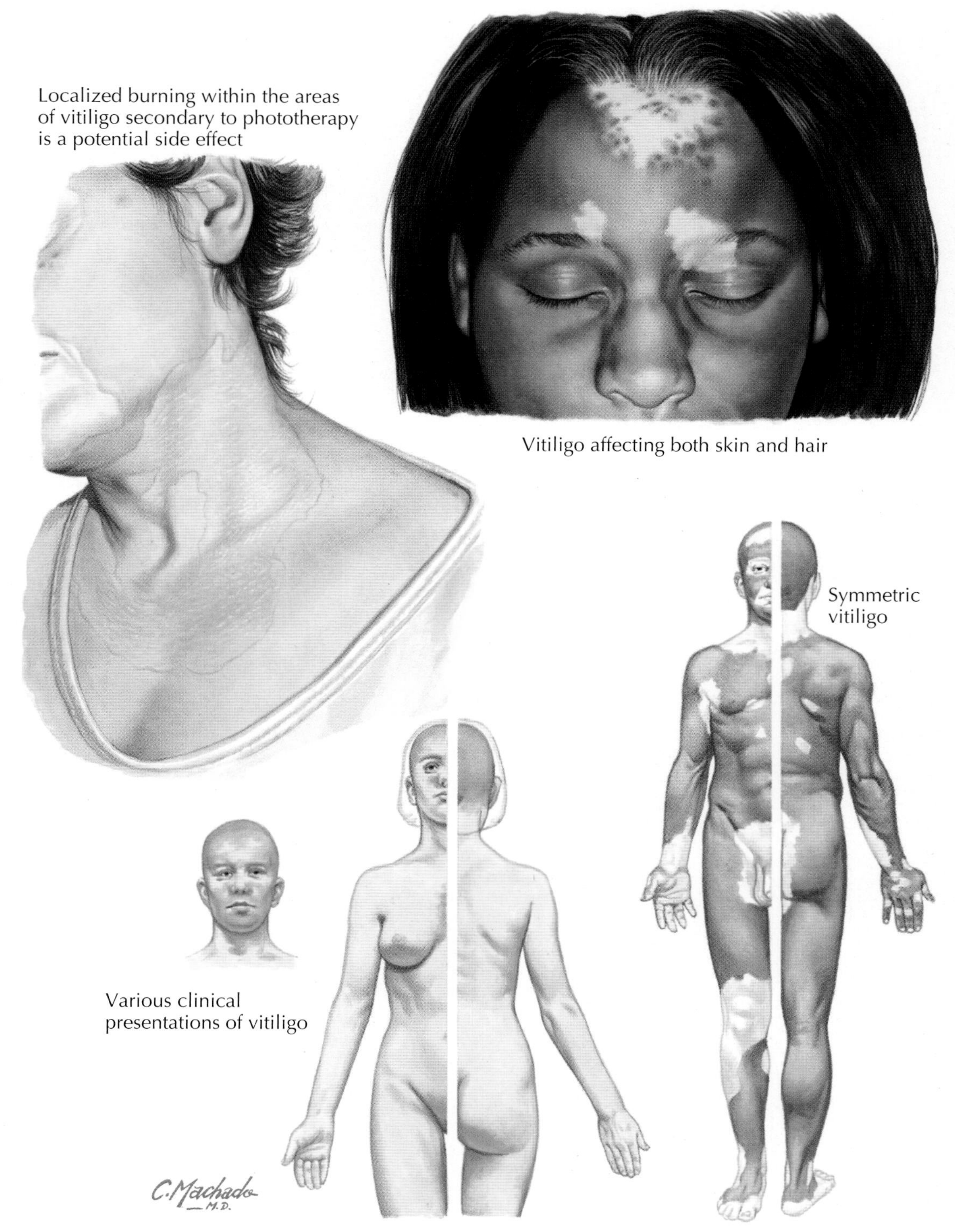

Treatment: Patients with vitiligo should be screened for underlying autoimmune conditions such as diabetes and thyroid disease. Treatment of these conditions has not been shown to help the vitiligo. No therapy is needed. For patients who seek treatment, many therapies are available, mostly on an anecdotal basis. Potent topical corticosteroids and topical immunomodulators such as tacrolimus and pimecrolimus have been used. Phototherapy with narrow-band UVB light and PUVA has been used successfully. The risk of burning is very high in the affected regions, and care should be used when starting this treatment. Small areas have been treated successfully with surgical techniques involving autotransplantation of skin from unaffected regions. If the therapy works, melanocyte rejuvenation typically occurs in a speckled pattern centered on the hair follicles. The hair follicle is believed to be a reservoir of melanocytes for repopulation of areas that are devoid of their normal complement of melanocytes. JAK inhibitors have been reported to improve vitiligo.

Rarely, complete depigmentation is undertaken for those who are severely affected to allow for a uniform skin tone. Monobenzyl ether of hydroquinone is used to eliminate any remaining melanocytes and depigment the skin. Care must be taken because the depigmentation is permanent.

AUTOIMMUNE BLISTERING DISEASES

BASEMENT MEMBRANE ZONE, HEMIDESMOSOME, AND DESMOSOME

BASEMENT MEMBRANE ZONE

The basement membrane zone (BMZ) of the epidermis is a beautiful and complex structure and a marvel of biologic engineering. The zone acts to attach the overlying epidermis to the underlying stromal tissue, in this case the papillary dermis, which is made predominantly of collagen bundles. A plethora of unique and specialized proteins play critical roles in the proper functioning of the BMZ. Any defect or abnormal antibody that can cause disruption of the normal architecture can result in fracturing of the BMZ and blister formation.

The BMZ can be appreciated on routine hematoxylin and eosin staining as an eosinophilic band below the basilar keratinocytes. The components of the BMZ are produced in two locations: the epidermal keratinocyte and the dermal fibroblast. These cells act to produce the required proteins in the correct ratio to maintain a functional basement membrane. The basement membrane's most important function is to keep the epidermis firmly attached to the underlying dermis. This is necessary for life. This specialized structure also acts to encourage migration of cells and repair of the epidermal-dermal barrier after trauma. Many other critical processes and physiologic roles depend on the proper functioning of the BMZ, including permeability of water and other chemical substrates, proteins, and cellular elements. The BMZ is a highly organized structure that is consistent from person to person.

The structure of the BMZ can be subdivided into individual compartments for study, with the understanding that the entire unit functions as one. These are the epidermal basilar cell cytoskeleton, hemidesmosome, lamina lucida, lamina densa, and sublamina papillary dermis. Each of these components is made up of unique proteins that act in harmony to preserve the functional role of the BMZ. The basilar keratinocytes contain intracellular cytoskeleton components made of keratin intermediate filaments, predominantly keratin 5 and keratin 14. The keratin intermediate filaments are interwoven into the hemidesmosomal plaque to firmly adhere the basilar cell to the hemidesmosome.

The keratin intermediate filaments interact with bullous pemphigoid antigen 1 (BP230) and plectin. These two proteins are the main components of the hemidesmosomal plaque. Plectin and BP230 are bound tightly together. Plectin and bullous pemphigoid antibody 1 also bind to the integrin class of proteins and to bullous pemphigoid antigen 2 (BP180). Integrins and BP180 are transcellular proteins that bind to the intracellular molecules, plectin, and BP230; they also extend out from the basilar keratinocyte and interact with the laminin 5 and collagen IV molecules in the lamina lucida and lamina densa.

BASEMENT MEMBRANE ZONE AND HEMIDESMOSOME

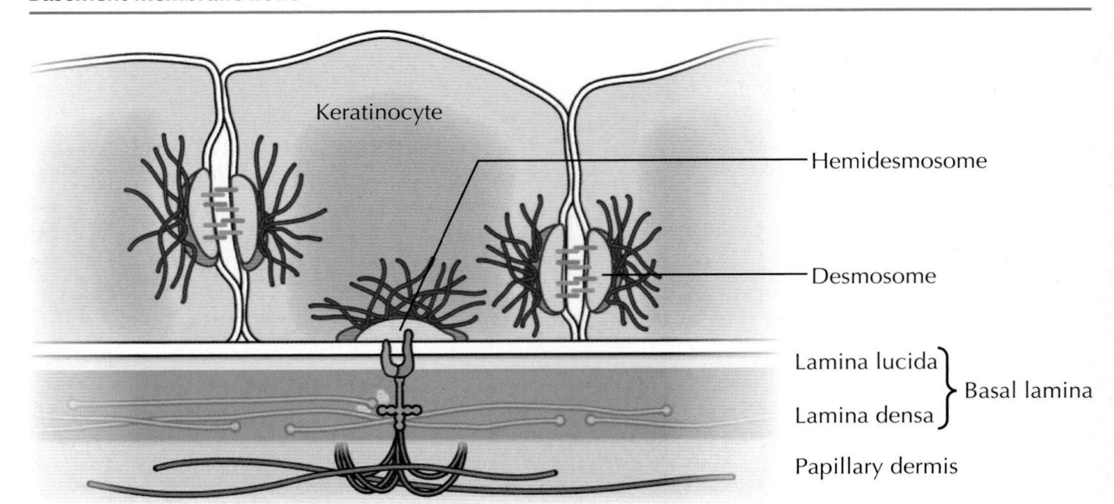

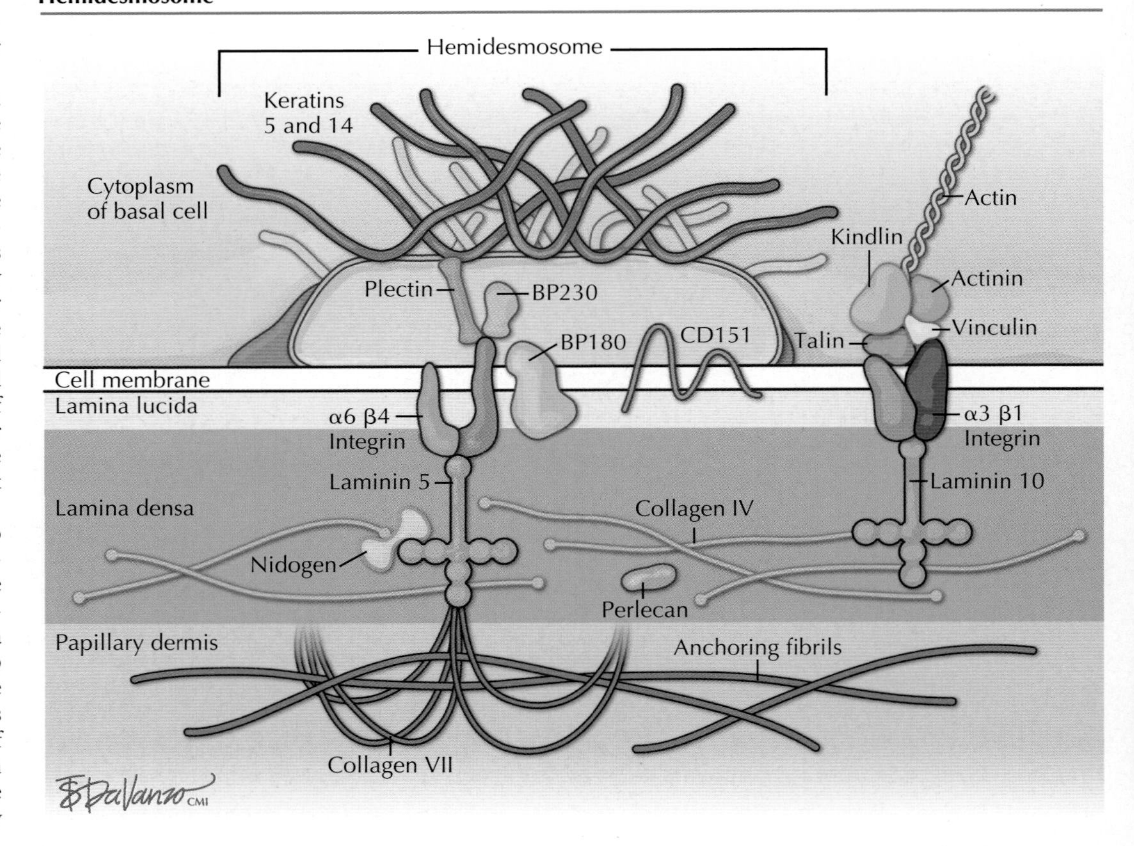

The lamina lucida is so named because of its translucent appearance on electron microscopy. In comparison, the lamina densa is an electron-dense region that lies just below the lamina lucida. The lamina lucida is composed of the transversing parts of the integrin and BP180 proteins. These two molecules attach to the laminin class of proteins in the lamina densa. The lamina lucida is considered to be the weakest part of the BMZ, and it is the blister plane in suction blisters, junctional epidermolysis bullosa, and salt-split skin. The lamina densa is composed of a latticework of type IV collagen. Type IV collagen is found only in the lamina densa. It is unique in that it retains its globular regions on either end. These form attachments to other type IV collagen molecules to create the lattice. Collagen type IV binds strongly to a dumbbell-shaped protein named *nidogen*. This nidogen protein is critical in attaching to the laminin proteins in the lamina densa. Nidogen locks the type IV collagen to the laminins, which are bound to the overlying integrin and BP180.

Basement Membrane Zone, Hemidesmosome, and Desmosome (Continued)

The laminin proteins appear as inverted crosses and serve to attach the aforementioned proteins to the papillary dermis that underlies the lamina densa by interacting with type VII collagen. Type VII collagen, which is made up of three identical alpha chains, is also known as the *anchoring fibril.* These fibrils interweave among the type I and type II collagens of the papillary dermis and attach either end to the laminin proteins in the lamina densa, thus firmly anchoring the entire overlying epidermis and BMZ to the papillary dermal collagen.

Many blistering diseases are caused by genetic abnormalities in the BMZ proteins; these are classified as the epidermolysis bullosa group of blistering diseases. Each of these diseases is unique due to different protein defects that lead to the various phenotypes. Autoimmune blistering diseases of the pemphigoid class target the BMZ and its components, including the hemidesmosome. Autoimmune diseases in the pemphigus class of diseases target the desmosome.

HEMIDESMOSOME

The hemidesmosome is one of the main components of the BMZ. Its purpose is to attach the basilar layer keratinocytes to the underlying stroma—that is, the papillary dermis. The hemidesmosome is made up of many unique and highly integrated groups of protein-to-protein connections. The main proteins in the hemidesmosomal plaque are the bullous pemphigoid antigens BP180 and BP230, integrin, plectin, and laminin. Their interactions and how they connect the keratinocyte cytoskeleton to the underlying collagen have already been described. Antibodies directed against the components of the hemidesmosome can be seen in the pemphigoid group of disease states.

DESMOSOME

The desmosome provides the major connection between one keratinocyte and another. It is the most complex of the keratinocyte connection points, which also include tight junctions, adherens junctions, and gap junctions. Desmosomes are present on all keratinocytes from the stratum basalis through the stratum granulosum. Once they reach the stratum corneum, the desmosomes start to degrade and break apart as the corneocytes are desquamated off the surface of the skin. The main purpose of desmosomes is to connect the actin cytoskeleton of one keratinocyte to that of the adjacent keratinocyte. They achieve this goal through a series of highly coordinated protein connections. The main proteins that allow for the connection between adjacent cells and the strength of the connection are the cadherin proteins, desmoglein and desmocollin. These are calcium-dependent adhesion molecules. Desmoglein and desmocollin are transmembrane proteins. A desmocollin protein from one keratinocyte interacts with a desmoglein protein from the adjacent keratinocyte in a 1:1 ratio. There are multiple types of desmogleins and desmocollins, but they all interact similarly. Some of the subtypes are expressed at slightly different rates in various locations, such as mucous membranes and the different levels of the epidermis. Each desmoglein or desmocollin molecule is anchored within the keratinocyte to plakoglobin, which in turn is bound to a group of proteins named *desmoplakins.* The desmoplakin proteins ultimately connect with the intercellular actin cytoskeleton.

The pemphigus group of diseases are autoimmune blistering diseases caused by the formation of autoantibodies against desmoglein and, in some cases, also against desmocollin. These autoantibodies interrupt the cell-to-cell adhesion process, resulting in superficial blistering of the skin and mucous membranes.

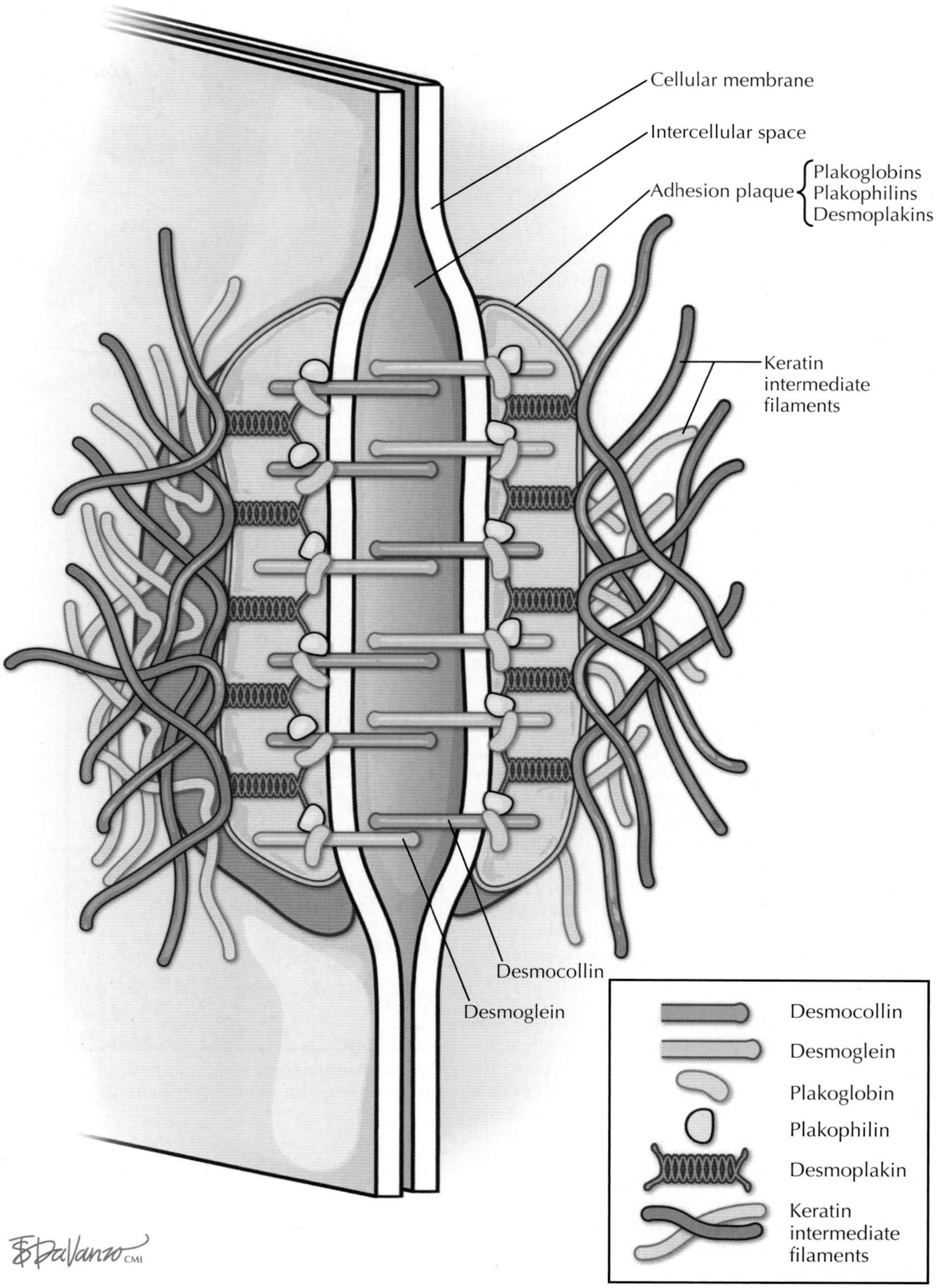

Bullous Pemphigoid

Autoantibody-mediated blisters: location of cleavage plane

PF (Dsg 1)

PV (Dsg 3)

BP (BP180, BP230)
CP, HG, LABD

EBA (Col VII), LABD

BP, bullous pemphigoid; Col VII, type VII collagen; CP, cicatricial pemphigoid; Dsg 1, desmoglein 1; Dsg 3, desmoglein 3; EBA, epidermolysis bullosa acquisita; HG, herpes gestationis; PF, pemphigus foliaceus; PV, pemphigus vulgaris; LABD, linear immunoglobulin A bullous dermatosis

Bullous pemphigoid is the most frequently encountered of all of the autoimmune blistering diseases. It is directly caused by the formation of autoantibodies directed against two hemidesmosomal proteins, BP180 and BP230. These two proteins are critical for stabilization of the hemidesmosomal plaque. If the hemidesmosomal plaque is interrupted or destroyed, the end result is subepidermal blistering of the skin.

Clinical Findings: The hemidesmosomal plaque is the main anchoring system of the dermal-epidermal junction. It is a complex apparatus with a multitude of proteins that interact to bind the epidermis to the underlying dermis. If it is interrupted, the pemphigoid complex of diseases may occur. These conditions include bullous pemphigoid, herpes gestationis, and cicatricial pemphigoid. Of these, bullous pemphigoid is the disease state most frequently encountered. It most commonly occurs in the fifth to seventh decades of life, with no race or sex predilection.

Clinically, patients often have a prodrome of intensely pruritic patches and plaques on the trunk, particularly the abdomen. Soon thereafter, they begin to develop large, tense bullae. The bullae can range from 1 cm to 10 cm in diameter, with an average of 2 cm. The blisters are tense to palpation and are not easily ruptured. If they do rupture, a fine, clear to slightly yellow serous fluid drains, and the underlying dermis is exposed. Reepithelialization is fairly rapid. Patients have continuous formation of new bullae, followed by healing and then repetition of the blistering pattern, until treatment is obtained. Scarring is minimal unless secondary infection has occurred. Oral involvement can occur, but most patients with pemphigoid do not have oral lesions; this is in direct contrast to those patients with the pemphigus class of diseases.

Bullous pemphigoid can spontaneously remit and relapse over time. Most patients seek therapy and are treated with a host of agents. Patients typically respond well to therapy and overall have an excellent prognosis. Secondary infections and side effects from therapy can lead to morbidity and mortality. Laboratory testing reveals immunoglobulin G (IgG) antibodies against BP180 or BP230 or both.

Pathogenesis: Bullous pemphigoid is caused by IgG and IgE autoantibody production. The autoantibodies produced attack the BP180 and BP230 proteins, which are integral components of the hemidesmosomal plaque. BP180 is a transmembrane protein, and BP230 is an intracellular protein that lies within the keratinocyte and binds to BP180 and keratin filaments. The reason for the development of these autoantibodies is unknown. Once they have formed, they attach to the hemidesmosomal proteins. This activates a plethora of pathogenic mechanisms that act to induce separation of the epidermis from the dermis. Critical in the pathogenesis is activation of the complement cascade by the IgG_1 antibodies. IgG_1 autoantibodies are able to fix complement, starting its inflammatory cascade. Complement activation may lead to further recruitment of inflammatory cells, which can be activated and thereafter release cytokines and enzymes that perpetuate the response. IgG_4 is the second most frequent form of IgG found and is has been shown to activate leukocytes.

Histology: Routine hematoxylin and eosin staining reveals a cell-poor subepidermal blister with scattered eosinophils. The histologic differential diagnosis can be between bullous pemphigoid and epidermolysis bullosa acquisita (EBA). Immunofluorescence staining can be used to help differentiate the two. IgG and complement C3 localize to the BMZ and appear as a linear band. The salt-split skin technique can also be used to differentiate the two diseases. This is achieved by incubating skin in a 1 M NaCl solution to split the skin through the lamina lucida. When immunofluorescence staining is used on salt-split skin, the immunoreactants localize to the blister roof in bullous pemphigoid and to the dermal base in EBA.

Treatment: The severity of bullous pemphigoid varies. Therapy needs to be tailored to the individual. Many patients are older and have comorbidities that must be considered. Mild, localized disease can be treated with high-potency topical steroids. Severe disease is treated initially with oral steroids, and then the patient is transitioned to a steroid-sparing agent. The medications that have been routinely used include mycophenolate mofetil, azathioprine, and the combination of tetracycline and nicotinamide. Intravenous immunoglobulin (IVIG), rituximab, dupilumab, and omalizumab have been used for severe refractory disease.

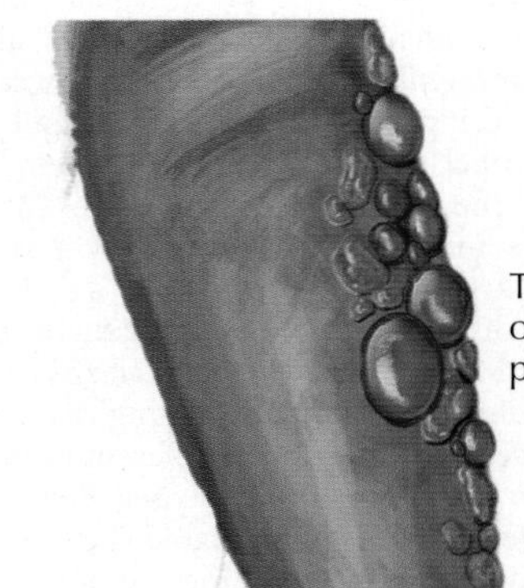

Tense bullae of bullous pemphigoid

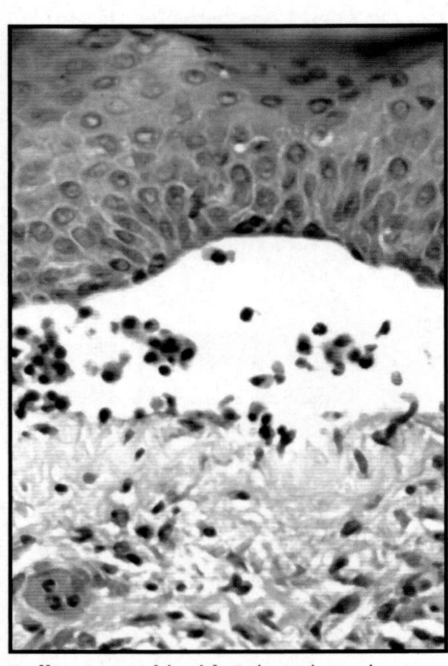

Bullous pemphigoid. Subepidermal blister cavity with multiple eosinophils.

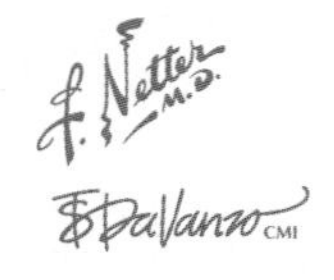

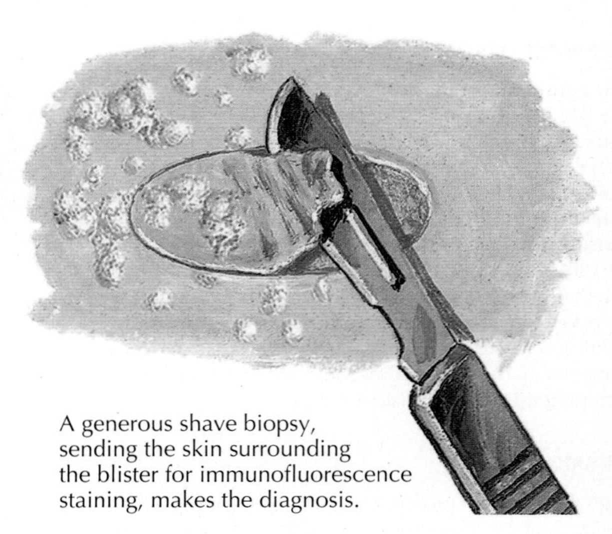

A generous shave biopsy, sending the skin surrounding the blister for immunofluorescence staining, makes the diagnosis.

Mucous Membrane Pemphigoid

Mucous membrane pemphigoid goes by other names, including cicatricial pemphigoid, Brunsting-Perry pemphigoid, ocular pemphigoid, and benign mucous membrane pemphigoid. The last name should not be used because this is a chronic progressive, disabling disease with severe morbidity and mortality. The term *cicatricial* inherently states that the disease is associated with scarring, but this is not always the case. Hence one patient without scarring may be referred to as having ocular pemphigoid and another with scarring may be said to have cicatricial ocular pemphigoid. Most patients will have some form of scarring, albeit very mild in some cases, if monitored for a long enough period. In reality, these are names given to a heterogeneous group of autoimmune blistering diseases that express a unique phenotype and have been shown to have small variances in the BMZ autoantibodies they produce.

Clinical Findings: Mucous membrane pemphigoid can be seen in any racial group and affects females more often than males, in a 2:1 ratio. It is a disease of older persons and is most commonly seen in the seventh and eighth decades of life. Mucous membrane pemphigoid is a severe, chronic autoimmune blistering disease with grave consequences. It is a major cause of morbidity and mortality, and therapy can be difficult. Up 25% of these patients have eye involvement, which can lead to decreased vision and blindness. Mucous membrane disease is typically the initial sign; patients present with painful erosions in the nasal passages, oropharynx, conjunctiva, genitalia, and pulmonary tree. Patients complain of pain and difficulty eating secondary to severe discomfort. Erosions are the most common clinical findings, but vesicles and bullae may also be seen. Pulmonary and esophageal involvement may lead to strictures that result in difficulty with breathing or eating solid food. Weight loss typically ensues, as do malaise and fatigue.

The skin can also be affected, leading to blister formation that heals with scarring and milia. If blisters develop on the scalp, they heal with a scarring alopecia. This form of the disease has been given the name *Brunsting-Perry pemphigoid.* This term is typically reserved for cases involving only the scalp and skin that do not affect the mucous membranes.

Ocular pemphigoid is a chronic symmetric disease. The initial symptoms are inflamed conjunctiva, discomfort, pain, and increased tear production. Scarring soon develops and forms fibrous adhesions between the palpebral and bulbar conjunctivae. This scarring is termed *symblepharon*. The scarring is progressive, and it may cause the eyeball to become frozen in place. Entropion is common, and as it progresses the eyelashes turn inward (trichiasis) and are forced against the cornea, which causes severe pain, irritation, and corneal ulceration. Patients cannot entirely close their eyelids because of the severe scarring. The damaged cornea undergoes keratinization, leading to opacity of the cornea and blindness.

Pathogenesis: Autoantibody formation against proteins of the BMZ has been linked to cicatricial pemphigoid. Many different antibodies against these proteins exist, including antibodies against the laminins, BP180 and BP230, and epiligrin. The heterogeneity in antibody production likely accounts for the varying clinical phenotypes that are expressed.

Histology: Subepidermal blistering that heals with scar formation is the hallmark of this disease. The blistering takes place just below the keratinocyte, within the lamina lucida. Immunohistochemical staining with collagen type IV shows that the blister plane is above the level of the lamina densa. Immunostaining and routine hematoxylin and eosin staining show a picture very similar to that of bullous pemphigoid. Linear IgG and complement C3 immunofluorescent staining are present along the BMZ.

Treatment: Prednisone is the drug initially used to treat the disease. After the disease is under some control, the addition of a steroid-sparing immunosuppressant should be initiated. Immunosuppressant medications used include azathioprine, cyclophosphamide methotrexate, mycophenolate mofetil, and rituximab. Dapsone and sulfapyridine, a similar medication that can be used in place of dapsone, have had some success treating this disease. Some individuals with very mild disease may be able to be treated with topical steroids alone. IVIG has been used with success in refractory cases. Trichiasis is treated with removal of the eyelashes.

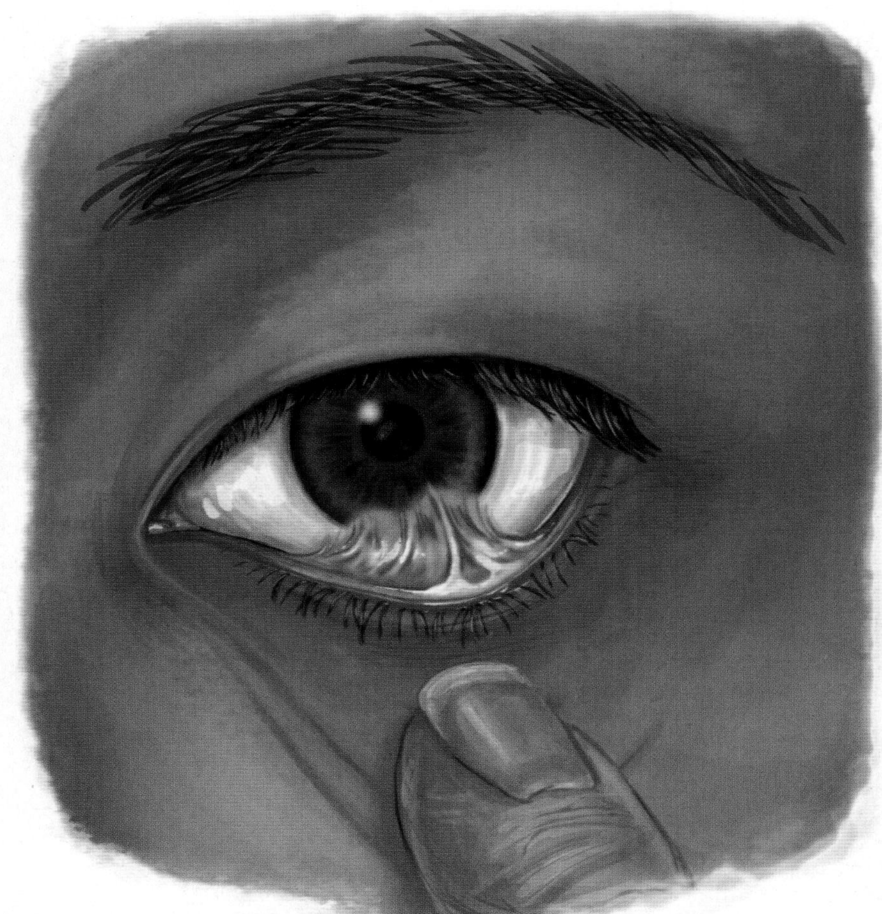

Ocular cicatricial pemphigoid. Scarring can become so severe as to cause vision loss. Symblepharon is commonly seen.

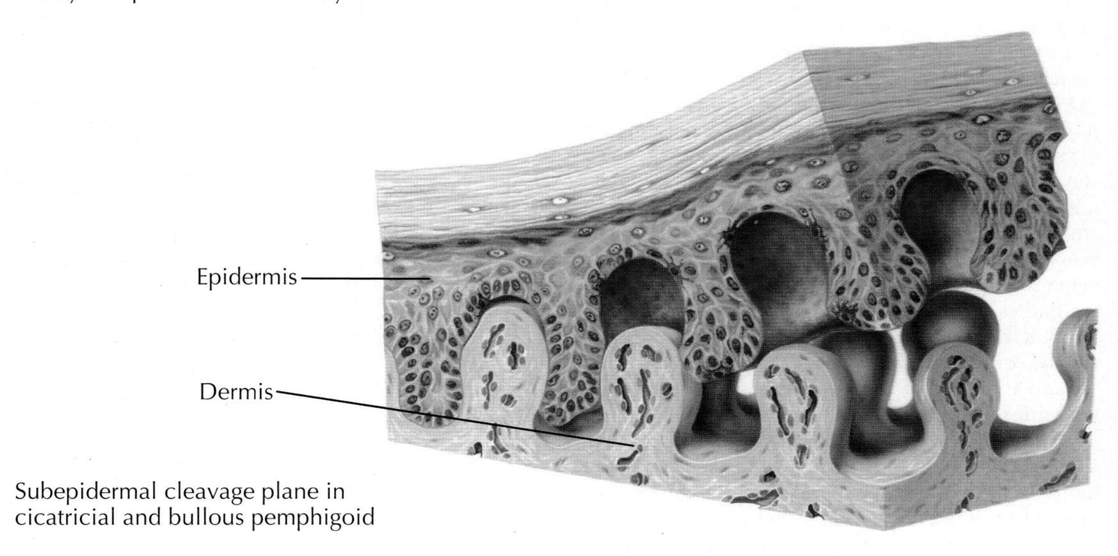

Subepidermal cleavage plane in cicatricial and bullous pemphigoid

Dermatitis Herpetiformis

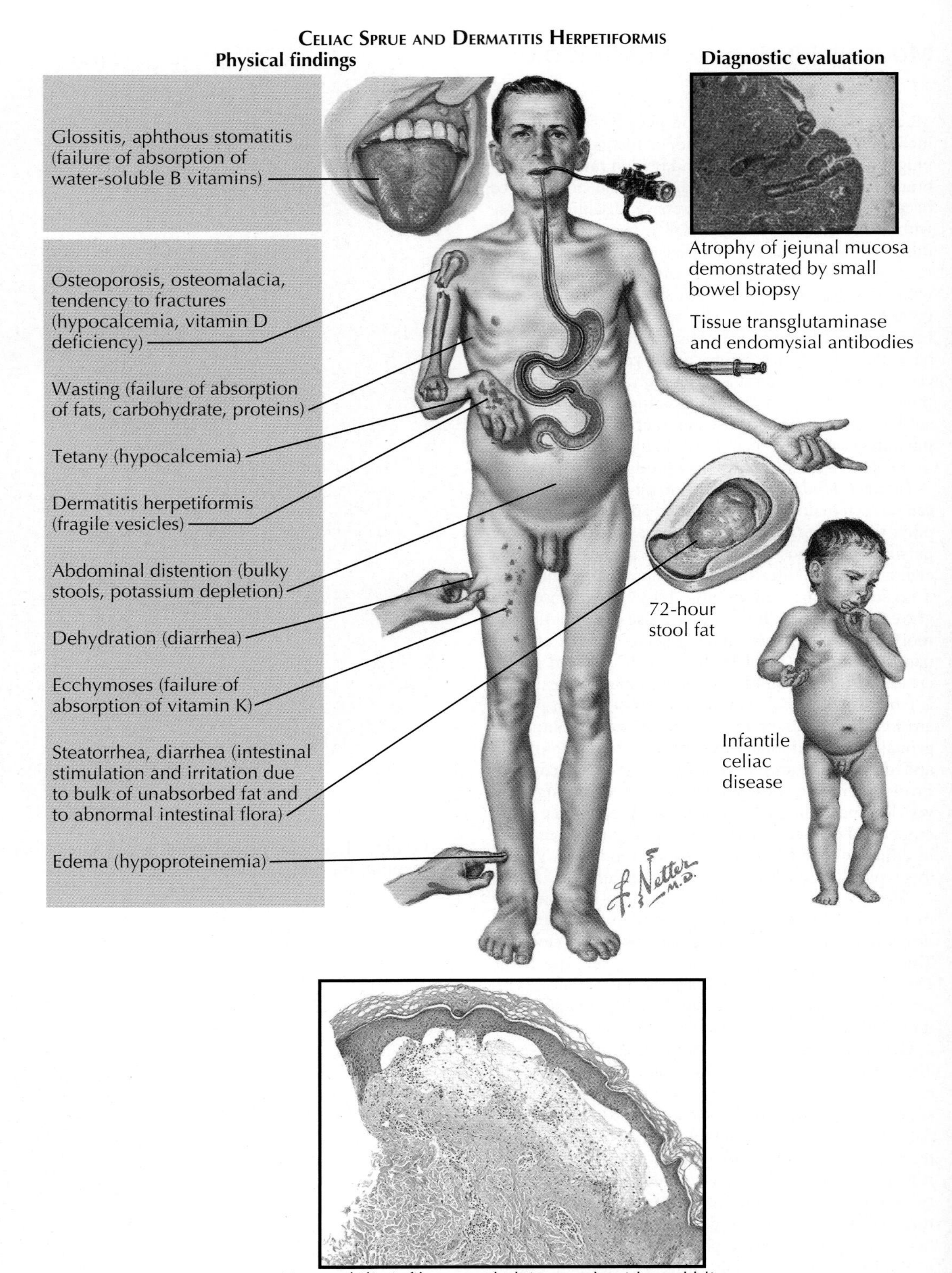

Neutrophilic infiltrate underlying a subepidermal blister

Dermatitis herpetiformis is a unique chronic blistering disease that can be seen in isolation or in conjunction with celiac sprue. Dermatitis herpetiformis is the cutaneous manifestation of underlying gluten sensitivity. Patients with a genetic predisposition seem to be at risk for development of IgA autoantibodies that cross-react with gluten proteins and specific components of the skin and gastrointestinal tract. Dermatitis herpetiformis is always associated with small bowel disease, and in some cases celiac sprue coexists. Patients with dermatitis herpetiformis are at increased risk for development of lymphoma of the gastrointestinal tract, potentially caused by the chronic inflammation and stimulation of the gastrointestinal-associated lymphatic tissue. Following a gluten-free diet cures the disease in both the skin and gastrointestinal locations.

Clinical Findings: Dermatitis herpetiformis is most frequently seen in the fourth and fifth decades of life, with a higher prevalence in the White female population. The reason for this preference may be that dermatitis herpetiformis has associations with the human leukocyte antigen DQ2 and DQ8 haplotypes. It is uncommon in children. Dermatitis herpetiformis manifests as a symmetric vesicular eruption, which is often preceded by a burning sensation or pruritus. The extensor surfaces of the elbows, knees, and lower back, as well as the scalp, may be involved. The vesicles are fragile and break easily. Erosions and excoriations are frequently seen. Diarrhea can be a recurrent complaint secondary to involvement of the small bowel. Patients frequently report a flare of the rash and abdominal pain and diarrhea after eating certain foods.

Laboratory testing is frequently performed. High levels of IgA anti–tissue transglutaminase (antitTG) antibody and antiendomysial antibodies (EMAs) are commonly found and are highly specific for dermatitis herpetiformis. In cases of suspected sprue, an upper endoscopy can be performed, with a biopsy of the small bowel to evaluate for the characteristic villous atrophy.

Pathogenesis: Dermatitis herpetiformis is an autoimmune blistering disease caused by the development of specific antibodies, notably antitTG and EMAs. Tissue transglutaminase (tTG) is very similar to epidermal transglutaminase, and it is believed that the anti-tTG antibodies attack both proteins. This disruption of the epidermal transglutaminase is thought to be responsible for the blistering skin findings. Once the antibodies attach to the epidermal transglutaminase protein, the complement cascade and various cytotoxic cellular events are activated. The anti-EMA test is the most specific of the antibody tests for dermatitis herpetiformis.

Histology: Early lesions of dermatitis herpetiformis show subepidermal clefting with a neutrophil-rich infiltrate in the papillary dermis. As the lesions progress, subepidermal blistering becomes prominent, and the papillary dermis is filled with neutrophils. The histologic findings of dermatitis herpetiformis can be difficult to differentiate from those of linear IgA bullous dermatosis on routine hematoxylin and eosin staining. Direct immunofluorescence is required to differentiate the two diseases. The direct immunofluorescence staining pattern in dermatitis herpetiformis is that of a speckled or granular arrangement of IgA within the papillary dermis. In linear IgA bullous disease, as the name implies, a linear pattern along the BMZ is seen. Small bowel biopsies show atrophy of the intestinal villi and crypt hyperplasia.

Treatment: The treatment of dermatitis herpetiformis is twofold. The first aspect of therapy is to control the itching and blistering. This can be rapidly achieved with dapsone or sulfapyridine. The response to these two medications is remarkably quick, with most patients noticing near resolution of their symptoms within 1 day. In cases of suspected dermatitis herpetiformis that has not been confirmed histologically, dapsone can be used as a therapeutic test; if the patient sees a rapid response after the first day of dapsone therapy, the diagnosis is most certainly dermatitis herpetiformis. Dapsone or alternative medications can treat the blistering and pruritus, but they do not decrease the long-term risk of small bowel lymphoma. The only means of decreasing and removing the risk of lymphoma is to have the patient adhere to a strict gluten-free diet. This requires nutritional education. If patients are able to entirely avoid gluten-containing products, not only will the rash resolve but the gastrointestinal abnormalities will resolve as well, and the risk of lymphoma will return to that of the general population.

EPIDERMOLYSIS BULLOSA ACQUISITA

Epidermolysis bullosa acquisita (EBA) is a rare chronic autoimmune blistering disease that is caused by autoantibodies against type VII collagen. EBA has many features in common with the dominantly inherited form of the blistering disease dystrophic epidermolysis bullosa (DEB). DEB is caused by a genetic defect in collagen VII that leads to a reduced amount or total lack of this type of collagen. Collagen VII serves as the anchoring fibrils that attach the epidermis via a series of protein connections to the dermis. Any defect in the production of collagen VII or abnormal destruction of this protein leads to blistering of the skin. EBA has been shown to be associated with a number of underlying systemic conditions, including inflammatory bowel disease, leukemia, tuberculosis infection, and other autoimmune diseases.

Clinical Findings: EBA is an extremely rare disease that affects 1 in 2 to 3 million people. It is almost always seen in the adult population, with the peak incidence in the fifth decade of life. A small number of cases of children affected by EBA have been reported. There is no race or sex predilection. The classic mechanical bullous form of EBA is the most common variant and manifests with blister formation or with fragile skin and erosions from slight trauma. When located on the dorsal hands, this can have a similar clinical appearance to porphyria cutanea tarda. The blistering is most frequently located in regions that experience mechanical friction or trauma. The dorsal surfaces of the hands are almost always involved, and patients complain of skin fragility and blister formation after slight trauma. The blisters heal slowly with scarring, and on close inspection, milia are found in the region of the healed blister. The mucous membranes are frequently involved, and oral disease can lead to weight loss. Other clinical variants of EBA have been described that typically mimic the clinical appearance of other autoimmune blistering diseases. Bullous pemphigoid-like EBA is the second most common variant seen. For this reason, the only method to correctly diagnose any blistering disease is by correlation of clinical and pathologic findings.

Pathogenesis: EBA is caused by the production of autoantibodies directed against type VII collagen. The noncollagenous portions of type VII collagen are the most antigenic sections. Type VII collagen is the main component of the anchoring fibrils found within the dermis. The antibodies that have been found are in the IgG subclass. They activate complement, which results in inflammation and destruction of the anchoring fibrils, eventually leading to fractures within the dermal-epidermal junction and, ultimately, to blistering. The etiology of antibody formation is not fully understood.

Histology: Biopsy specimens of EBA show a cell-poor subepidermal blister. The amount of inflammation is often minimal, but in some subtypes of the disease a lymphocytic infiltrate can be appreciated. The histologic differential diagnosis includes bullous pemphigoid, and only with immunostaining can the correct diagnosis be decisively made. Linear Ig and complement staining along the basement membrane are detected. With immunohistochemical staining for collagen IV, the main component of the lamina densa, the blistering can be localized to the plane above the lamina densa in bullous pemphigoid or below the lamina densa in EBA. The salt-split skin method has also been used to split skin through the lamina lucida by incubating the skin specimen in 1 M NaCl. Immunofluorescence staining of the split skin shows staining below the split in EBA and above the split in bullous pemphigoid in a serrated pattern.

Treatment: Therapy is difficult. Treatment of any underlying infection, autoimmune disease, or malignancy may help keep the blistering disease under control. Even with therapy, EBA tends to run a chronic waxing and waning course with frequent flares. Immunosuppressive agents have been used in EBA with varying success. Azathioprine, methotrexate, prednisone, IVIG, rituximab, mycophenolate mofetil, cyclosporine, and cyclophosphamide have all been used. Dapsone and colchicine have had anecdotal reports of success as well.

Supportive care is critical. Protection of the skin from trauma can help decrease blister formation. Early detection of infection and intervention to treat superinfection are critical. Even with all of the current treatment strategies that have been attempted for EBA, the disease tends not to enter remission and remains chronic in nature.

Formation and composition of collagen

Fibroblast, chondroblast, or osteoblast

Nucleus

Endoplasmic reticulum cistern

Ribosome

Cell membrane

Hydroxylation of certain prolyl and lysyl amino acid residues begins as pre-pro-α chains enter cistern. This requires vitamin C, Fe^2, O_2, and α-ketoglutarate.

Glycosylation involves enzymatic addition of galactose to certain hydroxylysine residues by galactosyltransferase.

Three pro-α chains assemble into triple helix, bonded by OH groups.

Golgi apparatus

Disulfide bonds

Procollagen released to extracellular space by pinocytosis

Terminal propeptides split off by procollagen peptidase

Collagen

Assembly into fibrils (quarter staggered)
Cross-links formed under influence of lysyl oxidase and copper

Gal galactose
Glc glucose
Gly glycine

Structure of α chains

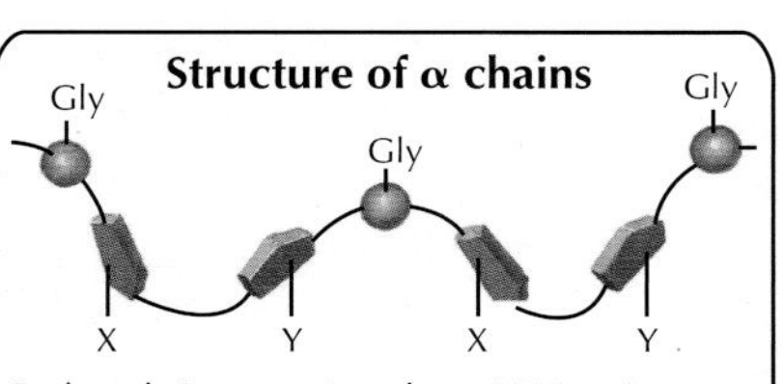

Each α chain comprises about 1000 amino acids. Every third amino acid in chain is glycine, smallest of amino acids. Glycine has no side chains, which thus permits a tight coil. X and Y here indicate other amino acids (X often proline; Y often hydroxyproline). Proline and hydroxyproline, respectively, constitute about 10% and 25% of total amino acids in each α chain.

Types of collagen
(based on a chain composition of fibrils)

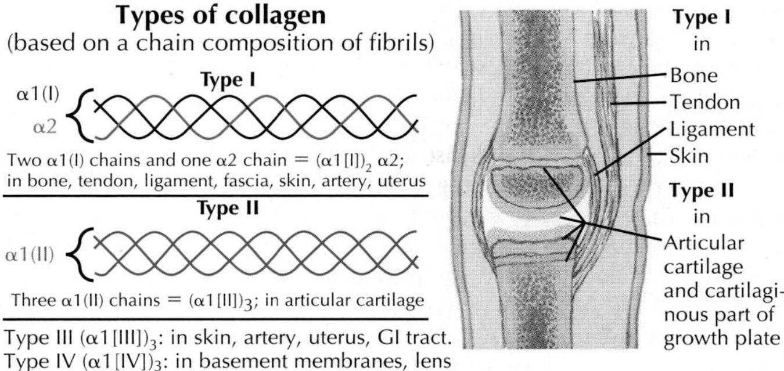

Type III $(\alpha 1[III])_3$: in skin, artery, uterus, GI tract.
Type IV $(\alpha 1[IV])_3$: in basement membranes, lens capsule. Type V $(\alpha B)_3$ or $(\alpha B)_2\ \alpha A$: in basement membranes, other tissues. At least 12 different collagen molecules have been identified.

Types of Collagen and Main Locations

Type	Main Location	Type	Main Location
Type I	Dermis, other tissue (most common form)	Type XII*	Dermis around hair follicles
Type II	Hyaline cartilage	Type XIII	Cell-to-cell adhesion
Type III	Skin and vascular tissue, fetal dermis	Type XIV*	Dermis, cornea
Type IV	Lamina densa of basement membrane zone	Type XV	Basement membrane zone
Type V	Found in association with type I collagen	Type XVI*	Dermis, cartilage
Type VI	Cartilage, dermis	Type XVII	BP180
Type VII	Anchoring fibrils	Type XVIII	Basement membrane zone
Type VIII	Vascular tissue, eye	Type XIX*	Basement membrane zone
Type IX*	Articular cartilage	Type XX *	Unknown
Type X	Cartilage	Type XXI*	Extracellular vascular wall matrix
Type XI	Cartilage		

*FACIT collagen, fibril-associated collagens with interrupted triple helices.

Linear Immunoglobulin A Bullous Dermatosis

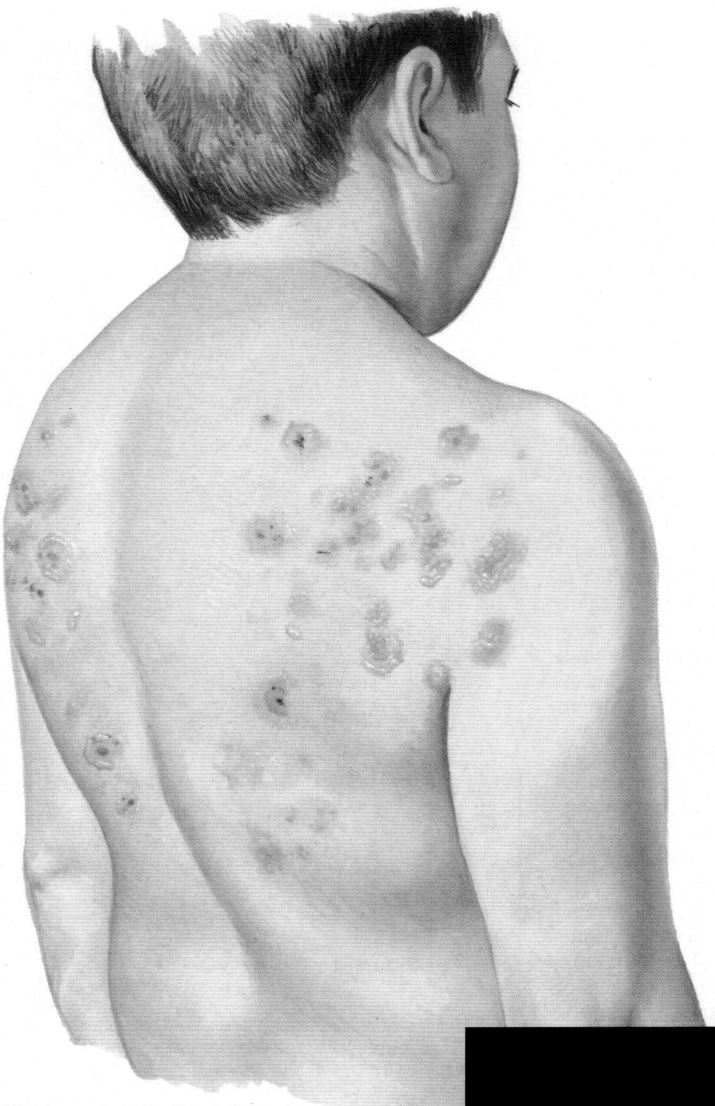

Linear IgA bullous dermatosis is an infrequently encountered autoimmune blistering disease that was originally described in 1979. This disease has a characteristic immunofluorescence staining pattern that is used to differentiate it histologically from other blistering diseases such as dermatitis herpetiformis. As the name implies, linear IgA is deposited along the length of the dermal-epidermal junction. Chronic bullous disease of childhood is considered by most to be the same disease, although there are a few clinical differences in age at onset and associations that can be used to justify separating them into two distinct, albeit very similar, entities. Most cases of chronic bullous dermatosis of childhood are idiopathic, whereas most cases of linear IgA bullous dermatosis are drug induced and occur in an older population.

Clinical Findings: Linear IgA bullous dermatosis is rare and is estimated to occur in 1 of every 2 million people. There is no race or sex predilection. It occurs most frequently in the adult population. The blistering disease has an insidious onset with small vesicles that may mimic dermatitis herpetiformis. The blisters are pruritic and do not have the same burning sensation as occurs in dermatitis herpetiformis, nor is there any relationship to dietary intake. The bullae in linear IgA bullous dermatosis are characteristically arranged in a "string of sausages" configuration. Each bulla is elongated and tapers to an end, with a small area of intervening normal-appearing skin before the tapered beginning of a new bulla. This string can be linear or annular in orientation. The blisters are tense and eventually rupture and heal with minimal scarring. Mucous membrane involvement is frequently seen and can resemble that of mucous membrane pemphigoid.

Chronic bullous disease of childhood manifests in early childhood (age 4–5 years). Although rare, this is the most common form of autoimmune blistering disease in children. The blistering is similar to that of linear IgA bullous dermatosis, and the histologic findings are identical. Blistering in chronic bullous disease of childhood is more often localized to the abdomen and lower extremities but may occur anywhere on the skin; it also commonly affects mucous membranes. Chronic bullous disease of childhood is most often idiopathic, whereas linear IgA bullous dermatosis can also be seen in association with the use of underlying medications, malignancies, or other autoimmune conditions. Many medications have been implicated in causing linear IgA bullous dermatosis, with vancomycin being the most common by far.

Pathogenesis: The exact target antigen in linear IgA bullous dermatosis is unknown. It is speculated that the IgA antibodies are directed against a small region of BP180. Other possible antigens exist and have been localized to the lamina lucida and lamina densa regions of the basement membrane. The reason for formation of these antibodies and how certain medications induce them are unknown. Once present, the antibodies target the BMZ and cause inflammation by various mechanisms, ultimately leading to disruption of the dermal-epidermal junction and blistering.

Histology: The immunofluorescence staining pattern is characteristic and shows linear IgA all along the BMZ. This is highly specific and sensitive for the diagnosis of linear IgA bullous dermatosis and chronic bullous disease of childhood. Routine hematoxylin and eosin staining demonstrates a subepidermal blister with an underlying neutrophilic infiltrate. This can be impossible to distinguish from dermatitis herpetiformis or bullous lupus, so immunostaining is required.

Treatment: The first line of therapy is dapsone. Patients respond quickly to this medication. Low doses of dapsone are usually all that is needed. Alternative substitutes for dapsone include sulfapyridine and colchicine. Oral prednisone can be helpful initially, but because of the long-term side effects, patients should be transitioned to one of the other medications mentioned. Drug-induced variants of this blistering disease are best treated by recognizing the common culprits and removing them immediately. Over a period of a few weeks, most patients who have discontinued the offending medication return to a normal state. If the disease is found to be associated with an underlying malignancy or other autoimmune condition, therapy with dapsone is warranted. Treatment of the underlying condition should also be undertaken. If the malignancy or the associated disease is put into remission, there is a good possibility that the blistering disease will remit as well.

Characteristic bullae of linear IgA disease, or chronic bullous disease of childhood. They are configured in an annular manner with small areas of intervening normal skin.

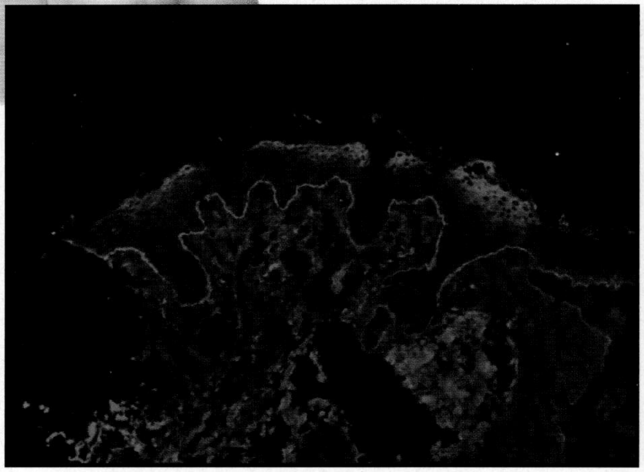

C. Machado M.D.
DaVanzo CMI

Linear deposition of IgA along the basement membrane zone

PARANEOPLASTIC PEMPHIGUS

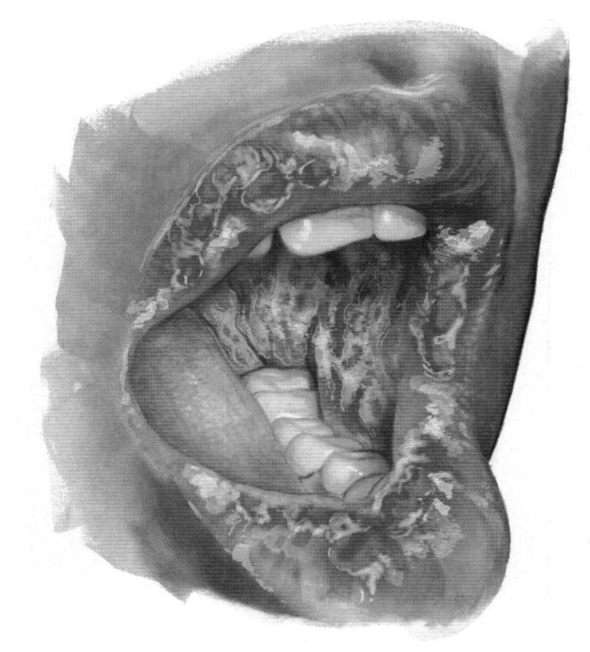

Severe involvement of the oral mucosa is the hallmark of paraneoplastic pemphigus.

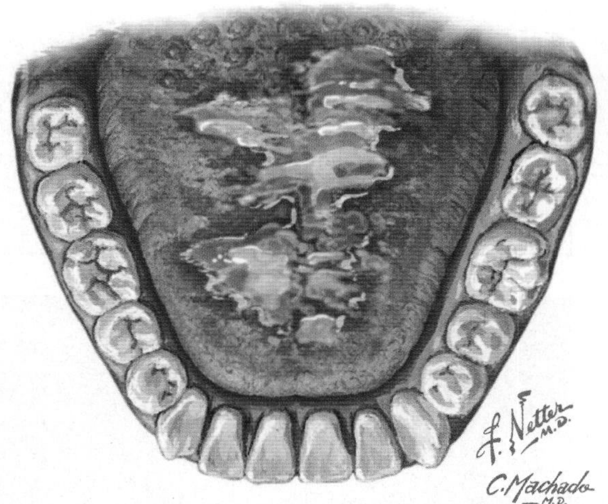

Diffuse erosions on the tongue

Antibodies Found in Paraneoplastic Pemphigus
BP230
BP180
Desmoglein 1
Desmoglein 3
Desmoplakin 1
Desmoplakin 2
Envoplakin
Periplakin
Plectin
Associations with Paraneoplastic Pemphigus
Hematologic malignancies (85% of cases)
Non-Hodgkin lymphoma
Hodgkin lymphoma
Chronic lymphocytic leukemia
Lymph node hyperplasia
Castleman disease
Solid tumors (15% of cases)
Thymoma
Sarcomas—predominantly retroperitoneal location
Adenocarcinoma
Breast
Pancreas
Lung
Prostate
Colon
Squamous cell carcinoma
Oral cavity
Melanoma

Paraneoplastic pemphigus was not described until the early 1990s. It is a rare subset of the pemphigus family of diseases that is associated with the synchronous occurrence of a systemic neoplastic process. The neoplastic disease may precede the diagnosis of paraneoplastic pemphigus. This disease has been differentiated from other forms of pemphigus by its unique antibody profile and staining patterns. Most cases have occurred secondary to hematologic malignancy, but solid tumors have also been seen with paraneoplastic pemphigus.

Clinical Findings: Paraneoplastic pemphigus is most likely to occur in the older population, usually during the fifth to eighth decades of life. It has also been reported to occur in young children with neoplastic disease. There is no sex or race predilection. Most patients develop paraneoplastic pemphigus after the diagnosis of an internal malignancy or at the same time as their diagnosis.

The oral mucosa is almost always the first mucocutaneous surface to be affected. Severe erosions and ulcerations occur throughout the oropharynx. This leads to significant pain and difficulty eating. Patients avoid eating because of the severe, unremitting pain. Weight loss and blistering, in combination with the underlying malignancy, result in a severe, life-threatening illness. The hallmark of this disease is the severe oral mucous membrane involvement. In fact, if the patient does not have oral involvement, the diagnosis of paraneoplastic pemphigus should be reevaluated, and the patient most likely has another form of pemphigus. Soon after the onset of oral disease, the patient's skin begins to break out in vesicles and flaccid bullae. These blisters are identical to those seen in pemphigus vulgaris. Histologically, there are some subtle differences in immunofluorescence.

The bullae can spread, and large surface areas of skin may become involved. Other clinical morphologies of skin disease have been described, including an erythema multiforme–like eruption, a pemphigoid-like eruption, and a lichenoid eruption that can mimic both graft-versus-host disease and lichen planus. These variants are infrequently seen. The combination of paraneoplastic pemphigus and an underlying malignancy has led to poor outcomes; this condition can be refractory and very difficult to treat. The diagnosis is made by consistent clinical features in a patient with an underlying malignancy who also has serum autoantibodies against certain proteins, most frequently the plakin family of proteins.

Some individuals will develop bronchiolitis obliterans, which can be a life-threatening pulmonary disease.

Pathogenesis: Paraneoplastic pemphigus is caused by circulating autoantibodies directed against various intercellular keratinocyte proteins. The most commonly found antibodies are directed against the plakin family of proteins, which include envoplakin and periplakin. Many other autoantibodies have also been found. It is theorized that the underlying neoplasm stimulates the cellular and humoral immune systems to form these autoantibodies. The exact mechanism by which the tumor causes this to occur is unclear.

Histology: Acantholysis is the main histologic feature on routine staining. Varying amounts of keratinocyte necrosis are also appreciated. The blister forms within the intraepidermal space. Routine staining cannot differentiate among the various members of the pemphigus family of diseases. Direct immunofluorescence staining in these diseases shows a fishnet staining pattern caused by intercellular hemidesmosomal keratinocyte staining.

Paraneoplastic pemphigus is much more likely than any of the other pemphigus diseases to have a positive indirect immunofluorescence staining pattern when rat bladder epithelium is used, whereas it is routinely negative when monkey esophagus epithelium is used. The opposite pattern is seen with most other types of pemphigus. Enzyme-linked immunosorbent assay looking for antibodies directed against periplakin and envoplakin has shown good sensitivity and specificity for the diagnosis of paraneoplastic pemphigus. The unique histologic and immunofluorescence staining patterns seen in paraneoplastic pemphigus can lead to the diagnosis. Immunoblotting may also be done and has been shown to have a very high specificity.

Treatment: Therapy needs to be directed at the underlying neoplastic process. The overall outcome is poor. Supportive care to prevent superinfection of the skin is imperative. Immunosuppressants are used to help decrease the blistering, but they may have deleterious effects on the underlying neoplasm. If the underlying neoplasm can be cured, there is a better chance that this disease will go into remission, although this does not always happen. Corticosteroids, azathioprine, IVIG, rituximab, plasmapheresis, bone marrow transplantation, and a host of other therapies have been used.

PEMPHIGUS FOLIACEUS

Pemphigus foliaceus is a chronic autoimmune blistering disease. Pemphigus foliaceus can be seen in an isolated form or as an endemic form termed *fogo selvagem*. These diseases are caused by autoantibody production against desmosomal proteins. The endemic form of the disease is seen in small regions in rural South America, predominantly in Brazil. Pemphigus foliaceus is closely related to pemphigus vulgaris, and in some cases the clinical picture and antibody profile can shift from one disease to the other, leading to difficulty in classification.

Clinical Findings: Pemphigus foliaceus is a rare disease that most frequently affects patients who are about 50 years of age. There is no sex or race predilection. Blistering of the skin is prominent and can affect large body surface areas. The blisters tend to be more superficial than those of pemphigus vulgaris. The blisters are rarely found intact because of their superficial and fragile nature. Mucous membranes are rarely affected because the mucocutaneous surfaces do not contain high concentrations of the desmoglein 1 protein. Patients exhibit a positive Nikolsky sign. This sign is positive when exertion of pressure (rubbing) induces a blister or erosion on nonaffected skin.

Fogo selvagem (Portuguese for "wildfire") affects a younger population. It is believed to be transmitted by the bite of the black fly or the mosquito in patients who are susceptible to the disease. It has been postulated that the bite begins a cascade of immune system antibody production, resulting in formation of the pathogenic antibodies against desmoglein 1. An infectious agent transmitted by the flies has not been discovered. Antidesmoglein 1 antibodies have been shown to cross-react with sandfly saliva proteins. A fair percentage of patients have a family member who is also affected, which provides some clinical evidence for a genetic predisposition to the disease. The disease exhibits photosensitivity in the ultraviolet B range.

Indirect immunofluorescence testing of the patient's serum shows autoantibodies against desmoglein 1.

Pathogenesis: Abnormal antibody production is directed against the desmoglein 1 protein, which is a critical component of the desmosomal attachment between adjacent keratinocytes. Desmoglein 1 is found predominantly in the superficial epidermis. Desmoglein 3 is found deeper within the epidermis. Desmogleins are calcium-dependent adhesion proteins known as *cadherins*. As the autoantibodies attach to the desmoglein protein and are deposited within the epidermis, they activate complement. Complement activation, along with the cytotoxic effects of lymphocytes, leads to acantholysis of keratinocytes and the eventual blistering of the epidermis. The hemidesmosome is unaffected, and the basilar layer of keratinocytes stays attached to the BMZ.

Histology: The histologic findings of pemphigus foliaceus and its endemic form, fogo selvagem, are identical. Intraepidermal blistering is caused by acantholysis. The acantholysis is most prominent in the upper epidermis, usually starting in the granular cell layer and above. Typically, a mixed inflammatory infiltrate is seen within the dermis. Varying amounts of crust and superficial bacteria are seen in areas of chronic erosion. Immunofluorescence staining shows a fishnet pattern of intercellular staining with IgG and complement.

Treatment: Because mucous membrane involvement is almost nonexistent and the blistering is more superficial, the course of pemphigus foliaceus is typically less severe than that of pemphigus vulgaris; however, this is not always the case. Therapy is directed toward decreasing the antibody formation. Immunosuppressants are the mainstay of therapy, and combinations are occasionally required to get the disease under control. Oral corticosteroids are typically the first medications used, along with a steroid-sparing agent. Azathioprine, mycophenolate mofetil, cyclophosphamide, and rituximab have all been used with varying success. IVIG and dapsone are other options. Use of the nonimmunosuppressive agents tetracycline and nicotinamide has shown variable success. The same can be said of hydroxychloroquine. The treatment of pemphigus foliaceus requires chronic therapy because this is a chronically relapsing and remitting disease. Supportive care is required to avoid excessive trauma and friction to the skin as well as to avoid sun exposure, which can all induce blistering. Bacterial superinfection needs to be treated promptly.

Therapy for fogo selvagem is similar in many respects. The use of mosquito and fly control measures may be of help in the endemic regions because these insects are believed to be the vectors of transmission to susceptible humans.

Endemic locations

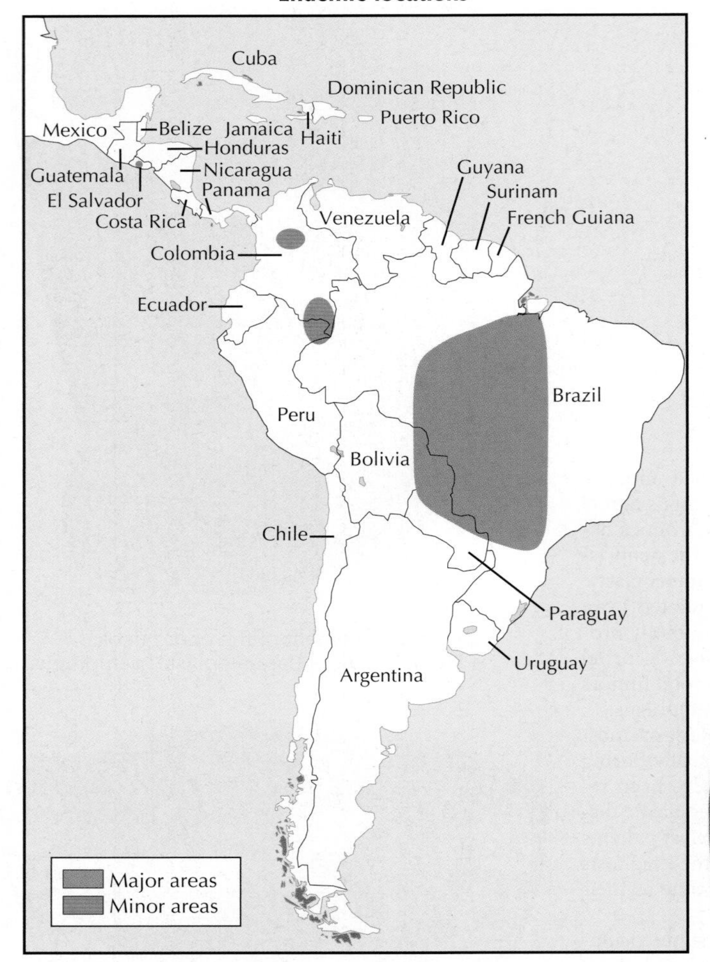

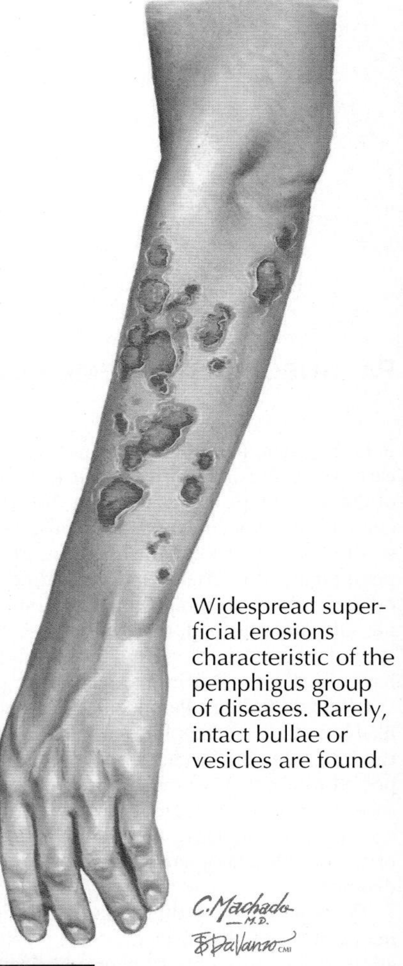

Widespread superficial erosions characteristic of the pemphigus group of diseases. Rarely, intact bullae or vesicles are found.

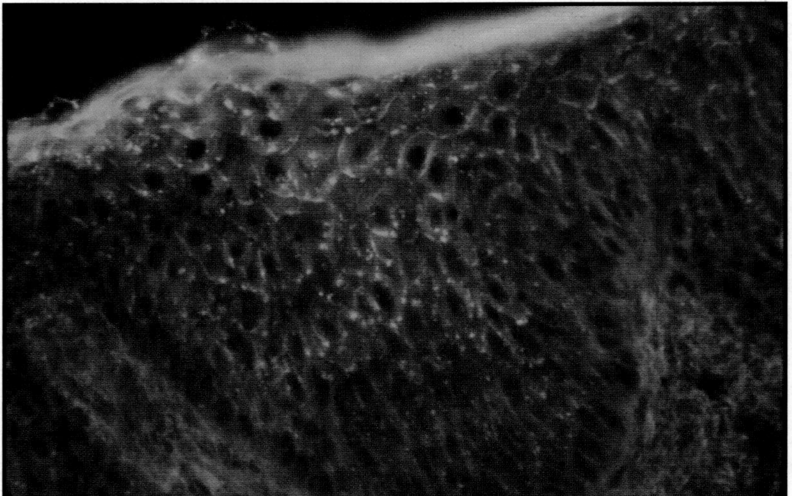

Direct immunofluorescence showing uniform staining between keratinocytes in the dermis. The antibody is directed against the desmoglein 1 protein.

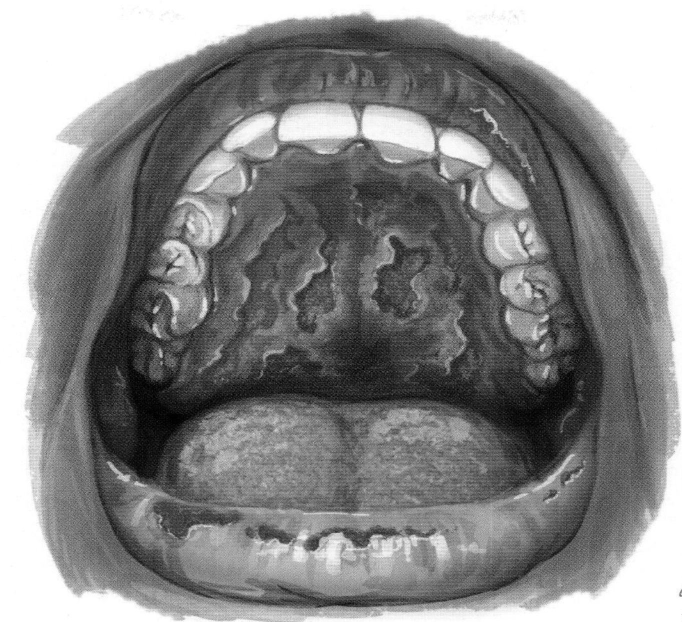

Oral erosions can be the first mucocutaneous sign of the disease pemphigus vulgaris.

Pemphigus Variants

- Pemphigus vulgaris
- Pemphigus foliaceus
- Endemic pemphigus
- Pemphigus erythematosus
- Paraneoplastic pemphigus
- Pemphigus vegetans
- IgA pemphigus

Blister formation via acantholysis is the hallmark histologic finding in pemphigus vulgaris.

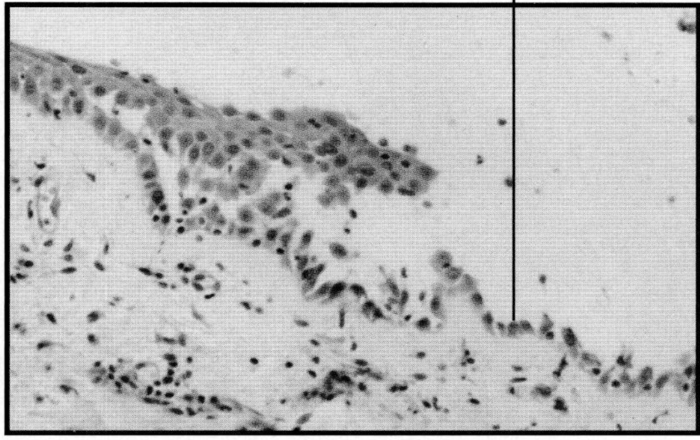

Pemphigus vulgaris. Severe acantholysis with "tombstoning" along the basement membrane zone (BMZ). This is caused by uninvolved hemidesmosomes, which adhere the basilar keratinocytes to the BMZ.

PEMPHIGUS VULGARIS

Pemphigus vulgaris is the prototypical acantholytic autoimmune blistering disease. It is one of the most serious of all blistering diseases. Blister formation in this subset of skin diseases occurs secondary to intraepidermal acantholysis. The desmosomal plaque is the target of the autoantibodies found in this disease.

Clinical Findings: The mean age at onset is approximately 55 years. Patients present with rapid onset of vesicles and bullae that rupture easily. The flaccid bullae are rarely found intact. The disease often begins within the oral cavity, and the oral lesions can either precede the skin disease or occur independently of skin manifestations. Vesicles and bullae are almost never seen in the oral cavity because the blisters in pemphigus are superficial and rupture almost immediately after they are formed. The oral erosions are excruciatingly painful and are frequently misdiagnosed as a herpes simplex infection. Often, it is not until the erosions become chronic that the diagnosis of pemphigus is entertained. Patients eventually avoid eating because of the pain, and they often complain of weight loss, fatigue, and malaise.

If skin lesions are also present, the diagnosis can be made with more confidence based on the clinical findings. However, a biopsy must be performed to rule out the other pemphigus variants. Paraneoplastic pemphigus always starts in the mouth and tends to be much more severe and refractory to therapy than pemphigus vulgaris. This diagnosis should be considered in a patient who has a coexisting malignancy and treatment-refractory disease. Immunoblotting is a specific test to look for the exact autoantibody present in paraneoplastic pemphigus; it can be performed in highly specialized laboratories. In pemphigus vulgaris, indirect immunofluorescence almost always shows a high titer against desmoglein 3. The antibody titer correlates with the disease activity, and titers have been monitored to assess the treatment of the disease. Pruritus is uncommon in patients with pemphigus; the overwhelming complaint is skin pain. If left untreated, the disease is progressive and carries a mortality rate of 60% to 65%.

The skin blisters of pemphigus vulgaris rupture early in the course of their formation. The remaining erosions can become quite large, however. Weeping of serous fluid occurs, and bleeding from the erosions can also be seen. Secondary superinfection is common and may cause an increase in autoantibody production.

Pathogenesis: Pemphigus vulgaris is a chronic autoimmune blistering disease in which autoantibodies are directed against the desmosomal plaque. The desmosomal plaque is the most crucial element that holds adjacent keratinocytes in place and juxtaposed to one another. There are other intercellular connections between keratinocytes, including gap junctions, adherens junctions, and tight junctions. The desmosomal plaque is composed of various proteins that act to connect the intracellular actin cytoskeleton of one keratinocyte to that of another; these include various desmoglein, desmocollin, desmoplakin, plakophilin, and plakoglobin proteins. The central portion of the desmosome contains the proteins desmoglein and desmocollin. They are responsible for the tight binding of adjacent keratinocytes. There are many members in each of the desmoglein and desmocollin families.

Autoantibodies to the desmoglein family of proteins, specifically desmoglein 3, are responsible for the formation of pemphigus vulgaris. Antibodies against desmoglein 1 have also been found in patients with pemphigus vulgaris and pemphigus foliaceous.

Histology: Skin biopsies of pemphigus vulgaris display intraepidermal blister formation. The blisters are formed by acantholysis, and keratinocytes appear to be free-floating within the blister cavity. "Tombstoning" may be present. This is the designation given to basilar keratinocytes that stay attached to the BMZ by their unaffected hemidesmosomes. The basilar keratinocytes appear to be standing up in a row, mimicking tombstones. Immunofluorescence demonstrates IgG staining in a fishnet pattern throughout the epidermis. Each intercellular connection between keratinocytes is highlighted.

Treatment: Appropriate therapy must be instituted as soon as the diagnosis is made. Oral corticosteroids in conjunction with intravenous rituximab have become the first-line therapy. Many immunosuppressive medications have been used to treat pemphigus vulgaris. The more common ones are azathioprine, methotrexate, mycophenolate mofetil, cyclophosphamide, and cyclosporine. IVIG and dapsone are other therapeutic options. Morbidity and mortality have been dramatically reduced since the introduction of steroids and steroid-sparing agents.

SECTION 6

INFECTIOUS DISEASES

Actinomycosis

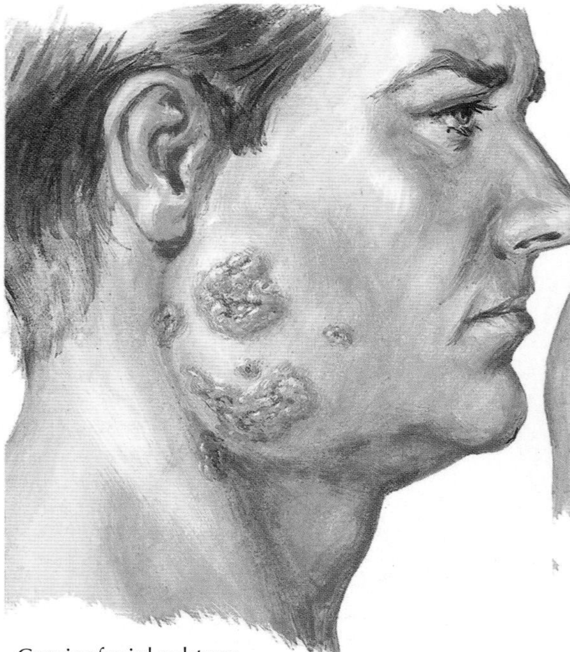

Many species of the bacterial genus *Actinomyces* cause disease in humans. The infection tends to run a chronic course that leads to suppurative granulomatous abscesses in the skin. The diagnosis may be suspected if there is clinical evidence of painful draining of suppurative material and histologic evidence of granuloma formation. The exact diagnosis is based on tissue culture or culture of the suppurative material. These infections are frequently polymicrobial in nature. The disease is progressive if appropriate therapy is not instituted. The organisms responsible for these infections are normally found within the oral cavity and are commensal organisms. They can also be found throughout the gastrointestinal tract.

Clinical Findings: Males are much more likely to develop this infection than females, with an estimated ratio of 3:1. Most patients are between 30 and 50 years of age. Predisposing factors include poor dental hygiene. The infection is believed to be endogenous in origin. It is a rare infection in the United States. There are several clinical pictures of actinomycosis. The most common form seen is the cervicofacial subtype, which accounts for more than 50% of cases. It is related to oral trauma, such as recent dental work. The area that has been traumatized provides a portal of entry for the bacteria, and there is a progressive induration of the underlying tissue. With time, the firm swelling begins to break through the skin and drain through multiple cutaneous fistulas. Pain can be intense and is relieved as the fistulas spontaneously drain. The designation "lumpy jaw" signifies the induration and fistula formation seen in patients with actinomycosis cervicofacial disease.

The next most prevalent form of the disease is the pulmonary form. This is believed to be caused by aspiration of the causative bacteria. Patients often report hemoptysis and low-grade fever. Chest radiographs can show features similar to those of tuberculosis infections. Any lobe of the lung may be involved, but the right lower lobe is most frequently affected because the infection is caused by aspiration. If the disease goes unrecognized, sinus tracts eventually form through the lung lining, muscle, and skin to the thoracic cutaneous wall. Skin abscess and a draining sinus in this location suggest pulmonary involvement, including the development of empyema. Abdominal forms of the disease are believed to occur after trauma to the bowel. This has been reported most frequently after appendectomy, in which for unknown reasons the bacteria localize to that area. The last form of the disease is the disseminated form, which is rare and can occur after any form of the disease that is not appropriately treated. Any organ system may be involved.

Pathogenesis: Actinomycosis is caused by one of the gram-positive anaerobic filamentous bacteria of the *Actinomyces* genus: *A. israelii*, *A. turicensis*, *A. lingnae*, *A. graevenitzii*, *A. meyeri*, *A. naeslundii*, *A. radingae*, *A. europaeus*, *A. viscosus*, *A. neuii*, or *A. odontolyticus*. *A. israelii* is most frequently observed to cause disease. These are anaerobic, acid-fast bacteria that have a filamentous morphology with varying amounts of branching. The definitive diagnosis is made by culture of the organism.

Histology: Biopsy specimens show a suppurative granulomatous reaction pattern. Neutrophils, histiocytes, and lymphocytes make up the majority of the inflammatory infiltrate. Basophilic granules (sulfur granules) are surrounded by a predominantly neutrophilic infiltrate. The sulfur granules have a rich yellow color.

Anaerobic culture of the purulent material or a portion of the tissue is critical for proper identification of the responsible organism and ultimately for choosing the appropriate therapy. Material should be immediately sent anaerobically to the laboratory, although even in the best circumstances these are difficult-to-culture bacteria. Yellow to white sulfur granules form as the culture material grows. Evaluation of the sulfur granules with the use of an oil immersion microscope shows the filamentous bacteria. rRNA sequence analysis and mass spectrometry tests have been shown to be helpful in identifying species of bacteria.

Treatment: The drug of choice to treat this bacterial infection is penicillin. Therapy needs to be maintained for months to be certain of complete cure. Abscesses should be incised and drained surgically. If the infection is treated promptly, almost all patients have a full and complete recovery.

Cervicofacial subtype of actinomycosis ("lumpy jaw")

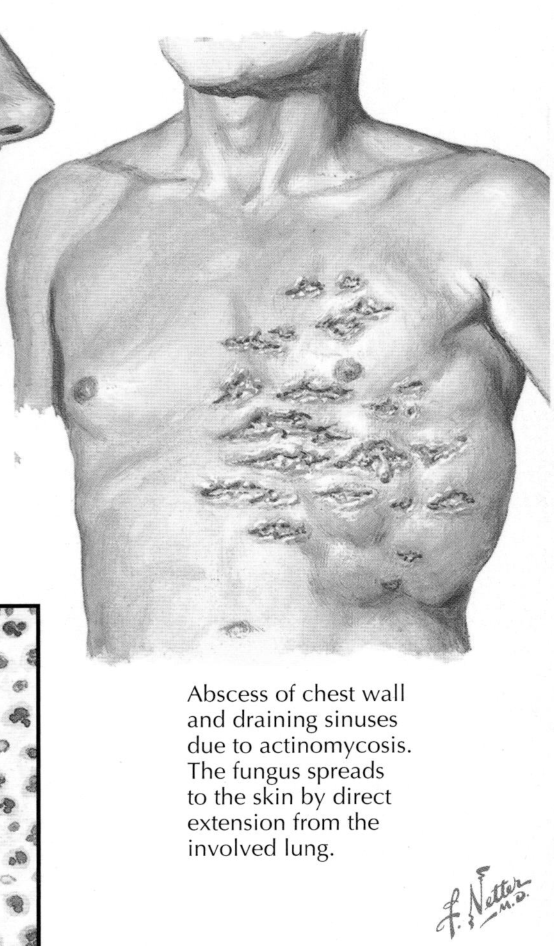

Abscess of chest wall and draining sinuses due to actinomycosis. The fungus spreads to the skin by direct extension from the involved lung.

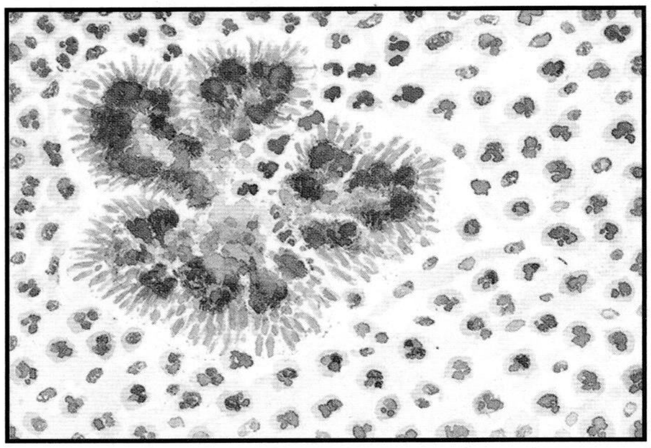

The "ray fungus" as it appears in H&E-stained tissue section with surrounding neutrophilic infiltrate

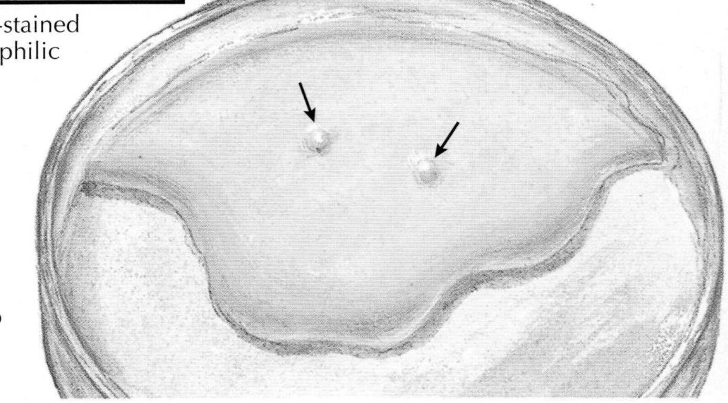

Pus in a Petri dish showing two sulfur granules (small lumps indicated by *arrows*)

BLASTOMYCOSIS

Blastomycosis is a fungal infection found predominantly in North America. This disease is also known as *North American blastomycosis* or *Gilchrist disease*. However, because it has also been reported in Central and South America, the preferred name of this disease is *blastomycosis*. It is endemic in the areas of the United States and Canada that border the Great Lakes, the Saint Lawrence Riverway, and the Mississippi River Valley. The highest number of cases have been reported from Wisconsin and Ontario. The infection is common in other mammals such as dogs. Dogs have been found to have an incident rate nearly 10 times that of humans. Most cases are isolated and sporadic in nature; however, outbreaks of the infection have occurred in which many people who came into contact with the same environmental source were infected.

Clinical Findings: The organism is first inhaled into the lungs, where it quickly reverts to its yeast state. Most infections are controlled by the local immune response, and minimal to no symptoms occur. The disease most frequently stays localized within the pulmonary system. It can, however, spread to any other organ system in an immunosuppressed host. After the conidia (spores) are inhaled, the most frequent symptoms are coughing, fever, pleurisy, weight loss, malaise, arthralgias, and hemoptysis. The symptoms may initially mimic those of an influenza infection. Approximately half of patients with symptomatic disease have only pulmonary findings; the other half have both pulmonary and other organ system findings. Traumatic implantation of the fungus directly into the skin has also been shown to cause disease.

Cutaneous findings are nonspecific and have been classified as verrucous or ulcerative. The verrucous lesions can range from small papules and plaques to large nodules with sinus tract formation. The central face and nose are common locations of involvement. Ulcerated lesions can occur anywhere and are associated with underlying abscess formation and drainage. The skin lesions can mimic those of skin cancers, and biopsy is required to make the appropriate diagnosis.

Pathogenesis: Blastomycosis is directly caused by infection with the dimorphic fungus *B. dermatitidis*. This organism inhabits soil and vegetation in its mold or mycelial form. When the environment that contains the fungus is disrupted, the spores of this fungus may gain entry into a human (or other mammal) by direct inoculation or by inhalation. Once the fungus has entered the human body, the increase in temperature causes it to convert to its yeast form. The yeast form is not contagious, and the human acts as a host for reproduction but is unable to transmit the disease to any other human. The normal host is able to contain the inhaled spores within alveolar macrophages and granulomas in the lung, but the yeast form of the fungus is much more resistant to killing by natural host responses. If the host is immunocompromised, the fungus may disseminate to other organs, particularly the cutaneous surface. Dissemination occurs via vascular spread of the yeast organisms.

Histology: Biopsies of blastomycosis show pseudoepitheliomatous hyperplasia of the epidermis. Within the dermis is a granulomatous infiltrate of predominantly noncaseating granulomas. Neutrophils and macrophages are prominent. The yeast can be appreciated on routine hematoxylin and eosin (H&E) staining. They appear as oval cells with a thick, refractory wall. Often, broad-based budding is noted. This form of solitary broad-based budding is specific for *Blastomyces dermatitidis*. Other special stains can be used to better highlight the fungus, including the periodic acid–Schiff and silver stains.

The best means of diagnosing this fungal infection is by culture on Sabouraud medium. The mold begins to grow quickly and forms white to gray, waxy colonies. Special DNA probes can be used to quickly identify the fungus growing in the medium. Antigen testing is available for testing urine and other tissue samples.

Treatment: Prompt treatment with amphotericin B is the therapy of choice for those with disseminated or severe disease or any evidence of immunosuppression. Milder cases can be treated with prolonged courses of the azole antifungal agents; amphotericin B is used if the disease fails to respond to this treatment. Itraconazole and voriconazole are the two antifungal agents most frequently used, although other options are available. Before antifungal therapy was available, more than 80% of cases were fatal.

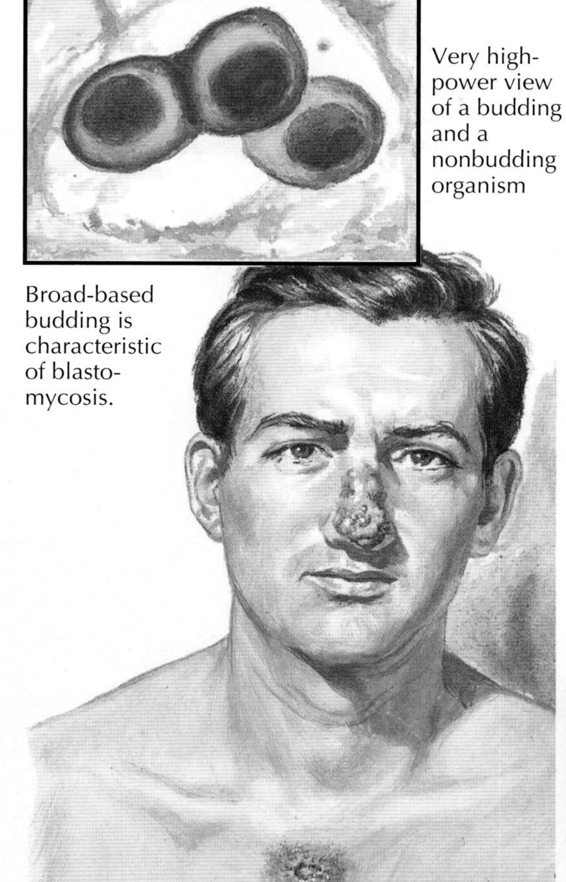

Very high-power view of a budding and a nonbudding organism

Broad-based budding is characteristic of blastomycosis.

Verrucous ulcerated plaques and nodules

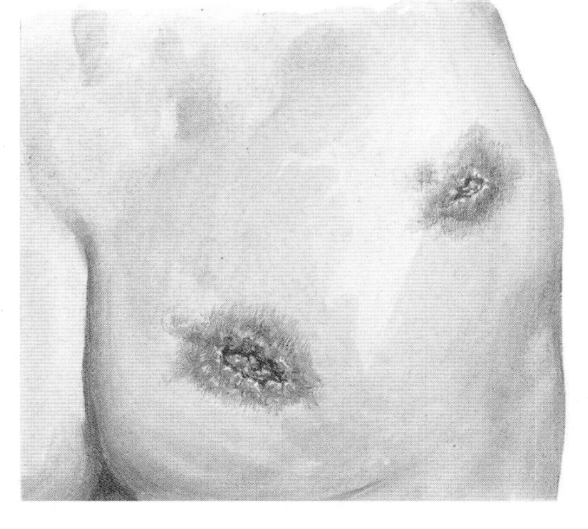

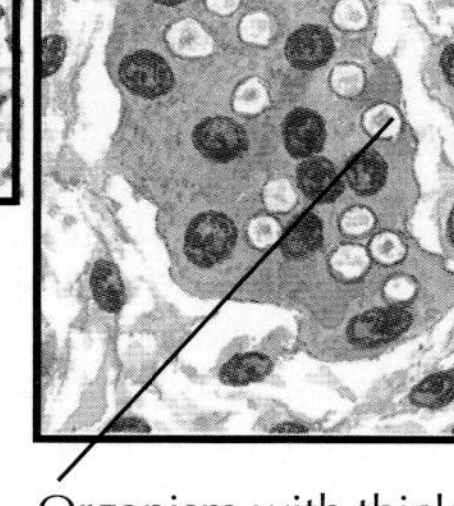

Granulomatous reaction with many giant cells containing organisms; high-power view *(inset)* of giant cell with organisms

Organism with thick, refractory cell wall

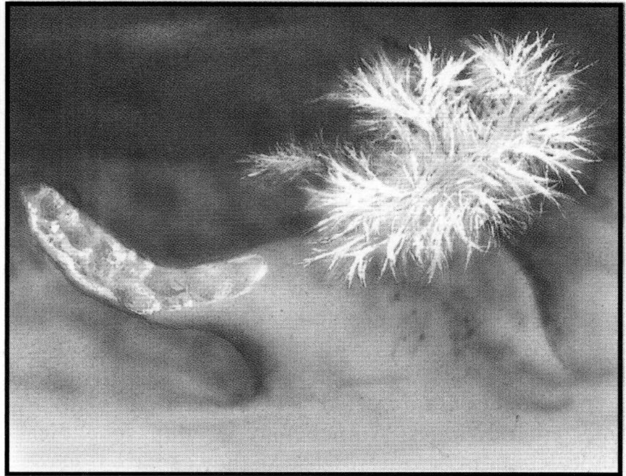

Organism in culture: free-living or infectious phase of *Blastomyces dermatitidis*. Sabouraud dextrose agar medium

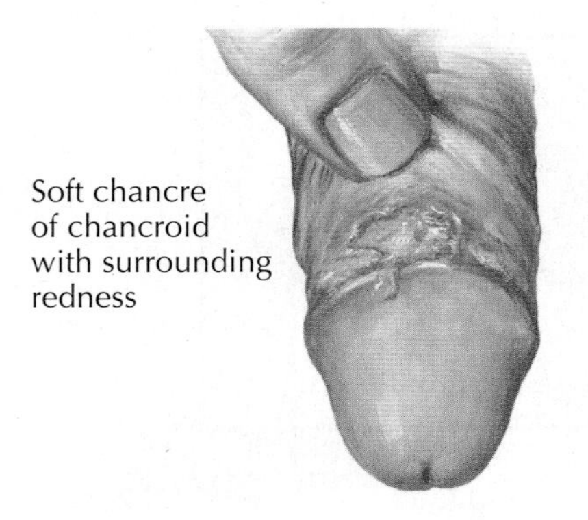

Soft chancre of chancroid with surrounding redness

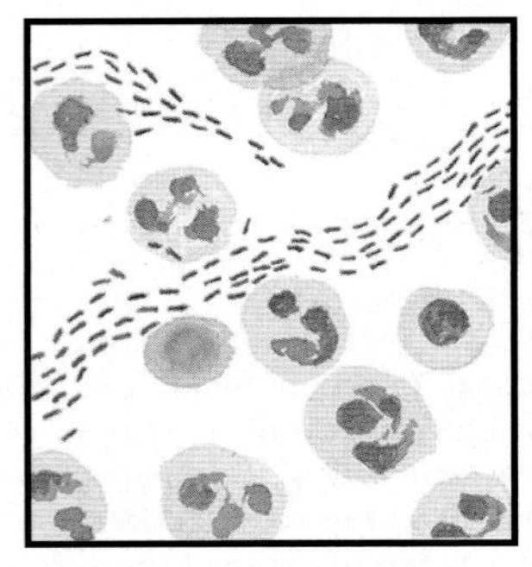

Haemophilus ducreyi in a "school of fish" pattern with surrounding neutrophils

CHANCROID

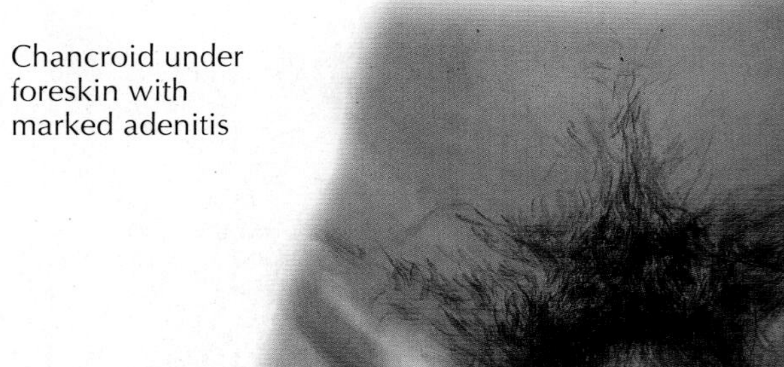

Chancroid under foreskin with marked adenitis

Swollen lymph nodes (buboes) can spontaneously drain to the skin surface.

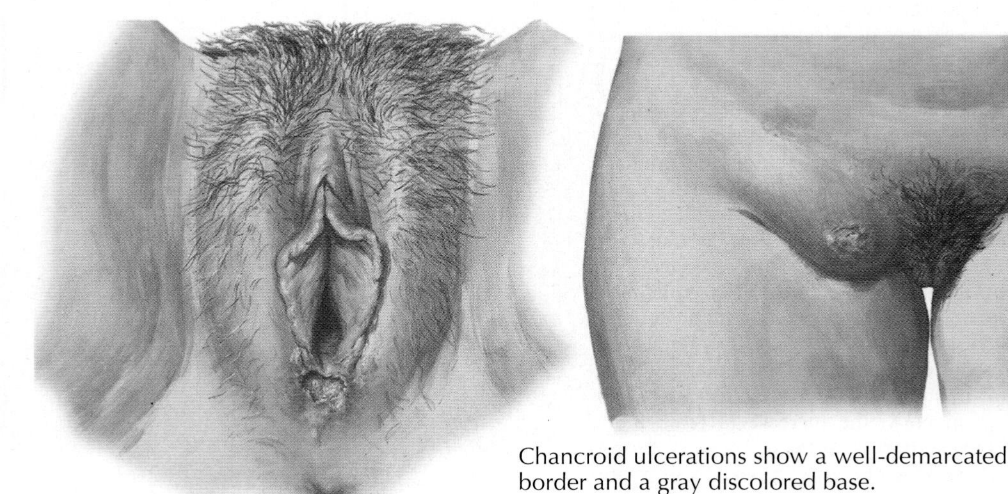

Chancroid ulcerations show a well-demarcated border and a gray discolored base.

Chancroid is a sexually transmitted infection (STI) caused by *Haemophilus ducreyi*. Infection with this bacterium is one of the most common causes of acute genital ulcerations in the world. Although it is most frequently encountered in Africa and Asia, it can be seen worldwide. Infection with this agent is frequently associated with other STIs. *H. ducreyi* infection has been shown to increase the likelihood of contracting human immunodeficiency virus (HIV) after exposure. Specialized serology testing and polymerase chain reaction (PCR) testing have been developed but are not commercially available. The diagnosis is based on the clinical history and physical exam in conjunction with the culture results.

Clinical Findings: *H. ducreyi* is transmitted via sexual contact, and the first sign of the disease is the formation of a papule at the site of inoculation. The papule occurs, on average, 3 to 5 days after exposure. The papule, which is often surrounded by a red halo, quickly turns into a vesiculopustule and then a painful ulceration. The ulcer is nonindurated and has undermined edges with a well-demarcated boundary. If left untreated, the ulcerations can become enormous and serpentine in appearance. The base of the ulcer has a gray appearance with granulation tissue present. The infection is associated with massive inguinal adenitis, termed *buboes*, in about 50% of cases. The disease is transmitted by unprotected sexual intercourse with an infected individual. Women may develop subclinical undetected disease, in which case they can act as carriers for transmission. Active disease is more frequently encountered in males, in a 4:1 ratio.

Pathogenesis: *H. ducreyi* is a gram-negative coccobacillus. The organism is transmitted from one human host to another by intimate physical contact. The bacterium requires a break in the integrity of the epidermis to gain entrance to the body. It then multiples locally and forms the initial papule, which soon becomes a pustule teeming with bacteria. Once the papulopustule ulcerates, the bacterial load is high and allows for further transmission. It has been shown that the bacteria can be shed from nonulcerated lesions. The formation of ulcerations on epidermis that opposes the original ulcer has been termed a "kissing ulcer" and is caused by direct autoinoculation of the bacteria. The bacteria cannot live long outside its human host, which can make it difficult to properly culture. Many virulence factors have been detected, including the cell surface lipooligosaccharide protein. The bacteria grow on chocolate agar culture medium.

Histology: A skin biopsy from the edge of the ulcer may be helpful in diagnosis. There are three zones of inflammation from superficial to deep. Zone 1 is the necrotic superficial tissue. The second zone is the largest and consists of a proliferation of freshly made blood vessels. The last zone is a deep layer consisting of an inflammatory infiltrate with many plasma cells. Detection of the bacteria is difficult on tissue biopsies unless the bacterial load is tremendous. If a high burden of bacteria is present, they may be seen on microscopy lined up in a "school of fish" pattern. This is rarely observed in skin biopsy specimens. Culturing of the bacteria is the best means to firmly make the diagnosis.

Treatment: Treatment can be accomplished with azithromycin, erythromycin, ceftriaxone, or ciprofloxacin. The clinician should also consider treating empirically for other STIs because they tend to congregate together. This is especially true of gonorrhea, which is often a coinfection with *H. ducreyi*. For some reason, the disease is more difficult to treat in patients who have a coexisting HIV infection. This may be because HIV-positive patients have a lowered cell-mediated immunity, and an intact cell-mediated immune system is needed to treat *H. ducreyi* infection. Surgical incision and drainage of fluctuant nodules should be considered as an adjunct to oral antibiotics. Drainage decreases the bacterial load and potentially makes antibiotic therapy more effective.

Coccidioidomycosis

Coccidioidomycosis, or Valley Fever, is endemic in the southwestern United States. Patients who breathe in spores (arthroconidia) from the fungus *Coccidioides immitis* or *C. posadasii* may become infected. Most patients do not develop active disease; instead, their exposure is confirmed by the presence of a positive delayed hypersensitivity test to the fungus. Primary cutaneous coccidioidomycosis is a rare entity caused by inoculation of the fungus directly into the skin. By far the most common form of cutaneous coccidioidomycosis is caused by dissemination to the skin from a primary pulmonary infection. The incidence in the United States has increased over the past 25 years.

Clinical Findings: This infection has a slightly increased incidence in the Black population. Males and females are equally affected. The incidence increases with age. Most individuals who inhale the spores do not develop active disease. Rather, the fungus lies dormant or trapped within pulmonary granulomas. About one-third of patients who are exposed to the fungus develop an acute pneumonitis. Fever, cough, malaise, and pleurisy are the main symptoms. The pneumonitis may be severe enough to bring the patient to the clinic to seek therapy, but many cases are mild and patients routinely dismiss the symptoms as the common cold. Reactivation later in life may occur secondary to acquired immunosuppression, pregnancy, or older age.

Cutaneous findings in coccidioidomycosis have a variable morphology. Papules, plaques, and nodules are the most frequent forms of disseminated coccidioidomycosis. These skin lesions have a predilection to affect the face and, in particular, the nasolabial skin fold. Multiple draining cutaneous abscesses with fistula and sinus formation can occur in late untreated disease. Chronic ulcerations have also been reported to be a manifestation of cutaneous disease.

Nonspecific skin findings attributed to fungal infection with *C. immitis* are well recognized. The best reported and most clearly associated finding is erythema nodosum. Erythema nodosum is a reaction that occurs in many internal and cutaneous disease states. Almost any deep fungal infection can induce erythema nodosum. Patients who have a history of travel to an endemic area should be screened for this fungal disease. Rarely, erythema multiforme and Sweet syndrome have been reported in association with coccidioidomycosis.

Pulmonary disease is almost always present and should be thoroughly searched for in patients presenting with cutaneous coccidioidomycosis. Chest radiographs may show many findings, including cavitary lesions, hilar adenopathy, pneumonitis, pleural effusions, and lobar disease.

Diagnosis is possible only by an appropriate tissue culture that shows growth of the causative fungus. The clinical examination and history are not as sensitive or specific as culture of the fungus. If there is a high index of suspicion for this disease, treatment should be instituted and then adjusted after the culture results become available.

Pathogenesis: Coccidioidomycosis is caused by the soil-dwelling fungi *C. immitis* or *C. posadasii*. Endemic to the Southwestern United States, Central America, and parts of South America, this fungus is found in the environment in its mycelial or mold phase. It produces white, light, and fluffy arthrospores. These arthrospores are highly infectious. Once inhaled, this dimorphic fungus turns into its yeast form. The yeast form is made of thick-walled spherules with multiple, centrally located endospores that can be released from the host by coughing or by drainage of an abscess. The resulting endospore readily converts back to its mycelial phase and can infect another host.

Histology: Punch biopsy or excisional biopsy specimens show a diffuse granulomatous inflammatory infiltrate. Pseudocarcinomatous epithelial hyperplasia often overlies the granulomatous infiltrate. Within the granulomatous portion of the dermal infiltrate are the characteristic spherules that contain endospores. The spherules are thick walled and can readily be seen on specimens routinely treated with H&E stain. The spherule can be highlighted with the use of a silver stain.

Treatment: The azole antifungals fluconazole and itraconazole are first-line therapies for coccidioidomycosis. Treatment typically lasts 6 to 12 months; prolonged therapy may be required in some cases. Voriconazole can also be used, but its higher side effect profile has limited its use to patients who do not respond to first-line therapy. Severe, life-threatening cases and those refractory to azole antifungal medications can also be treated with amphotericin B. Adjunctive surgical treatment can be used to debride abscesses and remove isolated pulmonary disease.

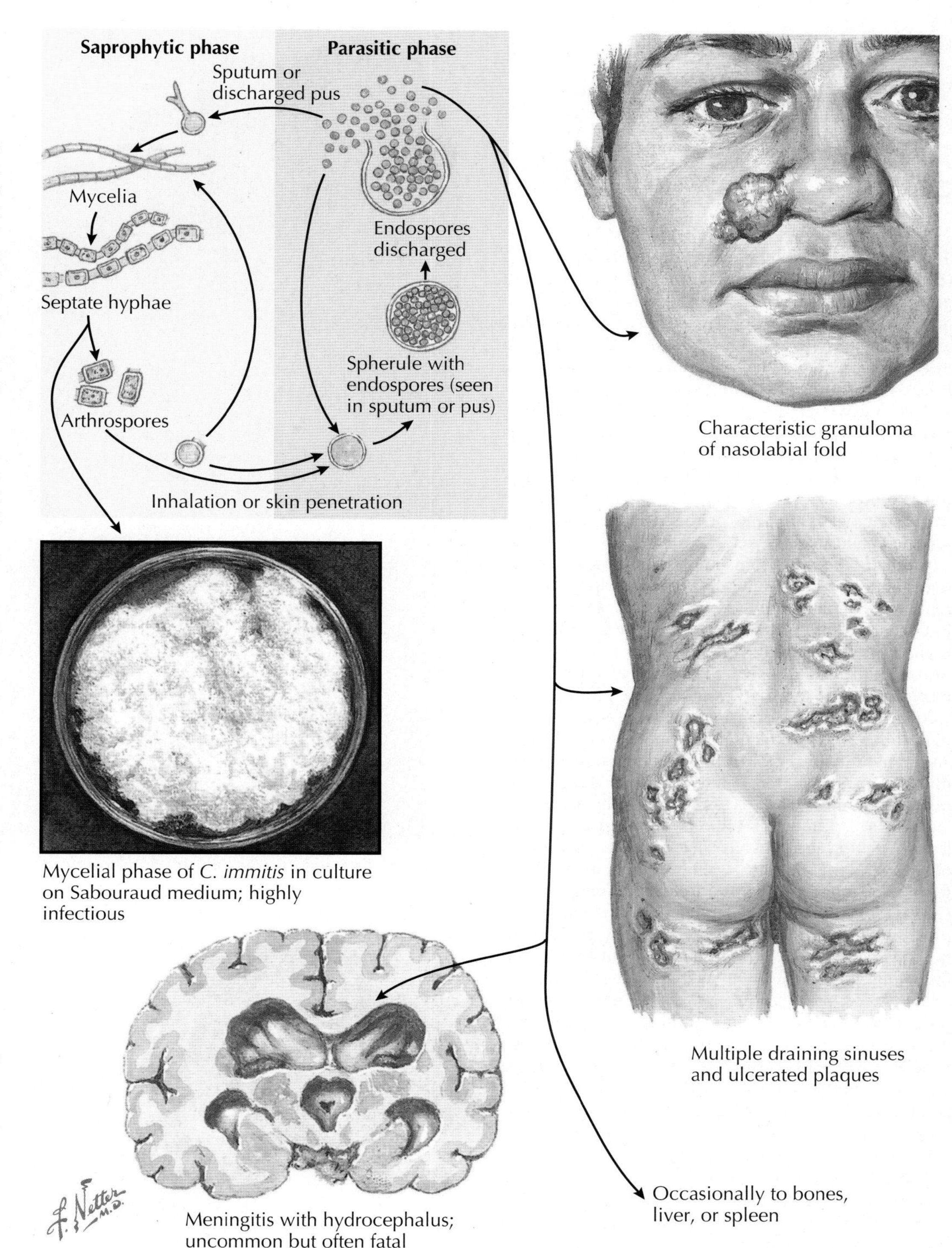

COVID-19

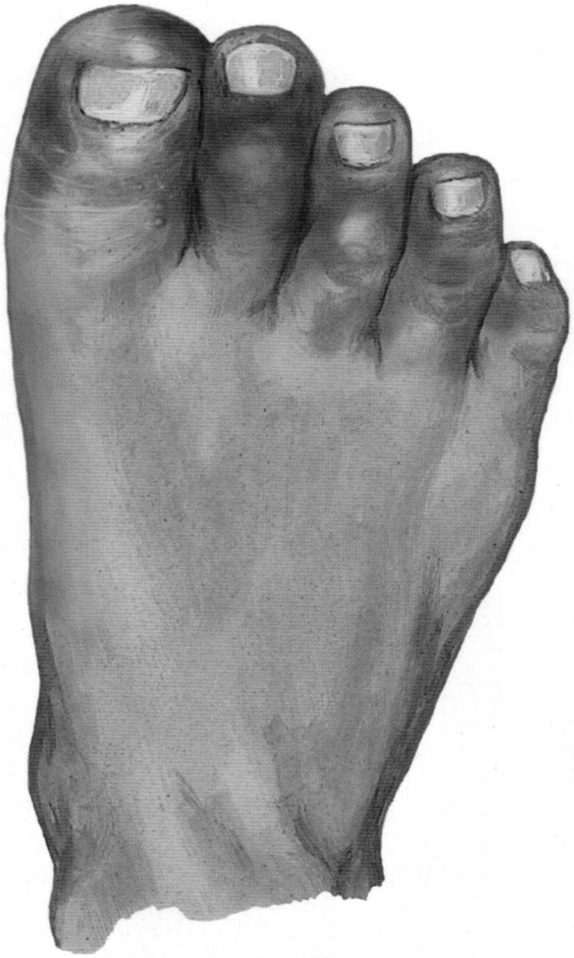

The severe acute respiratory syndrome coronavirus 2 (SARS-CoV-2) was first recognized in late 2019 and quickly spread worldwide, causing a significant pandemic resulting in millions of deaths. Coronaviruses are single-stranded RNA viruses with the ability to infect humans and other mammals as well as birds. Numerous pathogenic coronaviruses have been described and result in a spectrum of clinical disease. SARS-CoV-2 has been found to be highly contagious and pathogenic, causing more severe illness in the elderly as well as those with underlying medical conditions. Soon after the virus began to spread around the world, cutaneous findings of the viral infection were reported and categorized.

Clinical Findings: From a purely cutaneous perspective, SARS-CoV-2 infection has been shown to cause a number of clinical findings. Some findings are unique to this virus, but most are nonspecific and can be seen in other viral infections. "COVID toes," a form of pernio or chilblains, was one of the first cutaneous findings recognized and is one of the unique skin findings. Individuals presented with varying degrees of erythematous pink to red macules, plaques, and nodules on the toes and sometimes fingers. This finding is much more commonly seen in children. There is no sex predilection, unlike pernio, which is predominantly found in females. Most individuals are asymptomatic from the lesions. Itching and pain have been reported. Spontaneous resolution is the most common outcome within a few weeks. Interestingly, most individuals who develop COVID toes have a milder course of the systemic disease. COVID toes often present after the patient has cleared the respiratory part of the infection, and individuals often did not know they were infected.

Numerous other cutaneous rashes have been reported, including erythema multiforme, vesicular and maculopapular exanthems, urticaria, livedo reticularis, pityriasis rosea–like eruptions, and vasculitis. These cutaneous findings are more likely to be seen in the adult population. These other patterns of skin involvement are usually early in the course of infection.

Children are more likely to develop a multisystem inflammatory syndrome. This had originally been termed *Kawasaki disease–like inflammatory syndrome* because of its many similar features. It can be severe and life-threatening and presents with a persistent fever, exudative conjunctivitis, heart abnormalities, diarrhea, rash (both desquamative and nondesquamative), hand and foot swelling, and erythema. Heart abnormalities can include coronary aneurysm, valve damage, pericardial effusion, and decreased cardiac output.

Pathogenesis: Coronaviruses are able to infect and cause disease in humans and other animals. There are four well-known endemic coronaviruses that cause upper respiratory infections in humans. SARS-CoV-2 is a coronavirus in the genus *Sarbecovirus*. This virus is able to infect human cells via binding the angiotensin-converting enzyme-2 binding site on the epithelium of the lung. From there it is able to replicate and can cause a large spectrum of disease, from asymptomatic carriers to death from acute respiratory distress syndrome or thromboembolic events. The exact pathogenesis of how various skin manifestations are formed is currently a focus of study. The urticaria, erythema multiforme, and maculopapular-like eruptions are likely a form of a viral hypersensitivity. There are many theories on the underlying mechanisms that may cause COVID toes, including a strong interferon response, a thrombosis, or lymphocytic vasculitis.

Histology: Chilblain-like lesions of COVID toes show a dense superficial and deep lymphocytic infiltrate as well as perieccrine inflammation. Dermal edema and epidermal spongiosis are present. Lymphocytic vasculitis is present with varying degrees of red blood cell extravasation. Microthrombi and necrotic keratinocytes are present. Spike protein of the SARS-CoV-2 virus has been detected in the eccrine gland epithelial cells of skin biopsy specimens.

Treatment: The cutaneous findings of SARS-CoV-2 infections are typically not life-threatening and will resolve with time and therapy of the underlying viral infection if warranted. Pain control, control of itching, and care of cutaneous ulcerations are managed with analgesics, antihistamines, and wound care, respectively. Topical steroids have been used to decrease skin inflammation.

Discoloration of toes (red/purple) and/or with pus under skin in "COVID toes"

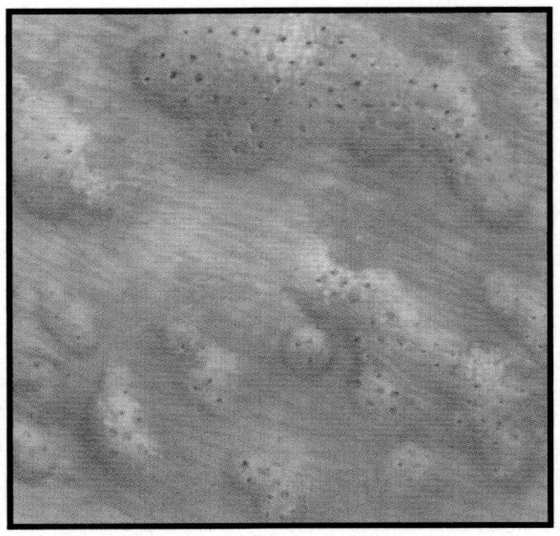

Urticaria: Pink edematous plaques with follicular accentuation caused by the dermal edema.

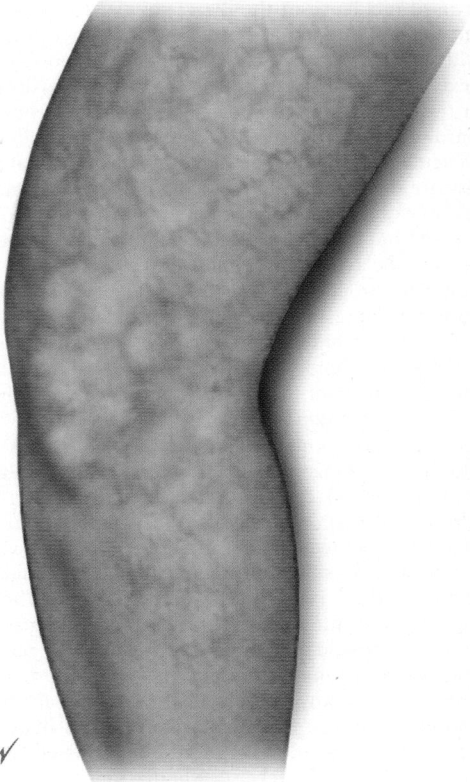

Livedo reticularis

Loss of smell

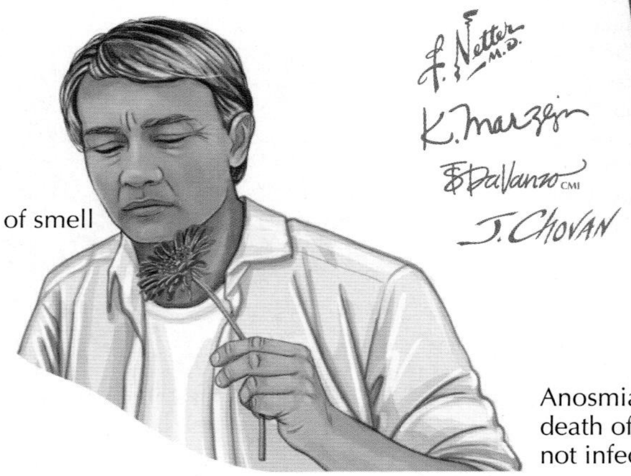

Anosmia is due to SARS-CoV-2 entry, infection, and death of olfactory sustentacular epithelial cells and not infection of the olfactory nerve.

CRYPTOCOCCOSIS

India ink preparation showing *C. neoformans*. No hyphae are seen.

A. Budding organism with thick capsule

B. Nonbudding organisms

C. Unencapsulated form (budding)

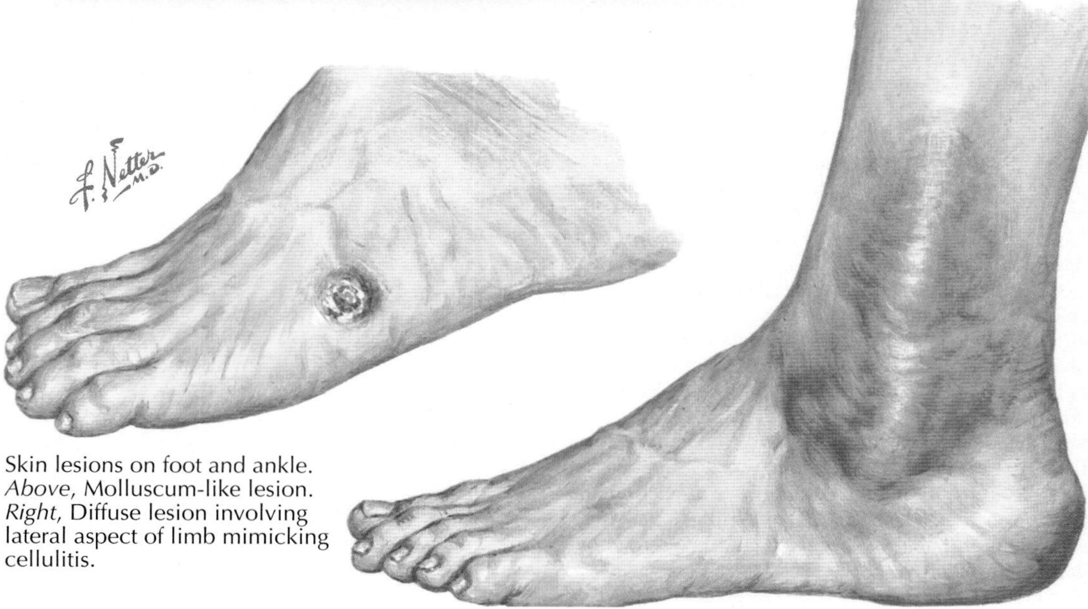

Skin lesions on foot and ankle. *Above,* Molluscum-like lesion. *Right,* Diffuse lesion involving lateral aspect of limb mimicking cellulitis.

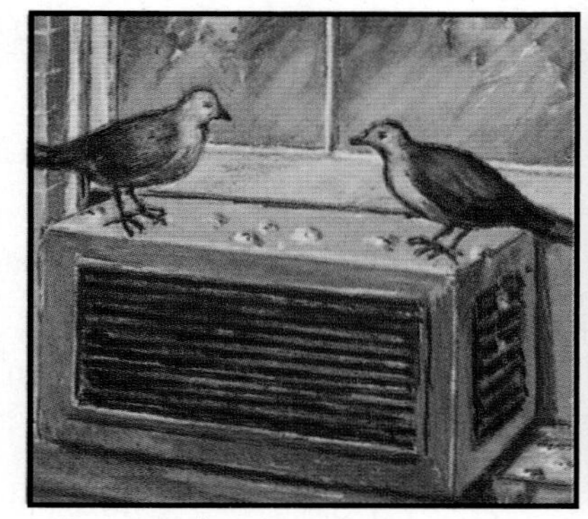

Infection is by respiratory route. Pigeon dung and air conditioners may be factors in dissemination.

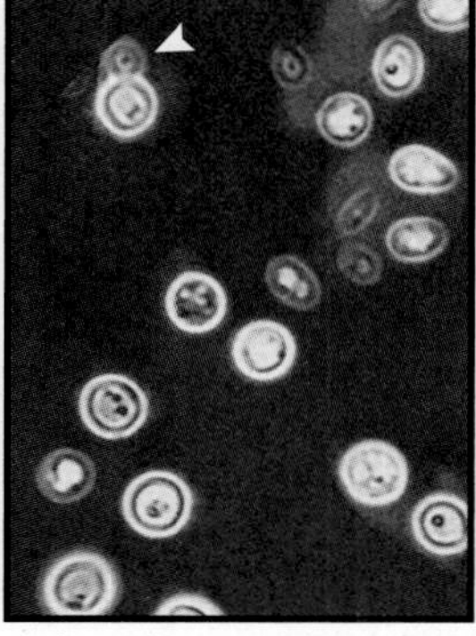

India ink preparation showing budding and capsule

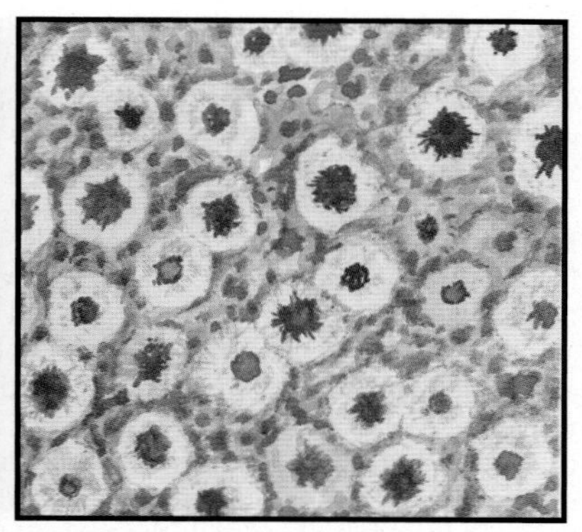

Accumulation of encapsulated cryptococci in subarachnoid space (PAS or methenamine-silver stain)

Cryptococcosis is an opportunistic fungal infection caused by *Cryptococcus neoformans* or, less frequently, by *Cryptococcus gattii*. It is seen primarily in immunosuppressed patients such as those taking chronic immunosuppressive medications and those with acquired immunodeficiency syndrome (AIDS). A diagnosis of cryptococcosis in a patient with HIV infection is considered an AIDS-defining illness.

Cryptococcosis is primarily a lung disease, but dissemination to the skin and central nervous system (CNS) is well described. Cryptococcosis has a higher propensity to affect the CNS than any other opportunistic fungi. Primary cutaneous cryptococcosis is a rarely seen condition caused by direct inoculation of the yeast into the skin.

Clinical Findings: A variety of infectious outcomes can occur after exposure to this encapsulated yeast. Immunocompetent hosts typically do not show any signs or symptoms. On occasion, the fungus can be found colonizing the oropharynx and upper airway; this has been shown to be transient and appears to cause no harm. Most of the population in North America show serologic evidence of exposure. If a colonized patient subsequently becomes immunosuppressed, the dormant fungus may cause disease. Cryptococcosis is ubiquitous in North America, and patients routinely come in contact with the fungus. Immunosuppressed patients who contact the fungus during routine outdoor environmental exposure may become infected. The fungus can be found in soil and is frequently found in bird droppings, especially those of pigeons. The fungus gains entry via inhalation. Once in the lung tissue, it is able to grow and reproduce. The host may develop signs of lung inflammation, including cough, hemoptysis, pain, pleurisy, and pneumonia. The fungus eventually disseminates through the bloodstream to infect various tissues.

The skin is affected in up to 25% of patients with disseminated disease, especially patients with AIDS. The lesions can appear as small white papules with a central dell that mimics molluscum contagiosum. The most commonly described morphology of cutaneous cryptococcosis is that of a red macule that can be large and imitate cellulitis. Many other cutaneous morphologies have been described in the literature. Cutaneous nodules with underlying abscess formation and overlying ulcerations are not uncommon. Clinical suspicion should lead the physician to perform an incisional or punch biopsy for histologic evaluation and microbiologic culture to ascertain the diagnosis.

Pathogenesis: *C. neoformans* and *C. gattii* are opportunistic yeasts that are encapsulated. The capsule is critical in that it helps the fungus avoid host defenses. Various serotypes of the species exist. The host inhales the organism or accidentally becomes inoculated through a penetrating skin wound. The yeast can overcome the host's cell-mediated immunity if the immune system is compromised. This can lead to fungal abscess and hematogenous spread of the fungus. *Cryptococcus* is a unique fungus that has a neurotrophic behavior and often causes CNS disease.

Histology: The histologic features are somewhat dependent on the immune status of the patient. In severely immunosuppressed patients, the biopsy specimen often shows a gelatinous appearance with numerous yeast cells and a mixed inflammatory infiltrate. Immunocompetent patients are more likely to have a granulomatous infiltrate with few yeast organisms and a vigorous host inflammatory response. The yeast capsule can be stained with Alcian blue, India ink, or mucicarmine. Periodic acid–Schiff stain can be used to demarcate the central portion of the yeast.

Cultures of the fungus reveal fast-growing, off-white, mucoid colonies. The fungus is unique in that it can grow at varying temperatures, including the routine culture temperature of 24°C to 25°C and body temperature of 37°C. Microscopic examination reveals round, budding, encapsulated yeasts without hyphae. *C. neoformans* has unique biochemical features, such as the inability to ferment sugars, that allow mycologists to study and differentiate this organism from other fungi and cryptococcal species.

Treatment: Patients with a diagnosis of cutaneous cryptococcosis need to be evaluated for CNS involvement because the therapy is very different. If a spinal fluid analysis shows evidence of fungal involvement, the treatment of choice is amphotericin B with or without flucytosine. If no CNS involvement is present, long-term use of itraconazole or fluconazole can be prescribed. Cutaneous abscesses should be incised and drained to decrease the fungal load. Treatment considerations should also include the immune status of the patient and appropriate screening and testing for HIV infection.

CUTANEOUS LARVA MIGRANS

Cutaneous larva migrans is a tropically acquired skin disease caused by the aimless wandering of a nematode larva. This disease has also been termed "creeping eruption" because of the slow, methodical movement underneath the skin, which subsequently manifests with classic cutaneous findings. The most frequent cause of cutaneous larva migrans is the larva of *Ancylostoma braziliense* or *Ancylostoma caninum*. The cutaneous findings are similar among the various species that can cause disease. Treatments are effective for this condition, which causes more psychological than physical harm. Establishment of the specific larva responsible for the disease is not routinely attempted, nor is it practical or cost-effective.

Clinical Findings: The larvae gain entrance into the epidermis through tiny abrasions, cuts, or any disruption of the normal epidermal layer. The larvae are frequently obtained during a barefoot walk on a contaminated beach or from a similar environment. Travelers to Central and South America often acquire the larvae on the beach while lying on or playing in the sand. The initial entry of the larvae goes entirely unnoticed. It is not until days to weeks later that the human host begins to develop cutaneous signs of the disease. The first evidence is a pink to red edematous eruption that begins to take on a serpiginous course. The involved skin appears as red, squiggly lines. If only one larva is present, only one serpiginous line will be present. The line meanders and slowly elongates over days to weeks until the patient seeks medical advice. Patients who are infected with multiple parasites have multiple serpiginous areas of involvement, with some in a crisscrossing pattern. Pruritus is universal, but pain is infrequent. The lesions are typically elevated and can become vesicular in nature.

Pathogenesis: Cutaneous larva migrans is caused by penetration of the epidermis by one of the various larvae known to cause disease. The larvae are derived from eggs that are laid in the intestines of an infected animal, such as a dog or cat, and then released in the stool. When the animal defecates, the eggs are readily passed into the soil, where they hatch into larvae. The human is an incidental or dead-end host because the larva is unable to replicate or complete its life cycle in humans. This is very much different than infections with the gastrointestinal parasites *Ancylostoma duodenale* and *Necator americanus*, which require the human host to replicate. The larvae wander around the epidermis, unable to penetrate the basement membrane zone and therefore unable to enter the dermis. If the condition is left untreated, the larvae die in the skin within a few months. The larvae have been shown to secrete enzymes that help them travel throughout the epidermis, but they lack an enzyme to penetrate the dermal-epidermal junction.

Histology: The histopathology is nonspecific unless the actual larva is biopsied. This is highly unlikely, because the larva is typically an estimated 2 to 3 cm ahead of the leading edge of the serpiginous rash, and most biopsies are taken from the serpiginous region. The biopsy specimen shows a lymphocytic dermal infiltrate with eosinophils. Occasionally, a space is seen within the spongiotic epidermis, which indicates the area through which the larva passed.

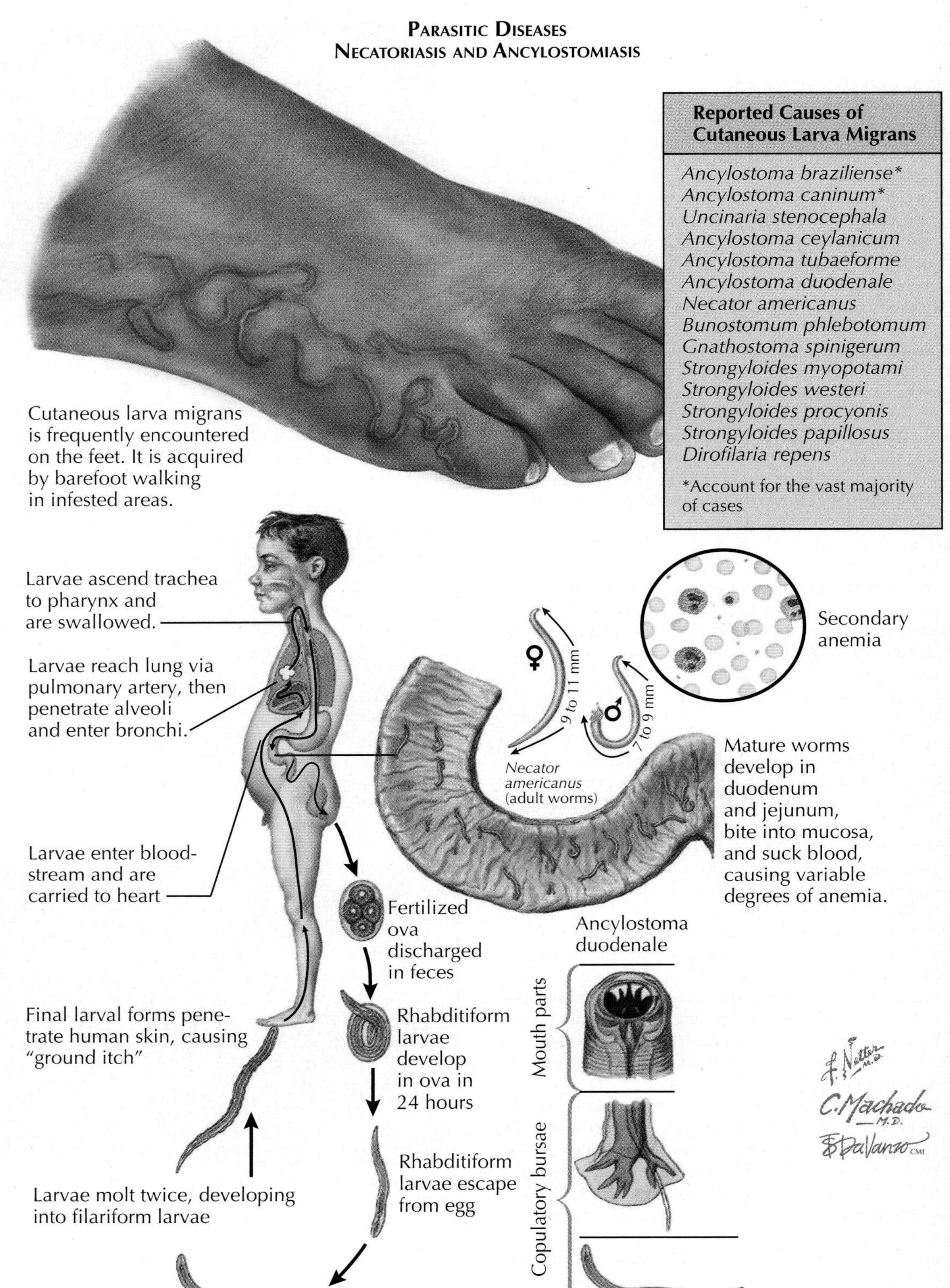

Reported Causes of Cutaneous Larva Migrans
*Ancylostoma braziliense**
*Ancylostoma caninum**
Uncinaria stenocephala
Ancylostoma ceylanicum
Ancylostoma tubaeforme
Ancylostoma duodenale
Necator americanus
Bunostomum phlebotomum
Gnathostoma spinigerum
Strongyloides myopotami
Strongyloides westeri
Strongyloides procyonis
Strongyloides papillosus
Dirofilaria repens
*Account for the vast majority of cases

Treatment: The mainstays of treatment are anthelmintic agents. Albendazole and ivermectin are the most frequently used medications. Oral ivermectin is well tolerated and works equally as well as the others. Ivermectin binds to glutamate-gated chloride channels in the parasites, allowing free passage of chloride and eventually death of the cell. Thiabendazole and albendazole work by inhibiting microtubule polymerization in the parasite, ultimately leading to its death. Thiabendazole and albendazole can cause severe gastrointestinal side effects, and they are best used topically. A pharmacist can compound these agents into a topical solution to apply to the affected area. Other therapies that have been attempted include cold therapy with topical liquid nitrogen, which is no longer advocated. The larvae have been shown to survive at subfreezing temperatures, and because the location of the larva cannot be predicted with high certainty, a large area of skin must be treated with liquid nitrogen for the treatment to be effective.

TINEA FACIEI AND TINEA CORPORIS

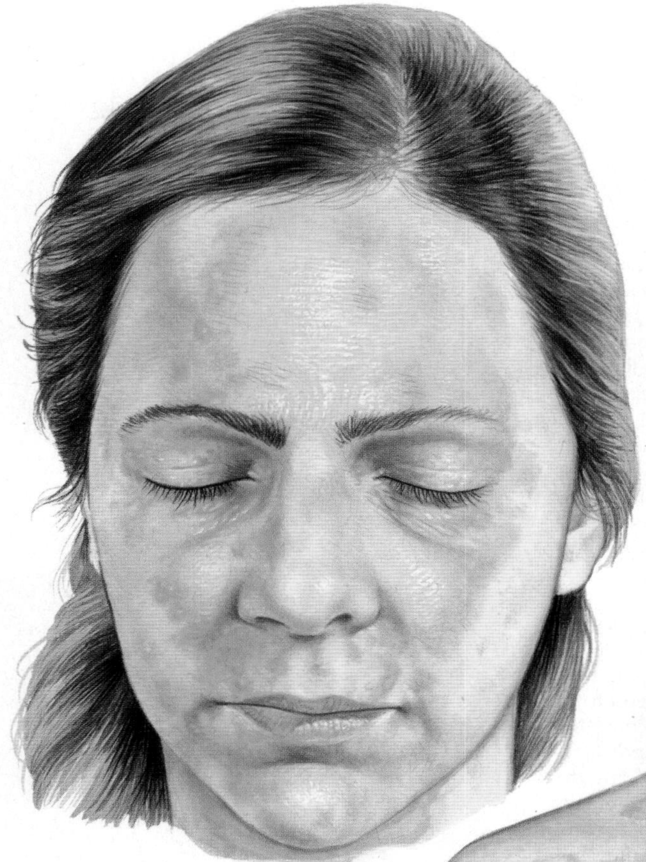

Tinea faciei. Annular patches occur in a diffuse pattern. Extensive disease may be caused by topical corticosteroid use.

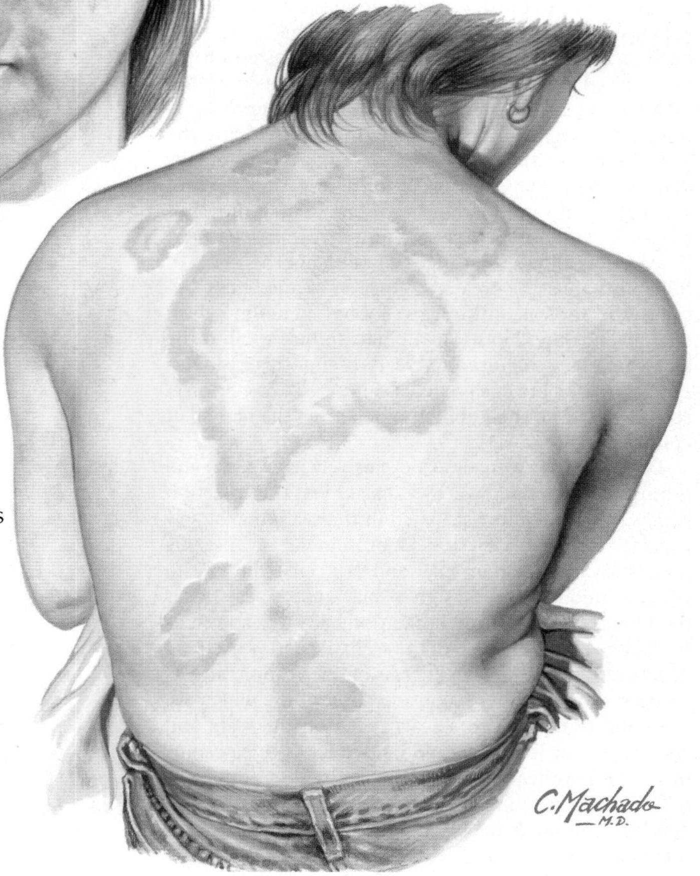

Tinea corporis. Annular scaly patches with a leading edge of scale.

C. Machado M.D.

DERMATOPHYTOSES

Dermatophytes are classified in many ways by mycologists and physicians. One of the simplest classification systems is based on the natural living conditions of the studied fungi. Fungi can be classified as zoophilic (affecting mammals only), anthropophilic (affecting predominantly humans with little transference to other mammals), or geophilic (predominantly soil fungi that are capable of affecting mammals under the correct living conditions). This classification is widely used by physicians because more complicated categorizations have minimal effect on the overall therapy and prognosis. Most of these infections are treated with topical antifungal agents that can be purchased over the counter and have very high success rates. Fungal infections of the hair shaft and nails require systemic therapy for the highest efficacy of treatment. Topical antifungal agents do not penetrate the deeper layers of the stratum corneum, the nail plate, or the hair shaft; in these cases systemic antifungals are required for therapy.

Clinical Findings: Superficial fungal infections have been around for millennia and have been reported under various names and descriptions. Most terms used for these infections are based on the location of the disease. An individual may be affected by more than one of these types. Immunocompetent individuals are less likely than those who are immunosuppressed to develop widespread disease.

Tinea corporis (ringworm) is a superficial dermatophyte infection of the skin of the trunk or extremities. It begins as a small red macule or papule and, over time, spreads in an annular or polycyclic nature. The primary morphology of tinea infections is the scaly patch with a leading trail of scale. On close examination, a random amount of hair loss can be observed within the affected area. Most cases are mild and affect only one or two areas, but some can be widespread and associated with other forms of tinea, such as tinea unguium. If tinea corporis is left untreated, the fungus will continue to spread out from the center of each lesion; lesions can merge into very large patches that may envelop the entire trunk or extremity.

Tinea faciei, as the name implies, occurs on the face. It appears as annular patches with a leading edge of scale. The scale is easily scraped off. In adult men, the term *tinea faciei* is used to describe disease in regions of the face other than terminal hair–bearing skin, such as the beard and scalp. The lesions may converge into polycyclic patches and are typically pruritic. This form of superficial fungal infection is commonly seen in children. Sleeping in the same bed as pets may increase the risk of exposure to the causative fungus and the chance of acquiring any of the superficial fungal infections. *Trichophyton tonsurans* is the most likely etiologic agent in North America.

Tinea barbae is a fungal infection in the beard region of postpubertal men. This infection often affects the skin as well as the hair follicles, and it can appear as red patches with follicle-based pustules. Many fungal species have been shown to cause this condition, with the zoophilic agents being more commonly responsible. *Trichophyton verrucosum* has been frequently reported, along with other *Trichophyton* species. The infection may form boggy, crusted plaques identical to a kerion of the scalp. If the lesions are plaque-like and affect the hair follicles, systemic therapy is needed.

Tinea cruris (jock itch) is one of the most easily recognized and prevalent forms of superficial fungal infections. The fungus prefers to live in dark, moist regions of the skin that stay at body temperature. The groin is a perfect location for fungal infections. The disease is often very pruritic, which is what gives it the vernacular name "jock itch." It is seen frequently in athletes but is not limited to them. *Trichophyton rubrum* and *Epidermophyton floccosum* are the most commonly reported etiologic agents.

Tinea pedis (athlete's foot) is probably the superficial fungal infection best known to the general public because of personal experience. This fungal infection is

DERMATOPHYTOSES (Continued)

seen in two predominant forms: the interdigital type and the moccasin type. The interdigital subtype forms macerated, red patches in the toe web spaces. The areas can become pruritic and can lead to onychomycosis. Moccasin-type tinea pedis involves the entire foot and is the less common of the two types. *T. rubrum* is the most frequent isolate in these cases.

Tinea manuum, also most frequently caused by *T. rubrum*, predominantly affects one hand only. It is commonly seen in association with bilateral tinea pedis and therefore has been called "one hand two feet disease." The reason that it affects only one hand is unknown. The most frequent complaint is itching and the appearance of the red annular patches.

Majocchi granuloma is a form of fungal folliculitis caused by one of the dermatophyte species. It is universally seen in patients with undiagnosed tinea who have been incorrectly treated with topical corticosteroids for a presumed form of dermatitis. As the patient continues to apply the steroid cream to the patch of fungal infection, redness spreads and pustules may form within the affected region. The pustules are based on a hair follicle, and the hair may be absent or easily pulled from the region with minimal or no discomfort. Removal of the hair and use of a potassium hydroxide (KOH) preparation allows the fungus to be seen. This form of folliculitis must be treated with a systemic agent because the topical antifungals do not penetrate deep enough into the depths of the hair follicle or into the hair shaft, as is required to treat an endothrix fungus. Fungal species are designated as endothrix or ectothrix species based on their ability to penetrate the hair shaft epithelium.

Tinea capitis is seen almost exclusively in children and is most commonly caused by *T. tonsurans*. This infection begins as a small, pruritic patch in the scalp that slowly expands outward. Hair loss is prominent because the fungus invades the hair shaft and can cause the hair to break. A frequent clinical sign is "black dot" tinea. This is the clinical finding of tiny, broken-off hairs that appear as black dots just at the level of the scalp. Posterior occipital adenopathy is always seen in cases of tinea capitis, and its absence should trigger reconsideration of the diagnosis. If a child presents with a scaly patch on the scalp and associated hair loss, it should be treated as tinea capitis until proven otherwise. A KOH examination of the hair or of a scalp scraping often, but not always, shows evidence of a dermatophyte. A fungal culture can be used in these cases to confirm the diagnosis if the KOH examination is negative. The culture sample is easily obtained by rubbing the scaly patch with a toothbrush and collecting the scale that is removed in a sterile container. The cultures are grown in the laboratory on dermatophyte test medium, and growth is often seen in 2 to 4 weeks. Tinea capitis requires at least 6 weeks of systemic oral therapy to clear, and all of the patient's pets, especially cats, should be evaluated by a veterinarian for evidence of disease.

A kerion is a boggy plaque found on occasion in tinea capitis that results from a massive immune inflammatory response to the causative fungal agent. The fungi most likely to cause this reaction are in the zoophilic class. The kerion often appears as a large, inflamed, boggy-feeling plaque with alopecia. Serous drainage and crusting are also present. These plaques are very tender to palpation, and children complain of pain even when the lesions are not manipulated. Alopecia overlies the plaque, and if it is severe, a kerion can lead to permanent scarring alopecia. Posterior occipital and cervical adenopathy is present and tender to palpation. The kerion often become impetiginized with bacteria, especially *Staphylococcus* species. Treatment is based on the use of systemic oral antifungals in association with an oral corticosteroid to decrease the massive inflammatory response. Any bacterial coinfections must be treated at the same time. Scarring alopecia may be permanent and may lead to morbidity for the child.

Tinea unguium, or onychomycosis, is clinically recognized by thick, dystrophic, crumbling nails. One or all of the nails on a foot or hand may be involved. Toenail

TINEA CRURIS AND TINEA CAPITIS

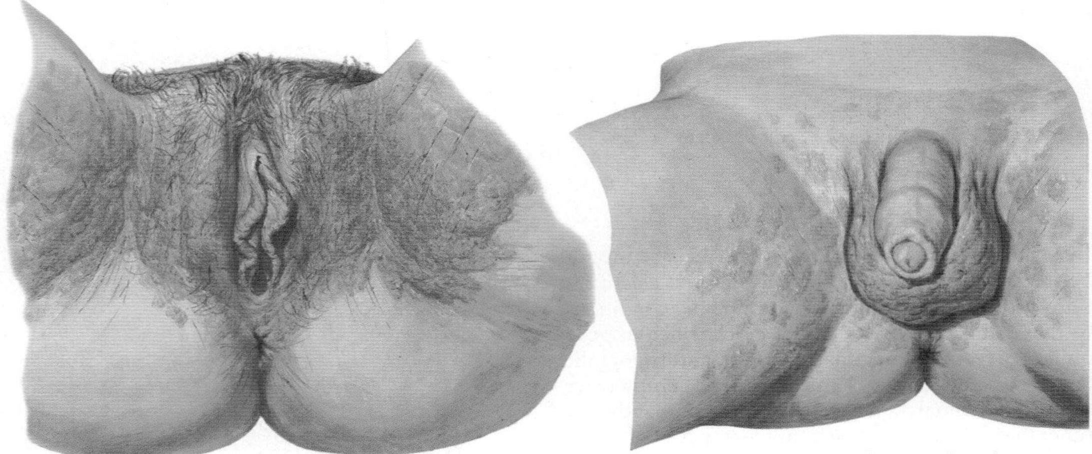

Tinea cruris (female)

Tinea cruris (male), "jock itch," a very common infection in males

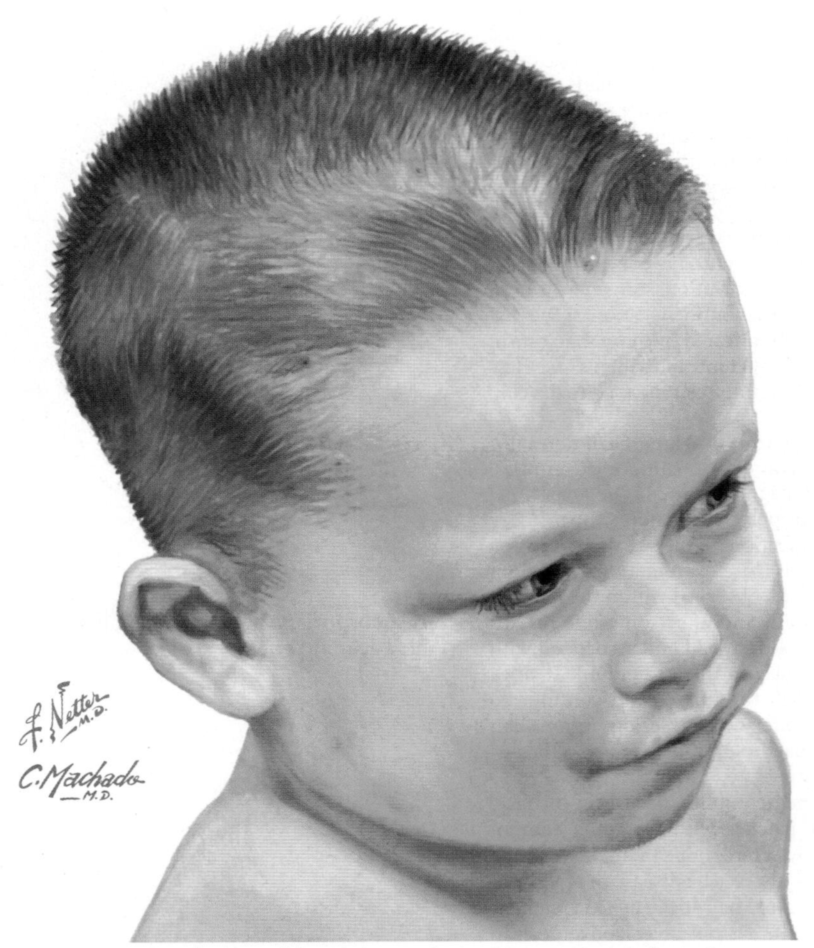

Tinea capitis. Scaly patches with associated alopecia.

DERMATOPHYTOSES (Continued)

infection is much more common than infection of the fingernails. Most patients start with tinea pedis, after which the fungus spreads to infect the nail plate. This results in yellowing of the nail. Over time, the nail becomes thickened with subungual debris that is easily removed with a blunt instrument such as a curette. The nail plate may become onycholytic and fall off the nail bed. Patients are most frequently asymptomatic, but some report discomfort and difficulty clipping their nails. Patients with diabetes and those with peripheral vascular disease are at risk for bacterial cellulitis. The dystrophic nails serve as a nidus for infection with various bacteria. Nail disease requires the use of systemic oral medications to get the best therapeutic response. Topical agents have shown some benefit but only for very mild nail involvement. A deep green discoloration under the nail is an indication of *Pseudomonas* nail colonization. The bacteria create a bright green pigment that is easily visible. Soaks in acetic acid (vinegar) diluted 1:4 in water are effective in clearing up the secondary *Pseudomonas*.

Dermatophytid reactions can occur with any dermatophyte infection. They are infrequently seen. They manifest as monomorphic, pink-red, scattered papules. They are typically pruritic and are most commonly seen in patients with tinea capitis or kerion infection. Another manifestation of dermatophytid reactions is a deep vesicular reaction on the palms or soles. This can closely mimic dyshidrotic dermatitis. Treatment of the underlying fungal infection clears the dermatophytid reaction. Topical or oral corticosteroids may be used for relief until the fungal infection is cured.

The easiest, most sensitive, and most specific means of diagnosing the infection is by KOH examination. A scraping of the leading edge of the rash is taken and placed on a glass slide; KOH is added, and the preparation is heated for a few seconds. It is then viewed under a microscope for the characteristic branching and septated fungi of a dermatophyte. This method does not allow speciation of the fungus, which requires growth of cultures on fungal growth media. Each fungus has characteristic growth requirements and appears slightly different on microscopic evaluation of the cultured colonies.

Pathogenesis: Dermatophyte infections are predominantly caused by three fungal genera: *Trichophyton*, *Microsporum*, and *Epidermophyton*. Multiple species within each of the first two genera have cutaneous effects; *Epidermophyton floccosum* is the only known species in the last genus to cause skin disease. Other genera have been implicated, but 99% of dermatophyte infections are caused by these three genera of fungi.

Histology: Tinea corporis infections are rarely biopsied. When they are, fungal hyphae within the stratus corneum are seen on close inspection. Hyphae can be demonstrated with various staining methods. Neutrophils are the predominant cell type seen in the stratum corneum.

Treatment: Topical antifungal agents are the mainstay of treatment for tinea corporis, pedis, manuum, and cruris. Terbinafine is a topical fungicidal agent that has excellent efficacy against dermatophytes. The topical azoles are used equally as often and also show excellent therapeutic results. Twice-daily treatment for 2 to 4 weeks usually is an effective treatment course. The importance of cleaning and drying the involved skin thoroughly cannot be understated. The fungi do not like to live in dry environments, and these simple steps can help treat and prevent the disease. Immunosuppressed individuals with widespread disease are candidates for oral antifungal agents.

Tinea capitis, tinea barbae, Majocchi granuloma, and onychomycosis all require oral systemic treatment. Topical antifungals are ineffective in these cases because they do not penetrate deeply into the hair shaft or into the nail plate. Topical antifungals may be used in conjunction with the oral agents. The two most commonly prescribed oral antifungals are terbinafine and griseofulvin. The azole antifungal agents have also been used with excellent efficacy rates. Nystatin, although good to treat *Candida* infections, is not used to treat dermatophyte infections.

TINEA PEDIS AND TINEA UNGUIUM

Tinea pedis

The two most common forms of tinea pedis are interdigital and moccasin.

Area typically affected by interdigital tinea pedis

Area typically affected by the moccasin form of tinea pedis

Moccasin form of tinea pedis

Tinea unguium

Proximal subungual onychomycosis (PSO)
Proximal white subungual onychomycosis
Fungus infection reaches the nail plate via the cuticle, eponychium, or ventral face of the proximal nailfold.

PSO secondary to paronychia
Fungus from the lateral and/or proximal nailfolds reaches the nail plate through the injured cuticle.

Superficial white onychomycosis (SWO)
The fungus infects the dorsal surface of the nail.

Distal and lateral subungual onychomycosis (DLSO)
The most common form of onychomycosis. The fungus invades under the free edge of the nail and migrates proximally to involve the nail bed.

C. Machado M.D.

Onychomycosis. Classification by portals of entry.

Onycholysis, subungual hyperkeratosis, splitting, crumbling, and yellow longitudinal spikes are clinical features of distal and lateral subungual onychomycosis.

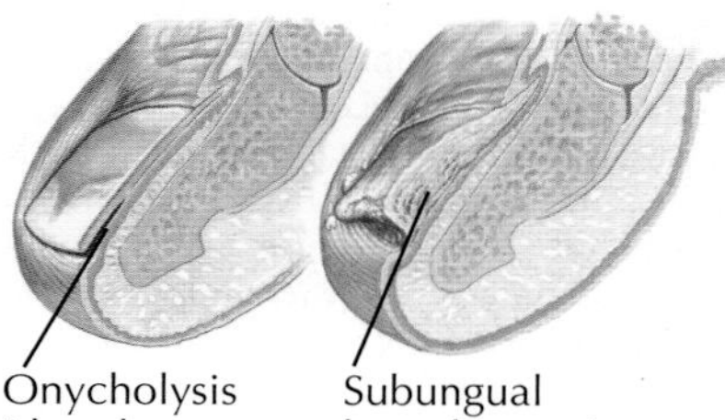

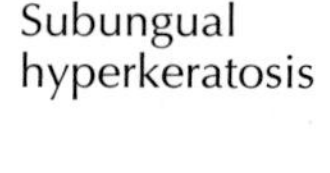

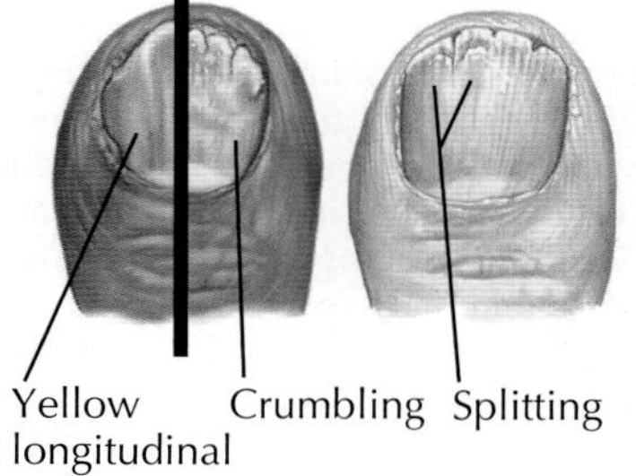

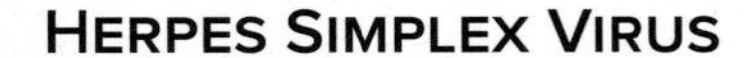

HERPES SIMPLEX VIRUS

Herpes simplex virus types 1 (HSV1) and 2 (HSV2) are responsible for the production of both mucocutaneous and systemic disease. Mucocutaneous disease is overwhelmingly more common than systemic disease such as HSV encephalitis. HSV infections are ubiquitous in humans, and almost all adults develop antibodies against one of these viruses. Most infections are subclinical or so mild that they are never recognized by the patient. HSV infections are predominantly oral or genital. The virus becomes latent in local nerves and can be reactivated to produce future outbreaks. Currently, there are eight known herpesviruses that infect humans, including HSV1 and HSV2. HSV infections can cause severe, life-threatening CNS disease in immunocompromised patients and in neonates. Many unique cutaneous forms of HSV have been described with their own clinical characteristics.

Clinical Findings: HSV can be spread from infected to uninfected individuals by close contact (e.g., kissing, sexual contact). The virus is shed from the infected host both when active lesions are present and when no clinical evidence of disease can be seen. It is believed that subclinical shedding of the virus is responsible for a great deal of transmission. HSV can cause oral labial disease (gingivostomatitis or herpes labialis) or genital disease, the main mucocutaneous forms of the disease. Most cases of oral labial disease are caused by HSV1, and genital disease is caused predominantly by HSV2. This is not always the case, and the viral type should not be assumed from the clinical location of disease. HSV infections in other areas of the body are becoming more common, and recurrent bouts of disease on the buttocks is one of the most frequently seen presentations.

The initial HSV infection can be subclinical, mild, or severe. Subsequent reactivation of the virus typically never approaches the severity seen in the initial primary infection. The exception occurs with immunosuppressed patients, in whom a widespread or chronic localized version of the infection may occur. Primary infection manifests with severe, painful mucocutaneous blistering and erosions. Primary oral labial herpes can lead to weight loss, fever, gingivitis, and pain. This is most commonly seen in children and is associated with tender cervical adenopathy. The infection spontaneously resolves within 2 to 3 weeks. If treated, the disease may be slightly decreased in length and severity, but this is highly dependent on the timing of diagnosis and initiation of therapy.

Herpes labialis is the term given to recurrent episodes of oral labial herpes. The episodes are milder than the primary infection and often start with a prodrome. Most patients report a tingling or painful sensation hours to a day before the appearance of herpes labialis. Patients can use this knowledge to their advantage and begin antiviral therapy at the first indication of recurrence to decrease the severity of the episode or stop it all together. Herpes labialis, also known as a *cold sore* when it appears on the face, appears as a vesicle or bulla that quickly breaks down and forms an erosion and crusted papule or plaque. The lesions last for a few days to 1 week and can cause significant psychological issues.

Herpes infection of the genital region is spread by sexual contact and is one of the most common of all STIs. Initial episodes of genital herpes infection manifest with fever, adenopathy, and painful ulcerations and blistering of the affected region. The primary episode is always more severe than subsequent reactivations of the virus. The ulcerations are grouped vesiculopustules on an erythematous base. They are extremely tender and easily rupture to form shallow ulcerations that appear "punched out" with an overlying serous crust. The cervix is often involved, and scarring can occur. Genital herpes infection almost universally causes dysuria and inguinal adenopathy that is tender.

Recurrent episodes of genital herpes produce a milder version of the primary infection. The systemic

LESIONS OF HERPES SIMPLEX

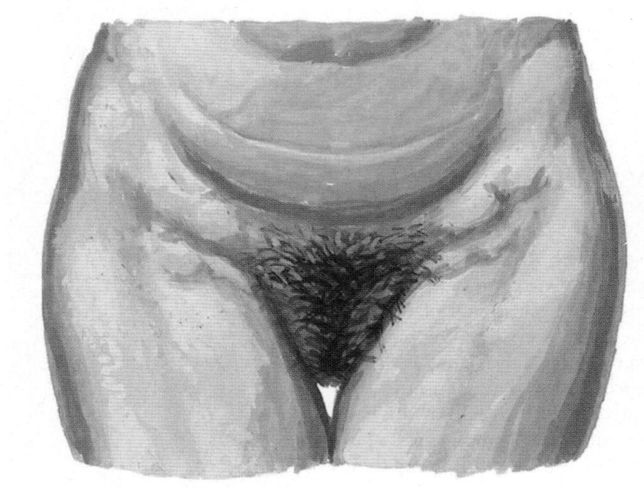

Regional tender lymphadenopathy is commonly seen in genital herpes.

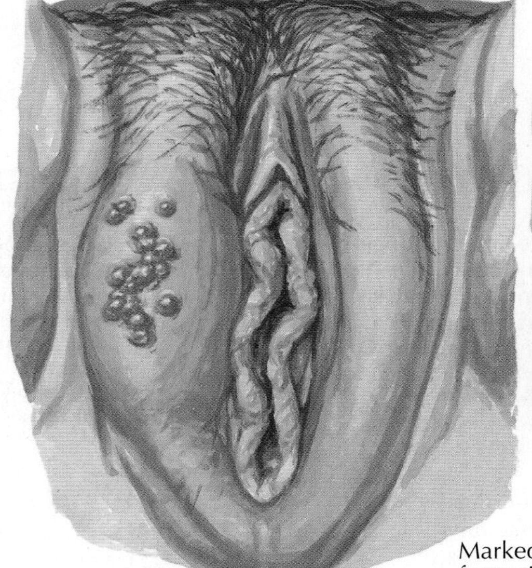

Grouped vesiculopustules on a tender red base

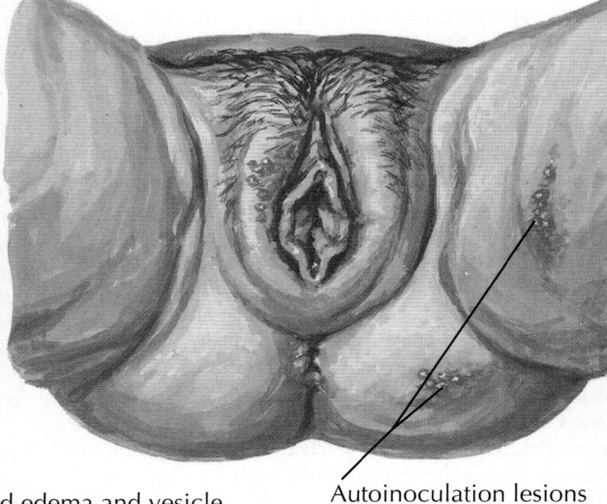

Marked edema and vesicle formation in primary herpes

Autoinoculation lesions

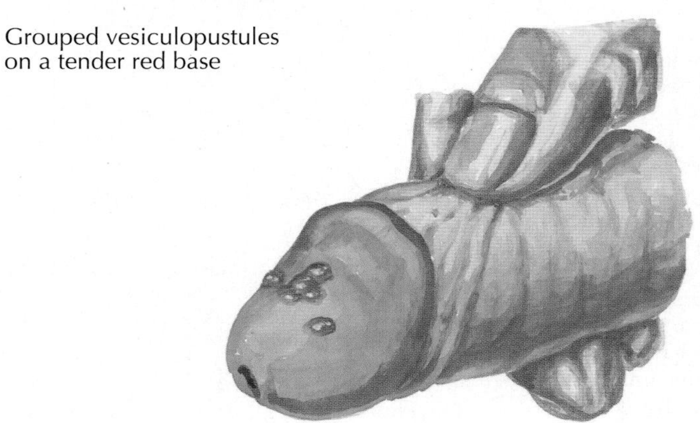

Primary HSV disease is almost always more severe than reactivation of HSV.

JOHN A.CRAIG—AD

HERPES SIMPLEX VIRUS (Continued)

constitutional symptoms are often absent, but the grouped vesicles and ulcers can cause excruciating pain and social stigma. The frequency and severity of recurrent episodes in an individual patient are variable and impossible to predict. A generalization can be made that those who have more severe primary infections tend to have more relentless recurrences.

Herpetic whitlow is the name given to a specific form of infection most commonly seen in medical laboratory workers and healthcare providers. It occurs from accidental inoculation of the herpesvirus into the skin. The finger is the area most commonly involved because of accidental needle sticks. A painful primary viral infection may occur at the site of inoculation.

Eczema herpeticum, also termed *Kaposi varicelliform eruption*, is often encountered in a young child with severe atopic dermatitis who is exposed to the herpesvirus. Because of the widespread skin disease, the virus is able to infect a large surface area of the body. This results in extensive skin involvement with multiple vesicles and punched-out ulcerations.

The transmission of HSV from mother to child during the birthing process is of significant concern, and mothers with active HSV disease at the time of delivery most likely should undergo cesarean section to help decrease the risk of transmission. Neonatal HSV infection is a life-threatening disease. The neonate may have widespread multiorgan disease, with CNS involvement being the major cause of morbidity and mortality. Temporal lobe involvement can lead to seizures, encephalitis, and death. The skin is always infected, and this is a clue for the clinician to search for other organ system involvement, especially involvement of the CNS and the eye. Ocular infection can lead to severe corneal scarring and blindness.

HSV encephalitis is a life-threatening disease that causes necrotizing encephalitis. Patients report an acute onset of fever and headache, with rapidly evolving seizures and focal neurologic deficits. Without treatment, coma and death occur in three-fourths of affected patients. The temporal lobes and insula are almost always affected. Prompt recognition and therapy have decreased the mortality rate to 15% to 20%.

A Tzanck preparation is a bedside procedure that takes only a few minutes to perform and is positive in cases of HSV1, HSV2, or varicella zoster virus (VZV) infection. The procedure does not differentiate among the three viruses. However, HSV infection can be clinically distinguished from varicella. The procedure is done by unroofing a vesicle and scraping its base with a No. 15 blade. The scrapings are placed on a glass slide and allowed to air dry for 1 to 2 minutes. A blue stain such as Giemsa or toluidine blue is applied for 60 seconds and then gently rinsed off. The slide is dried, mineral oil is applied, and the preparation is covered with a microscope cover slip. Multinucleated giant cells are readily seen throughout the sample, confirming the viral etiology of the blister.

LESIONS OF HERPES SIMPLEX (CONTINUED)

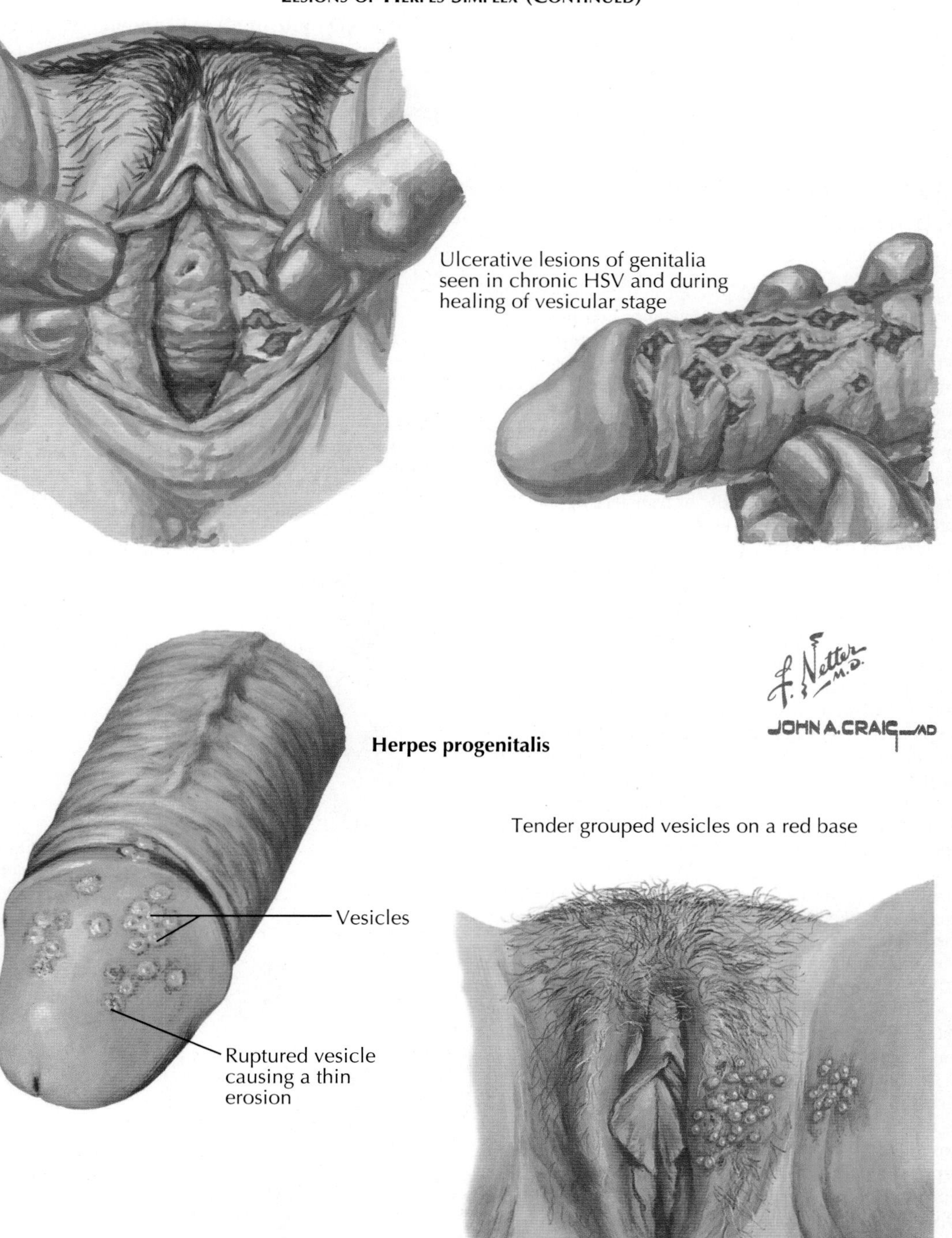

Herpes genitalis. Regional adenopathy is often appreciated.

Rapid immunostaining is available and can be used with high sensitivity and specificity to diagnose and differentiate the various herpesvirus types. This form of direct fluorescent antibody testing is similar to the Tzanck preparation. As in the Tzanck preparation, scrapings of the blister base are placed on a glass microscope slide. The slide is stained with antibodies corresponding to the various herpesviruses. The sample is viewed under fluorescent microscopy, and a positive sample fluoresces with one of the specific viral strains. This test takes 1 to 2 hours to perform.

Viral tissue cultures can also be performed to differentiate the HSV types, but the results can take days to 1 week to obtain. This is the most sensitive and specific test for the infection. Serum IgG and IgM testing can be done to look for evidence of current or past infection.

Pathogenesis: HSV1 and HSV2 are double-stranded DNA viruses encased within a lipid envelope. Along with VZV, they are classified in the subfamily *Alphaherpesvirinae*. The five other human herpesviruses are classified slightly differently. The virus attaches to the

HERPES SIMPLEX VIRUS (Continued)

host cells via specialized glycoproteins expressed on its lipid envelope. The lipid envelope then fuses with the host cell, allowing the virus to gain entry to the cytoplasm. Many glycoproteins are responsible for this attachment, fixation, and entrance to the host cell. The HSV capsid, which is an icosahedron-shaped structure, migrates from the cytoplasm to the nucleus of the cell. The viral capsid attaches to the nuclear membrane through the interaction of various membrane proteins and is capable of transferring its DNA into the cell nucleus.

Once the HSV DNA has gained entrance into the nucleus, it can become latent and quiescent or actively replicate new virus particles. When they are actively replicating, HSV particles often have a cytotoxic effect on the affected cell after viral replication has occurred; this ensures production of viral progeny and their release from the host cell. HSV is capable of hijacking the host cell's replication protein apparatus. HSV uses the host cell DNA polymerase to replicate its DNA and the cellular machinery to produce proteins required for viral replication. The virus carries various DNA genes that can be expressed early during the course of infection or later when the virus is ready to produce progeny. The early gene products are important for replication and regulation of the viral DNA genes. The late gene products encode the viral capsid. Once the viral elements have been produced in sufficient quantity and in the proper ratio, the viral particles spontaneously converge to produce a capsid, which encapsulates the viral DNA. This occurs within the host cell nucleus. The virus then passes through the nuclear membrane and the cytoplasmic membrane, acquiring its lipid bilayer. At this point, the virus can infect another host.

Alternatively, after it enters the cell's nucleus, the virus may become latent. This is particularly the case in neural tissue. The viral DNA inserts itself into the host DNA, where it lies dormant and hidden from expression until reactivation occurs at some later time. It accomplishes this by specialized folding of the DNA and histone complex so as not to allow for viral gene expression. When the virus is reactivated and ready to produce viral particles, this mechanism of latency is somehow deactivated, allowing for viral reproduction.

Histology: Examination of a biopsy specimen of a blister shows ballooning degeneration of the epidermal keratinocytes. This degeneration forms the blister cavity. There is a mixed inflammatory infiltrate around the superficial and deep dermal vascular plexus. Multinucleated giant cells are found at the base of the blister pocket. The skin biopsy findings are unable to differentiate HSV1 from HSV2 or from VZV infection.

Treatment: Therapy and its efficacy are highly dependent on the timing of administration. Antiviral medications work by inhibiting viral synthesis, and they work best when used early in the course of disease. All primary infections should be treated with one of the antiviral agents in the acyclovir family. These closely related medications include acyclovir, famciclovir, valacyclovir, and topical penciclovir. Recurrent episodes of the disease can be treated at the time of outbreak or with a chronic daily suppressive regimen. Widespread eczema herpeticum, CNS infection, or infection in an immunosuppressed patient is probably best treated with intravenous antiviral medication. The acyclovir family of medications is converted to the active form by viral-specific thymidine kinase. After conversion, this metabolite is a potent inhibitor of viral DNA polymerization. These medications are highly specific for the viral enzymes and have an excellent side effect profile. Acyclovir-resistant HSV has become well recognized and is best treated with foscarnet. Foscarnet does not require modulation by thymidine kinase to become an active inhibitor of HSV replication, thereby bypassing the HSV resistance mechanism. No medication to date has shown activity against latent viral infection.

HERPES SIMPLEX VIRUS ENCEPHALITIS

Possible route of transmission in HSV encephalitis

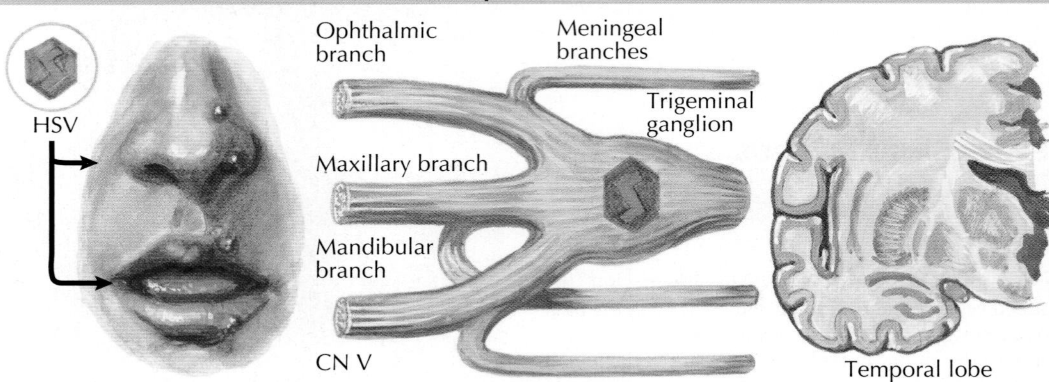

Primary infection — Virus enters via cutaneous or mucosal surfaces to infect sensory or autonomic nerve endings with transport to cell bodies in ganglia.

Latent phase — Virus replicates in ganglia before establishing latent phase.

Reactivation (lytic phase) — Reactivation of HSV in trigeminal ganglion can result in spread to brain (temporal lobe) via meningeal branches of cranial nerve V.

Clinical features of HSV encephalitis

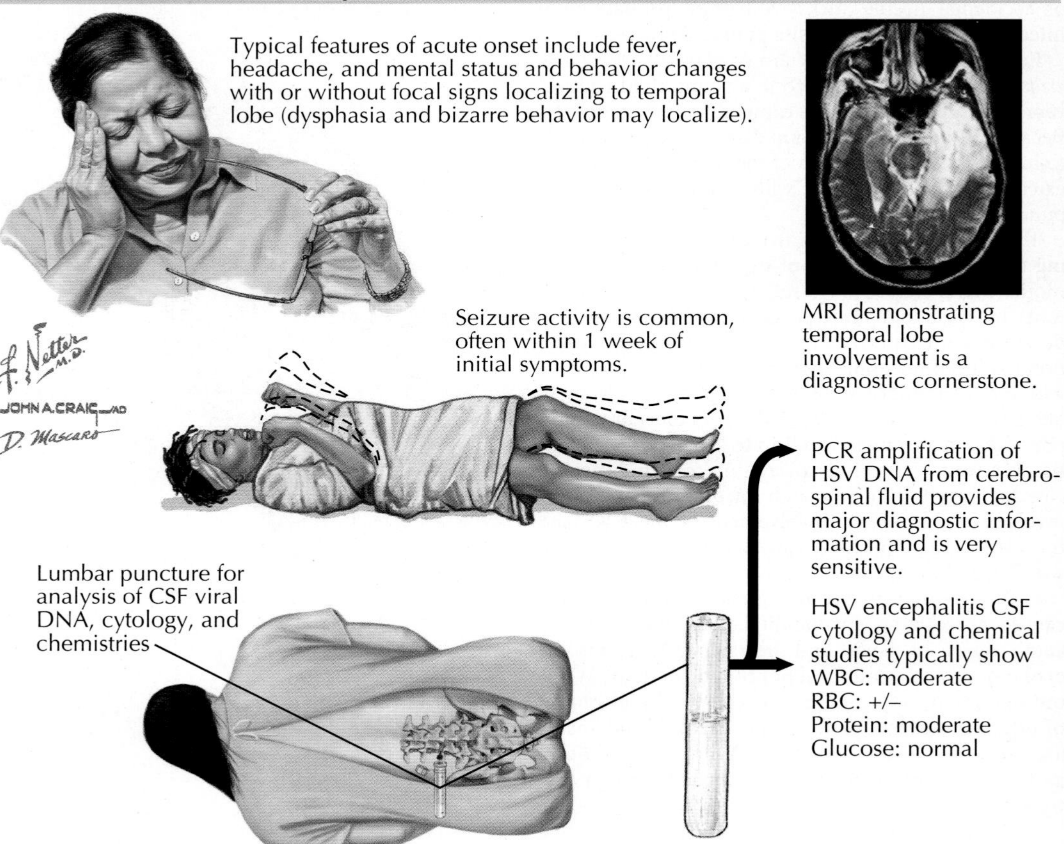

Histoplasmosis

Histoplasmosis is endemic in the Ohio and Mississippi River Valleys but exists throughout North America and is also seen in Central and South America. It is a primary pulmonary disease, with the skin being secondarily involved in disseminated disease; however, isolated cutaneous disease can result from direct inoculation. Patients typically breathe in the infective spores, which lodge in the pulmonary tree. Most infections are subclinical.

Clinical Findings: The disease is seen primarily in immunocompromised patients. Other risk factors include occupations that include contact with bat or bird droppings in an endemic region. The fungus is not found in fresh bird droppings, but the droppings provide the perfect environment for the soil-based fungus to grow and reproduce. Patients inhale the spores into the lungs. Most have no symptoms. Some have mild flu-like symptoms that go undiagnosed or misdiagnosed as an upper respiratory infection. The primary infection heals, and the lungs may have visible findings on chest radiography. Variable radiographic findings are seen. Small, symmetrically located areas of hilar miliary calcification are the most common finding. Other lung findings can mimic those of tuberculosis, lung cancer, or metastatic cancer. Bilateral hilar adenopathy may be seen, as may lobar pneumonia.

Dissemination of the disease to other organs can occur in the immunocompromised host. The skin is commonly affected in disseminated disease. The skin findings often appear as papules, plaques, or nodules with varying degrees of ulceration. Subcutaneous abscess formation may occur, and fistulas and sinus tract formation may be prominent. Surrounding redness may give the appearance of cellulitis. Adenopathy in the draining lymph nodes is commonly appreciated. The diagnosis depends on the histologic findings and the culture results.

Pathogenesis: *Histoplasma capsulatum* is a thermally dimorphic fungus responsible for a wide range of infections, including pulmonary, pericardial, and cutaneous diseases. The fungus is ubiquitous in nature and is found in soil, where it lives as a saprophyte. Spores from the mycelial phase of the fungus are inhaled or inoculated directly into the skin. Once they have entered the body, the change in temperature causes transformation of the spores into the yeast form of *H. capsulatum*. Most infections go unnoticed or induce a subclinical scenario or a mild, flu-like illness. Most cases are self-contained, and the only evidence of disease is the formation of granulomas within the lungs and a positive skin delayed hypersensitivity test. If a preexposed or newly exposed patient becomes immunosuppressed, the patient is at risk for disease reactivation and serious sequelae.

Ulcerating plaque of tongue due to histoplasmosis. Lesion may be identical in appearance to carcinoma of tongue.

Mycelial or free-living phase of *H. capsulatum* as it exists in nature or in culture

Spores of mycelial phase of *H. capsulatum*. Inhalation of these spores is the source of infection.

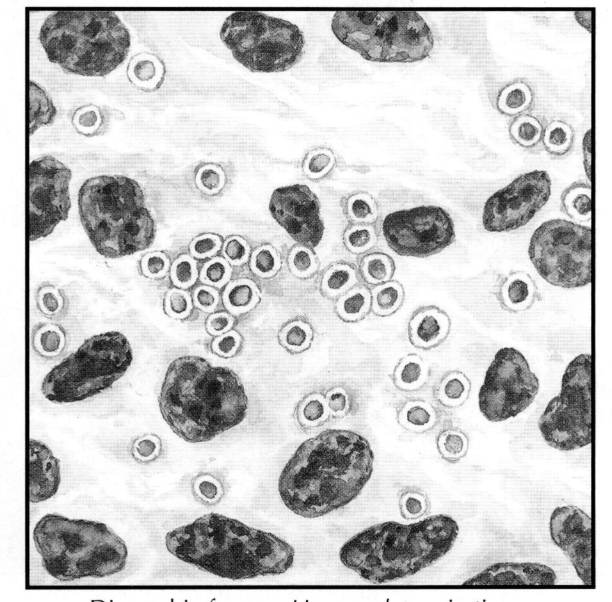

Dimorphic fungus; *H. capsulatum* in tissue

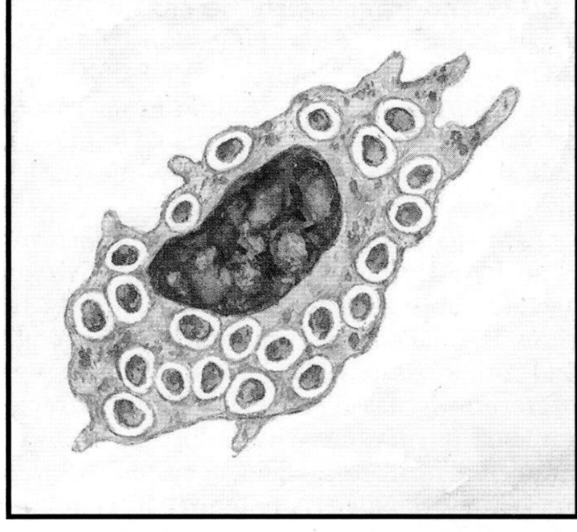

H. capsulatum in a macrophage, termed a *phagocytized histiocyte*. In this yeast or tissue phase, the organism is not transmissible from person to person.

Histology: Skin biopsy specimens show pseudocarcinomatous hyperplasia of the epidermis with an underlying granulomatous infiltrate. Ulceration and abscess formation are not uncommon with widespread necrosis. The yeast-like organisms can be appreciated in the cytoplasm of histiocytes. This is one of the few infections in which phagocytized histiocytes are seen. The yeast structures are round to oval, and there may be a clear region surrounding the yeast cell. Yeast organisms are also appreciated within the dermis, between and within the inflammatory infiltrate. They can be highlighted by use of special histology stains such as periodic acid–Schiff or Grocott silver stain.

Histoplasmosis is best cultured on Sabouraud medium. The fungus in its mycelial phase grows slowly. It appears as a brown, fluffy fungus on culture.

Treatment: Most cases of primary pulmonary disease go undiagnosed, and the patient's immune system contains the fungus. In patients with mild pulmonary symptoms who are not immunocompromised, therapy can be withheld because most cases resolve spontaneously. Patients who have more severe disease or are immunocompromised should be started on therapy with one of the three most efficacious and best-studied medications: fluconazole, itraconazole, or amphotericin B. Treatment may be prolonged. Patients who have AIDS benefit from directed therapy against HIV. Patients taking chronic immunosuppressants should have their medications discontinued or decreased, if possible.

LEPROSY (HANSEN DISEASE)

Leprosy is a chronic multisystem disease with cutaneous findings caused by the bacteria *Mycobacterium leprae.* It also goes by the name *Hansen disease.* Gerhard Hansen was the Norwegian physician who first described *M. leprae* as the cause of leprosy in 1873. Leprosy is most prevalent in regions of Africa, Southeast Asia, and South America, and it can be seen in isolated regions of North America.

Clinical Findings: Cutaneous findings often begin as a solitary hypopigmented macule. The area of involvement often has a loss of sensation and temperature discrimination. This initial phase has been termed *indeterminate* leprosy. At this point, it is unknown what type of overall immune response the host will mount. After a period of time, if the host's cell-mediated immune response is able to keep the bacteria in check, the patient develops tuberculoid leprosy or paucibacillary leprosy. Tuberculoid leprosy manifests with one to three patches or plaques. The border tends to be raised, with a central depression. Adnexal structures, such as hair, are lost, and the lesions are often hypopigmented. This form of leprosy tends to affect the peripheral nerves (e.g., median nerve, ulnar nerve). Palpation of the involved nerve demonstrates enlargement and irregularly spaced nodules. Nerve involvement leads to impairment of the innervated skin and muscle.

Patients who do not mount a strong cell-mediated immune reaction develop lepromatous leprosy or multibacillary leprosy. Up to hundreds of hypopigmented patches and plaques may be present. Hair loss may occur in the affected skin and along the eyelashes and eyebrows. This form of leprosy can affect many nerves in a widespread region, leading to neuropathy. There are varying degrees of cell-mediated immune response, and the disease is classified by the Ridley-Jopling system.

Pathogenesis: *M. leprae* is an acid-fast mycobacterium found in environments where the temperature averages approximately 29°C. Most likely, the bacterium is inhaled and subsequently invades the skin and other tissues by hematogenous spread. This bacterium is classified as an obligate intracellular organism. It survives within histiocytes, where it is protected from host defense systems. Several genes are being evaluated as potential susceptibility markers, as it appears that the organism is not highly contagious. It is estimated that only 5% of those exposed eventually develop disease. *M. leprae* is highly unusual in that it can infect peripheral nerves. The bacterium expresses a protein, phenolic glycolipid 1, that has the ability to bind to peripheral nerve cells. This allows initial entry into the host and provides the bacteria with a place to replicate. Many other tissue types can be infected.

Histology: Skin biopsy can be extremely helpful in confirming or making the diagnosis of leprosy. Biopsy findings are highly dependent on the type of leprosy the patient develops. Biopsies of paucibacillary leprosy show a granulomatous infiltrate with few bacteria present. The bacteria can be sparsely located, and the tissue must be stained with a modified acid-fast stain (Fite method) to appreciate the small, red, rod-shaped bacteria. These can be seen only with an oil immersion objective.

In multibacillary leprosy, there is a mixed dermal infiltrate with an overlying grenz zone. The dermal infiltrate is made up of plasma cells, lymphocytes, and foamy histiocytes. The histiocytes, when observed under oil immersion, show numerous bacteria. Bacteria are also seen scattered throughout the dermis.

Treatment: Guidelines for the treatment of leprosy have been established by the World Health Organization (WHO), and their most recent information should always be consulted when treating this disease. Treatment has historically been based on the bacillary load. In 2018, WHO recommended treating leprosy regardless of bacillary load to avoid undertreating individuals who have been misclassified. Paucibacillary and multibacillary are treated with a combination of dapsone, clofazimine, and rifampin for 12 months. Numerous alternative agents are available. Even after the bacterium has been killed, the skin lesions may take years to resolve.

Prevalence rates (per 10,000 population)
0 (no cases reported)
Less than 1
1.0–1.5
1.5–2.0
2 and above
No data

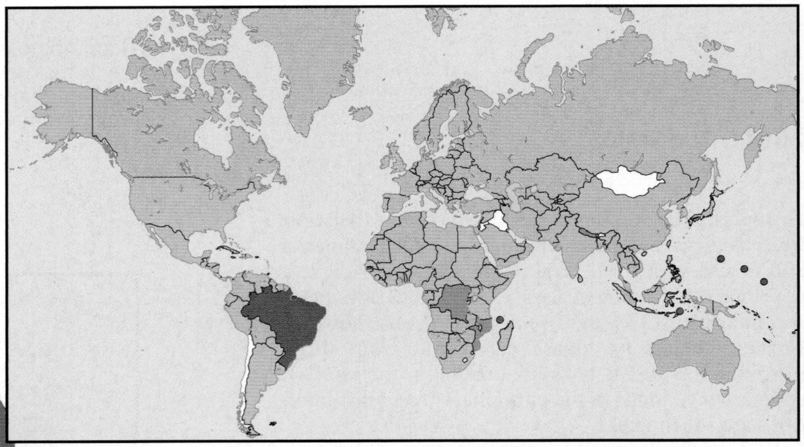

Based on leprosy prevalence, beginning of 2009. WHO.

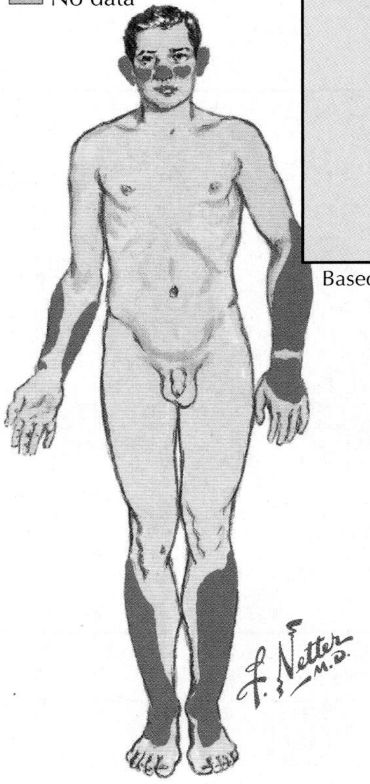

Typical early pattern of sensory loss in leprosy (Hansen disease) tends to affect cooler skin areas not following either segmental or nerve distribution; area kept warm by watchband is not affected.

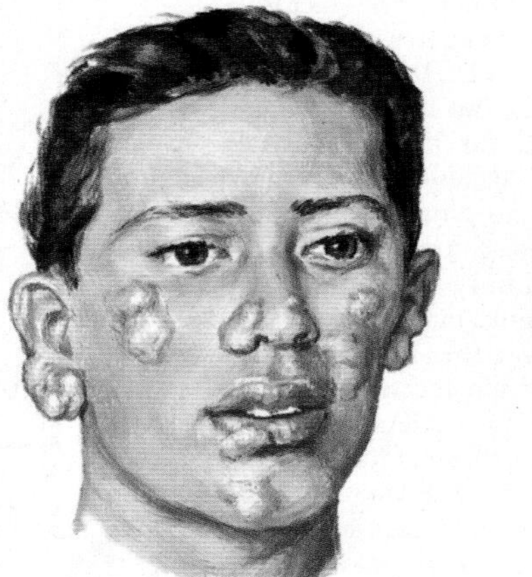

Patches and plaques on face and ears

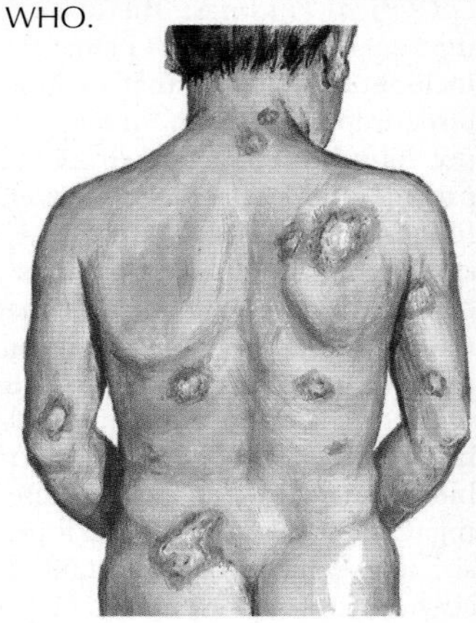

Multiple patches seen in lepromatous leprosy; central healed areas tend to be hypesthetic or anesthetic (dimorphous leprosy).

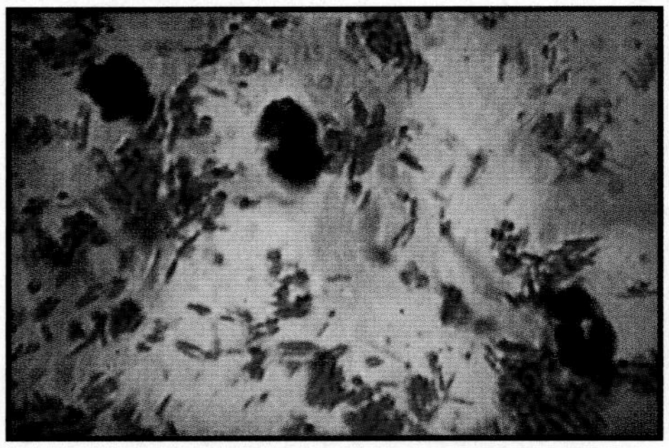

Biopsy specimen of nerve reveals abundant acid-fast bacilli *(M. leprae)*

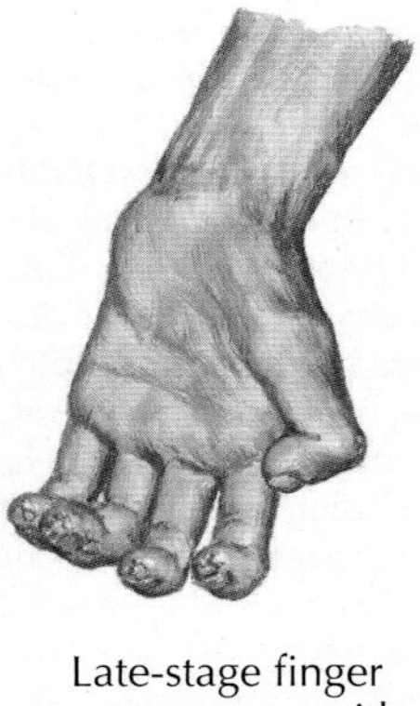

Late-stage finger contractures with ulcerations due to sensory loss

LICE

Lice are nonflying insects that live off the blood meal from a human host. They have been human pathogens for thousands of years and continue to cause millions of cases of disease annually. Three variants of the louse exist: the head louse, the body louse, and the pubic louse. For the most part, lice cause localized skin disease from the biting they do to secure their blood meal. However, some lice have been known to transmit other diseases to humans. The most important infectious agents transmitted by body lice are the bacteria that cause epidemic typhus, relapsing fever, and trench fever. These infections are uncommon in the United States and North America but are still seen, and clinicians should be aware of their causes and vectors.

Clinical Findings: Lice are capable of infesting any human, independent of age, sex, or race. Body lice are seen more frequently in patients of low socioeconomic status and especially in individuals experiencing homelessness. Underlying mental health issues in this subset may also predispose to conditions that are opportune for infestation. Pubic lice, or "crabs," is an STI seen more frequently in younger adults than in other age groups; however, it occurs in people of all ages.

Pediculosis capitis (head lice infestation) is probably the most common louse infestation in North America and Europe. The louse *Pediculus humanus capitis* preferentially locates to the scalp and lives between the hair shafts. These lice are transmitted by close contact and from fomites such as combs, pillows, and head rests. Patients report severe itching on the scalp and neck. On inspection, small (1–2 mm), red, excoriated papules are seen. Evidence of scratching becomes prominent as time goes on without a diagnosis. The diagnosis is confirmed by finding a louse, which is typically 2 to 4 mm long and light brown in color. On occasion, the abdomen of the louse can appear red directly after a blood meal. These insects are not particularly fast moving, nor can they fly or jump; as a result, they are easy to capture and identify. Egg sacks (nits) are firmly adhered to the hair. This is in contrast to the common hair cast, which can easily be moved up and down the hair shaft with minimal effort. The nits are laid in close proximity to the scalp, usually within 0.5 mm. The nits hatch within 2 weeks; therefore nits found more than 2 cm from the scalp are often nonviable because the larva has already emerged from the nit. Persistent infections can lead to bacterial superinfection and pyoderma with cervical adenopathy.

Pediculosis pubis (pubic lice infestation) is a commonly acquired STI. The pubic louse, *Phthirus pubis*, is structurally different from the body or head louse and can easily be distinguished. Affected individuals report itching and often note pinpoint drops of blood in their undergarments caused by small amounts of bleeding after the pubic lice feed. These lice have specialized arms that allow them to climb around the entire human body, and they may be seen at any location. They tend to affect the eyelashes and eyebrows. This is important to look for clinically in order to appropriately treat all affected regions.

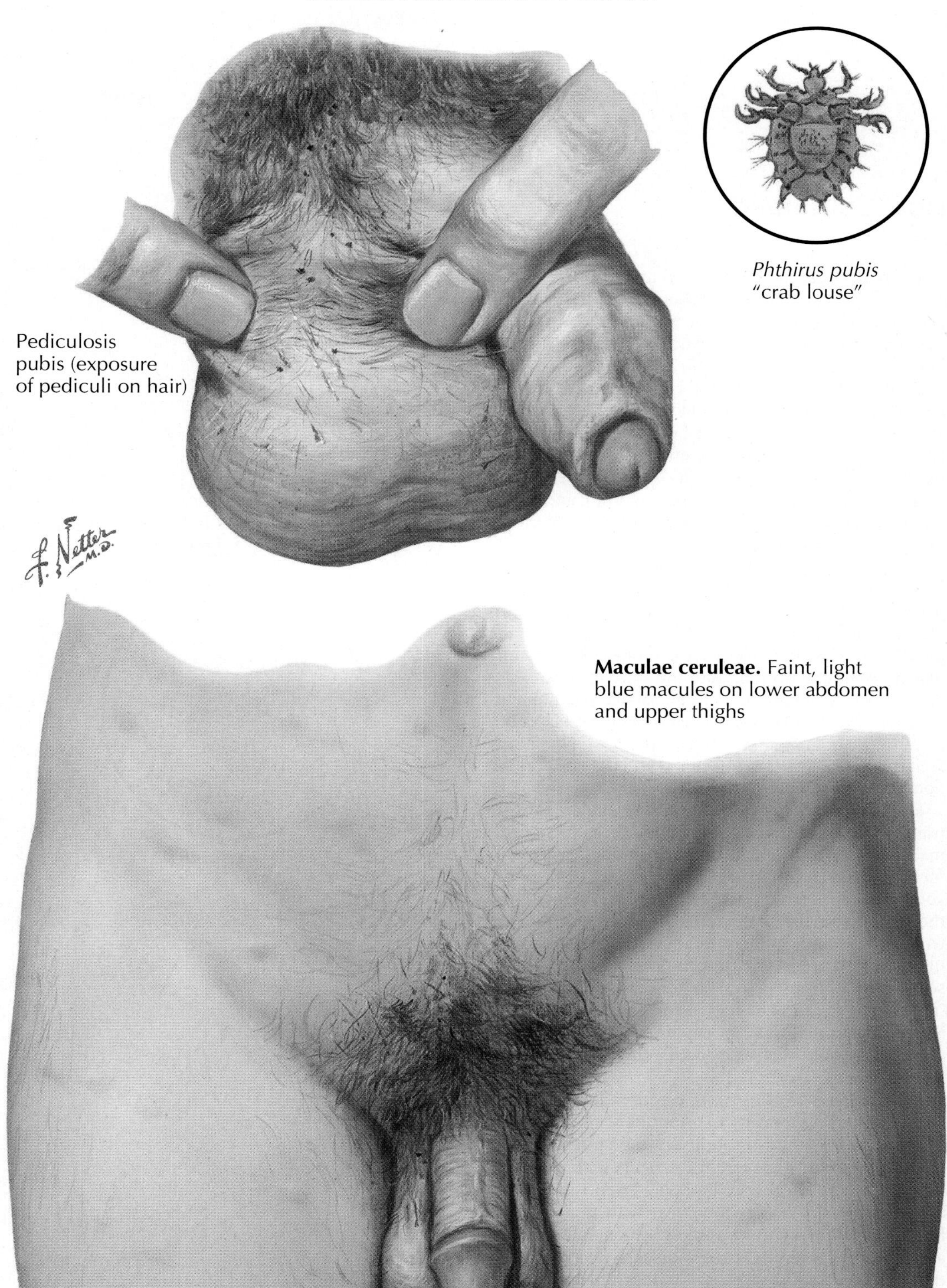

Pediculosis corporis (body lice infestation) is commonly seen in homeless individuals and in those with poor hygiene. Historically, body lice have been associated with epidemics during times of war because close contact for extended periods leads to easy transfer from one host to another. The body louse, *Pediculus humanus corporis,* is indistinguishable from the head louse on inspection with the naked eye. Entomologists trained in differentiating the species are capable of discerning the two. Body lice live on clothing and leave it to feast on human blood. Patients present with multiple pruritic, red to pink, excoriated papules anywhere on the body. On inspection of the skin, lice are not typically found. Only with close inspection of the clothing or bedding material does the infestation become apparent. Hundreds to thousands of lice may be present on the clothing, particularly in small hiding spaces such as the seams. Along with the lice, many eggs and larvae may be seen.

LICE (Continued)

The body louse has been shown to be a carrier of the bacterial agents that cause relapsing fever, trench fever, and epidemic typhus: *Borrelia recurrentis, Bartonella quintana,* and *Rickettsia prowazekii,* respectively. The louse carries the bacteria within its gut.

B. recurrentis is responsible for causing the disease relapsing fever. It is transmitted from one human to another when the fecal material of a human body louse gains entry to the bloodstream. This bacterium is unique in that it can rearrange its surface proteins. This is believed to be the reason for the relapsing and recurrent fevers: the host immune system reacts in a periodic manner to the changing surface of the bacteria.

B. quintana is transmitted through the feces of the louse. After a louse defecates on a patient's skin and the patient scratches, the stool and the bacteria are implanted into the skin, which causes infection. Also, the louse often bites after defecating and causes skin trauma that transfers the bacteria into the skin. *B. quintana* is the etiologic agent of trench fever, bacillary angiomatosis, and peliosis and has also been shown to cause endocarditis. *B. quintana* infections are most commonly seen in patients who are infected with HIV virus and in homeless individuals.

R. prowazekii is an obligate intracellular parasite transmitted to humans through the feces of the human body louse. The natural environmental reservoir for this bacterium is the flying squirrel *(Glaucomys volans)*. The infected louse feeds on the human, and the fecal material that contains the *R. prowazekii* bacteria is deposited into the fresh wound, allowing for infectious transfer. This infection is most frequently seen during times of war, when individuals are in close contact with one another for significant periods. Signs and symptoms of epidemic typhus include fever, rash, pain, delirium, and other constitutional symptoms.

Pathogenesis: *P. humanus capitis* affects humans and has a high propensity to infest the scalp. These lice live on the host and periodically take a blood meal from the scalp or neck area. In patients with very long hair, the blood meal may be taken from the back or any area of skin that is in contact with the hair. The lice are able to reproduce rapidly. The females, which are a bit larger than the males, lay eggs that hatch and develop into adults capable of reproducing within 4 weeks.

Histology: The histologic findings on skin biopsy are similar among all forms of louse bites. Histologic evaluation cannot differentiate a louse bite from any other insect bite with certainty. Skin biopsies are rarely performed in these cases because the diagnosis is made clinically. Biopsy specimens show a nonspecific, mixed superficial and deep inflammatory infiltrate with eosinophils. This may suggest a bite reaction. Unlike tick bites or scabies, in which occasionally tick parts or scabies mites are seen in a biopsy specimen, a biopsy from a patient with a lice infestation will never show mouth parts or other elements of the louse.

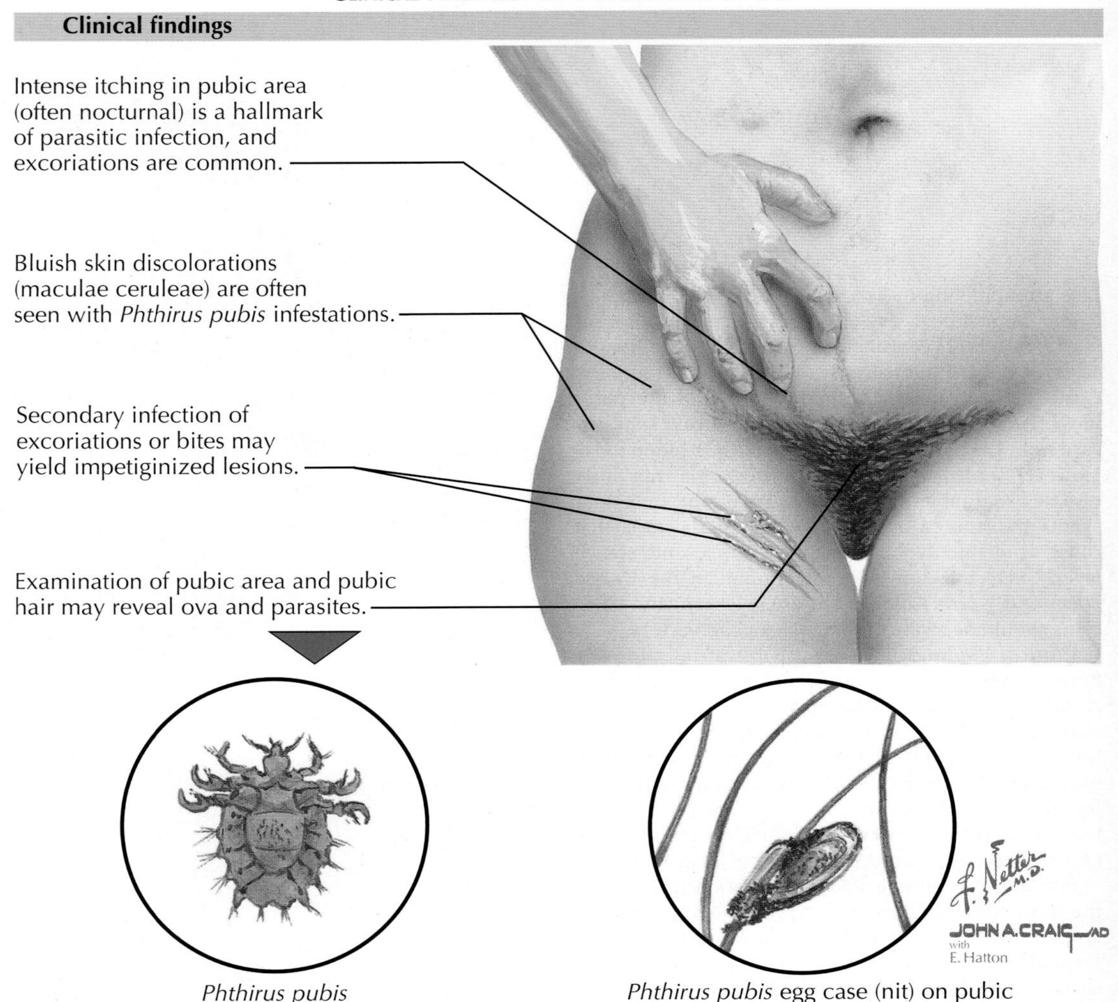

Phthirus pubis

Phthirus pubis egg case (nit) on pubic hair. The egg case is firmly attached.

Management

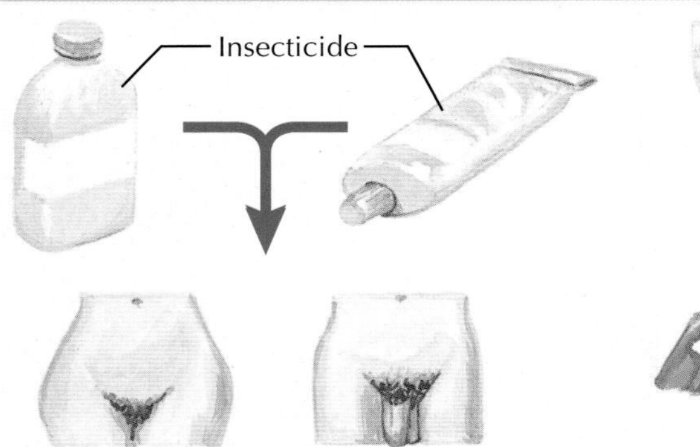

Increased general hygiene and treatment of household members and all sexual partners with insecticide shampoos and creams

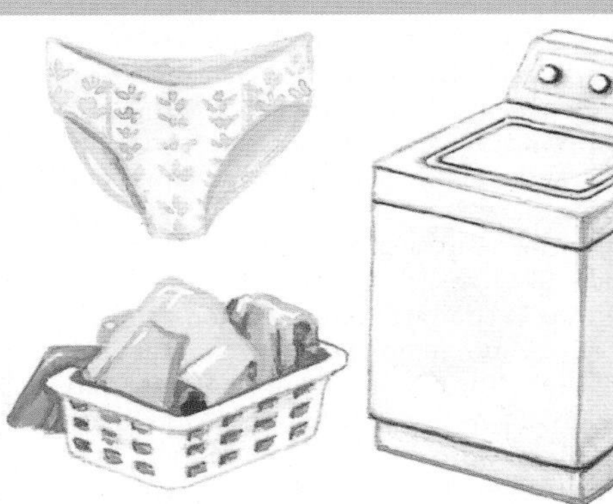

General house cleaning with emphasis on disinfection and laundering of underclothing and bedding

Treatment: Therapeutic agents to treat lice are similar among all species of human lice. The most commonly used therapies are based on permethrin; when used appropriately, they show good cure rates. These treatments should be used in conjunction with an agent that helps remove the nits from the hair shafts, and physical removal with a lice hair comb is a must. Therapy should be repeated on a weekly basis. Bedding and clothing need to be disinfected. The use of lindane has decreased because of its potential neurotoxicity. Malathion topically and oral ivermectin show excellent efficacy. Oral ivermectin needs to be repeated in 1 week because it does not kill the developing larvae within the nits. Other topical agents used to treat lice include benzyl alcohol and spinosad.

Therapy for body lice also requires complete disinfection of the household or living areas. Overtly infested clothing should be thrown away. Household contacts should be examined and treated if they have evidence of infestation. Professional fumigation should be considered.

Lyme Disease

Lyme disease is a tickborne infection caused by the spirochete bacteria *Borrelia burgdorferi*. The deer tick, *Ixodes scapularis,* is the main tick responsible for transmitting the disease to humans. Discovered in 1975 in the Connecticut town of Lyme, this disease has become the most common tickborne disease in the United States. Most cases are reported in the spring, summer, and early fall, correlating with tick activity. The disease also affects dogs, horses, and cattle.

Clinical Findings: Erythema migrans is the characteristic cutaneous rash of Lyme disease. Erythema migrans typically manifests as a solitary "bull's-eye" macule at the site of the tick bite. There is a central red macule surrounded by nonaffected skin, which is then entirely surrounded by an expanding erythema that blends in with the peripheral normal skin. The rash of erythema migrans is larger than 2 cm in diameter. The exanthem manifests soon after the tick has transmitted the bacteria into the skin. Occasionally, the central portion of the lesion forms a vesicle or bulla. Solitary skin lesions are the most frequent skin manifestation, but early disseminated Lyme disease also occurs, resulting in multiple areas of skin involvement. The numerous skin lesions are smaller than the original lesion, lighter in color, and not as fully developed as the bull's-eye lesions. This early dissemination of *B. burgdorferi* occurs in 25% of infected individuals. Most patients also exhibit constitutional symptoms at the time of diagnosis, including headache, fever, and malaise.

Erythema migrans occurs in approximately 75% of those infected with the spirochete. Individuals who do not exhibit the rash and those who go without treatment are likely to develop chronic disease, which manifests in many ways. Lyme arthritis is one of the most frequent manifestations of chronic Lyme disease; it is typically oligoarticular in presentation. Another frequently seen manifestation is Bell palsy, which is caused by involvement of the CNS. The cardiovascular, nervous, musculoskeletal, and hematologic systems may all be involved in chronic Lyme disease.

Pathogenesis: *B. burgdorferi* is a spirochete transmitted to humans via the bite of the deer tick *(I. scapularis).* The white-tailed deer and the white-footed mouse are two reservoirs for *B. burgdorferi*. These two animals are typically unaffected by the bacteria. The larval, nymph, or adult form of the *I. scapularis* tick takes a blood meal from one of these reservoirs and acquires the bacteria. The spirochete causes the tick no harm and can survive in the gut of the tick for prolonged periods. The tick can then transmit the bacteria to an incidental host such as a human. Transmission of the bacteria is increased the longer the tick is attached to the host. It is generally believed that a tick must be attached for 24 hours to transmit the bacteria.

Histology: Skin biopsies of erythema migrans show a lymphocytic superficial and deep dermal infiltrate. Numerous plasma cells may be seen in conjunction with eosinophils. Spirochetes are seen in fewer than half of specimens. The pathologic findings of erythema migrans are used to help confirm the clinical findings. However, the clinician should not wait for the pathology report to treat a patient with clinical evidence of Lyme disease.

Treatment: Treatment of erythema migrans consists of a course of doxycycline. The therapy is highly effective and has an excellent safety profile. Amoxicillin or cefuroxime can be used for patients who cannot take doxycycline and for young children. CNS involvement requires intravenous therapy with ceftriaxone or penicillin. Prevention is critically important. Permethrin-based insect repellants are effective at repelling deer ticks. Clothing impregnated with permethrin can be useful for those who spend time outdoors in endemic areas.

After being in a wooded region, people should check their skin for the presence of ticks and remove them immediately because the transmission of the spirochete requires approximately 24 hours of attachment. This inspection method works for adult ticks, but the larvae and nymphs are too small to see routinely and are almost always overlooked.

Early disseminated Lyme disease with multiple bull's-eye lesions of erythema migrans. This is seen in up to 25% of patients who develop Lyme disease.

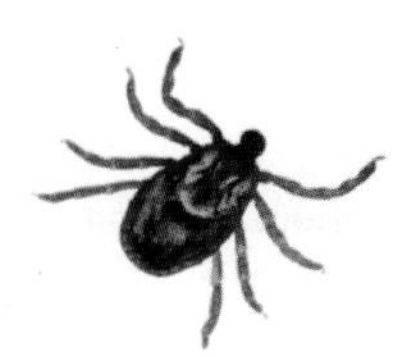

Lyme disease is spread by a bite from an *Ixodes scapularis* tick that is infected with *Borrelia burgdorferi.*

Bell Palsy: Common Manifestation of Chronic Lyme Disease

Hyperacusis

This may be an early or initial symptom of a peripheral CN VII nerve palsy: patient holds phone away from ear because of painful sensitivity to sound. Loss of taste also may occur on affected side.

Left peripheral CN VII facial weakness

Attempt to close eye results in the eyeball rolling superiorly, exposing sclera (Bell phenomenon), but no closure of the lid per se.

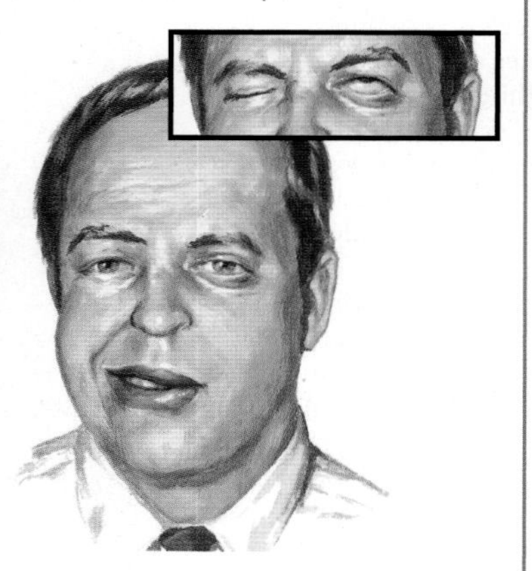

Patient is unable to wrinkle forehead; eyelid droops very slightly; cannot show teeth at all on affected side in attempt to smile; and lower lip droops slightly.

Left central CN VII facial weakness

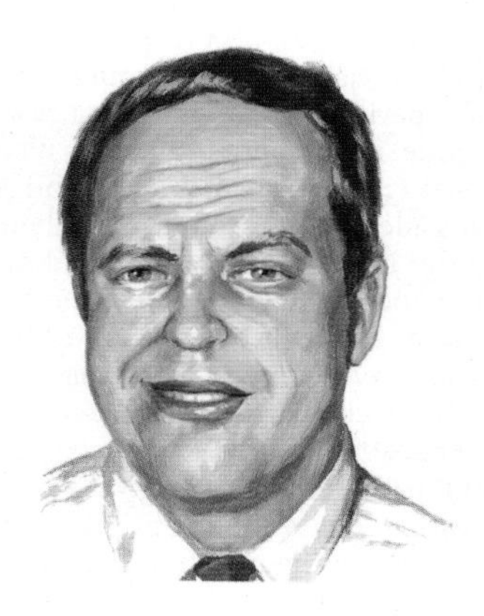

Patient has an incomplete smile with very subtle flattening of affected nasolabial fold and relative preservation of brow and forehead movement.

Lymphogranuloma Venereum

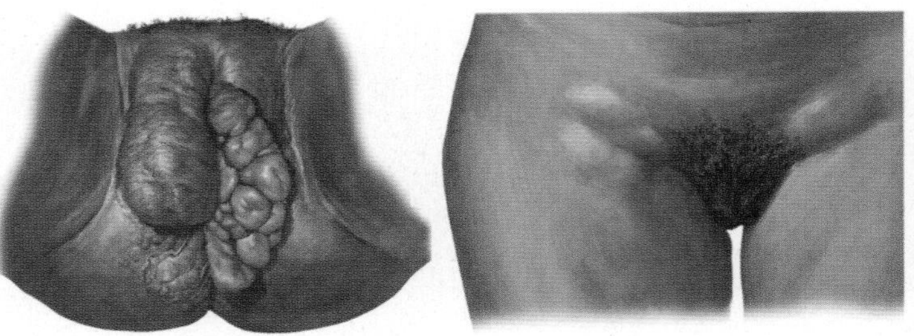

Lymphogranuloma venereum causing chronic lymphedema *(left)* and inguinal adenopathy *(right)*

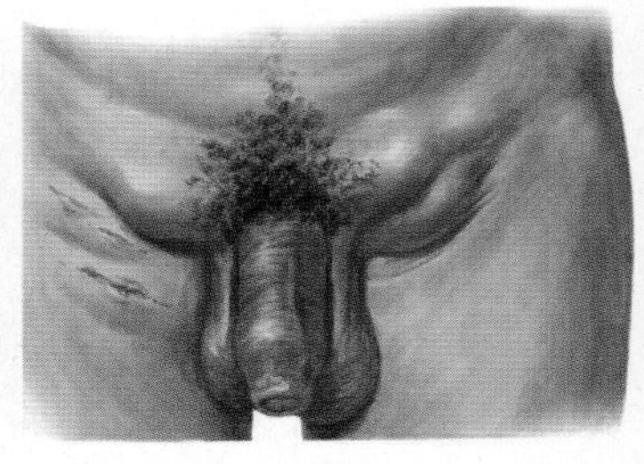

Groove sign seen in a male patient with lymphogranuloma venereum caused by massive adenopathy on either side of Poupart's ligament

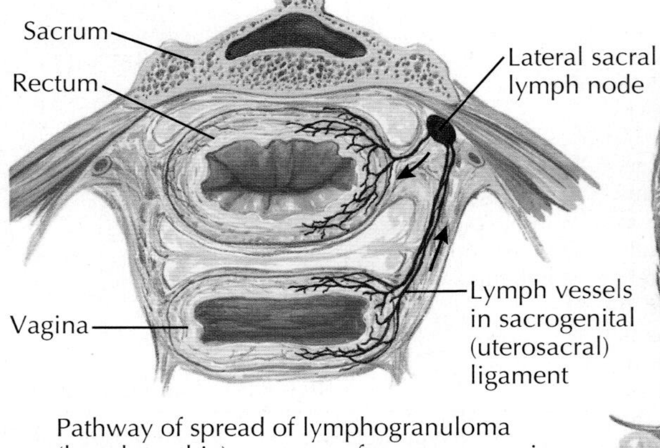

Pathway of spread of lymphogranuloma (lymphopathia) venereum from upper vagina and/or cervix uteri to rectum via lymph vessels

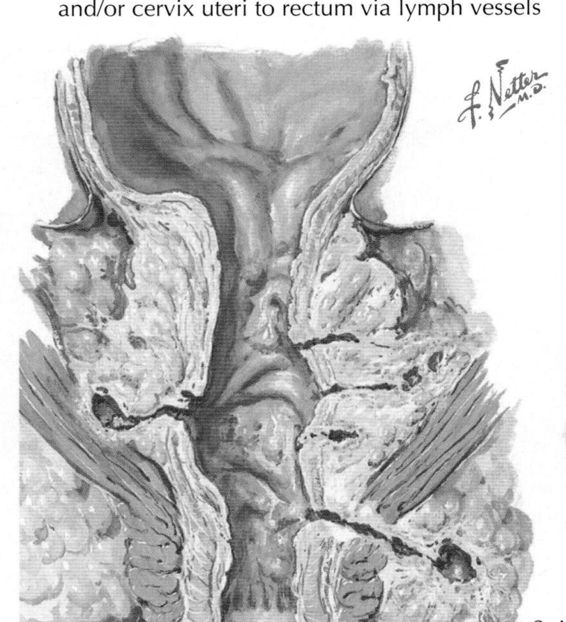

Stricture of rectum with multiple blind sinuses; strictures cause chronic pain and are a significant source of morbidity.

Long tubular stricture of rectum

Lymphogranuloma venereum (LGV) is an STI produced by infection with *Chlamydia trachomatis* serotypes L1, L2, and L3. LGV progresses through three distinct phases of transmission. This bacterial disease was once limited to tropical regions, but with the ease of worldwide travel, it is now seen globally. The skin manifestations are found predominantly in the groin and genital region. This infection is often seen in conjunction with other STIs, and screening for other STIs should be done routinely in patients diagnosed with LGV.

C. trachomatis has also been shown to be responsible for many infectious complications, including pneumonia, urogenital infections, proctitis, conjunctivitis, and trachoma. Trachoma, which often starts as conjunctivitis, results in chronic intense inflammation of the bulbar and eyelid conjunctiva that causes scarring and eventually blindness if left untreated. Trachoma and conjunctival disease are caused by the A, B, and C serotypes of *C. trachomatis*.

Clinical Findings: LGV is a rare disease in the United States and Europe but should be considered in the differential diagnosis of all anogenital ulcerations. The disease is seen more frequently in patients with a low socioeconomic status and in those with multiple sexual partners. LGV is passed from one individual to another via sexual intercourse. After a short incubation period (a few days to a few weeks), a painless papule forms and ultimately ulcerates. The ulcer is small (≤1 cm in diameter) and without induration. This ulceration is often described as painless, but it causes the patient irritation and discomfort with pressure and manipulation. This primary stage of the disease spontaneously resolves without therapy. The ulcer heals, leaving only a slight scar.

The secondary stage of disease begins with inguinal adenopathy. The inguinal lymph nodes become enlarged and painful. Initial involvement occurs within 2 to 3 weeks after healing of the ulcer and typically results in discrete, painful lymph nodes on each side of the inguinal crease. The lymph nodes coalesce over time and mat together into a large mass of tissue called buboes. If both sides of the inguinal ligament (Poupart's ligament) are involved, this can lead to a characteristic clinical finding named the *groove sign*. This name denotes the massive adenopathy on each side of the inguinal ligament; the groove is the area overlying the ligament with no adenopathy. The massive adenopathy may become necrotic, and suppurative lymph nodes are frequently seen. Sinus tracts from the adenopathy to the surface of the skin form and drain. This second stage is associated with fever and constitutional symptoms.

The third, or late, stage of LGV is less frequently seen and consists of scarring and fibrosis as well as elephantiasis of the genitals. If the primary and secondary diseases have affected the rectum, rectal fissures and strictures may be present, leading to chronic pain. Rectal disease and involvement are most frequently encountered in males who have sex with other males.

Pathogenesis: *C. trachomatis* is a gram-negative obligate intracellular bacterium. It is unique in that it has no ability, or only limited ability, to produce its own adenosine triphosphate energy source. This inability to create a steady source of energy forces the bacterium to reside within a host cell. The infectious form of the bacterium, called the *elementary body,* gains entry to a host cell. Within the cell, it forms a larger, actively reproducing reticulate body. The reticulate body undergoes binary fission to produce progeny (elementary bodies), which are then released from the cell to infect other cells or hosts.

Histology: A skin biopsy of a primary ulcer of LGV shows epithelial necrosis with a mixed, nonspecific inflammatory infiltrate. There are no pathognomonic histologic findings in LGV. A tissue culture (McCoy cell culture) is a reliable means of diagnosis. Nucleic acid amplification and PCR can be used to identify LGV. These tests are not universally available. The finding of iodine-staining, glycogen-containing inclusion bodies is sensitive and specific for the presence of *C. trachomatis*. Various serologic tests are available, but they cannot reliably differentiate between past and present disease.

Treatment: The routine application of erythromycin to the eyes of newborns has dramatically decreased the risk of trachoma. LGV is treated with oral antibiotics such as doxycycline or azithromycin. All sexual partners should also be treated, even if they do not exhibit overt signs of disease.

MENINGOCOCCEMIA

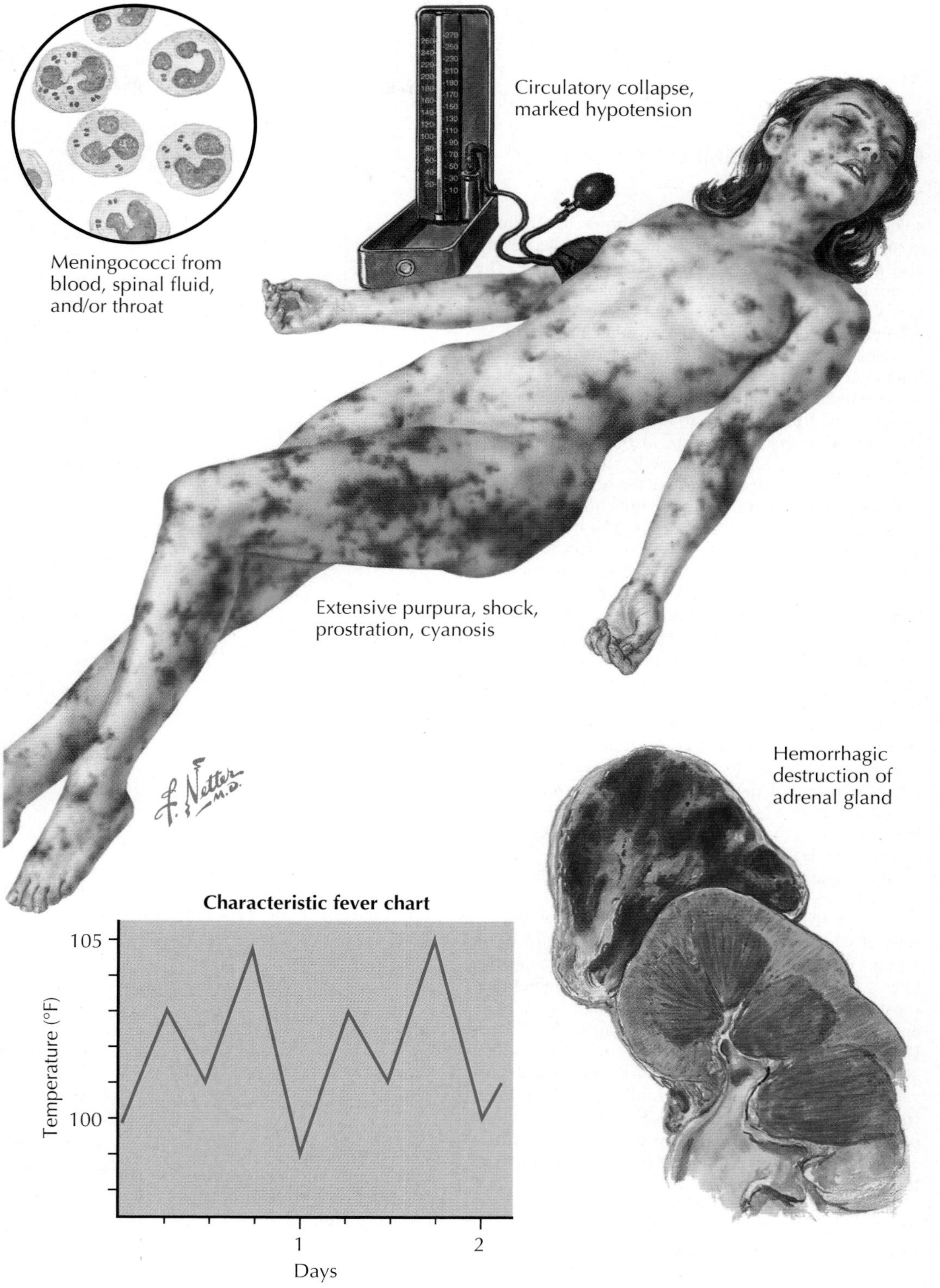

Neisseria meningitidis can cause a wide range of clinical diseases, of which neisserial meningitis is the most severe and life-threatening. The bacteria is capable of causing septicemia, pneumonia, and meningitis. These are all relentless diseases that can be fatal if not promptly treated. The bacteria has been known to cause severe disseminated intravascular coagulation (DIC) and Waterhouse-Friderichsen syndrome. The latter syndrome, also known as *acute adrenocortical insufficiency*, is directly caused by hemorrhagic destruction of both adrenal glands. This syndrome can result from a wide range of conditions, including infections both bacterial and viral. *N. meningitidis* was the first bacteria described to cause this syndrome. Waterhouse-Friderichsen syndrome has been shown to occur more commonly in individuals treated with blood thinners.

Clinical Findings: Children younger than 1 year are most likely to develop disease from *N. meningitidis* infection. They are more susceptible to infection after their maternal antibodies have dissipated. Boys may be at a slightly higher risk than girls, but there is no race predilection. One risk factor appears to be the presence of a smoker in the household. It is theorized that the secondhand smoke damages the child's respiratory epithelium just enough to allow the bacteria to penetrate the mucous membranes and enter the bloodstream. Other notable risk factor includes a deficiency of the complement components C5, C6, C7, and C8. Asplenia also increases risk because the spleen is extremely important in removing encapsulated bacteria from the bloodstream. Chronic immunosuppression increases the risk, as does living in crowded conditions. This is why military barracks and college dormitories are often sources of outbreaks.

Patients who develop meningitis have fever, headache, agitation, vomiting, photophobia, stiff neck, and meningeal physical signs, including the Kernig sign and Brudzinski sign. The Kernig sign is positive when placing a patient's hips and knees in 90-degree flexion and extending the knee joint elicits pain. The Brudzinski sign is more sensitive for meningitis and is positive when flexing of the patient's neck causes flexion of the hips and knees. These signs have long been used to help diagnose meningitis clinically. As the disease progresses, seizures or coma may occur.

Cutaneous findings include nonblanching palpable purpura, ecchymosis, widespread macular purpura, and necrosis of the skin with secondary vesiculopustules. The rash typically starts on the lower extremities. The purpura can be angulated with an irregular border. Centrally within the purpuric region, there is often a dusky gray discoloration of the skin. Patients often report skin pain. Necrosis may progress to cause gangrene of the digits or distal extremities. In severe cases, entire limbs can become gangrenous. If DIC sets in, the clinical skin findings of DIC may be seen on top of the initial skin findings. The presence of DIC is a poor prognostic indicator. Lesions heal with scar formation.

Fulminant meningococcal septicemia may lead to hemorrhagic necrosis of the adrenal glands; this is termed Waterhouse-Friderichsen syndrome. It leads ultimately to acute adrenal dysfunction. This syndrome is seen in fewer than 5% of patients with *N. meningitidis* septicemia, but it occurs in more than 50% of the fatal cases. Patients present with skin findings of widespread purpura and cyanosis. They have signs and symptoms of hemodynamic collapse, hypotension, acute renal failure, and a biphasic fever. The skin findings are caused by small-vessel embolization or endothelial destruction from the septicemia. Blood extravasates through the damaged endothelial walls and produces massive purpura. The more extensive the cutaneous purpura in meningococcal septicemia, the higher the incidence of Waterhouse-Friderichsen syndrome.

Laboratory testing can be used to diagnose the disease, but therapy should begin before receiving the results if there is a high clinical suspicion of *N. meningitidis* infection. Culture of *N. meningitidis* from blood, cerebrospinal fluid (CSF), or tissue is diagnostic. The gram-negative diplococcal bacteria grow on the chocolate agar plate and appear as small, round, moist, gray

Bacterial Meningitis
Sources of infection

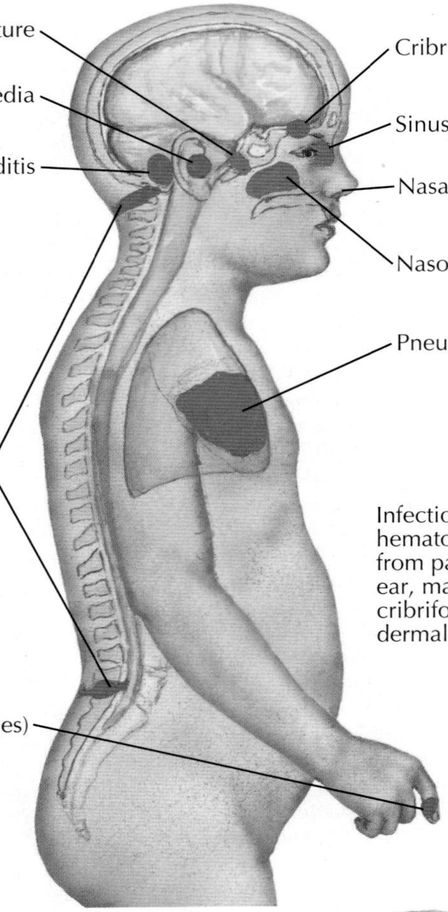

Basal skull fracture
Otitis media
Mastoiditis
Cribriform plate defect
Sinusitis (ethmoiditis)
Nasal furuncles
Nasopharyngitis
Pneumonia
Dermal sinuses
Skin (furuncles)

Infection of leptomeninges is usually hematogenous but may be direct from paranasal sinuses, middle ear, mastoid cells, or CSF leak due to cribriform plate defect or via dermal sinuses.

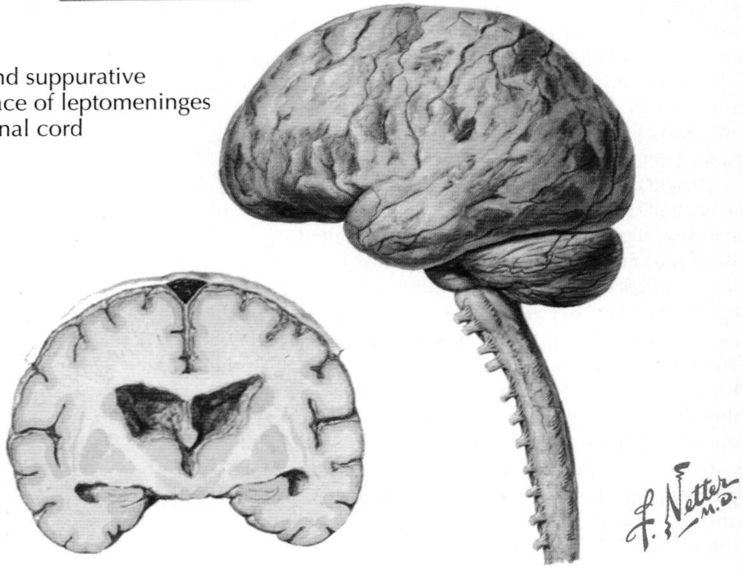

Inflammation and suppurative process on surface of leptomeninges of brain and spinal cord

Thrombophlebitis of superior sagittal sinus and suppurative ependymitis, with beginning hydrocephalus

Meningococcemia (Continued)

colonies. Gram staining of CSF shows intracellular gram-negative diplococcal bacteria. This bacterium also grows well on the Thayer-Martin agar plate. The bacterium is oxidase positive and is able to acidify certain sugars. These laboratory data can be used to help differentiate *N. meningitidis* from other bacteria. CSF samples can be used for PCR testing for the bacteria, but this is not routinely done in these cases. All cases of *N. meningitidis* infection should be reported to state and national health organizations.

A very rare chronic form of meningococcemia has been described and presents with recurrent chronic fevers and blood cultures positive for *N. meningitidis*.

Pathogenesis: Meningococcal infections, including septicemia and meningitis, are caused by the anaerobic gram-negative bacteria *N. meningitidis*. This is a diplococcal bacterium that requires an iron source for survival. Because of this unique metabolic requirement, humans are the only known host. The meningococcus bacteria can be found as a transient colonizer in the oropharynx of up to 10% of sampled individuals. These carriers express no sequelae but serve as a potential reservoir for meningococcal disease. The organisms are spread by close contact (respiratory droplets) and sharing of saliva. If the bacterium is able to reproduce to such an extent as to cause bacteremia, it then becomes a potential pathogen. Bacteremia can quickly lead to septicemia (meningococcemia). This is a severe, life-threatening disease that can kill quickly. Meningeal involvement leads to neisserial meningitis. The bacteria exhibit a neurotrophic behavior and attack the lining of the CNS.

At least 13 serotypes of *N. meningitidis* are known, nine of which have been conclusively shown to cause human disease. Currently, two vaccines are available. One, MenACWY, protects against the serotypes that most frequently cause disease: serotypes A, C, W-135, and Y. The other, MenB, protects against the B serotype. Currently there is no vaccine for the remaining serotypes, which can affect any individual regardless of vaccination status. The bacterium expresses a toxin (lipooligosaccharide) on its surface that causes many of the systemic symptoms of disease. *N. meningitidis* is an encapsulated bacterium, which helps protect it from the host's immune system.

Histology: Most skin biopsy specimens show evidence of vascular injury with neutrophils, fibrinoid necrosis, and extravasated red blood cells. Endothelial necrosis and thrombi are universally found. Varying degrees of vessel damage can be seen including all layers of the blood vessel. The inflammation fulfills the criteria for vasculitis. Varying numbers of *Neisseria* organisms can be found in the endothelium and within neutrophils. Organisms can be best appreciated on tissue Gram stains. Embolism of capillaries and small venules is often seen, and necrosis and ulceration can be secondary findings.

Treatment: Treatment requires prompt recognition of symptoms and immediate intravenous antibiotic therapy. Any close contacts of the patient should be screened for evidence of disease and given prophylactic oral therapy to decrease the potential of an epidemic. The main intravenous antibiotic of choice is ceftriaxone, followed by penicillin or by chloramphenicol in penicillin-allergic patients. Patients with Waterhouse-Friderichsen syndrome need adrenal gland replacement therapy.

Close contacts should be treated with ciprofloxacin, rifampin, or ceftriaxone. This prophylactic therapy, as well as intravenous therapy, should be started immediately if clinical suspicion is high enough; delaying therapy for even a few hours to wait for laboratory confirmation can be the difference between life and death.

Immunization is helping to keep the disease incidence low, and guidelines have been established for high-risk groups. Although the vaccine protects against only five of the 13 serotypes of *N. meningitidis*, it has the potential to decrease the incidence of this disease and save many lives. Prevention through vaccination is the single most important method to decrease the incidence of this disease.

Molluscum Contagiosum

As its name implies, molluscum contagiosum is a highly contagious viral infection that has little morbidity. This infection is most commonly encountered in children. The diagnosis is made on clinical grounds after inspection of the characteristic skin findings. When seen in the genital region of adults, molluscum contagiosum is considered an STI. This infection rarely occurs in immunocompetent adults outside sexual transmission. In adults with no clear evidence of transmission, an evaluation for an immunosuppressed state should be undertaken. Patients taking chronic immunosuppressive medications and those with AIDS are more prone to infection with molluscum contagiosum.

Clinical Findings: Young children are often affected by this common viral infection. Children pass the virus from one to another through close contact. The incubation period is 2 to 4 weeks. The characteristic finding is of small (3–5 mm), dome-shaped papules with a central dell. The coloration can be pink-red to slightly whitish. Solitary lesions may be appreciated, but clusters of lesions are often encountered. They may appear on any part of the body. Slight pruritus may accompany the lesions, but otherwise there are no symptoms. Molluscum lesions tend to become inflamed. When this occurs, they can become tender to the touch. Inflamed lesions are bright red and can bleed if the child scratches or traumatizes them. The more inflamed a lesion becomes, the more likely it is to leave scarring after healing. Scarring can also occur if the lesion becomes secondarily infected. Most noninflamed lesions spontaneously resolve within 6 months. Mollusca can be spread by scratching and/or shaving over the lesions.

Young and older adults who present with molluscum contagiosum in the genital region are believed to have acquired the infection through sexual contact. The number of lesions in these cases tends to be increased, and the lesions tend to be localized to the groin. These also spontaneously resolve over time with no therapy. Immunosuppressed individuals, especially those with HIV infection, have a high incidence of molluscum contagiosum viral infections. These infections tend to be widespread and can be larger than the typical version acquired in childhood.

Pathogenesis: Molluscum contagiosum is caused by an enveloped, large, double-stranded DNA poxvirus, of which there are four unique types. Humans are the only known species to be infected by this virus. The virus has been designated *molluscum contagiosum virus* (MCV), and the four types are MCV1 through MCV4. The virus is spread by close physical contact, and transmission on fomites has also been established. The virus attaches to the glycosaminoglycans on the surface of the targeted cell. The viral DNA gains entry into the cell cytoplasm, where it replicates itself. The virus carries with it a viral RNA polymerase, which acts to transcribe the viral genes, as well as a viral DNA polymerase for replication of its DNA. Early and late proteins are produced. The early proteins are generally for viral replication, and the late proteins are for production of the structural shell of the virus. These processes all occur within the cytoplasm of the infected cell. Once the virus has replicated, the infected cell typically dies, and the brick-shaped viral particles are released.

Histology: Skin biopsies of molluscum contagiosum are very characteristic, and the infection is easily diagnosed histologically. However, biopsies usually are not obtained because the disease is diagnosed clinically. The virally infected cells have molluscum bodies. The molluscum bodies transform from small, eosinophilic cytoplasmic bodies in the stratum basalis into larger basophilic bodies in the outer epidermis. As they enlarge, they often compress the nucleus of the infected cell. These intracytoplasmic eosinophilic inclusion bodies have been termed *Henderson-Paterson bodies*.

Treatment: In children a watch-and-wait approach is often the best therapy because most cases resolve spontaneously. Physicians need to recognize and treat secondary infections promptly to minimize scarring. Many destructive methods are available. Liquid nitrogen cryotherapy is highly effective, but most children have difficulty tolerating the pain it can cause. Many other therapies have been used, including tretinoin cream, salicylic acid, cantharidin, and curettage. Patients who are immunosuppressed can be treated with any of these modalities. Attempts to decrease immunosuppressive medications should be coordinated through the patient's transplant surgeon or primary care physician. Patients with widespread molluscum contagiosum and coexisting HIV infection have benefited from highly active antiretroviral therapy.

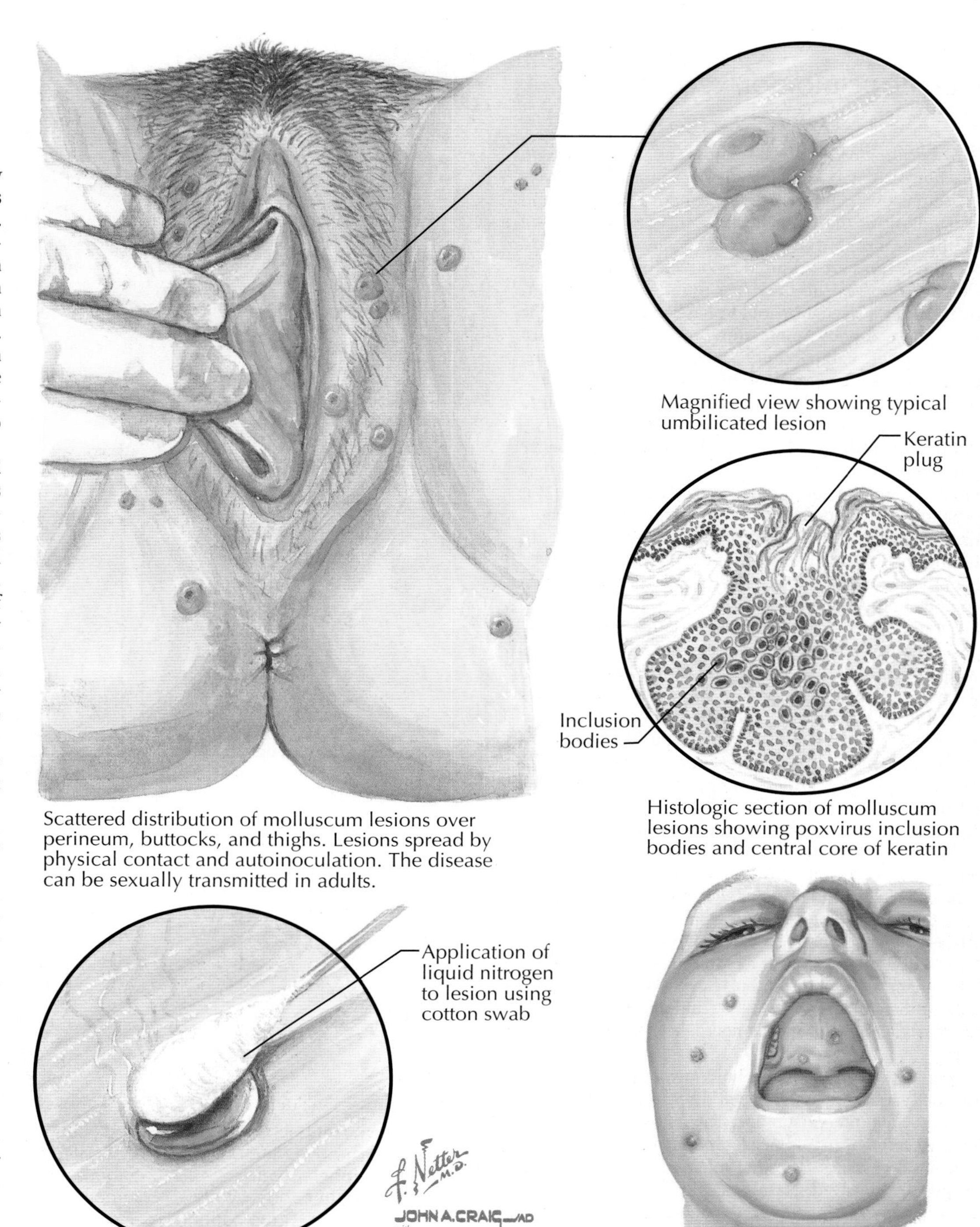

Magnified view showing typical umbilicated lesion

Scattered distribution of molluscum lesions over perineum, buttocks, and thighs. Lesions spread by physical contact and autoinoculation. The disease can be sexually transmitted in adults.

Histologic section of molluscum lesions showing poxvirus inclusion bodies and central core of keratin

Local eradication of lesions can be obtained with desiccation, cryotherapy, laser ablation, chemical cautery, or curettage.

Molluscum contagiosum is commonly encountered in children.

PARACOCCIDIOIDOMYCOSIS

Paracoccidioidomycosis, also known as *South American blastomycosis*, is a disease that is seen almost exclusively in regions of Central and South America. Humans and armadillos are the main hosts of disease. It is caused by the dimorphic fungus *Paracoccidioides brasiliensis*. Most infections are acquired by direct inhalation of the chlamydospores. The fungus is found in the environment in the mycelial or mold phase; it converts to the yeast phase at body temperature. Brazil has the highest incidence of paracoccidioidomycosis. Primary lung infection may lead to disseminated disease, with the skin being secondarily infected. Direct inoculation into the skin causes primary cutaneous disease.

Clinical Findings: In children there is equal incidence of infection in males and females. In adults, this fungal infection is more common in men than in women, for reasons poorly understood. It may be that men are more likely to have occupational exposures (most commonly, farming). A protective effect of estrogen also has been hypothesized. There is no race predilection. Immunocompetent hosts who are exposed to the fungus are likely to develop a subclinical infection; either the fungus becomes walled off in the form of granulomas within the lung or the patient goes on to develop clinical disease. Serologic testing may show evidence of past exposure in healthy subjects with no clinical findings. Some hosts have a constellation of flu-like symptoms that include malaise, weight loss, fatigue, fever, pneumonitis, and pleurisy. Progressive pulmonary lesions may occur regardless of immune status, but they are more severe in patients who are immunosuppressed.

Bilateral pulmonary infiltrates are seen on chest radiography and are similar to the radiographic findings of tuberculosis. The infiltrates often form consolidated areas with cavitations that heal with emphysematous changes. Almost all cases of paracoccidioidomycosis affect the lung. Hilar adenopathy is commonly present. Once a pulmonary nidus of infection is established, the fungus is able to disseminate to the skin, draining lymph nodes, adrenal glands, CNS, peritoneum, and gastrointestinal tract.

Skin lesions in paracoccidioidomycosis come in two distinct varieties. Disseminated disease is the more frequently encountered subtype. The lesions are predominantly on the head and neck, especially around the oral and nasal passages. The oral mucosal membranes and tongue are involved. Nasal and pharyngeal ulcerations are so frequently encountered that they have been given a name, *Aguiar-Pupo stomatitis*. The mucosal lesions are often peppered with pinpoint hemorrhagic areas. The skin findings may include papules, nodules, or fungating plaques. Ulceration is almost universal, and patients report pain and swelling. Cervical lymph nodes are enlarged. The infected lymph nodes often form sinus tracts to the skin and drain spontaneously.

The second form of cutaneous paracoccidioidomycosis is caused by direct inoculation of the fungus. The fungal elements are normally found in the soil, and piercing of the skin with a contaminated object can lead to primary cutaneous paracoccidioidomycosis. These lesions appear as papules or draining tender nodules with or without overlying ulceration. Some may spontaneously resolve, but most slowly enlarge. Intradermal and serologic testing are available in some centers.

Pathogenesis: The fungus *P. brasiliensis* has unusual living requirements, and its growth in the environment is dependent on the soil pH, the altitude, and a consistent temperature, with almost all cases seen within 20 degrees of either side of the equator. Alterations in the optimal growing conditions decrease the survivability of the organism. The host response to this fungus depends on an intact T helper 1 T-cell response.

Histology: Skin biopsy specimens show pseudocarcinomatous hyperplasia of the epidermis with varying degrees of ulceration and abscess formation. There is a mixed inflammatory infiltrate. Suppurative granulomatous inflammation is seen within the underlying dermis. The fungus can be seen on routine H&E staining with close inspection. The cells of the yeast phase are thick walled and refractile. They can be seen in the shape of a "mariner's wheel," which is highly characteristic and specific for *P. brasiliensis*. The fungus can be highlighted with a multitude of special staining methods, including periodic acid–Schiff and silver stains. The fungus is easily cultured on Sabouraud medium and shows fluffy white colonies.

Treatment: Treatment with itraconazole has had great success and has drastically altered the prognosis of this disease. As with all systemic fungal infections, treatment courses last for months to a year. Historically, sulfonamides were used. If left untreated, this disease has a significant mortality rate. Ketoconazole and fluconazole have also been used successfully, and amphotericin B is now reserved for the most severe cases and for those who do not respond to azole or sulfonamide therapy.

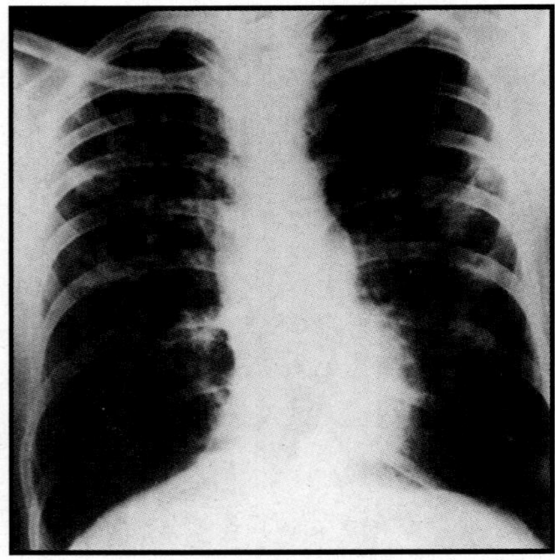

Bilateral pulmonary infiltrates, which closely resemble tuberculosis. Pulmonary lesions may range from minimal to very extensive.

Plaques on lips, nose, and tongue with cervical lymphadenopathy

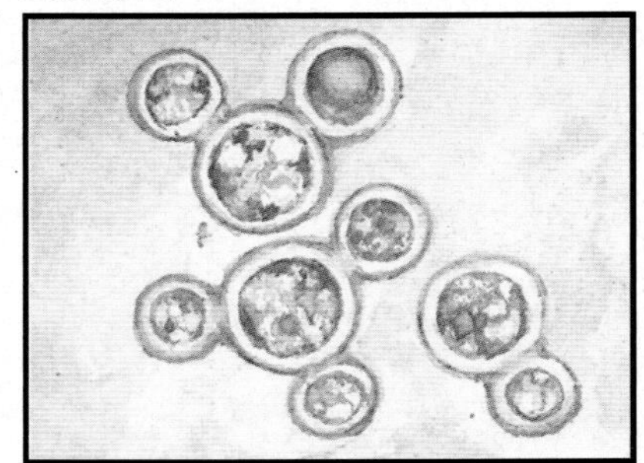

Yeast phase of *P. brasiliensis* in fresh unstained sputum prepared with 10% NaOH, showing double walls with single and multiple budding

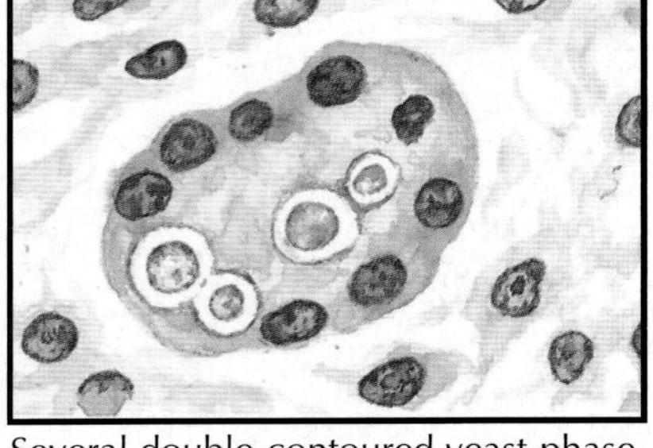

Several double-contoured yeast-phase cells with single buds in a giant cell from a skin lesion

F. Netter M.D.

JOHN A.CRAIG MD with E. Hatton

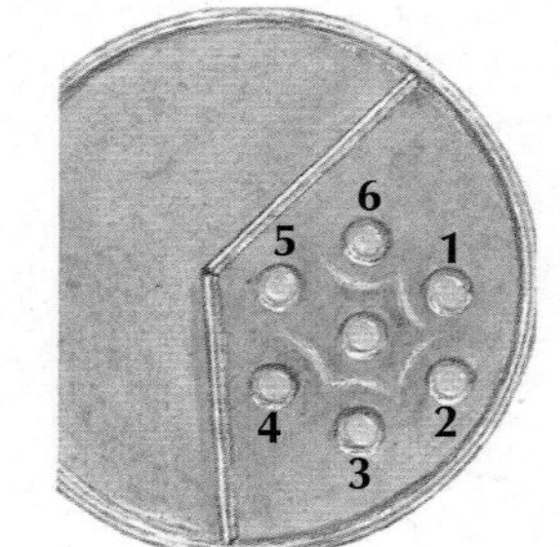

Precipitin test. Antigen in central well; serum from five different patients in peripheral wells showing precipitin bands. Wells *4* and *5* are from the same patient before and after treatment, evidencing response.

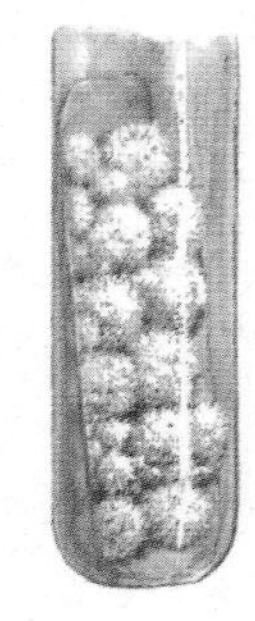

Mycelial colonies of *P. brasiliensis* grown on Sabouraud medium at room temperature. Downy appearance is caused by filamentous hyphae with intercalated or terminal chlamydospores.

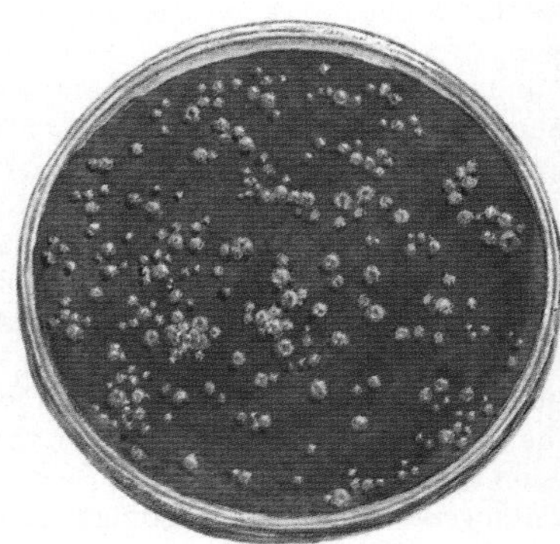

Colonies of yeast form of *P. brasiliensis* grown on blood agar at 37°C

Scabies (*Sarcoptes scabiei* in *circle*)

Inflammatory excoriated papules (note penile involvement). Involvement of genitalia, umbilicus, and finger webs is characteristic for scabies.

SCABIES

Human infection with the parasite *Sarcoptes scabiei* var. *hominis* causes scabies. Humans are the only known host, and the parasite is transferred from one person to another by close physical contact.

Clinical Findings: Scabies mites can affect any human. Men and women are equally affected, and there is no race predilection. The rash of scabies is highly pruritic. Patients often scratch in front of the examining physician and cannot stop themselves from doing so. Patients often state that it is the worst itching sensation they have ever experienced. The itching sensation is worse in the evening, especially when trying to sleep. Cutaneous findings are variable. Burrows are the hallmark of scabies and are pathognomonic for the disease.

Burrows consist of a fine, 0.5- to 1.0-mm-wide, 0.5- to 1.5-cm-long area of undulating or serpentine regions with a tiny black speck at one end. This tiny black speck is the pregnant scabies mite that is burrowing along the skin laying its eggs. Scraping the area of the burrow where the mite is located and examining the scraping under the microscope would reveal the mite. The mite may also be seen in association with eggs and scybala (mite feces). Any of these findings confirms the diagnosis. Burrows are most commonly appreciated along the sides of the fingers and the wrists.

The palms are commonly affected with tiny (1-mm) patches within the skin lines. They are intensely pruritic and are associated with excoriations. Scabies mites avoid the areas of the body that contain numerous sebaceous glands and for this reason are almost never seen on the face of anyone past the age of puberty. They may be found on the face of infants and children, who have not yet formed mature sebaceous glands. Scabies also has a propensity to affect the genitalia. The scrotum is almost always affected in cases that are more than a few weeks old. Very few rashes cause papules or nodules on the scrotum, and the presence of itchy nodules on the scrotum should be considered a sign of scabies until proven otherwise.

Crusted or Norwegian scabies is a rare form of scabies seen in immunosuppressed individuals. The crusted lesions represent the actions of hundreds to thousands of scabies mites. Patients are often covered from head to toe, and the lesions are extremely pruritic. A scraping shows the presence of numerous mites. Individuals with crusted scabies should be treated with a multimodal approach.

Scabies can cause outbreaks in long-term care facilities. These outbreaks can affect many individuals within the facility and are difficult to eradicate.

Pathogenesis: *S. scabiei* is spread from one human to another by close physical contact. The pregnant mite burrows into the epidermis but is unable to penetrate the basement membrane zone. Its presence sets off a massive inflammatory response. The female mites lay eggs as they burrow through the skin. Each egg hatches within 2 to 3 days and releases a larva. The female mite can lay three eggs per day. The larvae quickly grow and form nymphs and then mature adult mites. This process occurs within 1 weeks' time. The mites have a life span of 2 months.

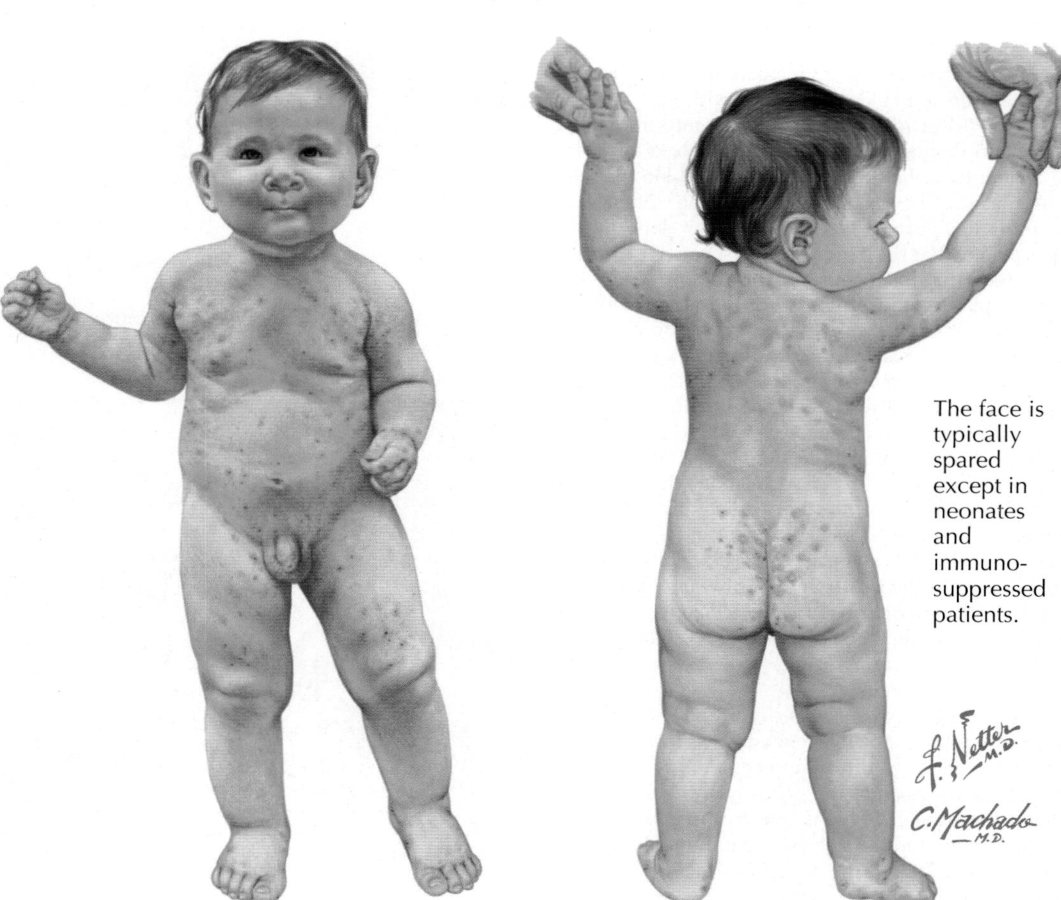

Child with scabies, ventral view

Child with scabies, dorsal view

Histology: Skin biopsies are rarely performed but would reveal a mixed inflammatory infiltrate in the dermis with many eosinophils. This is a nonspecific finding and can be the result of any bug bite reaction. If the actual mite is biopsied, scabies parts will be present within the epidermis.

Treatment: Permethrin is currently the drug of choice to treat scabies. It should be applied overnight and repeated in 1 week because it is pediculicidal but not ovicidal. The second application makes sure that any recently hatched mites are killed before they can reach reproductive age. Colloidal sulfur may be used on pregnant women. It is efficacious and safe but has a terrible odor. Outbreaks in long-term care facilities are often treated with oral ivermectin, which has shown good efficacy. Lindane has fallen out of favor because of its potential neurotoxicity. The use of malathion is advocated if permethrin fails. Other options include topical benzyl benzoate, spinosad, and crotamiton.

SPOROTRICHOSIS

Sporothrix schenckii is an environmental fungus capable of causing human disease after direct inoculation into the skin. Inoculation is the cause of cutaneous sporotrichosis, which is considered a subcutaneous mycosis. Unusual cases of inhalation sporotrichosis have been described in the literature, as have cases of CNS disease. These cases occur almost exclusively in immunosuppressed hosts. Sporotrichosis has classically been associated with inoculation after the prick from a rose plant. The fungus can be isolated from rose plants but is also found on many other plants and in soil environments.

Clinical Findings: Gardeners, florists, and outdoor enthusiasts are at highest risk for infection from *S. schenckii*. These activities and occupations increase the likelihood of contact with the soil fungus. The fungus lives in the environment, and humans become infected by direct implantation of the fungus into the skin. Common methods of inoculation are the prick of a thorn or an injury contaminated with soil or plant material. Within a few days after entry into the skin, a papule and then a pustule form at the site of inoculation. Patients may initially be given an antibiotic in the belief that they have a bacterial infection. Often, it is not until the pustule ulcerates and develops into a larger plaque that the diagnosis is suspected or considered. Once this has occurred, the fungus enters the local lymphatics and proceeds to migrate proximally. As the fungus travels through the lymphatic system, it periodically causes draining sinus tracts to the surface, which appear as papules or nodules. This characteristic lymphangitic spread, also called *sporotrichoid spread*, is seen in most cases of cutaneous sporotrichosis.

Although a few other infections can manifest with lymphangitic spread, its presence along with a history of trauma suggests an infection with sporotrichosis. If lymphangitic spread is present, a skin biopsy and fungal, bacterial, and atypical *Mycobacterium* cultures should be performed. Less commonly, solitary plaques of sporotrichosis occur without any evidence of sporotrichoid spread. The disease manifests as solitary, nonhealing, slowly enlarging plaque with varying amounts of ulceration and drainage.

Pathogenesis: *S. schenckii* is a dimorphic soil fungus found throughout the environment. *S. schenckii* causes human infection by direct implantation of the mold form of the fungus into the skin. Once the fungus has entered the human body, it transforms into its yeast form in response to the stable temperature. Most infections stay localized in the skin. In rare cases of severe immunosuppression, *S. schenckii* becomes disseminated; this occurs most frequently in association with HIV infection. Other *Sporothrix* species have been identified to cause disease, including *S. brasiliensis*, *S. pallida*, and *S. mexicana*.

Histology: Findings from skin biopsy specimens of sporotrichosis are not diagnostic in many cases. The presence of a granulomatous infiltrate is often the main histologic feature. Periodic acid–Schiff and Gomori methenamine silver are two excellent stains that highlight the fungus and allow the pathologist to more readily appreciate the few cigar-shaped fungal elements that are present within the dense inflammation. Multiple fungal organisms are rarely seen; they are observed most frequently in patients with an underlying immunodeficiency.

S. schenckii is best cultured on Sabouraud medium at room temperature. In these conditions, a white to brown colony of mold forms readily. As time elapses, the fungus forms a brown pigment that turns the entire colony brown to black. Because of its dimorphic nature, *S. schenckii* can be grown at 37°C, although it grows much more slowly at that temperature. Culture is the best method to determine the diagnosis.

Treatment: Saturated solution of potassium iodide has been used for decades to treat cutaneous infections with *S. schenckii*. This medication has an unknown mechanism of action in treating fungal infections, but it is believed to interrupt protein synthesis of the fungus and to boost local host immune function. The treatment of choice is one of the azole antifungal medications. Itraconazole has been the most widely studied and used antifungal and is the preferred agent. All azole antifungal agents inhibit the fungal cytochrome P450 enzyme 14-α-sterol-demethylase. This inhibition prevents the fungus from producing ergosterol, a vital cell membrane component. High-dose terbinafine has shown success in treating this fungal infection. Patients with pulmonary or CNS involvement or disseminated disease should be treated with amphotericin B.

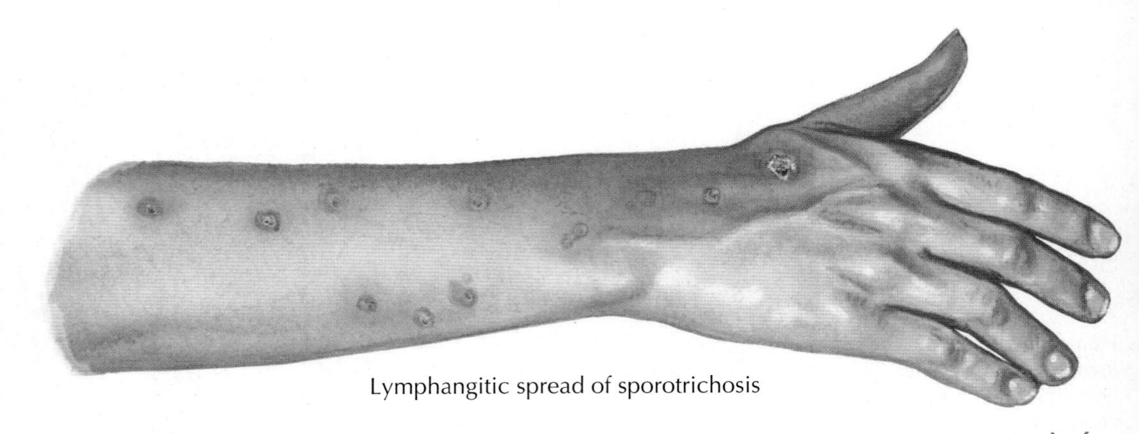
Lymphangitic spread of sporotrichosis

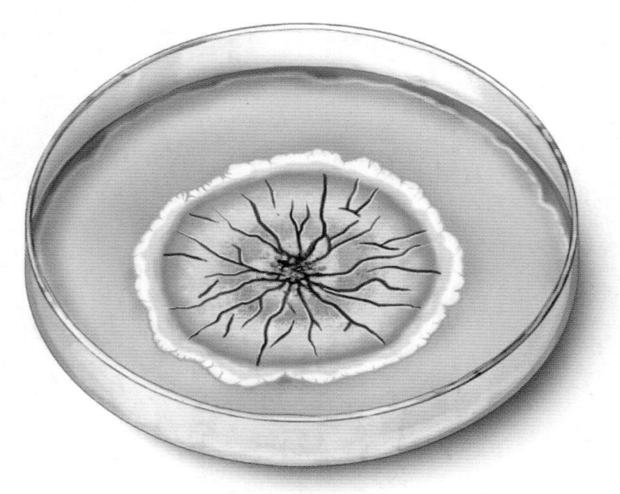
Sporothrix schenckii on Sabouraud plate

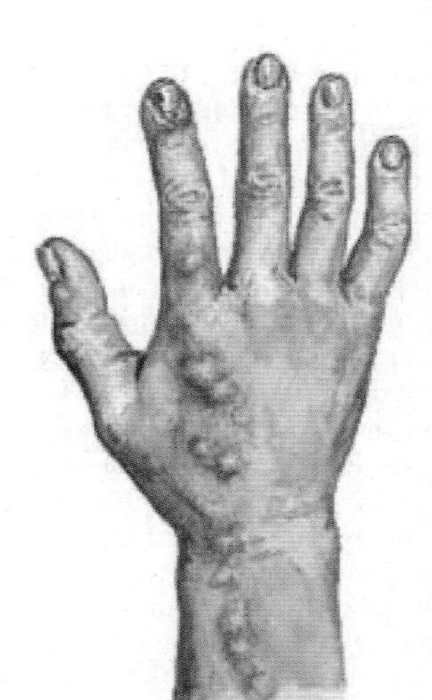
Begins as small nodule and spreads to hand, wrist, and forearm (even systemically). This and other mycotic infections are diagnosed with biopsy and culture.

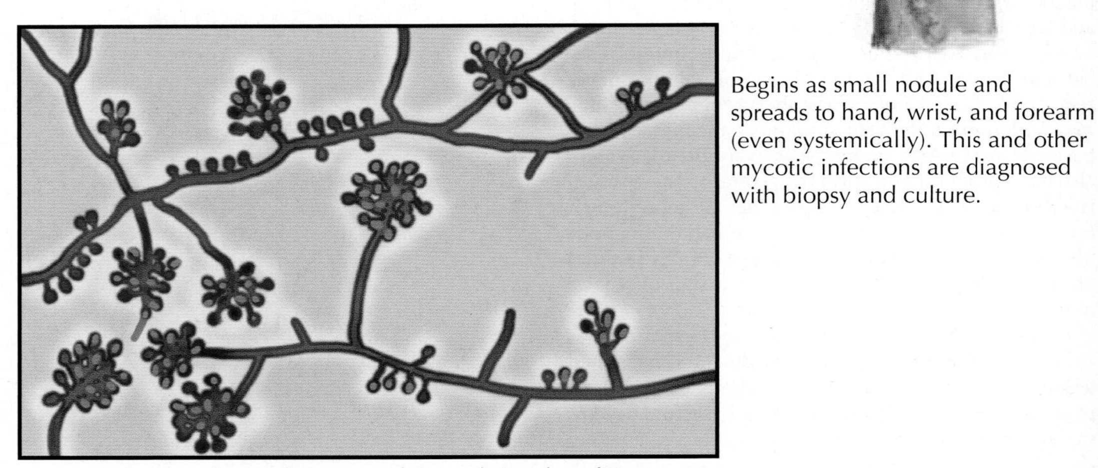
Structural growth pattern of *Sporothrix schenckii*

Types of Skin Infections

Cross section of the skin showing layers and types of infection

Folliculitis and furunculosis

Nasal furuncle

Carbuncle treated with incision and drainage

Felon. Line of incision indicated

Purulent drainage

Cross section shows division of septa in finger pulp

Pyoderma (subepidermal cellulitis) treated with oral antibiotics, not incision

Subcutaneous abscess. V-shaped line of incision indicated

STAPHYLOCOCCUS AUREUS

Cutaneous infection with *Staphylococcus aureus* can manifest in many ways. With the emergence of methicillin-resistant *S. aureus* (MRSA), these cutaneous infections have once again received the attention they deserve. Most cases of MRSA are community acquired, and they have entirely different sensitivity patterns than those of hospital-acquired MRSA infections. These cutaneous infections are increasing in incidence. They not only cause significant skin disease but have the potential to become systemic and cause septicemia, pneumonia, osteomyelitis, and other internal infections. *S. aureus* is a transient colonizer of the skin and nasopharynx. This bacterium has shown a remarkable ability to develop and acquire antibacterial resistance mechanisms. *S. aureus* and MRSA are major hospital-acquired infections, and community-acquired MRSA has become just as important. MRSA accounts for more than 50% of hospital-acquired *S. aureus* infections.

The emergence of community-acquired MRSA has led to an increase in the number of serious *S. aureus* infections. These community-acquired strains have been shown to cause an increased incidence of skin furuncles and abscesses as well as severe pneumonia. Most of these infections occur in young, previously healthy individuals.

Clinical Findings: *S. aureus* and MRSA can cause a wide range of cutaneous infections. The most superficial of all infections that this bacterium can induce is impetigo. Impetigo is often seen in children and in people with preexisting skin diseases, which increase the likelihood of cutaneous infections. The two most common causes of impetigo are *S. aureus* and *Streptococcus pyogenes* or group A *Streptococcus*. The disease often manifests on the face. Regardless of the location, the infection appears as small, superficial, honey-colored crusts with some weeping of yellow, clear serum. There is a bullous variant that manifests with superficial blisters that easily rupture. The disease is contagious and can be spread among children. Typically, topical therapy yields excellent results, and oral therapy can be avoided. Biopsy of an impetigo lesion would reveal a superficial infectious process in the stratum corneum. Neutrophils and bacterial elements would be found within the stratum corneum.

Infection of the hair follicle shaft, termed *folliculitis*, can occur with a wide variety of bacterial infections, including *S. aureus* and streptococcal species. Many forms of folliculitis have been described with etiologic agents. Hot tub folliculitis is caused by *Pseudomonas aeruginosa*, which grows in improperly disinfected hot tubs. Gram-negative folliculitis can be seen in patients receiving long-term antibiotic therapy for acne and other conditions. Regardless of the bacterial agent, the appearance of folliculitis is the same. A small (1- to 3-mm) pustule is present and surrounds a hair follicle. The pustule is easily broken and can be slightly itchy to slightly painful. The hair can easily be removed from the pustule with minimal effort. The pustule is surrounded by a millimeter or two of erythema, which in turn is surrounded by a blanched region extending out another few millimeters. Typically, entire regions of the body are affected, such as the legs or buttocks.

Folliculitis can lead to furuncles (boils) or carbuncles (large furuncles). However, most furuncles do not develop from a preexisting folliculitis. The furuncle is a deep-seated, red, inflamed, tender nodule. Furuncles can occur in any location and are commonly found within the nostril. The nostril is a location that *S. aureus* is known to colonize. Furuncles may become quite large and spontaneously drain to the surface. Before the drainage occurs, one can often appreciate the presence of a pustule developing within the central portion of the furuncle. Carbuncles appear to result from the coalescence of multiple furuncles. They can be large and can have multiple draining sinus tracts to the surface of the epidermis. Multiple pustules may precede the drainage. Pain and localized adenopathy are hallmarks of both furuncles and carbuncles.

STAPHYLOCOCCUS AUREUS (Continued)

Cellulitis develops from a bacterial infection within the dermis or the subcutaneous fat of the skin. The most frequent location is on the lower extremities. It occurs more commonly in people with diabetes, trauma to the skin, poor vascular circulation, or immunosuppression. Cellulitis starts as a small, pink-to-red macule that slowly expands and can encompass large portions of the skin. This is associated with edema and pain. The condition is almost always unilateral. The pain can be severe. Tender adenopathy of regional lymph nodes is present. Fever and systemic symptoms are almost always present. The redness is able to travel many centimeters a day. The presence of red lines is more indicative of lymphadenitis than cellulitis, but these conditions can coexist. Erysipelas is a more superficial form of cellulitis that occurs in the upper dermis. It manifests clinically as a well-demarcated, edematous red macule that is tender to the touch. The lower extremities and the face are common areas of involvement.

Toxic shock syndrome (TSS) is the name given to the development of fever, hypotension, and near-erythroderma. The rash can appear as widespread, red, blanching macules. If appropriately treated, the rash causes desquamation of the skin and return to normal within a few weeks. TSS was initially reported after the use of superabsorbent tampons that had been left in place for an entire menstrual cycle. These tampons are no longer available. The tampons provided an environment conducive to the rapid growth of *S. aureus*. Toxins produced by the bacteria are responsible for the symptoms. TSS can occur after any *S. aureus* infection but is much more likely with an abscess. The toxins act as superantigens and activate T cells without the normal immune system processing. This can lead to massive activation of the immune system.

Pathogenesis: *S. aureus* is a gram-positive bacterium found throughout the environment. In humans, it is most likely to be found colonizing the nares, toe web spaces, and umbilicus. The bacteria grows in grape-like clusters on blood agar cultures and is one of the most common bacterial causes of human infection.

Histology: The histologic findings are based on the form of infection biopsied. The common underlying theme is a neutrophilic infiltrate that can be present throughout the biopsy specimen. Bacteria are present and can be highlighted on tissue Gram staining. The inflammation in impetigo is often limited to the epidermis, with bacteria and neutrophils present within the stratum corneum. Superficial blistering may occur within the granular cell layer in bullous impetigo. Folliculitis shows edema and a neutrophilic infiltrate in and around the hair follicle. Furuncles, carbuncles, and abscesses show a massive dermal infiltrate with neutrophils and bacterial debris.

The pathology of cellulitis is more subtle, with neutrophils around blood vessels. Bacteria can be difficult to see or to culture from skin biopsies of cellulitis. Most cases of cellulitis are not biopsied. TSS shows a superficial and deep mixed inflammatory infiltrate. No bacteria are seen because the rash is toxin mediated.

TOXIC SHOCK SYNDROME

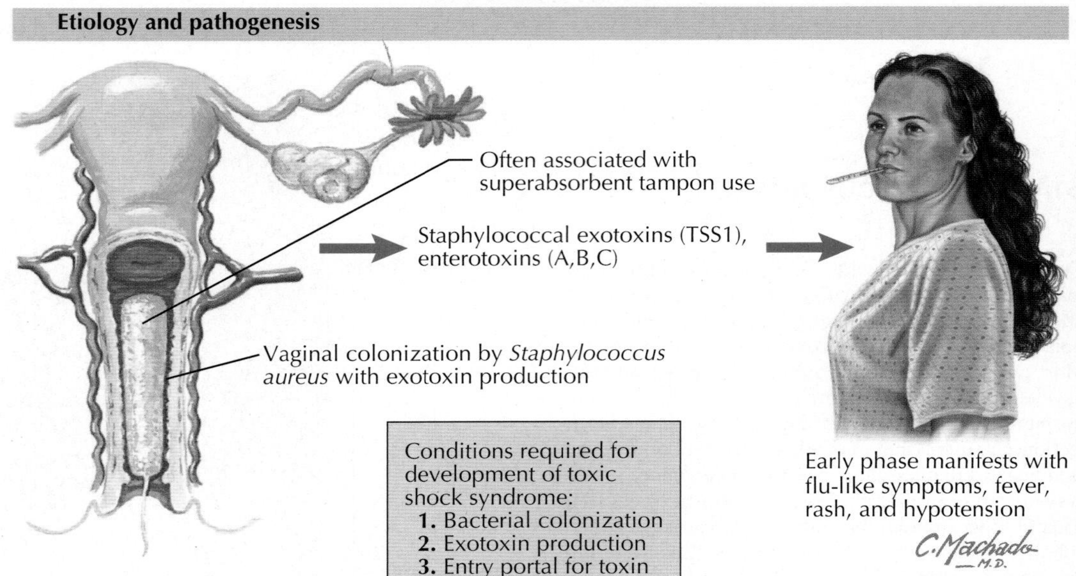

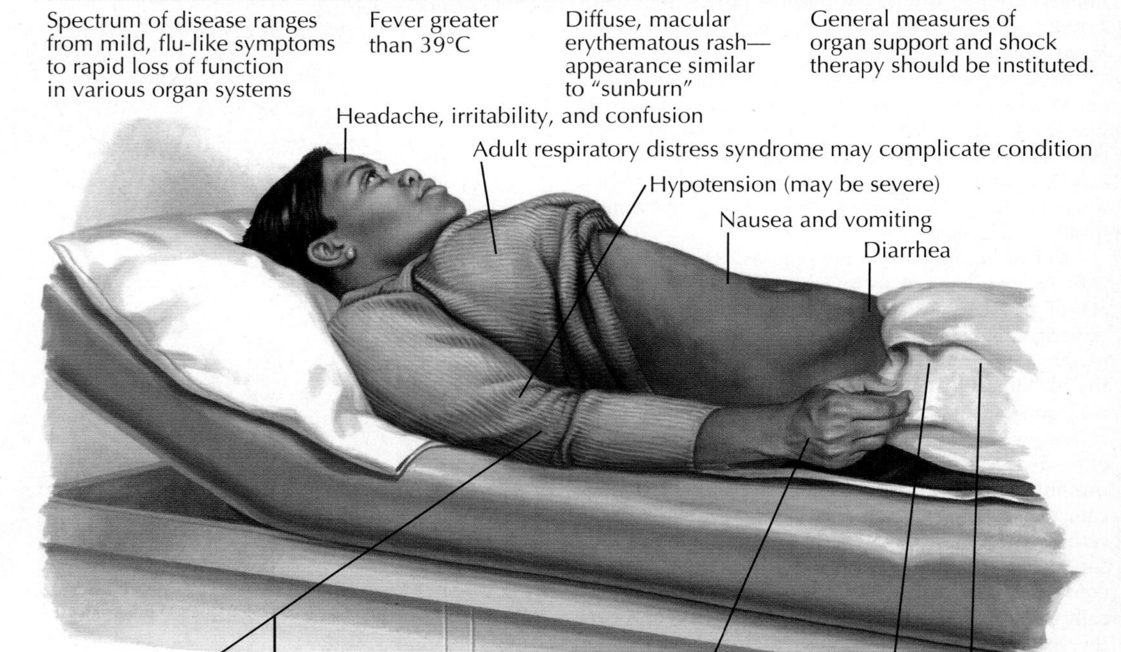

Treatment: Impetigo can be treated with topical antibiotic therapy directed against *S. aureus* and streptococcal species. Mupirocin is one such topical agent that is highly effective. The other forms of infection need to be treated with oral antibiotics. Cephalexin or dicloxacillin are good first-choice options. In areas with high rates of community-acquired MRSA, one should consider empirically treating for MRSA with a sulfa-based medication or a tetracycline derivative in adults. Options to treat MRSA include doxycycline, clindamycin, trimethoprim-sulfamethoxazole, and linezolid. Culturing of the bacterial agent should be done in all cases to select the most effective medication. Severe cases of cellulitis and all cases of TSS should be treated in the hospital in the appropriate setting. Intravenous antibiotics are always used, and vancomycin is the initial choice until the strain of *S. aureus* is isolated and sensitivities are assessed. Once the sensitivities of the bacteria have been determined, the antibiotic treatment can be tailored to the individual patient. Patients with TSS often require intensive care with pressure support and respiratory support.

Syphilis of Genitalia

Chancre with inguinal adenopathy
Primary syphilis

Condylomata lata
Secondary syphilis

Chancre of coronal sulcus; nontender ulcer

Chancre of glans: firm, rubbery, nontender ulcer

Multiple chancres (shaft and meatus)

Penoscrotal chancre with inguinal adenopathy

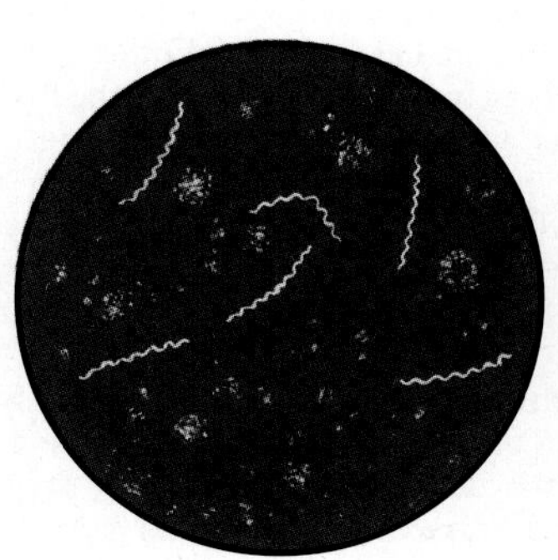

Spirochetes under darkfield examination

Syphilis

Syphilis has been well described in the literature since the late 1400s. The history behind the discovery and treatment of the disease is a story of perseverance and the willpower of many scientists working separately and together to help treat one the deadliest diseases of their time. Philippe Ricord, a French scientist, is given credit for describing the three stages of syphilis and differentiating it from other diseases such as gonorrhea. The infectious organism, *Treponema pallidum*, was described in 1905 by Fritz Schaudinn, a German zoologist, and Erich Hoffman, a German dermatologist. Soon after this discovery, the German scientist Paul Ehrlich developed the first specific therapy for syphilis. The oral medication he and his team discovered was initially called 606, because it was the 606th compound they had attempted to use to treat the disease. This organoarsenic molecule was soon renamed *salvarsan*. This medication is highly effective against *T. pallidum*.

T. pallidum is classified as a spirochete. Spirochetes are gram-negative bacteria that have a winding or coiled linear body. There are three subspecies of *T. pallidum*; the one responsible for syphilis is named *Treponema pallidum pallidum*. The other subspecies of *T. pallidum* cause endemic syphilis or bejel, pinta, and yaws. Syphilis is a highly infectious disease that is transmitted via sexual contact or vertically from an infected mother to her unborn child. Syphilis has been recognized to progress through three stages: primary, secondary, and tertiary. Not all cases progress through all of the stages, and only about one-third of untreated cases eventually progress to tertiary syphilis. The secondary and tertiary phases are interrupted by a latent phase of variable length.

Clinical Findings: Both historically and today, most cases of syphilis have been transmitted via sexual intercourse. The disease is often seen in conjunction with other STIs, especially HIV infection. The two infections may actually facilitate each other's infectious potential. There is no race or sex predilection, and the organism is able to infect any host with whom it comes in contact. The initial infection in most cases results in clinical findings in the genital region.

Primary syphilis is marked by a nonpainful ulceration that begins as a red papule and ulcerates over a period of a few days to weeks. The average time to onset of the ulcer is 3 to 4 weeks after exposure, but it can occur 3 to 4 months later. This primary ulcer, called a chancre, is firm to palpation. The ulcer can be found anywhere on the genitalia, including the labia, vaginal introitus, and mons in females and the glans, foreskin, and penile shaft in males. Lesions on the foreskin of males often show the "dory flop" sign. When grasping the area of the prepuce containing the ulcer and slowly retracting the proximal edge; after a critical angle has been achieved the entire ulcer flops over. This occurs because the ulcer is firm and does not bow under pressure. If left untreated, these ulcers self-resolve within 1 to 3 weeks. After this occurs, the bacteria hematogenously disseminate to other organ systems.

The timing of secondary syphilis is variable; it can occur immediately after primary syphilis or up to 6 months after the chancre of primary syphilis has healed. The average time frame is approximately 6 weeks after healing of the primary ulcer. Without treatment of primary

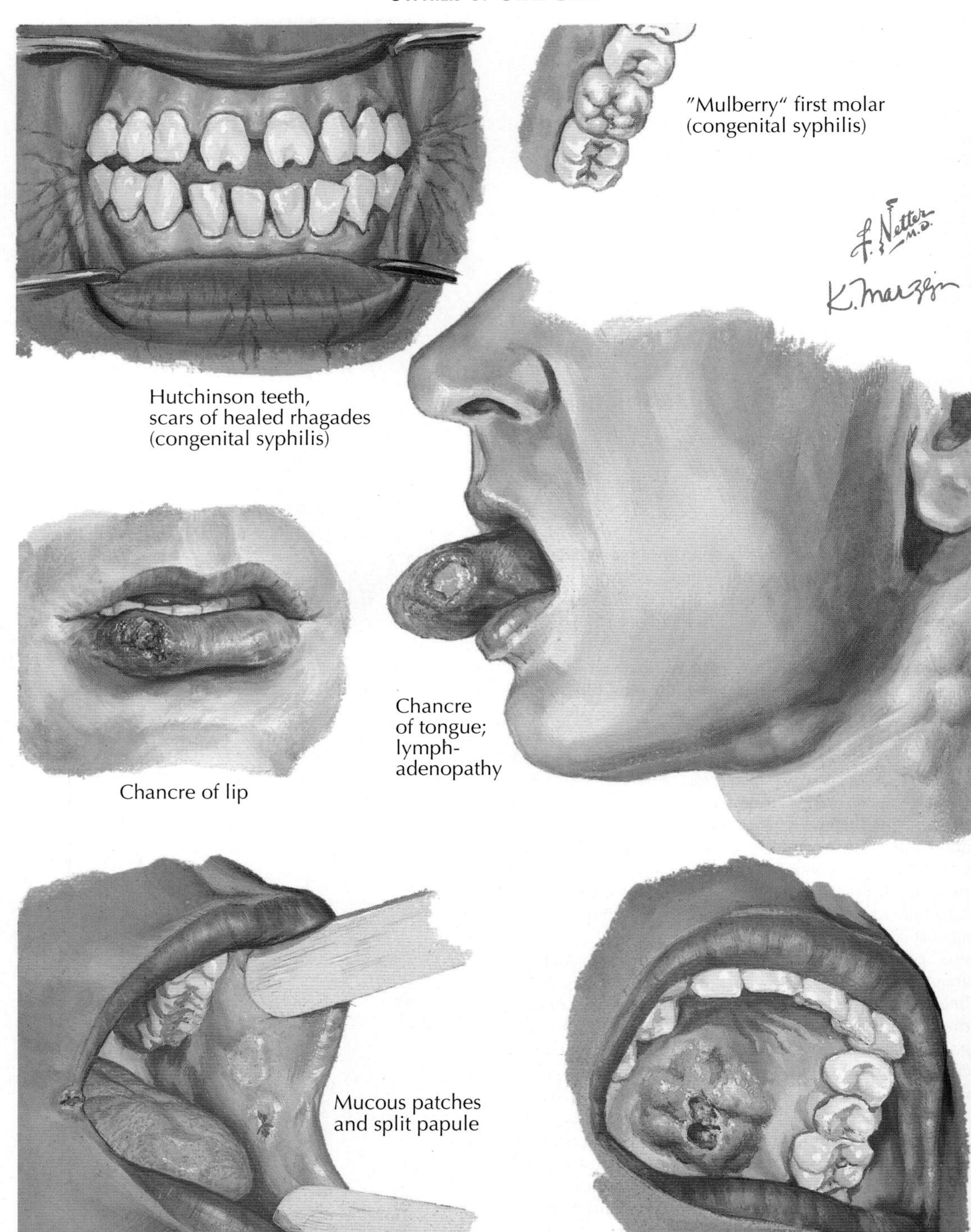

SYPHILIS (Continued)

syphilis, most if not all patients experience symptoms and skin lesions of secondary syphilis. Patients universally report constitutional symptoms such as malaise, fever, chills, fatigue, and weight loss. Cutaneous findings can be multifaceted. The most prevalent skin finding is that of skin-colored to red to slightly hyperpigmented papules and patches. The palms and soles are characteristically involved, which is a clue that the diagnosis of syphilis should be considered.

Condylomata lata is the name given to the moist plaques that develop in the groin region from secondary syphilis. These lesions contain numerous *T. pallidum* organisms. Adenopathy is almost always present. Some rare findings of secondary syphilis include ulcers in the mouth, which can mimic aphthous ulcerations, and a nonscarring alopecia. The alopecia has been described as having a "moth-eaten" appearance, in reference to the random arrangements of patches of alopecia. All lesions of secondary syphilis contain the bacteria, and samples can be taken and directly observed under darkfield microscopy. The organisms are seen as mobile spirochetes with a spiral configuration. Patients with secondary syphilis may have early CNS involvement and may report headaches and other meningeal signs. Approximately 3 to 4 months after the first signs and symptoms of secondary syphilis appear, they spontaneously resolve. This is the beginning of the latent phase, which is a phase of wide variability. Some patients never develop tertiary syphilis, and approximately one in five develop a recurrence of secondary syphilis.

Tertiary syphilis follows the latent phase of syphilis in 30% to 40% of untreated individuals. The average time from initial development to tertiary syphilis is approximately 4 years. Tertiary syphilis can affect the skin, bone, and mucous membranes. The characteristic skin finding is the gumma. Gummas appear frequently as individual lesions, although a multitude of gummas may occur at the same time. The gumma starts as a papule and then evolves into a nodule, which ulcerates over the course of a few days to weeks. The ulceration is caused by significant necrosis of the involved tissue. This leads to deep ulcers with well-defined borders. The surface of the ulcer may be covered with gelatinous exudates. Another form of tertiary syphilis is the nodular syphilid skin lesion. These lesions are red to red-brown nodules that slowly enlarge and can develop various configurations, including serpiginous and annular formations. These lesions rarely, if ever, ulcerate.

Unique forms of syphilis that do not fit neatly into one of the categories already described include neurosyphilis, congenital syphilis, and late syphilis. Involvement of the CNS by *T. pallidum* is termed *neurosyphilis*. Neurosyphilis can occur during any of the numerous forms and stages of syphilis. It is caused by direct infection of the CNS by the spirochete. Most patients with syphilis exhibit no signs of CNS involvement, even when the bacteria can be isolated from the CNS. However, almost all of these cases of asymptomatic neurosyphilis eventually progress to symptomatic clinical illness. Some of the common symptoms of neurosyphilis are headache, hearing difficulty, neck stiffness, and muscle weakness. As the disease progresses untreated, patients develop seizures, delirium, and tabes dorsalis. Tabes dorsalis results from degeneration of the posterior columns of the spinal cord.

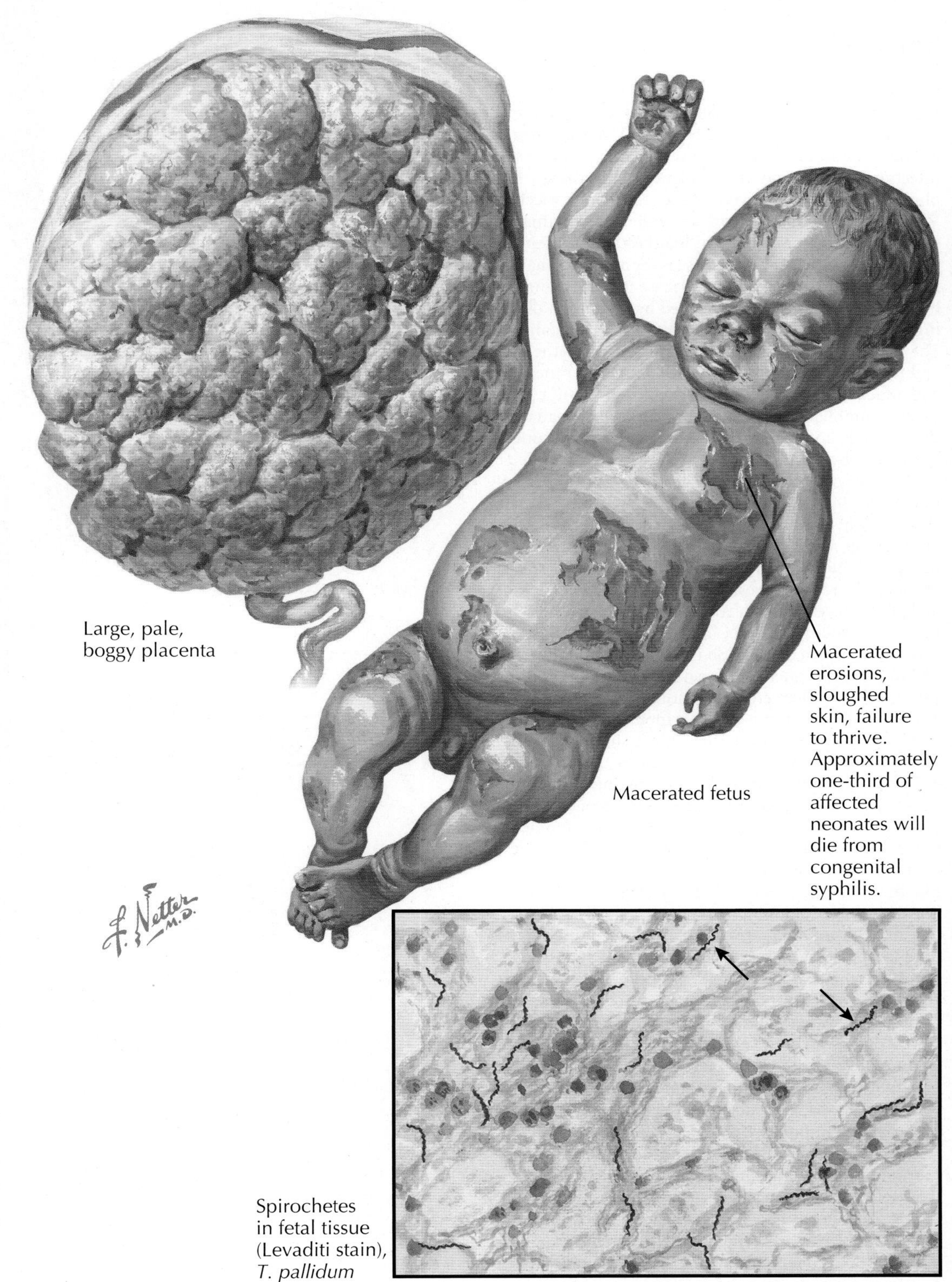

SYPHILIS (Continued)

The posterior columns are critical for proper sensation, and patients with tabes dorsalis develop gait disorders, diminished reflexes, proprioception abnormalities, pain, paresthesias, and a host of other neurologic symptoms. If neurosyphilis remains untreated, the patient dies of the disease. Therefore any patient who exhibits signs or symptoms of neurosyphilis should undergo a spinal tap to evaluate the CSF for involvement with *T. pallidum*.

Congenital syphilis occurs as the result of vertical transmission from an infected mother to her unborn fetus. Up to one-third of infected neonates die of the disease. In neonates who survive, the disease manifests in numerous ways. Neonates may present with macerated erosions associated with cachexia and failure to thrive. "Snuffles" is the term used to describe the chronic runny nose with a bloody purulent discharge. Rhagades are one of the most common signs seen in congenital syphilis; they appear as scarring around the mouth and eyes. Many bony abnormalities have been reported, including a saddle-nose deformity, the Higoumenakis sign (medial clavicular thickening), saber shins, and Clutton joints. Teeth abnormalities include Hutchinson teeth (notched incisors) and, less frequently, mulberry molars.

Pathogenesis: Syphilis is caused by *T. pallidum pallidum*. This bacteria is highly infective and is predominantly spread by sexual contact and by transmission from an infected mother to her unborn child.

Histology: Skin biopsies of syphilis evaluated with routine H&E staining show varying features depending on the stage and form of disease being biopsied. A universal finding in all forms is the presence of numerous plasma cells within the inflammatory infiltrate. Ulceration, granulomas, and vasculitis are often encountered. The spirochetes cannot be appreciated with routine H&E staining; special techniques are required. The Steiner stain and the Warthin-Starry stain are the two most commonly used stains. Immunohistochemical stains can also be used and have been shown to be highly sensitive and specific.

Treatment: The *T. pallidum* organism has very little antibiotic resistance, and the therapy of choice is still penicillin. To treat primary or secondary syphilis, a single intramuscular dose of benzathine penicillin G is recommended, and some now recommend a follow-up dose—the same as the initial dose—at 1 or 2 weeks. Three doses of benzathine penicillin G are given 1 week apart to treat tertiary syphilis. Patients who develop neurosyphilis need to be treated with intravenous penicillin for at least 2 weeks. Most patients who are treated for syphilis develop the Jarisch-Herxheimer reaction. This reaction is the result of the decimation of the *T. pallidum* organisms due to therapy with penicillin. As the scores of bacteria are killed, the dead spirochetes induce an inflammatory reaction. This reaction may manifest as fever, chills, fatigue, malaise, and rashes of varying morphology. It can often make the rash of secondary syphilis appear worse for a period of time. This reaction is not specific to *T. pallidum* and has been reported with other infectious agents. It is critical to follow patients long enough after therapy to ensure adequate treatment as measured by titers on rapid plasma reagin or Venereal Disease Research Laboratory testing. All patients with syphilis should be tested for HIV.

VARICELLA

Varicella zoster virus (VZV) causes two discrete clinical infections: chickenpox (varicella) and herpes zoster (shingles). Although chickenpox was once a universal infection of childhood, the incidence of this disease has plummeted since the advent of the chickenpox vaccine. VZV belongs to the herpesvirus family and is primarily a respiratory disease with skin manifestations.

Clinical Findings: The disease is seen predominantly in children and young adults. Disease in adults tends to be more severe. Varicella is caused by inhalation of the highly infectious viral particle from an infected contact. The virus replicates within the pulmonary epithelium and then disseminates via the bloodstream to the skin and mucous membranes. Most children do not have severe pulmonary symptoms. A prodrome of headache, fever, cough, and malaise may precede the development of the rash by a few days.

The rash of varicella is characteristic and is present in almost 100% of those infected. It begins as a small, erythematous macule or papule that vesiculates. After vesiculation, the lesion may form a small vesiculopustule and then quickly rupture and form a thin, crusted erosion. The resulting vesicle has a central depression or dell and is localized over a red base. This gives rise to the classic description of a "dew drop on a rose petal." The rash is more common on the trunk and on the head and neck, and it often is less severe when found on the extremities. A characteristic finding is an enanthem. The mucous membranes of the mouth are frequently involved with pinpoint vesicles with a surrounding red halo. A clinical clue to the diagnosis is the finding of lesions of multiple morphologies occurring at the same time. Most cases of varicella are self-resolving and heal with minimal to no scarring. Scarring can be significant if the vesicles or crusts become secondarily infected. Children are considered infectious from 1 to 2 days before the rash breaks out until the last vesicle crusts over. The diagnosis of chickenpox is made clinically. A Tzanck test, direct immunofluorescence, or viral culture can be used in nonclassical cases to confirm the diagnosis.

Adults who develop primary varicella infection are at risk for severe pulmonary complications and severe skin disease with a dramatically increased risk for scarring. Adults who are exposed to VZV for the first time are more likely to develop pneumonia and encephalitis. Children who develop pneumonia during an infection with chickenpox have most likely acquired a secondary bacterial pneumonia.

Since the universal adoption in the United States of routine childhood vaccination against varicella in 1995, the incidence of varicella has precipitously dropped. The VZV vaccine is a live attenuated vaccine that is highly effective in achieving protective titer levels. Individuals who develop chickenpox after vaccination have an attenuated course that is manifested by a few vesicles and more macules. This atypical variant of chickenpox is often misdiagnosed, or it may be so mild that the parents do not seek medical care.

Pathogenesis: Varicella is caused by VZV, a double-stranded DNA virus with a lipid capsule. It is spread from human to human via the respiratory route. Once inhaled, the highly infectious virus invades endothelial cells in the respiratory tract. The virus quickly disseminates to the lymphatic tissue and then to other organ systems. This virus is neurotrophic and can lie dormant in the dorsal root ganglion, with the potential to reactivate much later in the form of shingles.

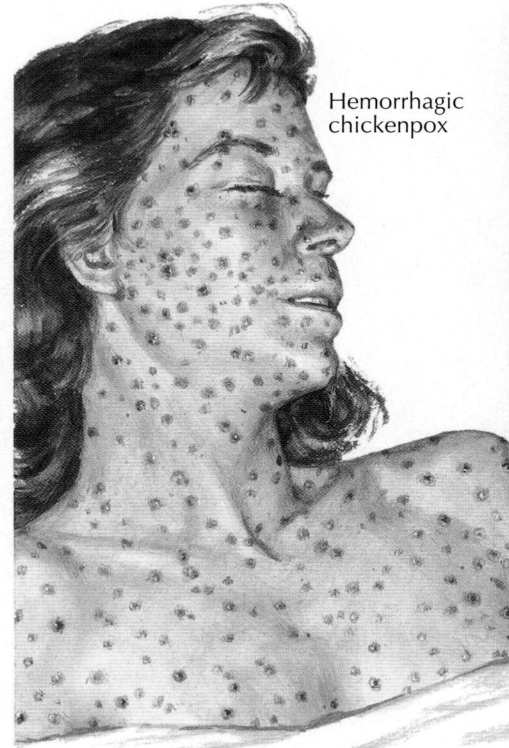

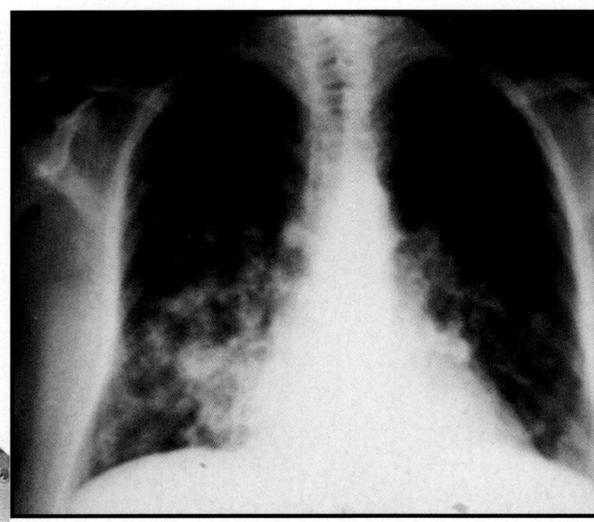

Varicella pneumonia. Nodular infiltrates in both lower lobes.

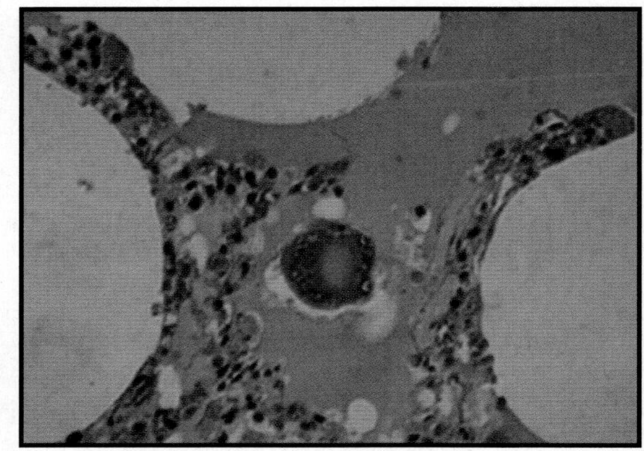

Multinucleated giant cell with massive edema of the alveolus

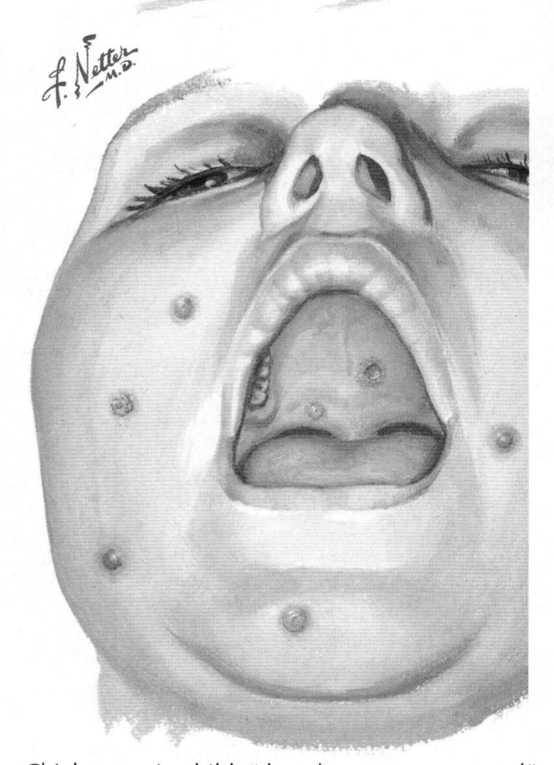

Chickenpox in child; "dew drops on a rose petal"

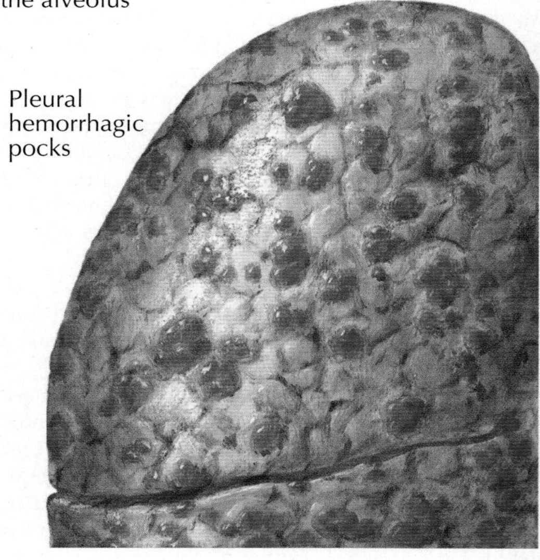

Histology: A skin biopsy of a vesicle shows an intraepidermal blister that forms via ballooning degeneration of the keratinocytes. There is a perivascular lymphocytic infiltrate in the dermis. Multinucleated giant cells can be seen at the base of the blister.

Treatment: Most childhood infections require no specific therapy other than supportive care and treatment of secondary bacterial infection. Immunocompromised individuals, including pregnant women, should be treated with an antiviral medication such as acyclovir. Neonates are also at high risk for serious disease and must be treated. The vaccine provides long-term effectiveness that has been shown to last for decades. More time is needed to firmly establish the need for and timing of any booster vaccinations. Vaccines are available to decrease the reactivation of VZV and, in doing so, decrease the risk for developing shingles.

Clinical Presentation of Herpes Zoster

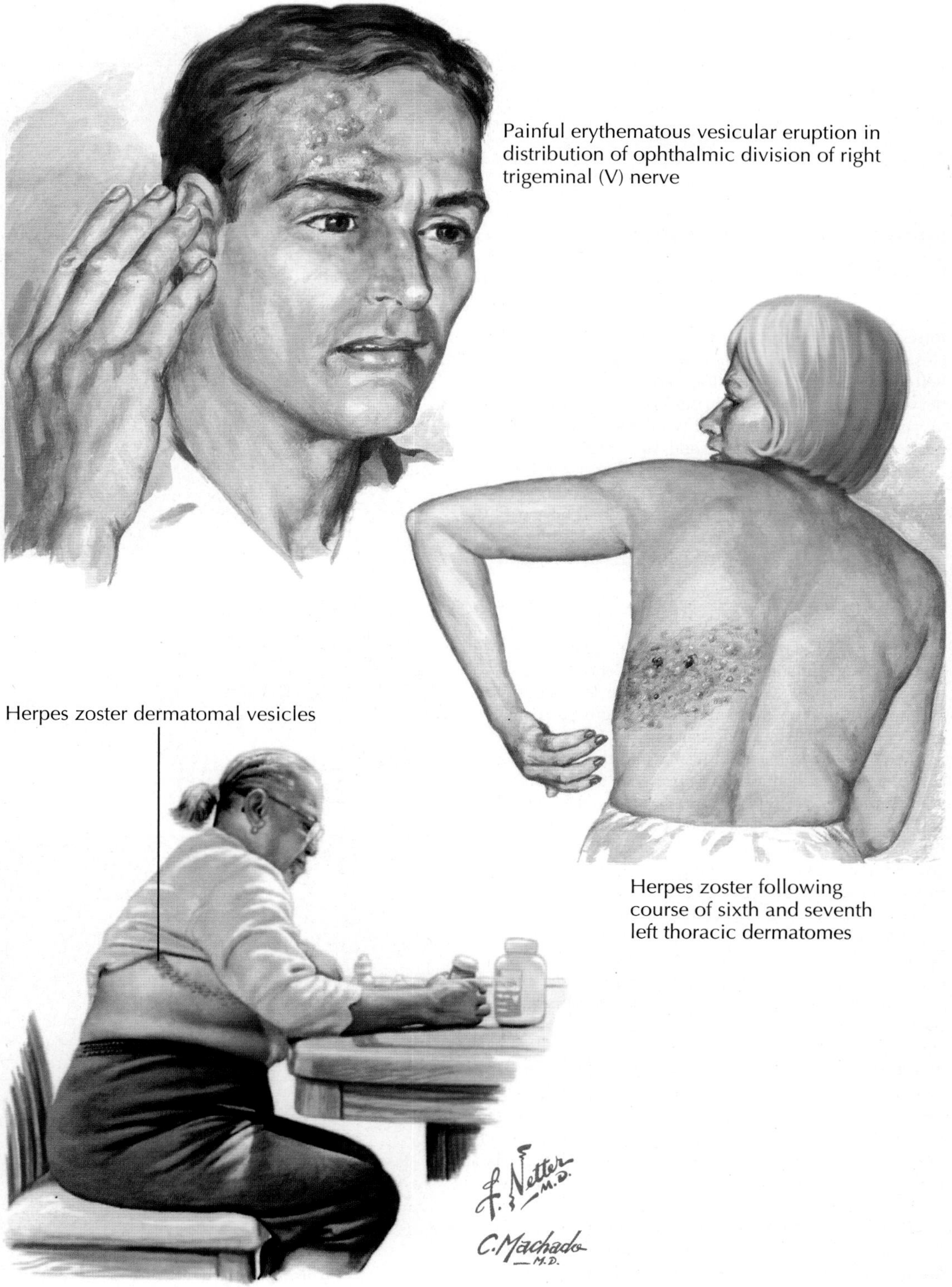

Painful erythematous vesicular eruption in distribution of ophthalmic division of right trigeminal (V) nerve

Herpes zoster dermatomal vesicles

Herpes zoster following course of sixth and seventh left thoracic dermatomes

F. Netter M.D.

C. Machado M.D.

Herpes Zoster (Shingles)

Varicella zoster virus (VZV) causes varicella (chickenpox) as well as herpes zoster (shingles). Herpes zoster is caused by reactivation of dormant VZV. Only hosts who have previously been infected with VZV develop herpes zoster. The incidence of shingles should decrease with the success of the current zoster vaccines in increasing immunity against the virus. The recombinant vaccine appears to have better efficacy than the live attenuated vaccine. The recombinant vaccine is currently recommended for individuals age 50 years and older who fulfill the criteria for receiving the vaccine, which is a two-part vaccine given 6 months apart. This age was chosen because the incidence of herpes zoster increases after age 50, possibly related to a waning immune response and antibody titer remaining from the patient's original VZV infection. Whether the VZV vaccine protects against herpes zoster will take years to determine. The United States introduced widespread childhood immunization against VZV in 1995, and none of these children have reached the age of 60 years. Whether future booster vaccinations or VZV revaccination will be required has yet to be determined.

Clinical Findings: Herpes zoster is caused by reactivation of previously acquired VZV lying dormant in the dorsal root ganglia of the spinal cord or the ganglia of the cranial nerves. Patients are typically older individuals. The incidence increases with each decade of life and peaks at about 75 years. Herpes zoster is infrequently encountered in children. Men and women are equally affected. The initial symptom typically is a vague pain, tingling, or itching sensation. This may precede the rash by 1 or 2 days. Constitutional symptoms are commonly seen in older patients. After this prodrome, the characteristic vesicular rash develops in a dermatomal distribution. The location most frequently affected is the thoracic spine region; however, the trigeminal nerve is the most frequently involved nerve. The vesicles spread out to involve almost the entire dermatome of the nerve that has been infected. The rash does not cross the midline, which is a clue to the diagnosis. Bilateral herpes zoster is very rare and is seen more frequently in immunosuppressed individuals.

The rash is exquisitely tender and can lead to significant sleep disturbances and significant morbidity. With healing, which usually occurs within 1 to 2 weeks, scarring is common. Pain typically dissipates over time, but a small subset of individuals, usually older than 50 years, develop postherpetic neuralgia. Postherpetic neuralgia can be a life-altering condition of abnormal sensation within the region affected by the herpes zoster outbreak. Patients often describe pain and paresthesias. Clothing or bedding rubbing against the skin can cause severe discomfort and pain. Postherpetic neuralgia can last for weeks to months or even years and can be devastating.

Although the thoracic dorsal ganglia, taken as a whole, are responsible for the most cases of herpes zoster, the trigeminal nerve is the most frequently involved single nerve. The severity of the infection depends on the branch or branches involved. Herpes zoster infections on the face are typically more severe than those on the trunk or extremities. Infections on the face can affect the eye and ear and can lead to blindness or hearing loss in severe cases. If the vesicles of herpes zoster affect the tip of the nose, the eye is likely to be involved. The nasociliary branch of the ophthalmic division of the trigeminal nerve innervates the nasal tip, and involvement of this region indicates that the infection is within the ophthalmic nerve. This involvement of the nasal tip with subsequent involvement of the globe is termed the *Hutchinson sign*. VZV infection of the eye is a medical emergency, and the patient must be evaluated by an ophthalmologist as soon as possible.

Simultaneous involvement of the facial and vestibular nerves is not infrequent and has been termed

VARICELLA ZOSTER WITH KERATITIS

Herpes zoster. Painful vesicles, erosions with an erythematous base

F. Netter M.D.
K. Marzen

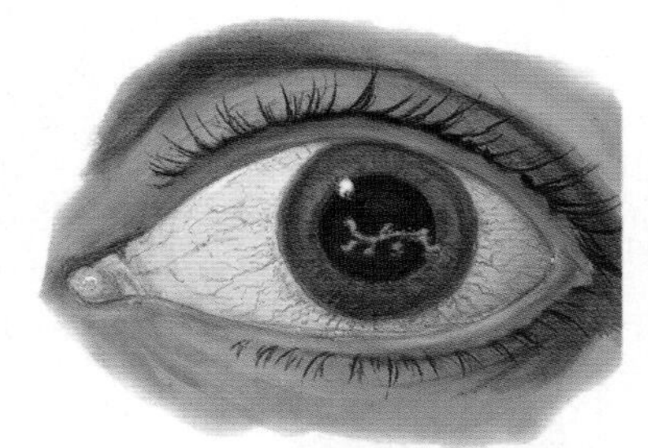

Dendritic keratitis (herpes simplex) demonstrated by fluorescein

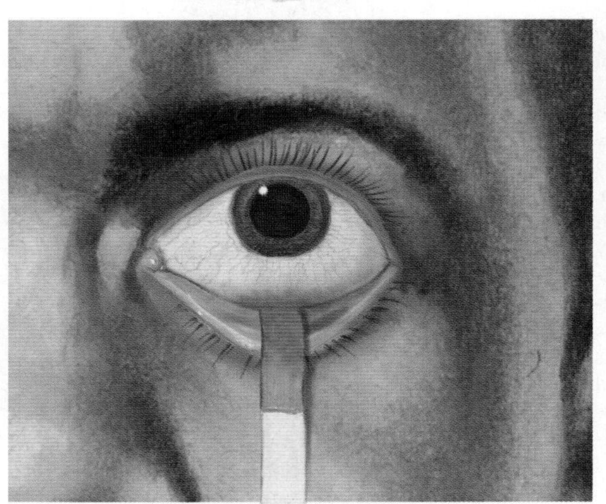

Technique of applying fluorescein strip in previously anesthetized eye

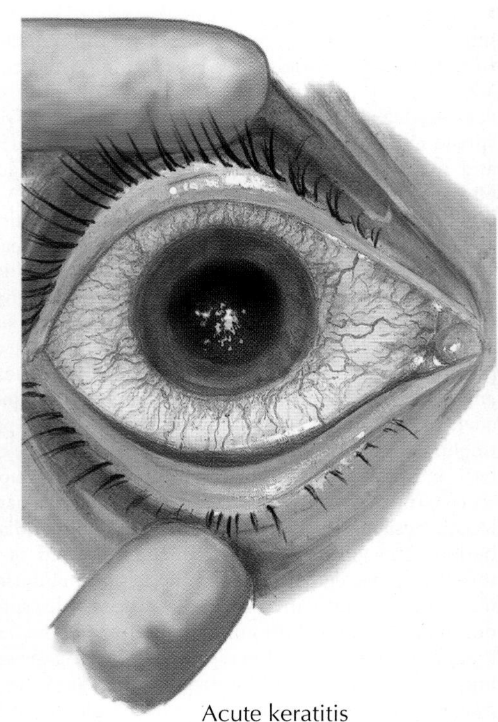

Acute keratitis (ciliary injection, irregular corneal surface)

HERPES ZOSTER (SHINGLES) (Continued)

Ramsay Hunt syndrome. These two nerves originate in close proximity to each other, and reactivation of VZV within the geniculate ganglion may involve both these nerves. This can lead to hearing loss and motor nerve loss due to involvement of the vestibular and the facial nerve, respectively. The ear and the anterior tongue develop the vesiculation seen in routine VZV infections. The motor loss may mimic Bell palsy, and hearing loss may be permanent. Other cranial nerves have been reported to be affected in Ramsay Hunt syndrome, but the seventh and eighth nerves are most frequently affected by far.

Scarring may be a severe sequela of this infection, which can be made worse by bacterial superinfection. The presence of any honey-colored crusting or expanding erythema outside the dermatome should suggest the possibility of secondary impetigo or cellulitis. Prompt recognition and therapy are required to help prevent serious, disfiguring scarring.

The diagnosis is made clinically, and the Tzanck test can confirm the diagnosis. The presence of multinucleated giant cells on a Tzanck preparation taken from a vesicular rash in a dermatomal distribution confirms the diagnosis. Viral culture can be performed but is not cost-effective. Direct fluorescent antibody testing is a rapid method to determine the viral cause, but it is expensive and is rarely needed in these cases.

Pathogenesis: Any individual previously infected with VZV in the form of chickenpox is predisposed to develop herpes zoster later in life. Most cases occur with advancing age because cell-mediated immunity tends to wane with time. The virus remains latent in the nerve ganglia until it reactivates. The ability to reactivate and the exact signal for reactivation are unknown. Once the virus reactivates, it begins to replicate and cause necrosis of the affected nerve cells. The virus travels along the cutaneous sensory nerves and eventually affects the skin that is innervated by the nerve root where the virus became reactivated.

Histology: Skin biopsies are not needed for diagnosis of this infection but would show ballooning degeneration of the keratinocytes. This ballooning degeneration leads to vesiculation and bulla formation. Multinucleated giant cells can be seen at the base of the blister. A mixed dermal inflammatory infiltrate is present.

Treatment: Treatment with antiviral medications from the acyclovir family should be instituted immediately. The sooner therapy is started, the better the chance of decreasing the length of disease. Therapy may also decrease the incidence of postherpetic neuralgia. The use of oral corticosteroids in conjunction with the antiviral medication has been advocated to help decrease the risk of postherpetic neuralgia, but large studies have thus far shown inconclusive data to support this approach. Therapy has the best chance of changing the course of the disease if given within the first 72 hours after the onset of disease symptoms.

A recombinant glycoprotein zoster vaccine for the prevention of herpes zoster is available to patients older than 50 years. This vaccine has been shown to boost natural immunity against VZV and to decrease the number of cases of herpes zoster and the frequency of postherpetic neuralgia in those who do develop herpes zoster after vaccination.

Currently, the treatment of postherpetic neuralgia is not optimal. Amitriptyline, gabapentin, pregabalin, anticonvulsants, serotonin-norepinephrine inhibitors, botulinum toxin, and opioids are all used with varying success. Milder symptoms may be treated with topical capsaicin and/or topical lidocaine.

VERRUCAE (WARTS)

Verrucae are one of the most frequently encountered viral infections in humans. They are capable of causing disease in any individual, but severe infections seem to be more likely in those who are immunocompromised. Warts can affect any cutaneous surface, and unique wart subtypes are more prone to cause disease in different clinical locations. By far the most important aspect of infection with the human papillomavirus (HPV) is the ability of the virus to cause malignant transformation. This malignant potential is specific to certain subtypes and is especially a concern in women, who are at risk for cervical cancer. Most cases of cervical cancer can be traced to prior infection with certain HPV strains. In June 2006 the US Food and Drug Administration approved the use of the first prophylactic HPV vaccine in prepubertal girls. That vaccine was a recombinant quadrivalent vaccine against HPV types 6, 11, 16, and 18. Types 16 and 18 are believed to have been responsible for up to 70% of cervical cancers. The indication was expanded to include males as well. Two other HPV vaccines are currently available: the HPV 9 valent vaccine that targets HPV types 6, 11, 16, 18, 31, 33, 45, and 52 and the HPV bivalent vaccine that targets HPV 16 and 18.

Clinical Findings: Verruca vulgaris, also called the *common wart,* is the most prevalent wart that infects the human. It can be located on any cutaneous surface. These warts often appear as small papules with a rough surface studded with pinpoint, dark purple to black dots. These dots represent the thromboses of the tiny capillaries within the wart. Most warts are between 5 mm and 1 cm in diameter, but some can become quite large and encompass much larger areas of the skin. The coalescence of multiple warts into one larger wart is called mosaic warts. These are most commonly seen on the plantar aspect of the foot. Verruca vulgaris can come in many sizes and shapes. Most lesions spontaneously resolve within a few years. A good rule of thumb is that 50% of verrucae will disappear spontaneously in 2 years. Many distinctive clinical forms of warts exist.

The filiform wart is represented by a small verrucal papule with finger-like projections extruding from the base of the papule. The projections are typically 1 to 2 mm thick and 4 to 7 mm long. They are commonly found on the face. The flat wart is frequently encountered and manifests as a 3- to 5-mm, flat papule with a slight pink to red to purple coloration. Flat warts are frequently seen on the legs of women and in the beard region of men, and they can be arranged in a linear pattern if the warts are spread during the act of shaving. Flat warts have been found to be highly associated with HPV types 3 and 10.

Plantar warts (myrmecia) are seen on the plantar aspect of the foot and are caused for the most part by HPV types 1, 2, and 4. They are deep-seated papules and plaques that may coalesce into large mosaic warts.

HUMAN PAPILLOMAVIRUS (HPV) INFECTION

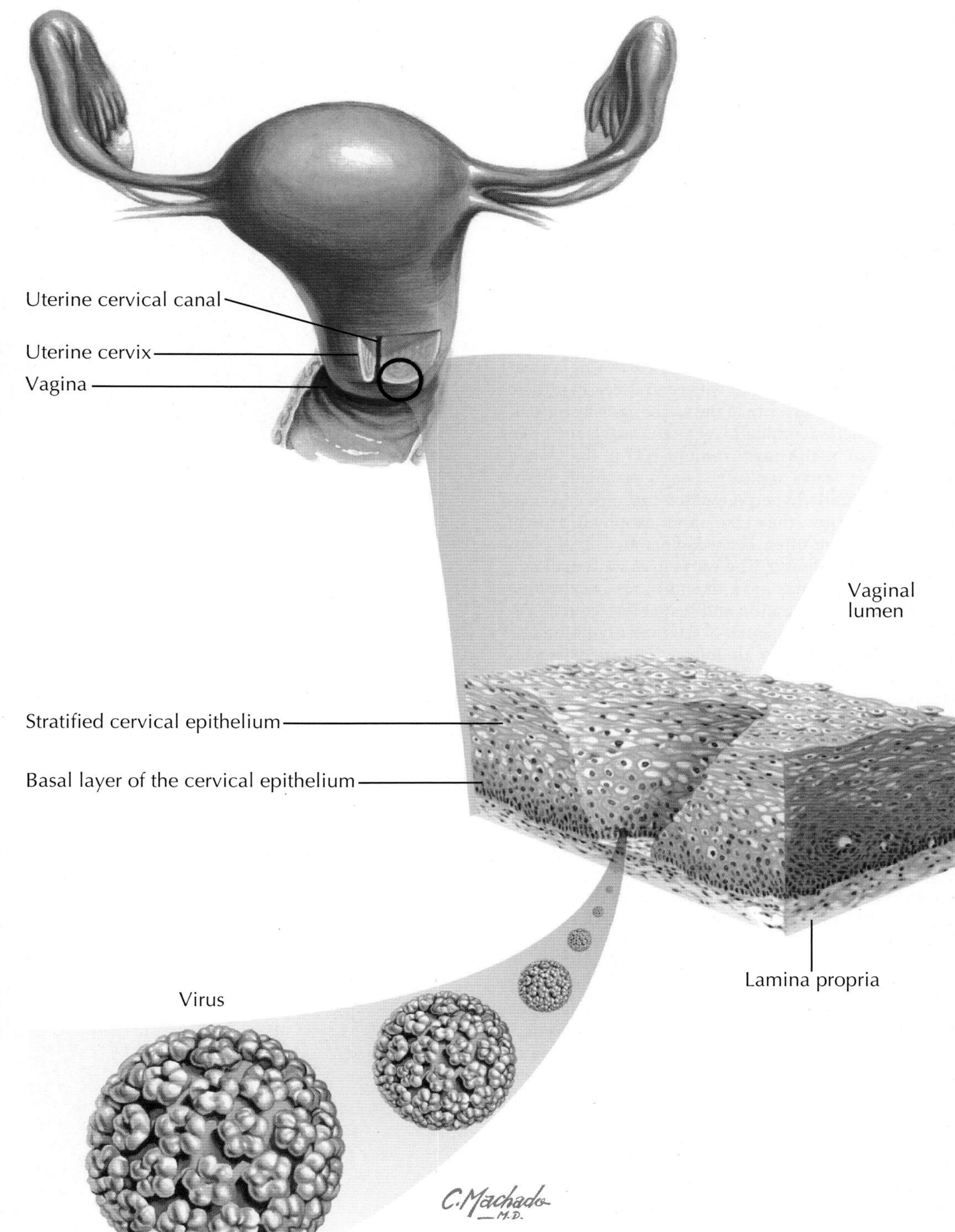

The warts are well defined and characteristically interrupt the skin lines. This is in contrast to a callus, in which the skin lines are retained; this sign can be used to differentiate the two conditions. Plantar warts can cause pain and discomfort if they are located in areas of pressure such as the heels or across the skin underlying the metatarsal heads. Palmar warts are very similar to plantar warts and have the same clinical appearance.

Subungual and periungual warts, a subclassification of palmar/plantar warts, are found around and under the nail apparatus. These warts can cause nail dystrophy and pain on grasping of objects. They tend to affect more than one finger and can be more difficult to treat than the common wart. Long-standing periungual or subungual warts that have a changing morphology should be biopsied to rule out malignant transformation into a squamous cell carcinoma. This is not infrequently encountered, and a high clinical suspicion should be used when investigating these types of warts.

VERRUCAE (WARTS) (Continued)

Ring warts are seen after various treatments of common warts, most frequently after liquid nitrogen therapy. The central portion of the wart resolves, leaving a ring-shaped or donut-shaped wart with central clearing. These warts can become larger than the wart originally treated.

Condylomata acuminata (genital warts) are often considered to be the most common STI in the United States. These warts typically begin as small, flesh-colored to slightly hyperpigmented macules and papules. As they grow, they take on an exophytic growth pattern and have often been compared with the appearance of cauliflower. The warts may stay small and localized, or they may grow to enormous size, leading to difficulty with urination and sexual intercourse. Females with cervical genital warts are asymptomatic and may not realize they are infected. Routine gynecologic examinations and Papanicolaou smears are the only reliable way to diagnose cervical warts. Diagnosis is extremely important because cervical HPV infection is the primary cause of cervical cancer.

Pathogenesis: Warts are caused by infection with HPV, of which more than 170 subtypes are known. They are small viruses with no lipid envelope, and they can stay viable for long periods. HPV has a double-stranded, circular DNA. A variety of subtypes are able to affect different regions of the body. HPV is capable of infecting human epithelium, including the keratinized skin and the mucous membranes. It gains entry through slightly abraded skin or mucous membranes. The virus does not actively infect the outer stratum corneum, but rather the stratum basalis cells. Like most viruses, HPV can produce early and late gene products. The early genes encode various proteins necessary for replication. These early gene products also play a role in malignant transformation of the infected cell. The exact mechanism is not completely understood. The late genes produce capsid proteins. At least eight early genes are present, and two late genes are included in the viral DNA.

Histology: Skin biopsies of wart tissue show the pathognomonic cell called the koilocyte. This cell, when present, is highly specific and sensitive for HPV infection. It is a keratinocyte with a basophilic small nucleus and a surrounding clear halo. There are few to no keratohyalin granules in the koilocyte. Other findings include varying amounts of hyperkeratosis, acanthosis, and striking papillomatosis.

Treatment: Common warts can be treated in a number of ways. Approximately 50% of the lesions spontaneously resolve. The others may or may not respond to therapy. This lack of universal treatment response is frustrating to patient and physician alike. Many destructive therapies are available, including liquid nitrogen cryotherapy, salicylic acid, trichloroacetic acid, cantharidin, podophyllin, fluorouracil, and bleomycin. Immunotherapy can be used to induce an immunologic response; these options include imiquimod, interferon, dinitrochlorobenzene, squaric acid, and *Candida* skin test antigen. No single therapy appears to work better than any other, and patients often need to undergo a variety of treatments until they find one that works.

Genital warts should be treated with imiquimod or one of the destructive methods to decrease the risk of transmission. Women who are sexually active should undergo routine gynecologic screening. The advent of the HPV vaccine has led to a decreased incidence of genital warts and cervical cancer.

CONDYLOMATA ACUMINATA (GENITAL WARTS)

In females

"Cauliflower"-appearing plaques

Cervical HPV infection is the leading cause of cervical cancer.

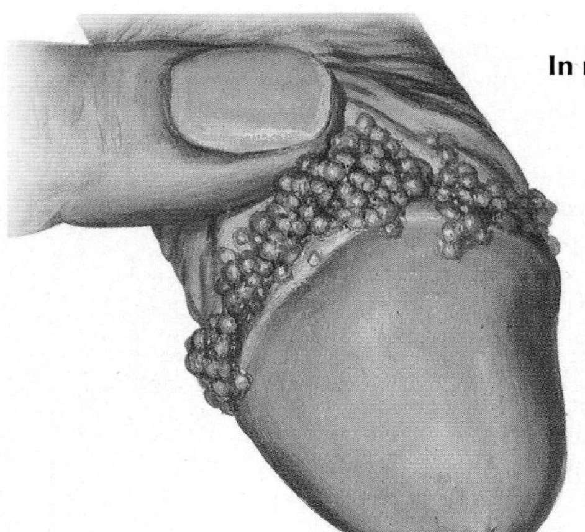

In males

HPV is one of the most common sexually transmitted infections.

HAIR AND NAIL DISEASES

Pilosebaceous unit

Epidermis
Hair shaft
Sebaceous gland and its duct
Arrector pili muscle
Hair cortex
Hair medulla
Hair cuticle
Huxley's layer
Henle's layer
Inner root sheath
Outer root sheath
Dermal papilla
Hair bulb

Schematic diagram of a pilosebaceous unit and innervation of skin

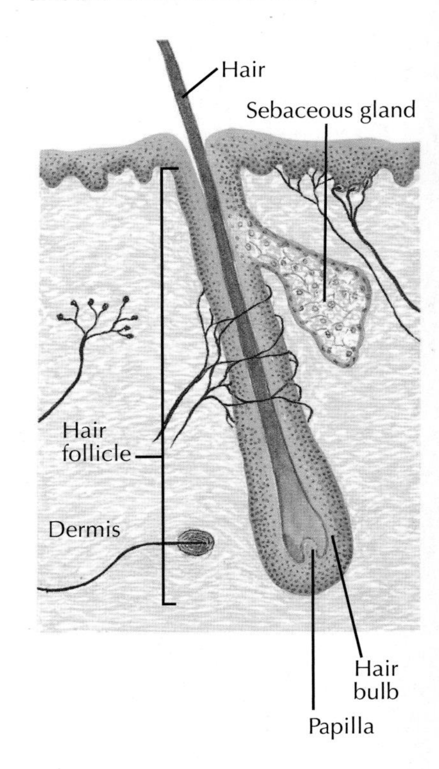

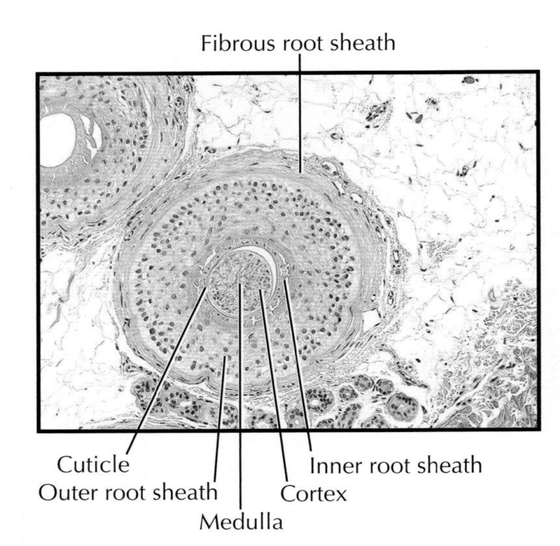

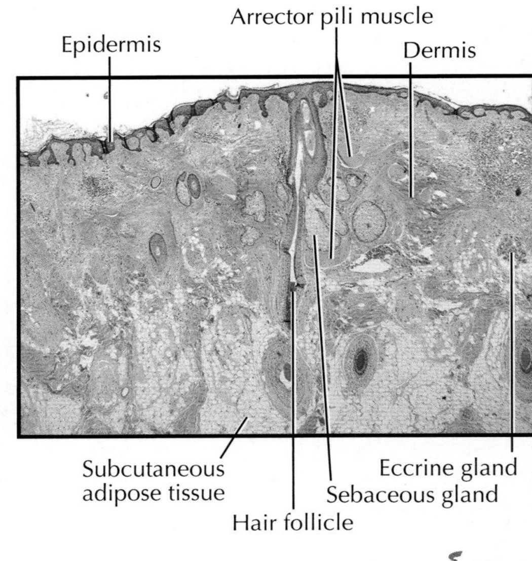

Normal Structure and Function of the Hair Follicle Apparatus

The pilosebaceous unit is a complex apparatus that is composed of a hair shaft and its follicle, sebaceous glands, arrector pili muscle, and, in some regions of the body, apocrine glands. Hair is a complex structure that is made of many different keratin proteins linked by disulfide bonds between neighboring cysteine amino acid molecules intermixed with cornified trichocytes. The keratin molecules come in acidic and basic forms. During hair formation, an acidic keratin fiber localizes with a basic keratin fiber and is cross-linked via disulfide bonds.

The exact function of hair is unknown, but it is theorized to act as an insulator for heat retention and to increase sensation perception, and it has been postulated to be important to attract a mate. No matter what the function, humans can live a normal life without the presence of hair with no ill effects.

Hair comes in a variety of colors. The amount of melanin or pheomelanin in the hair shaft determines the exact color of the hair. With time, the production of hair pigment decreases and the hair becomes dull gray or white. This process is unpredictable in a given individual, and even those within the same family may show striking differences in hair color change. As people age, the scalp hair usually tends to thin. This is considered to be a normal physiologic process.

There are two main types of hair in the adult. Terminal hair is thick hair that is present on the scalp, axilla, and groin and in the beard region in men. Vellus hair is the fine, thin, lightly pigmented hair that can be found in most areas of the body where terminal hair is not present. No hair is present on the lips, palms, soles, glans, or labia minora. Lanugo hair is present during fetal development and is predominantly seen in premature infants. This type of hair is shed in utero and replaced with vellus hair before delivery. Reversion of vellus hair and terminal hair back to lanugo hair is a sign of anorexia nervosa. Lanugo hair has a soft, fluffy white appearance.

The hair cycle is an extremely complex and highly coordinated process. The anagen phase is the growth phase. The anagen phase of the typical adult scalp hair lasts approximately 2 years. The cells at the anagen hair bulb proliferate at one of the highest rates in the human body. This growth phase is followed by the catagen phase, which is a short (2-week) transition period during which the hair follicle transforms from a growing, functioning hair into a club hair. This is followed by the telogen phase, which lasts approximately 2 months and ends with shedding of the club hair. Anagen hairs have a floppy, pigmented end that is easily distinguished from the telogen hair. Telogen hair is termed *club hair* because of its depigmented bulb at the proximal end. Catagen hairs are almost impossible to identify because they appear somewhere in the spectrum between anagen and telogen hair. The length of the anagen phase is responsible for the overall length of the hair: the longer the anagen phase, the longer the hair can grow. This process is preprogrammed and is different for all hair types on the body. The normal scalp can shed up to 100 hairs per day. The hair follicle is remarkably capable of regeneration after the hair has entered the telogen phase. An unknown signal causes the hair follicle stem cells, which are located in the bulge region, to differentiate and begin producing another hair, restarting the anagen phase. This is an extremely well-coordinated and complex process involving numerous cell types. The bulge region is an area found in approximation to the insertion of the arrector pili muscle into the hair follicle.

Histologic examination of a cross section of a terminal hair shaft reveals a complex architecture. The hair is made up of various concentric layers. The innermost layer is the medulla, which is pigmented. The next layer is the cortex, followed by the cuticle, the inner root sheath (Huxley's and Henle's layers), and the outer root sheath. The outer root sheath seamlessly blends into the epidermis. The hair follicle undergoes trichohyalin keratinization, which is different from the keratohyalin keratinization of the epidermis.

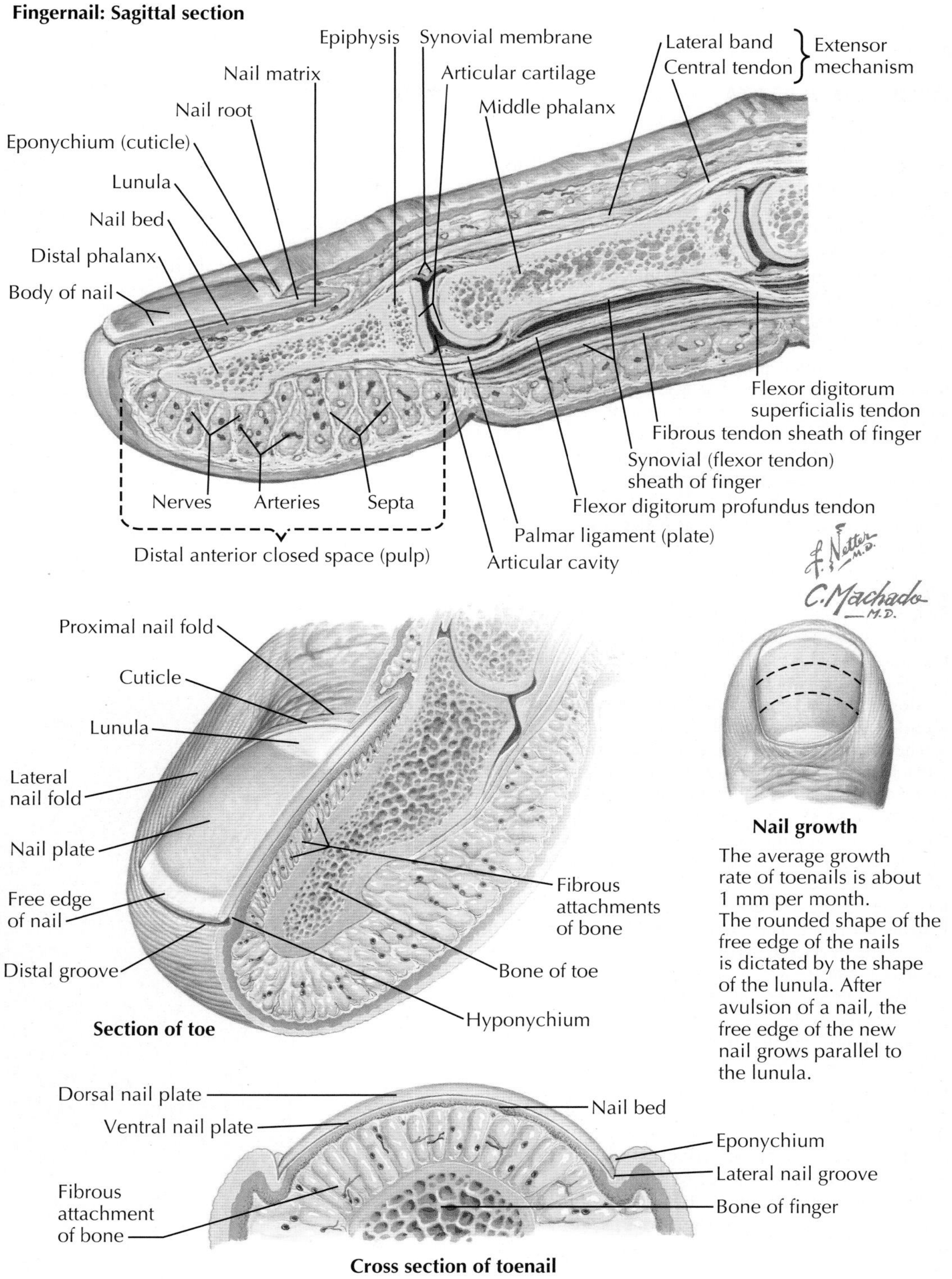

NORMAL STRUCTURE AND FUNCTION OF THE NAIL UNIT

The human nail is composed of various hard and soft keratin proteins as well as modified keratinocytes termed *onychocytes*. All 20 nails have the same chemical makeup; the only difference is in the size and thickness of the nail. The nail unit is made up of highly specialized structures. The nail matrix is the portion of the nail unit that is responsible for production of the nail plate. The matrix lies a few millimeters proximal to and beneath the proximal nail fold, which ends as the cuticle (eponychium), and extends under the nail bed. Under the proximal nail plate, the nail matrix can often be appreciated as a half-circle termed the *lunula*. The color of the lunula is often creamy white with a hint of pink. Any damage to the nail matrix can potentially cause a temporary or permanent nail dystrophy.

The distal nail matrix is responsible for producing the ventral portion of the nail plate. The proximal nail matrix is responsible for producing the dorsal surface of the nail plate. The nail plate is made of varying keratin proteins and is the hard portion of the nail. It has dorsal, intermediate, and ventral components. It is theorized to be protective to the underlying nail matrix and distal phalanx, as well as being helpful with grasping and dexterity of the fingertips. The nail plate is firmly attached to the underlying nail bed via tiny, vertically arranged interdigitations. These tiny undulations help lock the nail plate into the nail bed below. The nail plate is an avascular structure, and the underlying nail bed is highly vascular. Approximately one-third of the nail plate is located under the proximal nail fold.

The nail bed is attached to the epidermis via the proximal nail fold and the cuticle, as well as the lateral nail folds on either side of the nail. Damage to the cuticle, whether by accident or during manicures or pedicures, can increase the risk of bacterial or fungal infection within the nail or the skin of the nail folds. This can lead to acute or chronic paronychia or onychomycosis. Improper trimming of the lateral aspects of the nail plate may lead to an ingrown toenail (onychocryptosis). The distal nail plate is attached to the underlying epidermis by the hyponychium. Damage to this portion of the nail unit may allow for bacterial or fungal infections to take hold under or within the nail plate.

The nails grow continuously throughout a person's life span. Fingernails grow on average 3 mm per month, and toenails grow a bit more slowly, on average 1 mm per month. However, these growth rates are highly variable among individuals. Nails of younger individuals grow faster than nails of older individuals. Some medications (e.g., levodopa and itraconazole) and underlying health conditions (e.g., hyperthyroidism and psoriasis) can increase nail growth. Poor nutrition and various chemotherapeutics slow the growth rate. Both hair keratin and skin keratin types have been described to comprise the various portions of the nail unit. The hair keratin Ha1 and the skin keratins K5, K6, K14, K16, K17, and K31 make up the majority of the keratin types found in the adult nail. Other keratins have been identified during development of the nail.

Primary and secondary nail disorders are commonly encountered. Primary nail disorders include onychomycosis, onychocryptosis, onychoschizia (horizontal splitting), onychogryphotic nail ("ram's horn" nail), leukonychia, median nail dystrophy, and onycholysis. These disorders are most often seen in isolation, with no underlying systemic abnormalities. Secondary nail disorders are seen in the presence of an underlying systemic disease; examples include koilonychia (caused by iron deficiency), nail plate pitting (many conditions including psoriasis and alopecia areata), pterygium formation (lichen planus), longitudinal red and white streaks and distal V-shaped nicking (Darier disease), clubbing (pulmonary disease), and yellow nail syndrome (pleural effusion and lymphedema). All skin examinations should include evaluation of the nails because many systemic diseases can manifest with nail findings, and these clinical signs may be the first signs of underlying disease.

ANATOMY OF THE FINGERNAIL AND TOENAIL

The average growth rate of toenails is about 1 mm per month.
The rounded shape of the free edge of the nails is dictated by the shape of the lunula. After avulsion of a nail, the free edge of the new nail grows parallel to the lunula.

Alopecia Areata

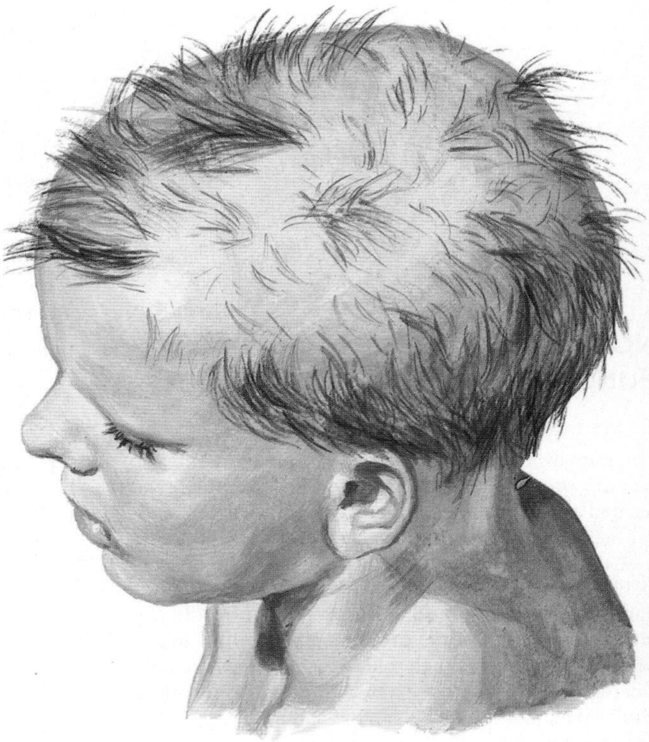

Alopecia areata is an autoimmune disease that causes discrete circular or oval areas of nonscarring alopecia. This form of alopecia has several clinical variants, including alopecia totalis, alopecia universalis, and an ophiasis pattern. Therapy is often difficult. The disease can have profound psychological effects, especially in young patients. It is critical to address this issue because the effects on the patient's psychological well-being are often more severe than the actual hair loss.

Clinical Findings: Alopecia areata can affect individuals of any age but is most frequently seen in children and young adults. It is estimated to affect 2% of the population. Both sexes are equally affected, and there is no race predilection. The first sign is hair loss in one specific area of the scalp. The hairs fall out in large numbers, especially when pulled. The patches of hair loss typically have an oval or circular pattern. There may be one or more than a dozen areas of involvement. The scalp hair is the most commonly affected region. The affected scalp is smooth without evidence of scarring or follicular dropout. Small, stubby hairs may be present at follicular openings and have been termed "exclamation point hairs." All hair regions may be involved, including the eyebrows, eyelashes, axilla, groin, and beard.

Alopecia areata has an unpredictable, waxing and waning course. Areas may begin to grow back as new patches form. It is not uncommon for a patient to have one solitary episode with spontaneous resolution and no future episodes. Some patients develop patches of alopecia intermittently over their lifetime. Complete loss of the scalp hair caused by alopecia areata is termed *alopecia totalis*. The rarest variant is alopecia universalis, which causes loss of all hair in all locations. These two forms of alopecia areata are very difficult to treat. Patients with both alopecia totalis and alopecia universalis should be offered psychological assessment because the loss of hair has severe social and self-esteem consequences. Patients often benefit from consultation with a professional psychologist or psychiatrist. Alopecia areata support groups can be extremely helpful.

The ophiasis pattern of alopecia areata is rare. It involves the parietal scalp dorsal to the occiput bilaterally. The diagnosis is typically made on clinical grounds. A skin biopsy is rarely needed. The hair pull test is a diagnostic test that can be performed at the bedside. It is positive when more than three hairs are pulled out in and around the patch of alopecia areata. If the hair is actively shedding, this test should be performed only once, because the number of hairs removed is large and can be very upsetting to the patient.

The hair that regrows is often lacking in pigment and appears white or gray. Over time, these white hairs are replaced with pigmented hairs as the hair pigmentation machinery begins to work again.

Individuals with alopecia areata have higher rates of atopic dermatitis, thyroid dysfunction, and vitiligo. Nail pitting and trachyonychia are nail findings commonly seen in association with alopecia areata.

Pathogenesis: Alopecia areata is believed to be an autoimmune inflammatory disease of T cells that, for unknown reasons, attacks certain hair follicles. It may be seen in association with other autoimmune diseases such as autoimmune thyroid disease. It is believed to be polygenic in nature.

Alopecia areata approaching the alopecia totalis stage. This patient has lost almost all of her scalp hair.

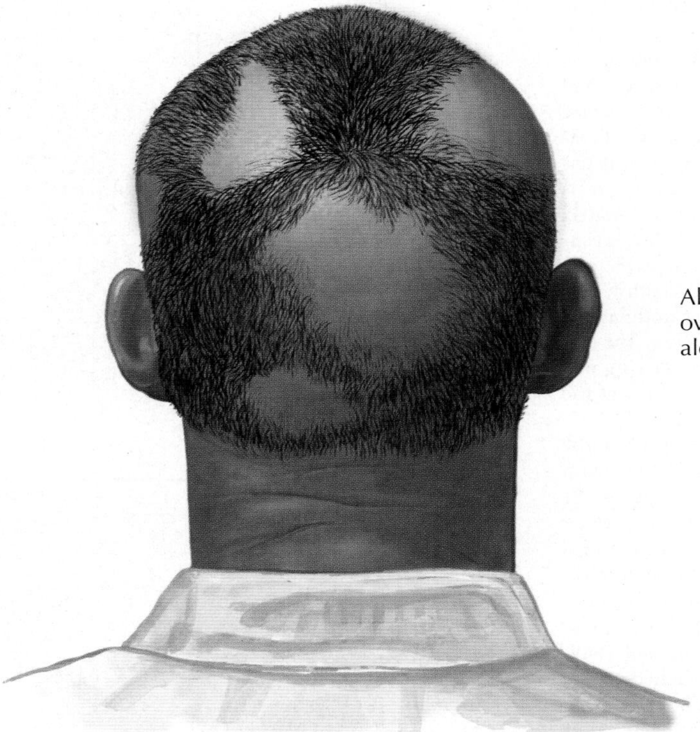

Alopecia areata with the characteristic oval and circular areas of nonscarring alopecia

Histology: Skin biopsies of the scalp of an affected area show a dense lymphocytic infiltrate surrounding all of the hair bulbs in what has been termed a "swarm of bees" pattern. There are increased numbers of catagen and telogen hairs. The epidermis is normal.

Treatment: Treatment consists of proper assessment of the patient and how the disease is affecting the patient's life in general. Some individuals tolerate the condition without adverse psychological effects; for them, the best treatment is a watch-and-wait approach. Others with mild disease may have severe self-esteem issues and should be offered therapy. No therapy has been shown to be uniformly effective. Topical retinoids and corticosteroids are used, as well as intralesional steroid injections if the areas are small. Contact sensitization with squaric acid has had equivocal results. Oral steroids should be avoided because the long-term side effects do not warrant their use. Most recently, oral and topical Janus kinase inhibitors have been found to be helpful.

ANDROGENIC ALOPECIA

Androgenic alopecia, also known as *male pattern baldness* or *female pattern hair loss*, is the most common form of hair loss. The age at onset is variable and likely has a genetic determination. Some men lose their entire scalp hair, resulting in baldness. Baldness is rare in women because their hair loss manifests as varying grades of thinning.

Clinical Findings: There are variable degrees of male pattern hair loss. The Hamilton-Norwood scale has been used to grade the degree of hair loss in men, and the Ludwig scale is used in women. Grade 1 is manifested by receding frontal hair. Grade 7 is near-total loss of the scalp hair with some sparing of the inferior occiput. The age at onset of androgenic alopecia in men can be any time from puberty into adulthood. Most men older than 50 years exhibit some form of androgenic hair loss. The White population is more prone to developing androgenic alopecia than Black or Asian populations.

Female pattern hair loss (androgenetic alopecia in females) is most frequently seen in the fifth to seventh decades of life but may be seen sooner. It is typically not as severe as in men, and most women will only develop thinning of the vertex. A characteristic finding in female pattern hair loss is the preservation of the frontal hair line.

Pathogenesis: Androgenic alopecia has been shown to follow an autosomal dominant pattern of inheritance. It is believed to result from an abnormal response of the hair follicle to androgens (i.e., dihydrotestosterone). Dihydrotestosterone has been shown to cause miniaturization of the terminal hairs over successive hair cycles. As the hair follicles miniaturize, they become smaller with a thinner caliber. This causes less scalp coverage, manifesting as hair thinning. The actual hair follicles are not scarred or lost. Inhibition of the production of dihydrotestosterone from its precursor, testosterone, is one therapeutic tactic.

Histology: Evaluation of a 4-mm punch biopsy specimen by the horizontal method is the best technique to evaluate hair loss. In androgenic alopecia, the follicles are normal in number, but they show evidence of miniaturization. Vellus hairs are increased. Whereas the normal scalp has been shown to have a vellus-to-telogen hair ratio of 1:7, the ratio in androgenic alopecia is 1:3.5. The hair shaft diameters of the terminal hairs are variable, which corresponds to the miniaturization affect. There is no scarring, and this is considered a nonscarring alopecia.

Treatment: Hair loss is made more difficult to treat because of the importance society places on appearance and the psychological effects that hair loss can have on men and women. Therapy for male pattern baldness includes use of the topical agent minoxidil 5%, applied twice daily, with or without the oral 5α-reductase inhibitor finasteride. 5α-Reductase is the enzyme responsible for converting free testosterone into dihydrotestosterone. Both of these agents have been shown in multiple randomized studies to decrease the rate of hair loss and increase the hair shaft diameter. These medications are well tolerated and have minimal side effects. Patients with prostate cancer should avoid the use of finasteride unless approved by their oncologist. The only US Food and Drug Administration–approved option at present for women with androgenic alopecia is topical minoxidil 2%. This has been shown to decrease the rate of hair loss.

HAMILTON-NORWOOD SCALE FOR MALE PATTERN BALDNESS

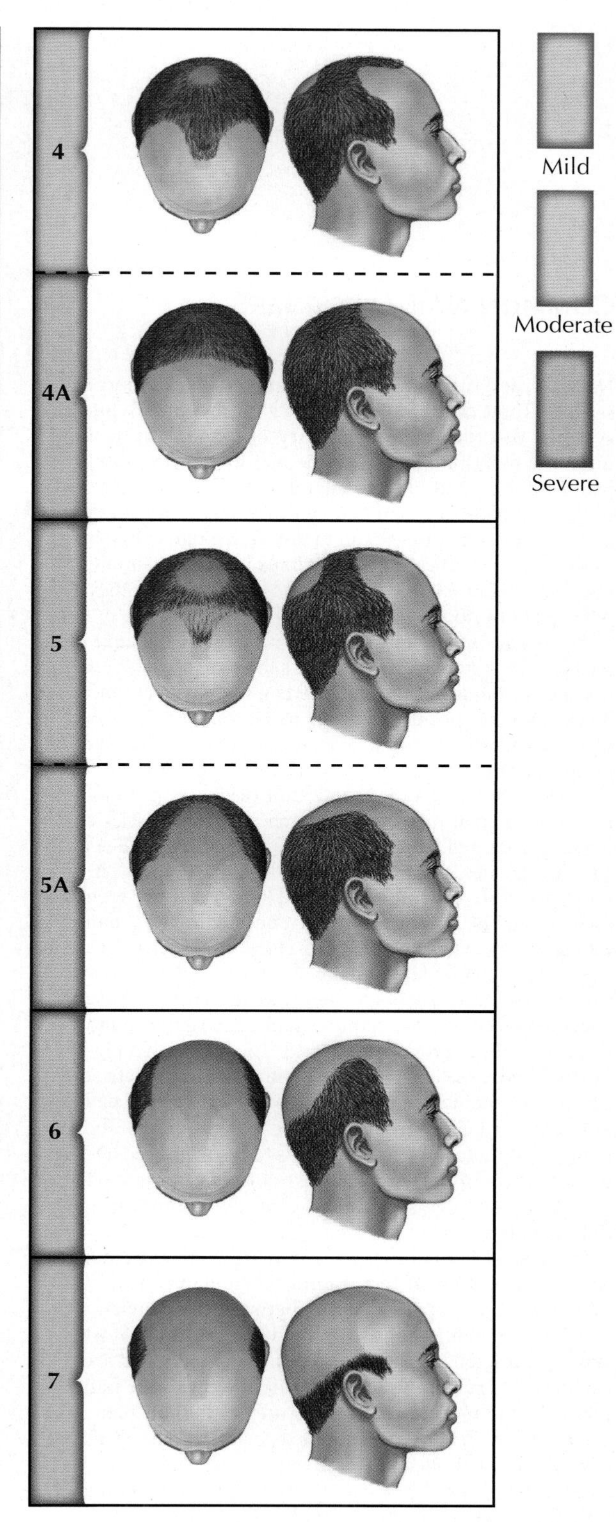

Most patients who use minoxidil experience a slowing of hair loss, and some see increased growth. It is critical to treat early in the course of disease to maximize the effects of the medication. Topical minoxidil may cause excessive hair growth on the forehead and temples if applied to these regions. This can be disconcerting for patients, and they need to be educated on the proper application of the medication.

Hair transplantation techniques continue to improve. The goal of surgery is a natural-appearing hair pattern. This is best accomplished with minigrafts of one to two follicles at a time. A strip of the patient's hair is removed from the occipital scalp, and each individual hair is dissected out. The separated hair follicles are then tediously inserted into the desired areas. Patients can have an excellent result, and the transplanted hair appear to be resistant to the effects of dihydrotestosterone. Low-level light therapy, prostaglandin analogs, and platelet-rich plasma have shown some efficacy.

COMMON FINGERNAIL DISORDERS

Acute paronychia. Tender red nail fold, commonly caused by *Staphylococcus aureus*.

Mees' lines. Mees' lines on fingernails and hyperpigmentation of the soles are characteristic of arsenic poisoning.

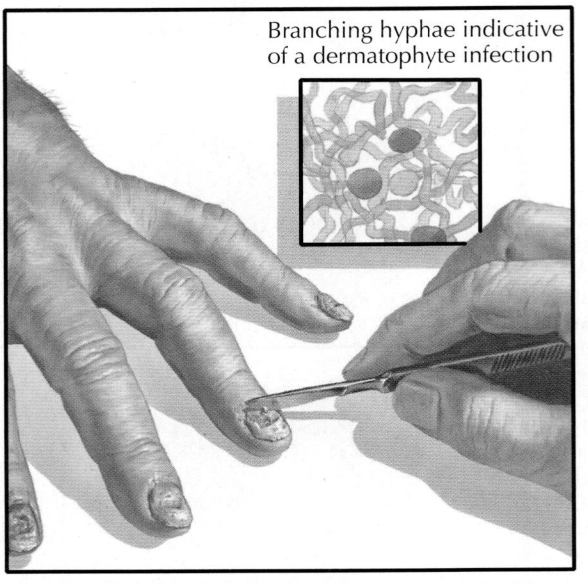

Onychomycosis of the fingernails. A KOH preparation is done by scraping the crumbling nail plate and examining it under the microscope.

Psoriatic arthritis with nail involvement. Sausage-shaped digits, psoriatic skin plaques, and nail changes.

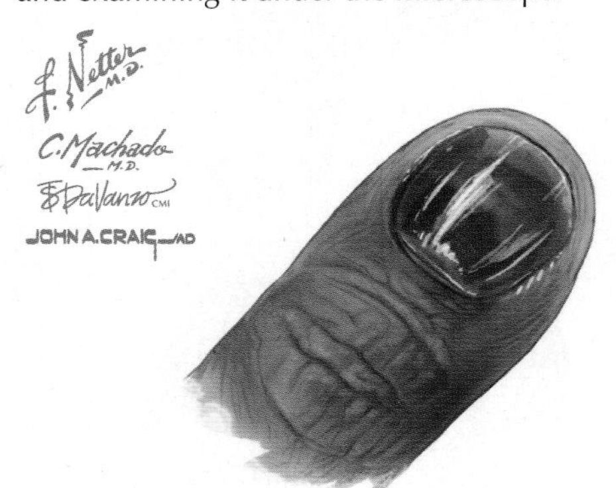

Subungal hematoma from trauma

Nail pits
Transverse ridges
Onycholysis

Psoriatic nail changes

COMMON NAIL DISORDERS

Nail disorders are frequently encountered in the clinical setting. They can occur secondary to an underlying systemic disorder or as a primary disease of the nail unit. The nail unit consists of the nail matrix, bed, and plate and the proximal and lateral nail folds. Disorders of the nail plate and nail bed can manifest in a variety of ways. Systemic disease can manifest through changes in the nail unit. The complete skin examination should also include an examination of the nails because they offer insight into the patient's health.

Beau's lines and Mees' lines of the nail are two nail findings seen in systemic disease. Beau's lines are caused by a nonspecific halting of the nail matrix growth pattern, and Mees' lines are specific for heavy metal toxicity. Dilation of the capillaries of the proximal nail fold or cuticular erythema can be a sign of connective tissue disease.

One of the most serious nail unit disorders is melanoma of the nail matrix. Melanoma may manifest as a linear, pigmented band along the length of the nail. As time progresses, the proximal nail fold and hyponychium may also become pigmented and involved with melanoma. The finding of pigment on the proximal nail fold and cuticle has been termed *Hutchinson's sign*. This sign is not seen in subungual hematomas. All new pigmented nail streaks should be evaluated and a biopsy considered. The biopsy requires nail plate removal and retraction of the proximal nail fold. The biopsy of a pigmented nail streak is performed within the nail matrix. Biopsies of the nail matrix may lead to a narrower nail or to chronic nail dystrophy because of disruption of the matrix. Subungual melanoma tends to be diagnosed late because these tumors are easily overlooked or passed off as a subungual hematoma. It is critically important to differentiate the two.

Subungual hematomas are frequently encountered. Most are caused by direct trauma to the nail plate and nail bed, which causes bleeding between the plate and bed. Acute hematomas can be very painful. Most acute subungual hematomas are on the fingers and are caused by a crush injury or by a direct blow to the nail plate. As the blood accumulates under the nail plate, the pressure created can cause excruciating pain. This can be easily treated by nail trephination. A small-gauge hole is bored into the overlying nail plate with a hot, thin metal object or small drill. Once the nail plate has been punctured, the blood that has accumulated under the nail freely flows out of the newly formed channel, and near-immediate pain relief is achieved. Most traumatic injuries to the nail unit do not cause these very painful hematomas but rather cause small amounts of blood to accumulate under the nail plate. Pain is absent or minimal. Most people remember some trauma to the nail, but others do not. This form of subungual hematoma can involve small portions of the nail or the entire nail. There is often a blue, purple, and red discoloration of the underlying nail. Occasionally, the nail plate has a black appearance and can be easily confused with subungual melanoma. The history can be misleading in these cases because many patients with and without melanoma remember some form of trauma to the nail that might lead the clinician to pass the lesion off as a subungual hematoma. If any doubt about the diagnosis exists, a nail biopsy should be considered. The nail plate is removed, and a subungual hematoma is easily distinguished from a tumor. Most subungual hematomas slowly grow outward toward the distal free edge of the nail. As the nail grows, its most proximal portion appears normal. The entire subungual hematoma eventually grows out and is shed or clipped off once it passes the hyponychium.

Onychocryptosis (ingrown nail) is almost universally seen in the great toenail. It is caused by burrowing of the lateral portion of the nail plate into the lateral nail fold. As the nail punctures the lateral nail fold, it sets off an inflammatory reaction that causes edema, redness,

COMMON NAIL DISORDERS (Continued)

pain, and occasionally purulent drainage. Secondary infection is common. Ambulation may become difficult because the pain forces the patient to avoid pressure. The exact etiology of onychocryptosis is not entirely known, but it is believed to be caused, or at least made more likely, by improper trimming or removal of the lateral portion of the nail. If the nail plate is cut at varying angles or torn from its bed by picking, this may allow for the lateral free edge of the nail plate to enter into the lateral nailfold. Tight-fitting shoes have also been implicated as increasing the likelihood of developing ingrown nails. This condition is seen more frequently in young men, but is seen in all age groups. The fingernails are rarely affected. Treatment consists of lateral nail plate removal with or without lateral nail matrixectomy. After anesthesia, a nail plate elevator is used to free the involved portion of the nail. A nail splitter is then used to remove the lateral third of the nail. The freed nail is grasped with a nail puller, and the nail is removed with a gentle rocking motion. The portion of the nail removed from under the lateral nail fold is often larger than expected. Recurrent ingrown nails should be treated with nail matrixectomy. This destroys the lateral third of the nail matrix, eliminating the ability to form that portion of the nail and preventing problems in the future. Application of phenol to the nail matrix after nail plate avulsion is one of the best methods for destroying the nail matrix. Bilateral nail fold involvement on the same toe is not infrequently encountered, and the entire nail can be removed in these cases. Onychocryptosis is not a primary infection of the nail unit, and any infection is believed to be secondary to the massive inflammatory response. This is in stark contrast to an acute paronychia.

Paronychia is a nail fold infection with either a bacterial agent (acute paronychia) or fungal agent (chronic paronychia). Acute paronychia manifests with redness and tenderness of the nail fold. The redness and edema continue to expand, causing pain and eventually purulent drainage. Removal of the cuticle or nail fold trauma lead to an increased risk for this infection. *Staphylococcus aureus* and *Streptococcus* species are the most frequent etiologic agents. Therapy is incision and drainage and appropriate oral antibiotics.

Chronic paronychia typically is less inflammatory and manifests with redness and edema around the nail folds. Many digits may be involved. At presentation, patients typically report that they have been having difficulty for longer than 6 to 8 weeks. Tenderness is much less significant than in acute paronychia. Chronic paronychia is usually caused by a fungal infection of the nail fold with *Candida albicans*. Individuals who work in occupations in which their hands are constantly exposed to water are at higher risk for chronic paronychia. Therapy includes topical antifungal and antiinflammatory agents.

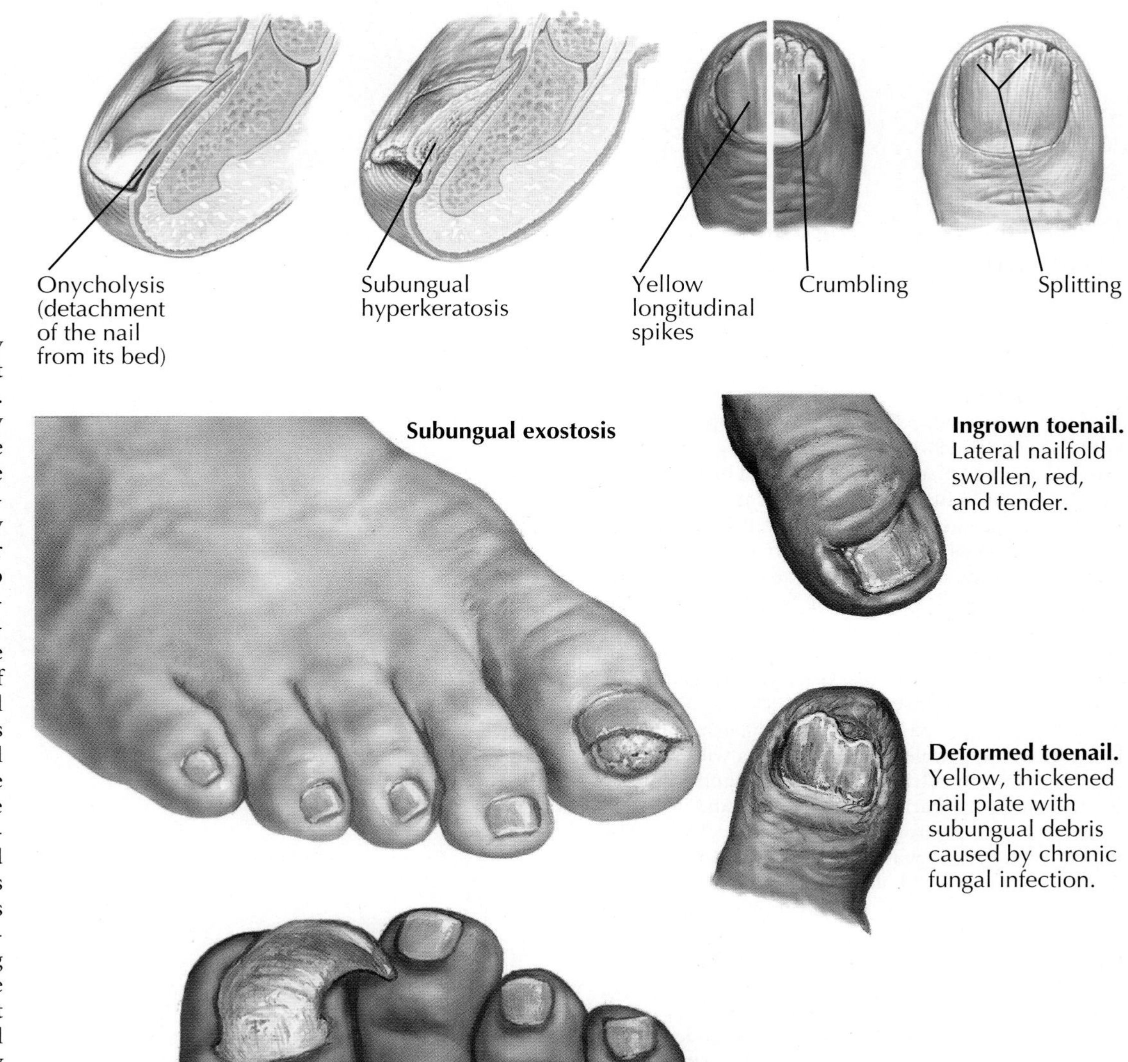

Onychogryphosis. "Ram's horn" nail. Nail plate is thick and curved.

A felon is often confused with acute paronychia, but it is a soft tissue infection of the fingertip pulp. It may arise secondary to an acute paronychia. The clinical finding is a swollen, red, painful finger pad. The treatment is surgical incision and drainage together with oral antibiotics to cover *S. aureus* and *Streptococcus* species.

Onychomycosis is seen in individuals of all ages, and its prevalence increases with age. Patients can present with different variants of onychomycosis. The most frequent type is distal and lateral subungual onychomycosis. Other variants include white superficial onychomycosis and proximal subungual onychomycosis. *Trichophyton rubrum* is the most frequent cause of all except white superficial onychomycosis, which is caused most often by *Trichophyton mentagrophytes*. Superficial white onychomycosis manifests with a fine, white, crumbling surface to the nail. When it is curetted off, the white areas are found to affect only the outermost portion of the nail plate. The material is a combination of fungal elements and nail keratin. Therapy includes curetting the white involved

Common Nail Disorders (Continued)

portion of the nail and applying a topical antifungal agent for at least 1 month.

Distal and lateral subungual onychomycosis manifests with thickened, yellow, dystrophic-appearing nails with subungual debris. There are varying amounts of onycholysis (nail plate lifting off the nail bed). One nail may be solitarily involved, but it is more common for several nails to be involved and for the surrounding skin to be involved with tinea manuum or tinea unguium. Fungal nail infections are more frequently seen on the toenails than on the fingernails. The nails can become painful, especially with ambulation. Occasionally, the entire nail is shed as a result of significant onycholysis, and the nail that regrows will again be involved with onychomycosis. The thick and dystrophic nails may become a passage for bacterial invasion of the body. This is especially true in patients with diabetes. Bacteria can gain entrance into the skin and soft tissue via the abnormal barrier between nail and nail fold, which can lead to paronychia, felon, and cellulitis. Distal and lateral subungual onychomycosis almost always needs to be treated with an oral antifungal medication. Topical agents may be helpful in limited nail disease, but their use is typically limited to an adjunctive role. Oral azole antifungals, griseofulvin, and terbinafine have all been used, with similar results.

Psoriasis can affect the nails in many ways. Nail involvement appears more frequently in patients with severe disease and in those with psoriatic arthritis. The nails can show oil spots, pitting, ridging, onycholysis, and onychauxis (subungual hyperkeratosis). Oil spots are brownish to yellowish discolorations under the nail plate with associated onycholysis. The discoloration is caused by deposition of glycoproteins into the nail plate. Nail pitting can be seen in other conditions besides psoriasis, such as alopecia areata; it is caused by parakeratosis of the proximal nail matrix, which is responsible for producing the dorsal nail plate. Ridging and onychauxis are caused by the excessive hyperkeratosis of the nail bed, which is directly caused by psoriasis. Therapy for psoriatic nails can involve intralesional steroid injections or use of systemic agents to decrease the abnormal immune response driving the psoriasis.

Onychogryphosis ("ram's horn" nail deformity) manifests with an unusually thickened and curved nail that takes the shape of a ram's horn.

A plethora of nail changes may be seen in response to systemic disease. Beau's lines are horizontal notches along the nails that may be caused by any major stressful event. The stressful event typically is induced by prolonged hospitalization, which causes temporary inadequate production of the nail bed by the nail matrix. It spontaneously resolves as the individual improves. Mees' lines are induced by heavy metal toxicity, most commonly from arsenic exposure. They appear as a single, white horizontal band across each nail. Mees' lines have also been reported in cases of malnutrition. *Terry nails* refer to nail changes seen in congestive heart failure and cirrhosis of the liver; more than two-thirds of the proximal nail plate and bed appear dull white with loss of the lunula. Half-and-half nails, also called *Lindsay nails*, are seen in patients with chronic renal failure. The proximal half of the nail is normal appearing, whereas the distal half has a brown discoloration. Yellow nail syndrome manifests with all 20 nails having a yellowish discoloration and increased thickness of the nail plate. This syndrome is almost always seen in association with a pleural effusion, often secondary to a lung-based malignancy. Koilonychia is one of the most easily recognized deformities of the nail; it is caused by iron deficiency. The nail plate develops a spoon-shaped, concave surface. Splinter hemorrhages may be a sign of bacterial endocarditis. Clubbing, which is defined as loss of Lovibond's angle, is typically caused by chronic lung disease. The nail unit can manifest disease in many ways, and awareness of the various nail signs can help the clinician diagnose and treat these conditions.

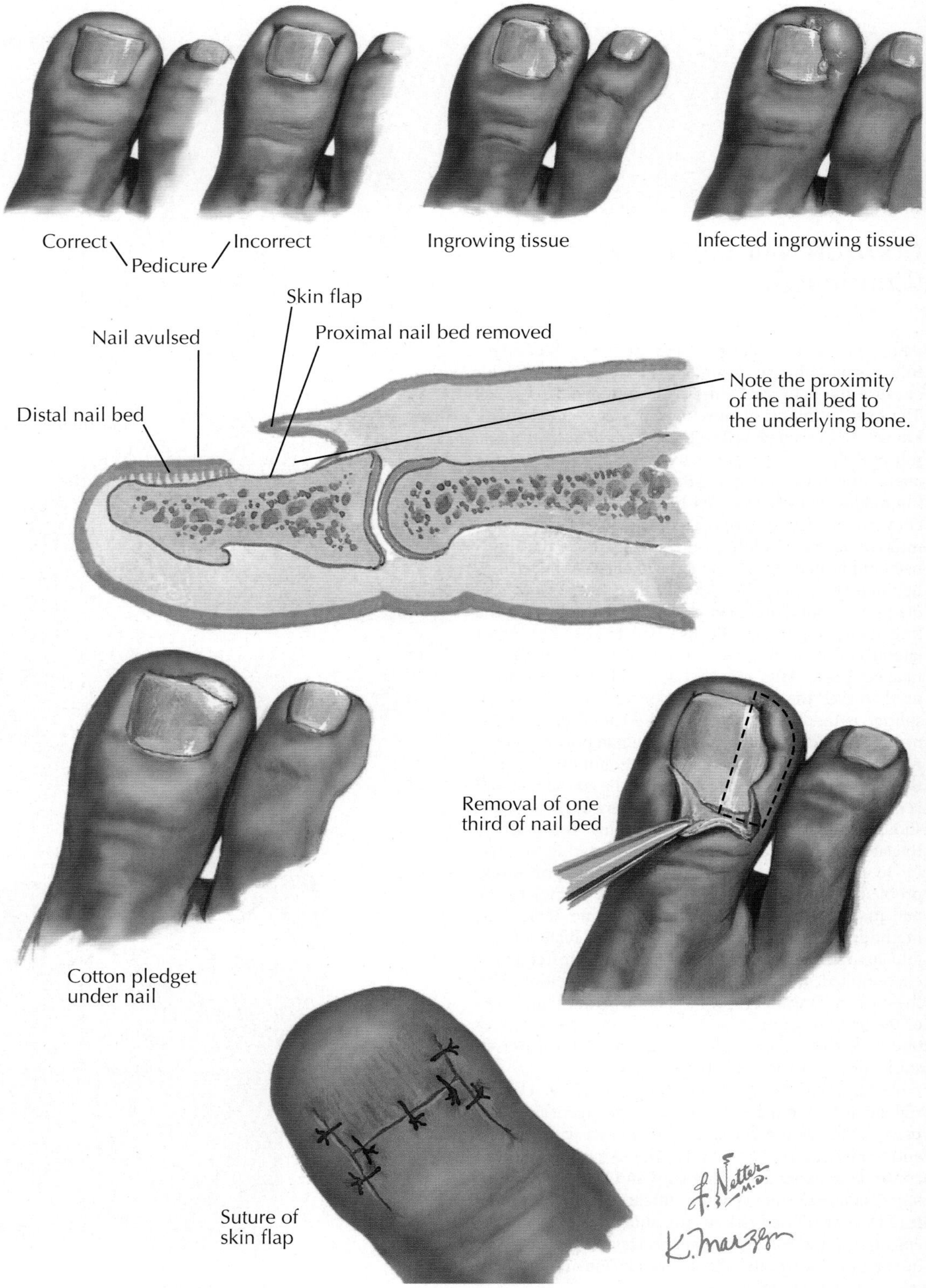

Hair Shaft Abnormalities

There are a wide variety of hair shaft abnormalities. Most are nonspecific clinical findings that can be seen in a multitude of underlying conditions as well as in healthy individuals. Trichoptilosis, known by the lay term "split ends," is probably the most common hair shaft abnormality in humans. It is nonspecific and is not associated with any particular underlying syndrome. Trichoptilosis is believed to be caused by excessive trauma to the distal hair shaft. Trichorrhexis nodosa is another hair shaft abnormality seen in individuals with no underlying disease state. A few highly specific hair abnormalities are indicative of particular disorders; for example, pili trianguli et canaliculi and trichorrhexis invaginata are seen only in uncombable hair syndrome and Netherton syndrome, respectively. Knowledge of hair shaft abnormalities helps form a differential diagnosis and in some cases confirm a diagnosis.

Pili torti is also known as "twisted hair" or "corkscrew hair." The hair twists on its axis in a corkscrew pattern. This twisting leads to increased pressure on the hair shaft, which results in early breakage and short, brittle hair. The involvement is almost exclusively on the scalp. Pili torti is nonspecific and can be found in a number of genetic skin conditions, including Björnstad syndrome, Menkes syndrome, and Crandall syndrome. It can also be seen as a primary hair disease with no underlying associations.

Monilethrix is a highly specific hair shaft abnormality. The hair has a beaded or undulating appearance, with nodes interspaced at regular intervals by abnormally thin hair. It is inherited in an autosomal dominant fashion and is caused by a mutation in the hair basic keratin 6 gene *(HB6)*, which is officially known as *keratin 86 (KRT86)*. The hair is fragile and breaks in the thinned internode regions. The internode regions are devoid of pigment, and this feature is used to discriminate this condition from pseudomonilethrix. There is no known therapy. Many afflicted individuals see improvement after puberty. It is almost never associated with systemic disease.

Trichorrhexis nodosa is a completely nonspecific finding that may be seen in healthy individuals. This hair shaft abnormality has been described as "broomstick hair" because of the appearance of the distal end of the broken hair, which resembles the bristles of a broom. Trichorrhexis nodosa is the most frequent reason for hair breakage. Trauma to the hair is causative. This trauma can be self-induced by rubbing or twisting, which results in fracturing of the hair and the appearance of trichorrhexis nodosa. This finding on microscopic examination can be helpful in evaluating hair loss secondary to trichotillomania or chemical-induced alopecia.

Pili trianguli et canaliculus, also termed "spun glass hair," is the diagnostic finding in uncombable hair syndrome. This rare and highly unusual syndrome is associated with no underlying ill effects on the afflicted individuals. The hair is uncontrollable and impossible to comb straight. This effect is related to the abnormal triangular shape of the hair shaft as well as changes in the direction of the hair, which occur at uneven intervals. The condition is inherited in an autosomal dominant or recessive pattern, and potential causative genetic mutations have been proposed. No therapy is needed, and most children with this condition spontaneously improve over time. The hair shafts appear triangular under electron microscopy.

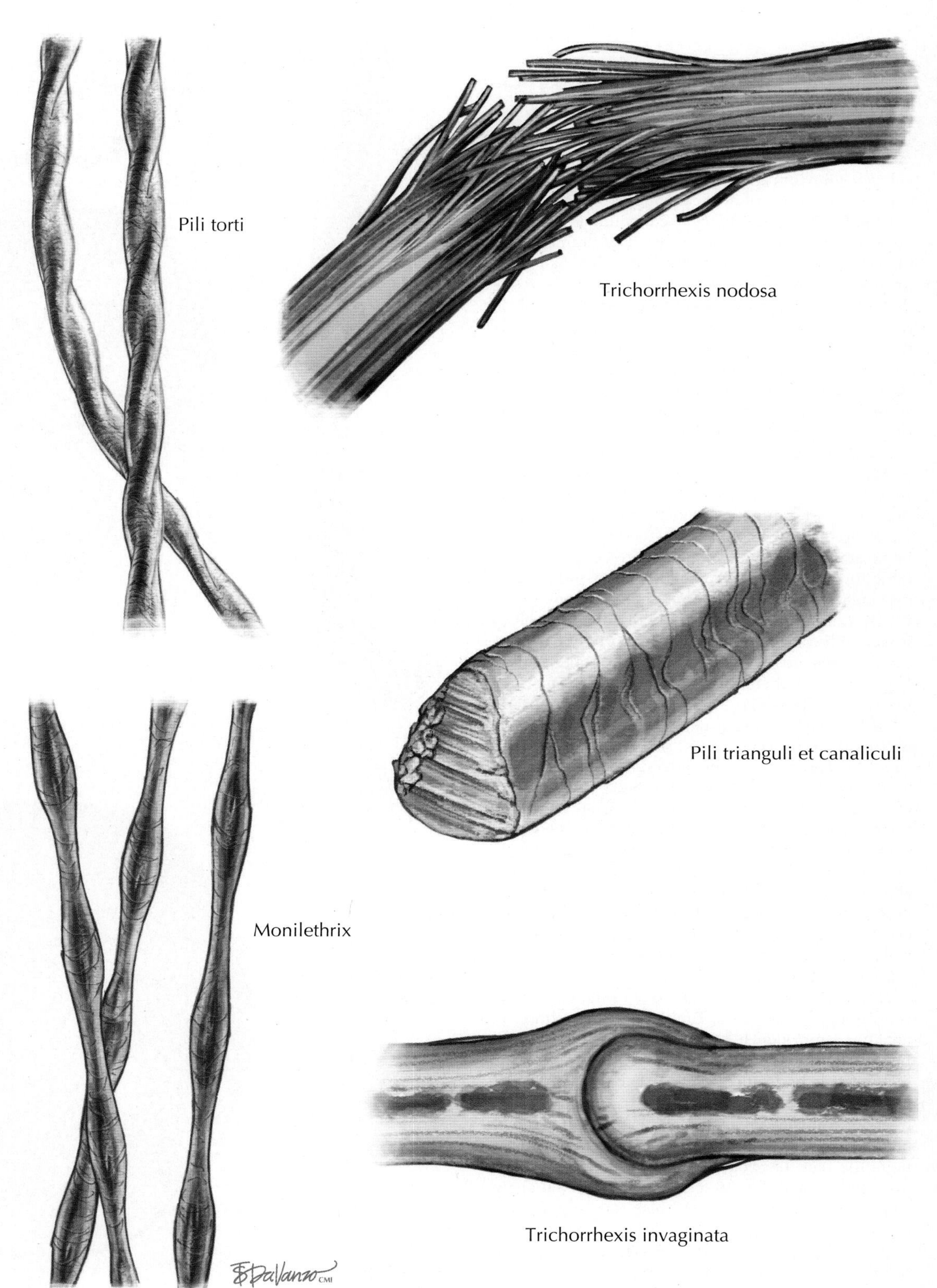

Trichorrhexis invaginata is seen only in patients with the autosomal recessive Netherton syndrome. This hair shaft abnormality has been termed "bamboo hair" because of its resemblance to the growth rings of a bamboo plant. Another descriptive term is "ball and socket hair," because it appears that the distal portion of the hair invaginates into the proximal hair cortex. The hair is brittle and breaks easily, leading to alopecia. The eyebrow hair is the best place to look for trichorrhexis invaginata. Netherton syndrome is a multisystem disease caused by a mutation in the *SPINK5* gene that is associated with erythroderma, alopecia, and elevated levels of IgE. Ichthyosis linearis circumflexa is the name for the migratory, irregular, serpiginous patches and plaques with a double-edged scale that are seen only in Netherton syndrome. *SPINK5* encodes the serine protease inhibitor, Kazal type 5 protein, which is important in epithelial desquamation.

Telogen Effluvium and Anagen Effluvium

Telogen effluvium and anagen effluvium are commonly encountered forms of nonscarring hair loss.

Clinical Findings: Telogen effluvium is a form of nonscarring alopecia that can result in dramatic thinning of the scalp hair but rarely causes total hair loss. It has been found to be induced by a number of stressors that cause the anagen hairs to abruptly turn into telogen hairs. This results in an abnormal number of hairs in the telogen phase and an increase in hair shedding. The hair loss can be profound and disconcerting to the patient. Causes include childbirth, major illness or stress, surgery, and medications. The hair loss is less rapid than in anagen effluvium.

Anagen effluvium is a specific form of alopecia that is typically induced by chemotherapeutic agents. Alkylating agents such as busulfan and cisplatin and the antitumor antibiotics (bleomycin and actinomycin D) are frequently responsible. Other agents have been implicated, including antimetabolites, topoisomerase inhibitors, and vinca alkaloids. Anagen-phase hair is particularly sensitive to these chemotherapy agents, which inhibit proliferation of rapidly dividing cells, as is seen in the anagen hair bulb. This form of hair loss is easier to diagnose because a history of taking one of the implicated chemotherapeutic agents is critical in making the diagnosis.

Pathogenesis: Telogen effluvium can almost always be traced to a recent illness, surgery, iron deficiency, childbearing, or other major stressor in the patient's life. Many medications have been reported to induce telogen effluvium, and the clinician should evaluate all medications taken. Dietary habits, especially crash dieting and anorexia nervosa, may lead to telogen effluvium. The hair follicles are not scarred and eventually grow back after the stressors have been resolved. Because the beginning of hair loss may be delayed after the stressful event, by 3 to 4 months on average, the patient may not realize the relationship. Anagen effluvium is directly caused by various chemotherapeutics.

Histology: Scalp biopsies are one of the best ways of confirming the diagnosis. The standard procedure is to obtain a 4-mm punch biopsy from the affected region. Instead of the routine vertical sectioning, horizontal sectioning is performed. The presence of scarring, the form of inflammation, and the ratio of anagen to telogen hairs are evaluated. In telogen effluvium, a normal number of hairs are present without evidence of miniaturization. The ratio of telogen to anagen hairs is increased from the normal 5 to 10 telogen hairs per 100 anagen hairs to more than 20 per 100. There is no scarring present. Biopsies of anagen effluvium show a normal ratio of anagen to telogen hairs, but the anagen hairs exhibit some evidence of abnormality, either broken shafts or apoptosis of the hair. No scarring is present in anagen effluvium.

Treatment: The treatment of telogen effluvium consists of determining the etiology and educating the patient. It is important to rule out an underlying disorder (e.g., iron deficiency, hypothyroidism) that may be triggering the hair loss. Once this has been accomplished, patients should be educated and reassured that telogen effluvium almost always resolves within 6 to 8 months, and they may expect full regrowth. Supplemental vitamins and topical minoxidil have not been vigorously tested as therapies for telogen effluvium, and their use cannot be scientifically advocated. Referral to a psychological counselor may be appropriate in situations such as eating disorders.

Anagen effluvium is related to the use of chemotherapeutic agents to treat systemic cancer. The therapy should not be stopped because of this side effect. After therapy has been completed, most patients regrow their hair. Patients have reported many changes in the color, texture, and curling of their newly grown hair. These changes have not been fully explained. Topical minoxidil may shorten the duration of anagen effluvium, but its prophylactic use has not been helpful in preventing it. More studies are needed to confirm these findings. At this point, education and reassurance are the most important therapeutic considerations. Most patients will regrow their hair, and for the few who do not, other options exist. The use of hair pieces has been expanded for many medically related forms of alopecia.

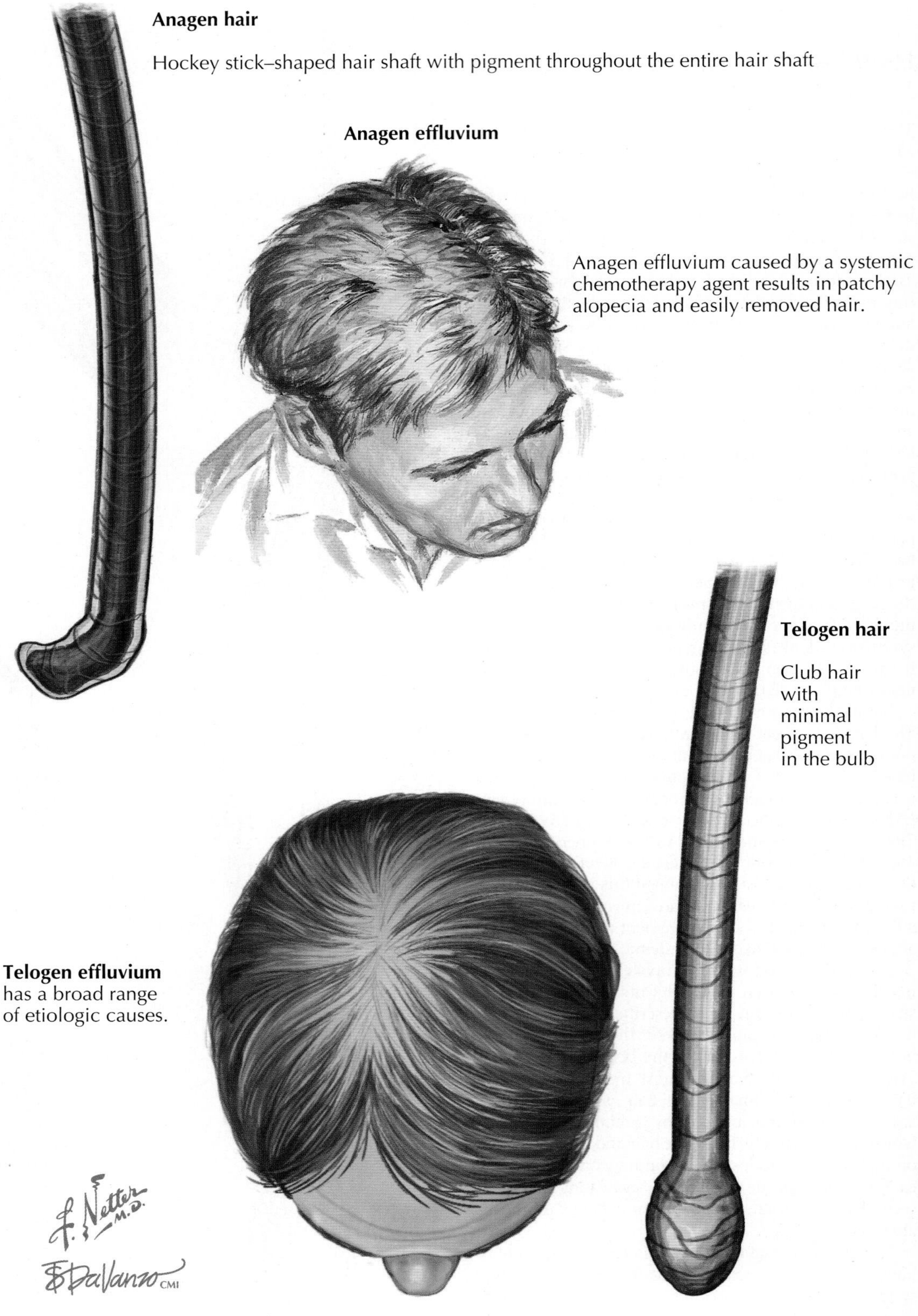

Anagen hair

Hockey stick–shaped hair shaft with pigment throughout the entire hair shaft

Anagen effluvium

Anagen effluvium caused by a systemic chemotherapy agent results in patchy alopecia and easily removed hair.

Telogen hair

Club hair with minimal pigment in the bulb

Telogen effluvium has a broad range of etiologic causes.

F. Netter M.D.

DaVanzo CMI

TRICHOTILLOMANIA

Trichotillomania is defined as the compulsive act of deliberate hair plucking, pulling, or twisting that causes hair breakage. There has been a push to rename this condition *trichotill* to remove the negative connotation of "mania" from the diagnosis. Two subgroups of patients with trichotillomania exist. The first is a younger population of mostly elementary school–aged children, and the second is the adult population. The younger the patient is at the time of diagnosis, the better the overall prognosis for a cure.

Clinical Findings: Patients present with bizarre configurations of hair loss. This is often the first clue to the diagnosis. On close inspection, the hairs are often broken off close to the surface of the skin. The broken hairs are of different lengths, which can be best appreciated when positioned against a white background, such as a white index card placed under the hairs. Hair shafts may show a twisting morphology. If the patient is evaluated soon after the hair pulling has been performed, pinpoint amounts of hemorrhage may be appreciated at the follicular openings. Microscopic examination of the ends of the hairs may show fracturing of the hair shaft and trichorrhexis nodosa. Most patients are not aware of the actions that are causing their hair loss. It is imperative to not be judgmental during patient visits, and the importance of developing a good rapport cannot be overestimated. One useful request that can be asked of patients is, "Show me how you manipulate your hair." Often patients unconsciously start to twist or tug at their hair during the examination. It is important to educate the parents to observe their child for any evidence of hair manipulation. After this form of education, the parents often become aware of the manipulation. It is important for them not to scold the child when this is taking place but rather to try to distract the child with positive reinforcement. Almost all children eventually outgrow the condition, and their hair then returns to normal.

Adults with trichotillomania have a much more chronic course. They typically have no insight into their condition. They commonly go from one doctor to another seeking therapy. In adults, biopsies are critically important to obtain objective diagnostic information. Referral to a psychologist or psychiatrist should be strongly considered for adult patients with trichotillomania.

Pathogenesis: Trichotillomania is a self-induced form of hair loss that is caused by intentional twisting, plucking, pulling, or other forms of direct damage to the hair shaft. This can be a conscious or an unconscious behavior. Most cases involve some form of emotional disturbance, and one must be cognizant of this when addressing the patient and family.

Histology: Histopathologic evaluation shows a noninflammatory, nonscarring alopecia. Characteristic to this diagnosis is the presence of trichomalacia, which is seen as follicular damage within the hair follicle. Varying degrees of follicular red blood cell extravasation are appreciated. Melanin pigment casts within the hair follicle are commonly seen. Overall, the number of hair shafts is normal. The performance of a scalp biopsy is advocated by many to give the patient or family objective information about the diagnosis.

Treatment: Trichotillomania may be considered in the spectrum of obsessive-compulsive disorders. Most children eventually abandon the actions that have caused their hair loss. Most cases in children are precipitated by emotional stress, and they tend to improve as that stress resolves. Positive reinforcement can help the child become aware of the hair manipulation. Punishment tends to be ineffective. In some cases, a child psychologist or psychiatrist can be extraordinarily helpful in treating these patients.

Adults with trichotillomania have an entirely different clinical course. Most cases are chronic, and most patients never develop insight into their disease. Underlying psychological conditions may be at the root of the issue, and cognitive therapy in the care of a psychiatrist or psychologist may be instrumental in helping these patients. The use of medications traditionally prescribed for obsessive-compulsive disorders may be warranted in the adult patient.

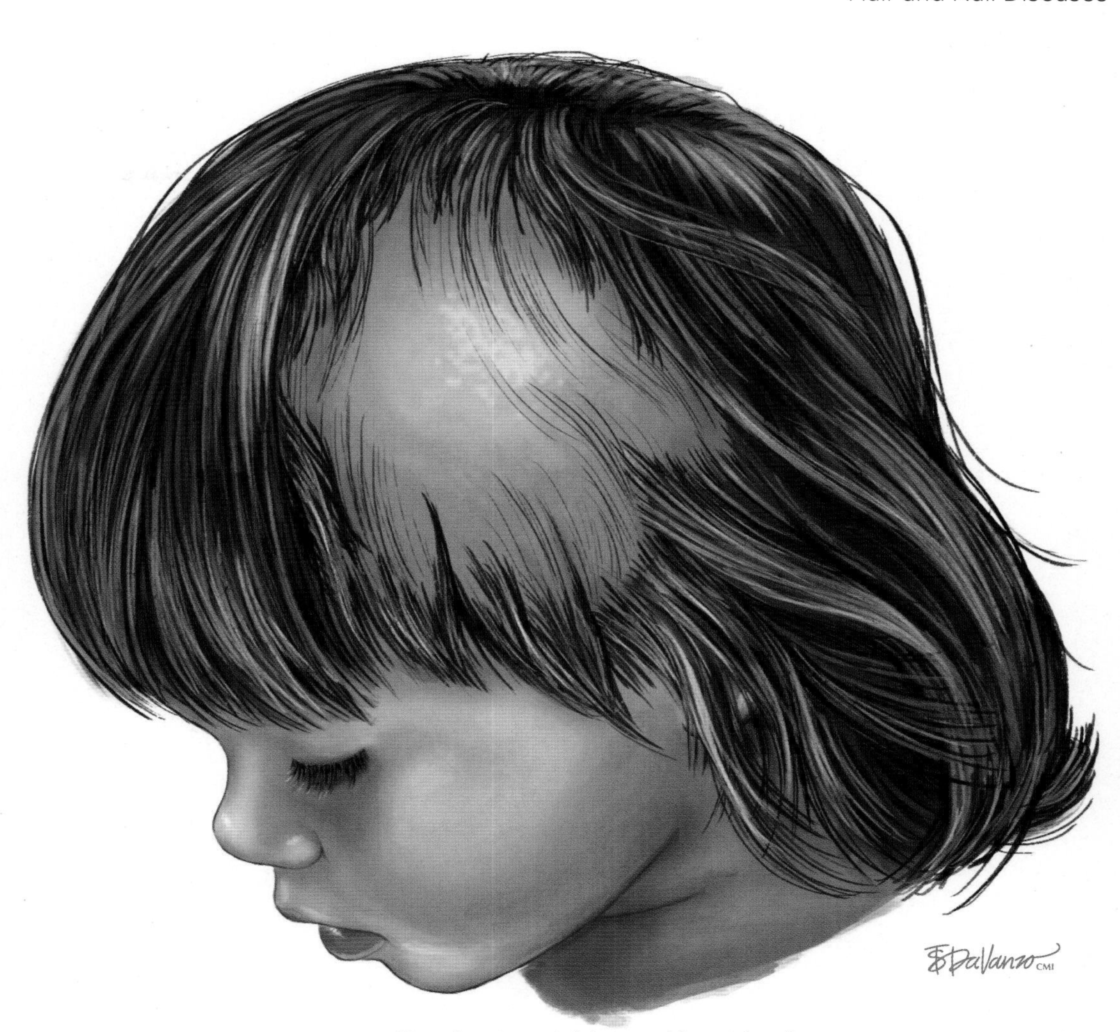

Bizarre area of hair loss in a child caused by trichotillomania

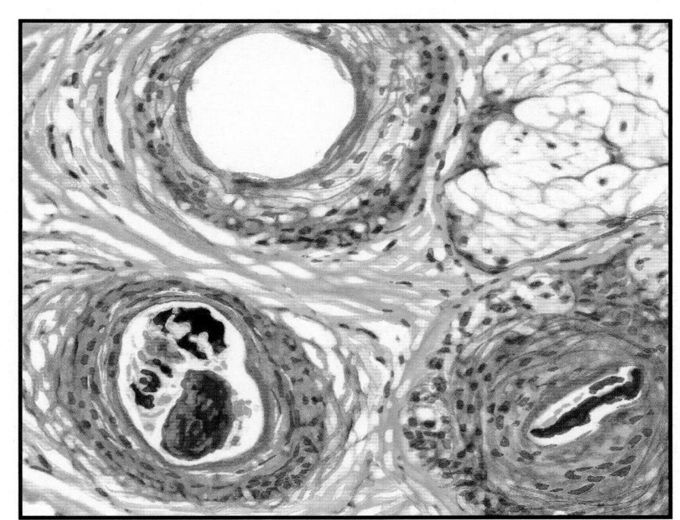

Trichomalacia is one of the histologic hallmarks of trichotillomania.

NUTRITIONAL AND METABOLIC DISEASES

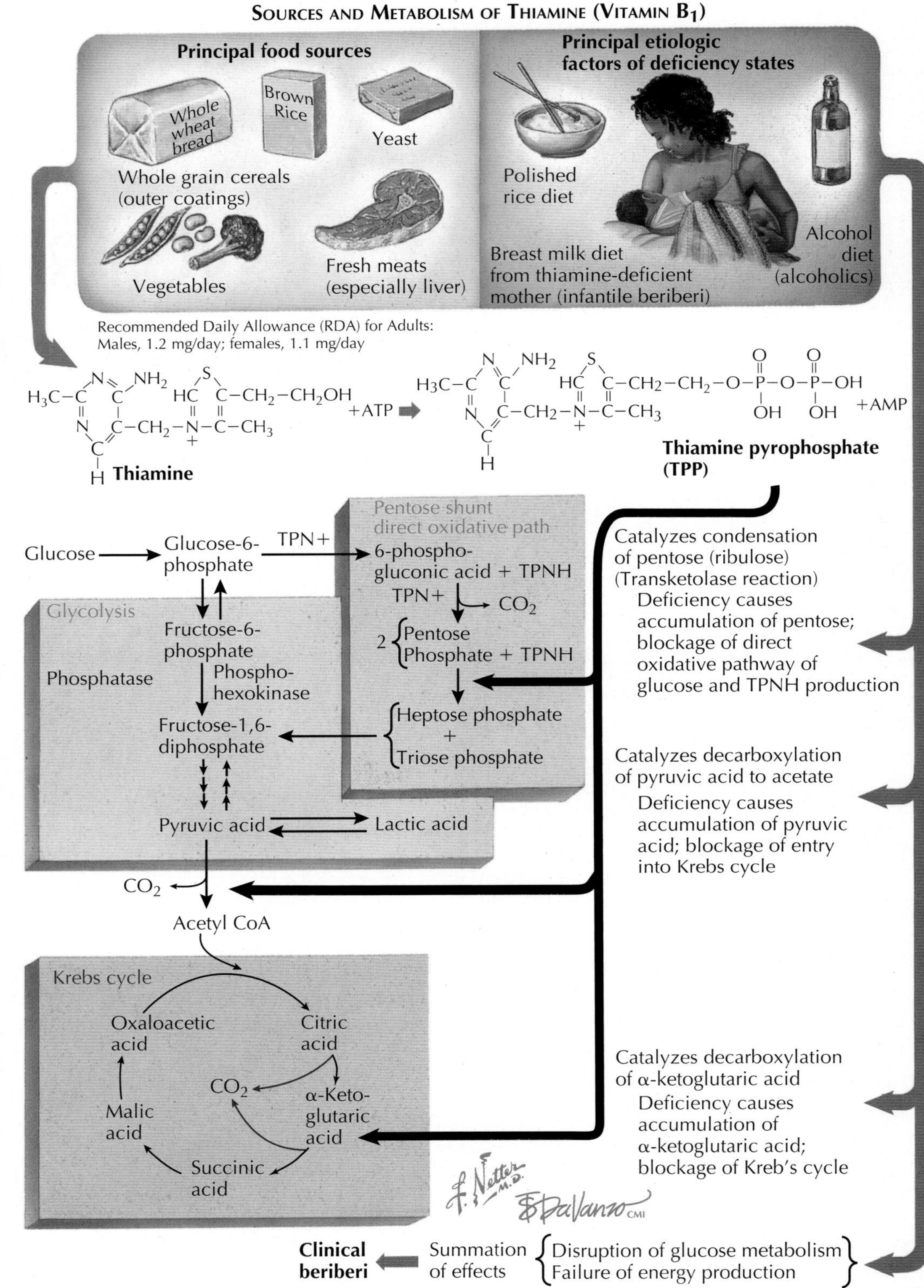

BERIBERI

Beriberi is a nutritional deficiency state caused directly by a lack of thiamine (vitamin B_1) in the diet or a lack of proper absorption of the vitamin. A rare form of acquired thiamine deficiency occurs after the ingestion of thiaminase, an enzyme that cleaves thiamine into a nonfunctional state. These cases are exceedingly rare and are considered to occur after an accidental poisonous ingestion of a source high in thiaminase. Thiamine deficiency is a rare occurrence in most of the world but is still seen in people whose food supply is based primarily on polished rice. The other major cause of the disease is alcoholism. Persons with alcoholism who obtain most of their caloric intake from alcohol may be deficient in a multitude of B vitamins, including thiamine. Thiamine deficiency may be seen in neonates and infants who are breastfeeding from mothers with borderline thiamine deficiency. The principal food sources of thiamine are fresh meats, liver, whole wheat bread, and vegetables. Nonpolished brown rice is also a good source of thiamine. Thiamine is absorbed in the gastrointestinal tract in the proximal jejunum.

Thiamine deficiency has been reported in cases of short gut syndrome and after bariatric surgery in which large parts of the jejunum are bypassed and absorption of thiamine is dramatically decreased. Most of these cases were complicated by the fact that patients were not following their prescribed diets. Beriberi has also been reported in patients with human immunodeficiency virus (HIV) infection and in some people taking long-term furosemide therapy without adequate thiamine intake. Furosemide has been shown to increase the rate of excretion of thiamine from the kidneys.

Thiamine is a water-soluble vitamin that is critical in the formation of the energy storage molecule adenosine triphosphate (ATP). Thiamine is crucial for the proper functioning of both glycolysis and the Krebs cycle. The US Nutrition Board of the Institute of Medicine, National Academy of Sciences, has designated 1.2 mg/day of thiamine as the normal recommended daily intake for men and 1.1 mg/day for women. This recommendation increases to 1.4 mg/day during pregnancy or lactation.

Clinical Findings: The disease is most frequently seen in areas of the world where polished rice is one of the main food sources. Persons with alcoholism are a unique population at very high risk for development of this vitamin deficiency. There is no race or gender predilection, and it can occur in all people. The clinical findings in beriberi are highly variable and depend on the level of deficiency and the patient's underlying comorbidities. The organ systems most commonly involved are the central nervous system (CNS) and the muscular system. Two major forms of beriberi occur, although there is much overlap. Dry beriberi is a form of the disease in which the CNS symptoms are most prevalent. Wet beriberi is the form in which the predominant symptoms are salt retention and congestive heart failure. Infantile beriberi is rare but is manifested by a combination of dry and wet beriberi with severe CNS depression and heart failure and can result in sudden death.

The first signs and symptoms of dry beriberi are typically those of a peripheral neuropathy and of muscle disease involving both skeletal and smooth muscle. Dry beriberi typically manifests with increasing fatigability, muscle weakness, paresthesias, a decrease in deep tendon reflexes, and loss of sensation. As the disease progresses, patients may develop a foot or wrist drop (flaccid paralysis). The lower extremity is typically affected before the upper. Loss of muscle mass may be prominent. Elevated levels of creatinine phosphokinase are seen, as well as creatinuria. Once loss of muscle mass has occurred weakness becomes profound.

Wet beriberi predominantly affects the muscle tissue and in particular the cardiac system. The end stage of beriberi results in high-output cardiac failure; without treatment, death follows. Beriberi rarely causes death if diagnosis is made and proper treatment is instituted before end-stage heart failure sets in. Patients with

BERIBERI (Continued)

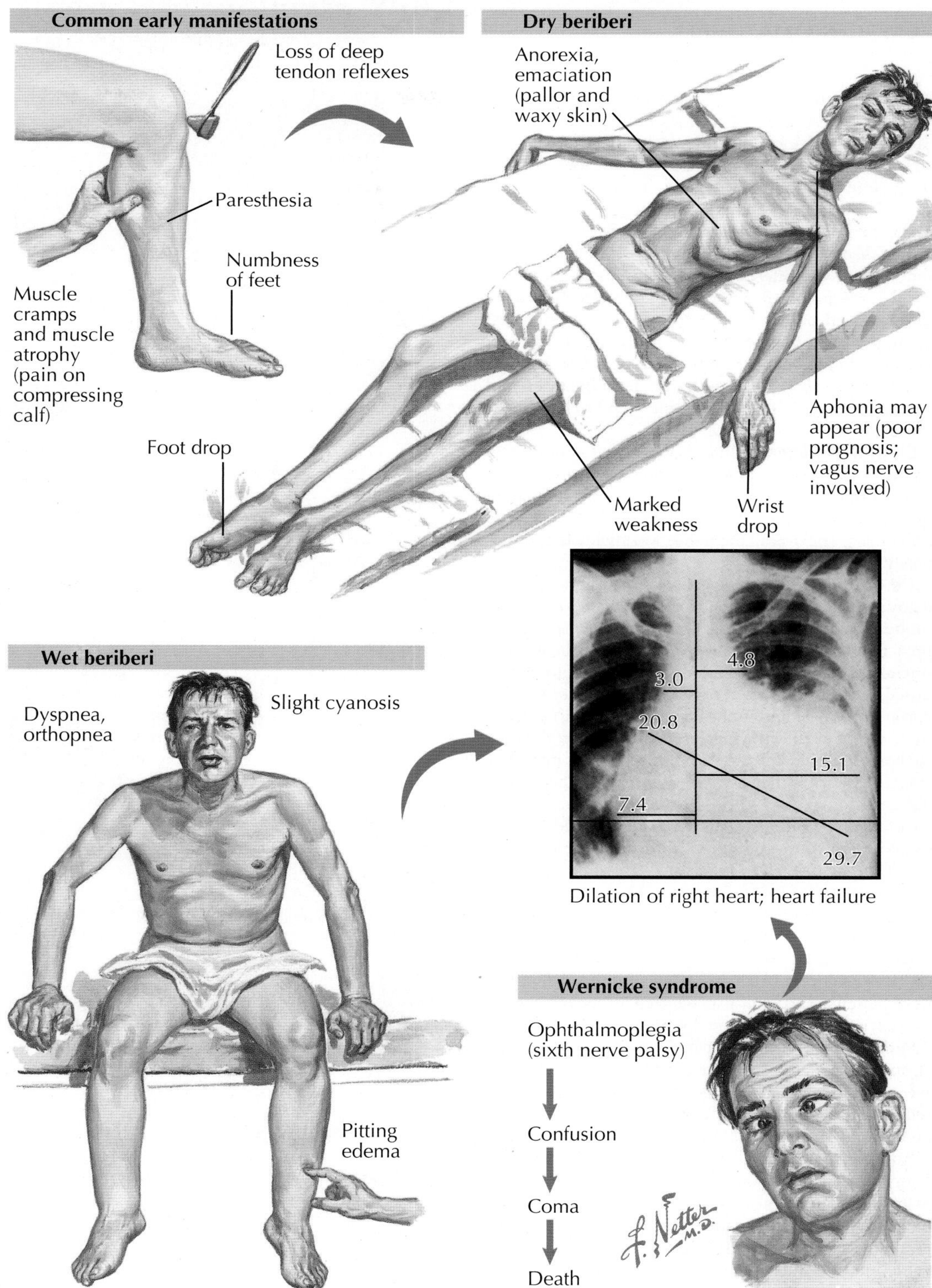

wet beriberi experience a decrease in diastolic blood pressure with a minimal change in systolic pressure, resulting in an overall increase in the pulse pressure. Tachycardia is prominent. As heart failure develops, pulmonary edema and fluid retention occur, causing dependent edema and difficulty breathing. Cyanosis may occur from poor oxygenation. Laboratory testing shows an increased QT interval on electrocardiography and increased serum levels of lactic acid, pyruvate, and α-ketoglutarate. Chest radiography shows an enlarged heart with dilation of the right side and pulmonary congestion, edema, or both.

The skin findings of beriberi are not specific, but when seen in conjunction with the rest of the clinical picture, they can definitely help make the diagnosis. The cutaneous findings of wet beriberi consist of cyanosis of the skin with variable amounts of peripheral edema. The skin has a waxy appearance and feel. Cutaneous pallor is prominent and, along with the cyanosis, gives the patient an overall ill appearance. Pallor is a common skin finding in dry beriberi as well. Patients may also present with accidental traumatic injuries to their extremities related to lack of sensation from the peripheral neuropathy. Hair loss has been reported, but most believe that this is secondary to a combination of niacin and thiamine deficiency.

The excretion of thiamine via the kidneys is markedly decreased in beriberi. Normally, 70 to 150 μg of thiamine is excreted per gram of creatinine. In beriberi, that level can drop to zero.

Pathogenesis: All forms of beriberi are caused by a nutritional deficiency of thiamine. Thiamine is a critical vitamin that is needed for carbohydrate metabolism. Thiamine is the precursor for thiamine pyrophosphate (TPP). It is converted to TPP by the addition of one ATP molecule. TPP is needed as a cofactor for the proper function of numerous metabolic pathways. TPP helps transfer an aldehyde group from a donor to a beneficiary chemical structure. Three major energy-producing pathways are modulated by TPP: glycolysis, the Krebs cycle, and the pentose shunt (hexose monophosphate shunt). The hexose monophosphate shunt is important in producing other cofactors that play important biochemical roles for the donation of hydrogen. The overall chemical state that occurs in patients with thiamine deficiency is a lack of ability to produce sufficient quantities of cellular ATP. This lack of the main source of energy for the cell results in the clinical findings. The nervous tissue and muscle tissue are particularly prone to damage from failure to produce sufficient ATP. It has been estimated that 3 to 6 weeks of a thiamine-free diet in an average human is sufficient to cause development of the initial signs and symptoms of beriberi.

Histology: Biopsy specimens of the skin in patients with beriberi are of no clinical usefulness. A skin biopsy from an area of cyanosis or pallor shows normal skin. A biopsy from one of the waxy areas may show variable mild degrees of acanthosis and parakeratosis. A muscle biopsy shows vacuolization and hyalinization of the muscle fibers. An inflammatory process may be present that can cause varying degrees of necrosis of the muscle. The muscle fibers may show diffuse or focal fiber necrosis. These changes are most prominent in the cardiac muscle. In patients who develop Wernicke syndrome, postmortem examinations of the brain have revealed small hemorrhages within the hypothalamus and upper brainstem. Peripheral nerve tissue shows noninflammatory degeneration of the neurons with atrophy and chromatolysis. This can occur in the neurons of the peripheral nervous system and the CNS.

Treatment: Therapy consists of supplementation of the patient's diet with 50 mg/day intramuscularly of thiamine until the symptoms resolve. Treatment should also include other B-complex vitamins because many patients who are deficient in one B vitamin also have low levels of the others. A nutritionist should be consulted to educate the patient on the need for a proper diet and how to achieve this. Persons with alcoholism are prone to recurrence of beriberi and should be encouraged to participate in alcohol abstinence programs and to take a daily multivitamin supplement. The symptoms rapidly reverse on replacement of thiamine.

HEMOCHROMATOSIS

Hemochromatosis is a fairly common autosomal recessive genetic disorder of iron metabolism that leads to excessive iron absorption and eventually iron overload. Iron progressively accumulates in various tissues throughout the body, with the liver most severely affected. Most cases are caused by a genetic mutation in the hemochromatosis gene, *HFE*. These cases are termed *hereditary hemochromatosis*. This gene mutation is seen in different frequencies throughout the world. For example, it is carried by approximately 7% of the European population but is very rare in the East Asian population. The disease signs and symptoms typically do not appear until after childbearing age, usually in the sixth or seventh decade of life. Men and women are equally affected, but men tend to have more serious disease.

Clinical Findings: White males are the most frequently affected, and there is variability of carrier rates among populations. For example, in Ireland the rate of homozygosity for the C282Y mutation in *HFE* is 1 in 85 individuals. The overall incidence worldwide is approximately 1 in 350.

The clinical manifestations of patients with hemochromatosis who are homozygous for the mutated *HFE* gene can be quite variable. Classic hemochromatosis includes three main components: liver cirrhosis, diabetes, and generalized skin pigmentation. These symptoms are caused, respectively, by a persistent chronic accumulation of iron in the liver and in the pancreas and by iron deposition in the skin with increased melanin production. Cirrhosis is the main cause of morbidity and mortality, and it dramatically increases a person's risk for hepatocellular carcinoma.

Cutaneous findings include a generalized bronze discoloration of the skin. This diffuse pigmentation is one of the first signs of the disease. This finding, along with diabetes, has led to the name "bronze diabetes" to describe the condition. Nails can be brittle and show varying degrees of koilonychia. There is widespread generalized hair thinning and loss, affecting all terminal hair locations. Arthritis is a common finding in these patients and can also be seen in asymptomatic heterozygous carriers of the disease.

Pathogenesis: *HFE* is located on the short arm of chromosome 6 and is mutated in this autosomal recessive genetic disorder of iron metabolism. The most frequently encountered genetic mutation is the C282Y mutation, with the H623D mutation the second most common. Normal iron regulation is dependent on absorption of iron from dietary sources and normal losses. Regulatory mechanisms allow for equalization of iron absorption to balance the iron losses in normal physiologic states. The defect in *HFE* leads to abnormal regulation of cellular uptake of iron as well as a loss of regulation of ferritin levels. The result of the excessive iron deposition is an increase in free radical oxygen species and their destructive interactions with various tissues. In the liver, this leads to fibrosis and eventually cirrhosis.

Histology: Histology of the skin is not useful for diagnosis. Liver biopsies show varying degrees of damage on a spectrum from fibrosis to cirrhosis. The Prussian blue stain is used to accentuate the iron within the hepatocytes and the cells of the biliary tract. There is less iron accumulation in the Kupffer cells, which is the direct opposite of the findings in states of iron overload.

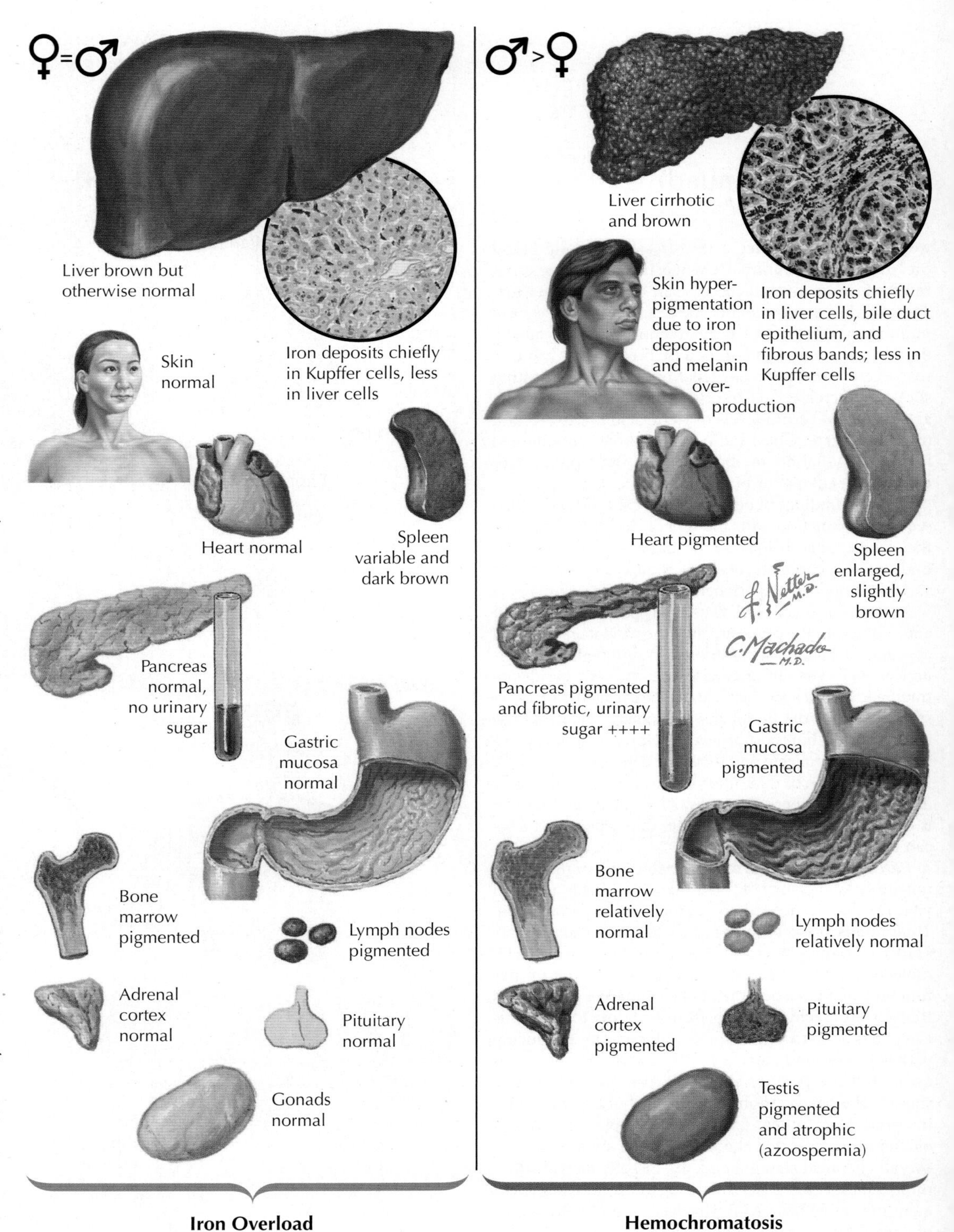

Treatment: Therapy requires removal of the excessive iron. This is best accomplished by routine scheduled phlebotomy. Phlebotomy decreases the concentration of iron stores and is used to attempt to prevent the progression to cirrhosis. Prevention of cirrhosis is the single best predictor of morbidity and mortality in these patients. The goal in most patients is to keep the hemoglobin in the range of 12 g/dL. Ferritin is another marker that is linked to morbidity and mortality and is routinely followed. Other methods to remove excessive iron include erythrocytapheresis and iron chelation therapy. Erythrocytapheresis is a method by which predominantly red blood cells are removed from the blood while the serum, white blood cells, and platelets are returned to the patient's bloodstream. Iron chelation therapy with intravenous deferoxamine has been helpful for patients who cannot tolerate blood removal procedures. Methods to try to decrease the absorption of iron from the gastrointestinal tract can also be attempted. In cases of end-stage liver disease, liver transplantation has been undertaken. These treatments have shown the best results if implemented before evidence of cirrhosis is present. The importance of genetic counseling cannot be overemphasized.

Metabolic Diseases: Niemann-Pick Disease, von Gierke Disease, and Galactosemia

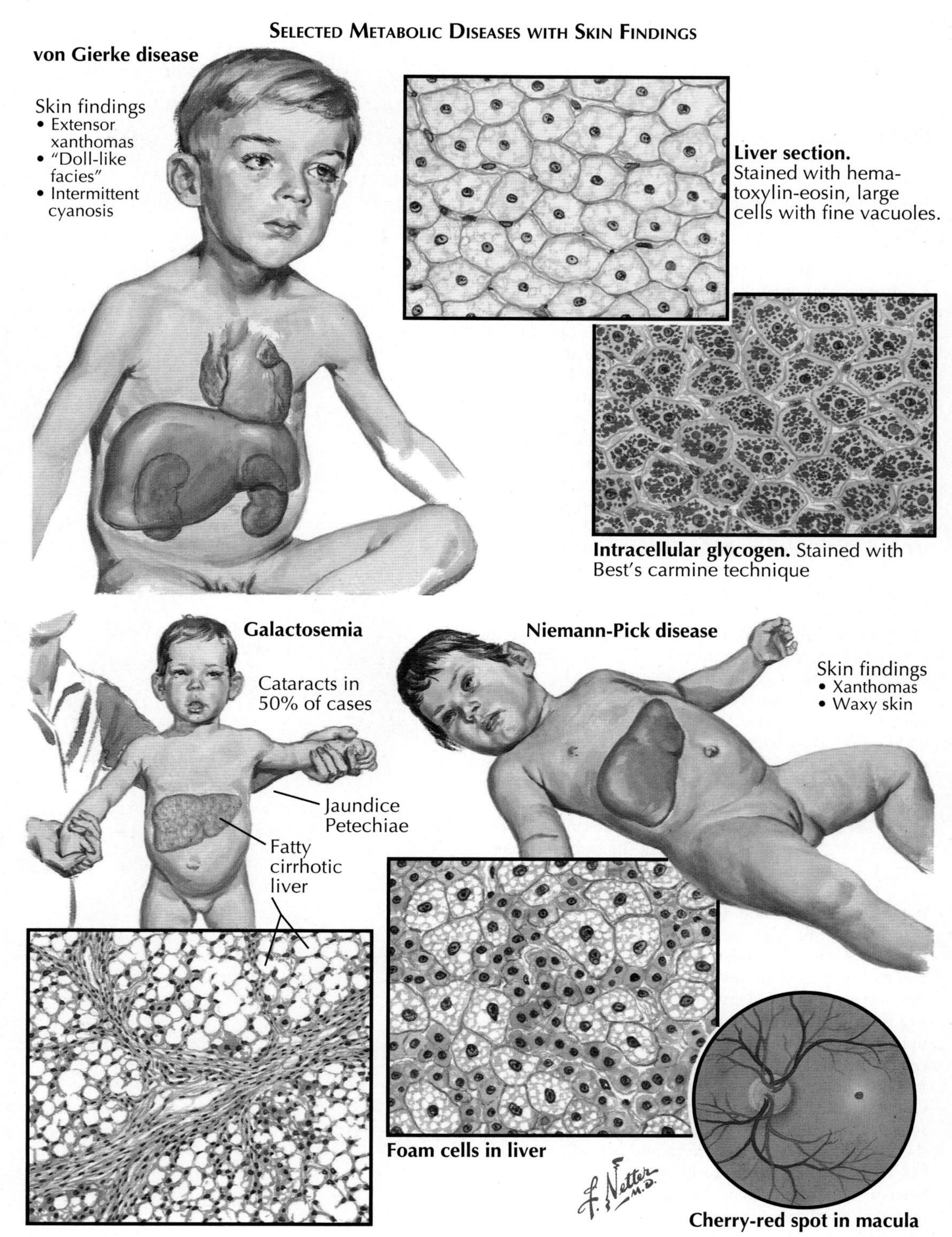

A plethora of metabolic diseases can have various cutaneous skin findings. These conditions, on the whole, are uncommon and are rarely encountered by the practitioner except in a tertiary referral center. However, knowledge of these uncommon diseases is important because prompt recognition and diagnosis can lead to proper referrals and a better outcome for all involved. Three such metabolic disorders are Niemann-Pick disease, von Gierke disease, and galactosemia.

Niemann-Pick disease is a heterogenous group of conditions resulting from the inability to properly metabolize sphingomyelin. There are three clinical variants designated types A, B, and C. They are all inherited in an autosomal recessive pattern, with the highest prevalence in people of Ashkenazi Jewish descent. Most cases are fatal in early childhood. Mental delay is profound. The disease results in massive hepatosplenomegaly caused by the excessive accumulation of sphingomyelin in various tissues. Niemann-Pick disease is caused by an abnormal lysosomal lipid enzyme degradation system and is therefore considered a lysosomal storage disease. Sphingomyelin is degraded into ceramide by the action of the enzyme sphingomyelinase. Type A and type B disease are similar in that the *ASM* gene, which encodes the acid sphingomyelinase enzyme, is mutated. This mutation leads to an inability of the lysosomes to metabolize sphingomyelin. Sphingomyelin accumulates in the liver and spleen. Severe neurologic disorders occur in type A disease but not in type B; this is the only factor differentiating the two. Patients present in infancy or early childhood. Skin findings include xanthomas and a waxy skin surface. Retinal examination reveals a cherry-red spot on the fovea. Niemann-Pick type C disease, which is caused by a mutation in the *NPC1* or the *NPC2* gene, does not involve any cutaneous findings. The cells are unable to normally process endocytosed cholesterol. Treatments are limited, with stem cell transplantation having been used with some efficacy. Miglustat is a drug that inhibits glucosylceramide synthase and has shown some help in delaying neurologic disease in type C disease.

von Gierke disease, also known as glycogen storage disease type I, can be subdivided into types Ia and Ib. These autosomal recessive diseases are caused, respectively, by defects in the enzymes glucose-6-phosphatase and glucose-6-phosphatase translocase. These defects prevent normal gluconeogenesis from glycogen stores. Patients develop profound hypoglycemia during periods of fasting because they are unable to break down glucose-6-phosphate into glucose within the liver. This leads to a fatty liver and increased glycogen storage. Glucose-6-phosphate is shunted into glycolysis, which results in increased lactate production.

Cutaneous findings in von Gierke disease include extensor xanthomas on the knees and elbows. Patients have a peculiar facies that has been described as a "doll-like face." This has been shown to be caused by an increased amount of fatty tissue deposited in the cheeks. Patients have frequent nosebleeds and severe gingivitis along with oral ulcerations. During periods of hypoglycemia, cyanosis may be very noticeable, and it may lead eventually to hypoxic brain injury. These patients are also at higher risk for skin infections because of an abnormal neutrophilic response to gram-positive bacteria. Treatment is based on a regular frequent diet of 60% to 70% carbohydrates to avoid episodes of hypoglycemia. Experimental gene therapy trials are underway.

Galactosemia is a rare autosomal recessive disorder that results from a defect in one of three enzymes: galactose-1-phosphate uridyltransferase, galactokinase, or uridine diphosphate galactose 4-epimerase. It most frequently caused by a mutation of the *GALT* gene on the short arm of chromosome 9. This mutation results in an increase of galactose-1-phosphate in various tissues. Nervous tissue, the lens, and the liver are areas of massive accumulation. This leads to the sequelae of the disease, predominantly mental delay, cataracts, and liver disease. The main cutaneous findings are jaundice secondary to liver disease and cutaneous signs of coagulopathy such as petechiae and hemorrhage. Cataracts are a well-known sign of galactosemia and are directly caused by the accumulation of galactitol in the lens, which results in edema and eventual cataract formation. Therapy requires the strict avoidance of galactose and lactose in the diet.

PELLAGRA

Pellagra is caused by inadequate dietary intake of niacin (nicotinic acid, vitamin B_3) or its precursor amino acid, tryptophan. It has also been discovered to occur on occasion in patients with carcinoid syndrome. In this syndrome, tryptophan is used entirely to produce serotonin, thus decreasing the ability to produce niacin. Pellagra was first identified as a unique disease in the early 1700s by a Spanish physician, Gaspar Casal, who observed it in Spanish peasants who ate diets almost entirely made of corn and corn-based foodstuffs. He named the disease "Asturian leprosy" after the region of Spain he was studying. An Italian physician, Francesco Frapolli, who studied the disease in endemic regions of northern Italy, later named it pellagra.

Pellagra has been dominant in regions of the world that rely heavily on corn as the main dietary staple. In the early 20th century, the Southern United States was inundated with cases of pellagra. Joseph Goldberger, a physician and epidemiologist studying the disease, discovered that pellagra was caused directly by a deficiency of vitamin B. He was unable at that time to isolate the specific B vitamin, but he has been given credit for discovering the cause of pellagra.

Clinical Findings: Pellagra can affect any individual regardless of race or sex. The incidence in North America and Europe is low, and cases are mainly caused by abnormal diets and alcoholism. The disease can still be seen in endemic regions of the world where corn is the main food source. The clinical cutaneous hallmark of pellagra is a severe dermatitis. The dermatitis is photosensitive, and exposure to the sun often brings out the rash or exacerbates it. Patients often present initially after having spent many hours outdoors on an early spring day. The dermatitis is symmetric and is manifested by eczematous patches and thin plaques that tend to be tender to the touch. There is a fine line of demarcation between abnormal and normal skin. The head, neck, and arms are the most involved regions because of their higher level of sun exposure. The dermatitis along the anterior neck and upper thorax has been termed *Casal's necklace*. This is represented by weeping pink and red patches and plaques in a distribution like that of a necklace touching the skin circumferentially around the neck. Because of its photosensitive nature, the dermatitis of pellagra often spares the skin directly behind the ears and beneath the chin. The nose, forehead, and cheeks are prime regions of involvement. Non–sun-exposed areas can also be involved, and the intertriginous regions are almost universally affected, including the perineum, axillae, and inframammary skin folds. The reason for the propensity to affect these non–sun-exposed regions is poorly understood but may be related to chronic friction that induces the dermatitis. In the areas of involvement, small vesiculations may occur because of separation of the epidermis from the dermis.

As time progresses, the dermatitis begins to desquamate. This process begins in the central portions of the dermatitis and spreads outward in a centrifugal manner. As the skin desquamates, it leaves behind red, eroded patches and plaques. Chronic involvement leaves permanent scarring and abnormal hyperpigmentation or hypopigmentation of the area. The epidermis over bony prominences (e.g., ulnar head) shows marked hyperkeratosis.

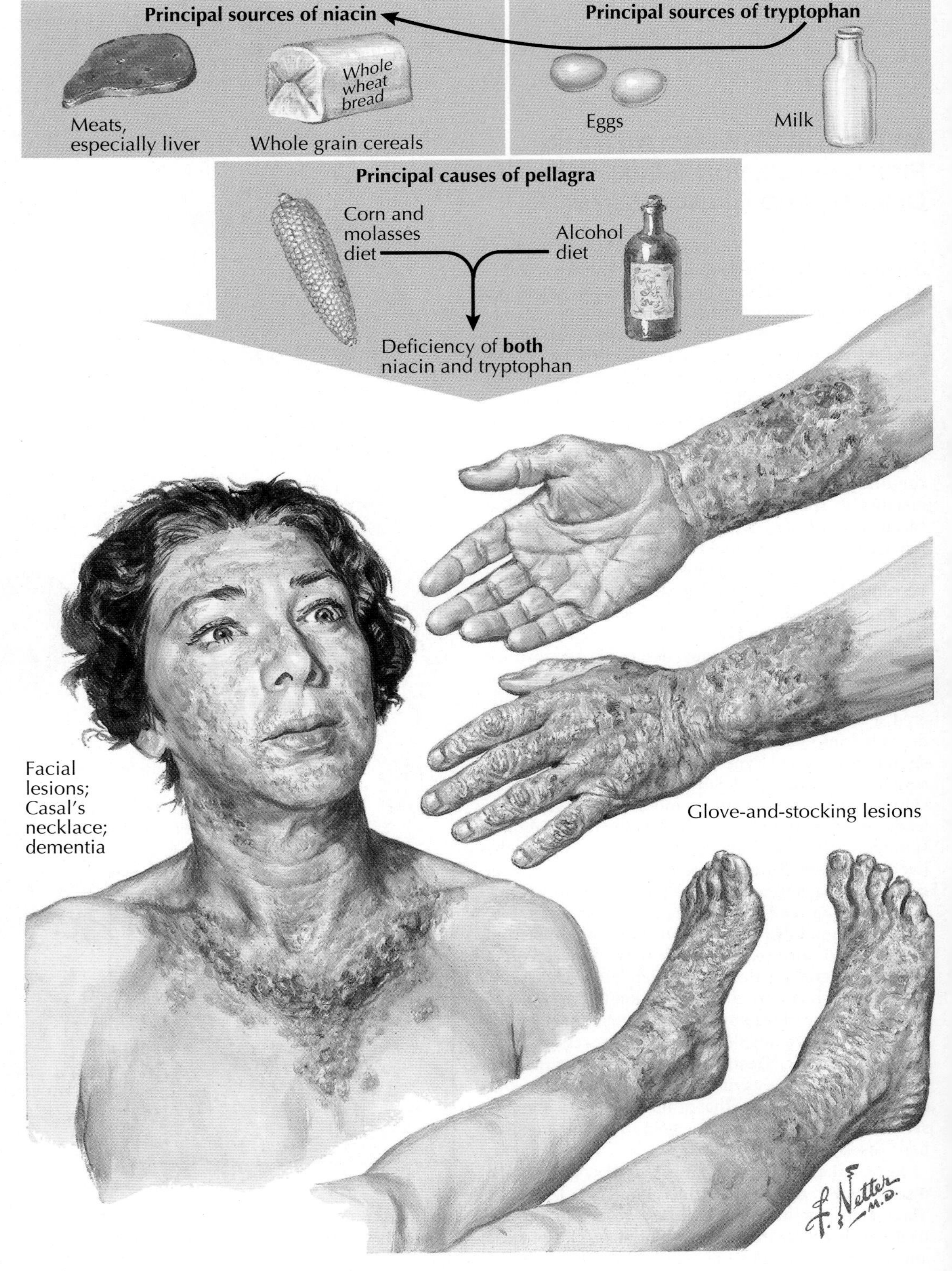

Mucous membrane involvement is common in all vitamin deficiency states, and pellagra is no exception. Angular cheilitis and a red, shiny, edematous tongue with atrophied papillae are seen routinely in patients with pellagra. The oral and gastrointestinal mucous membranes may be involved. Oral ulcerations are frequently seen. Patients routinely complain of a sore mouth and difficulty swallowing; these symptoms can lead to further lack of proper nutrition, exacerbating and compounding the disease.

Diarrhea is commonplace and is caused by the effect of niacin deficiency on the gastrointestinal tract. The diarrhea is watery and further complicates the patient's nutritional status and electrolyte and fluid balances. Blood and purulence may be present in the watery diarrhea as a result of ulceration and abscess formation. Ulcerations can be seen throughout the gastrointestinal tract, as can cystic dilation of the mucous glands. The colon may show small submucosal abscesses.

Mucosal and Central Nervous System Manifestations of Pellagra

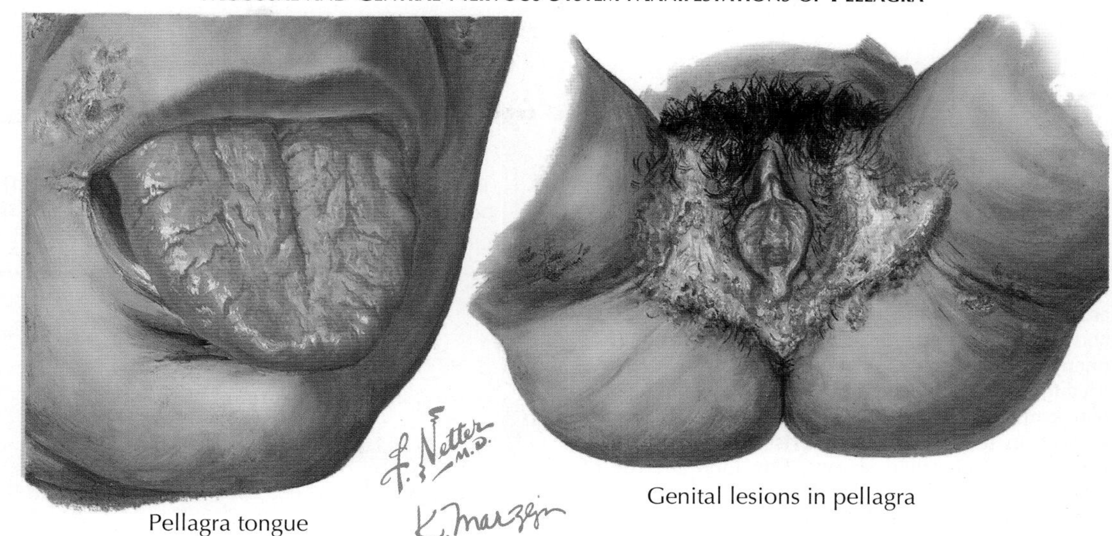

Pellagra tongue

Genital lesions in pellagra

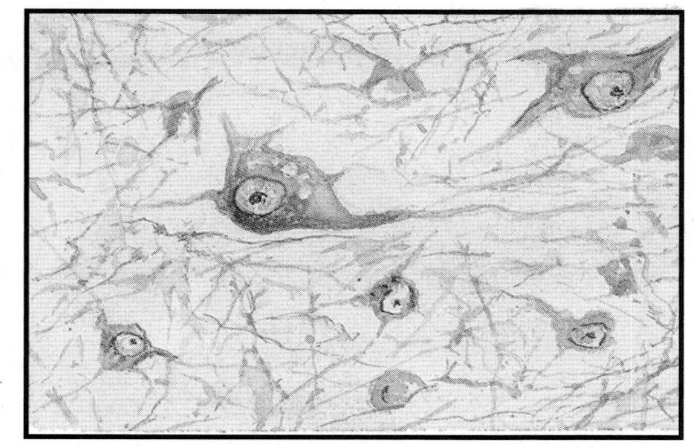

Degeneration of cells of cerebral cortex

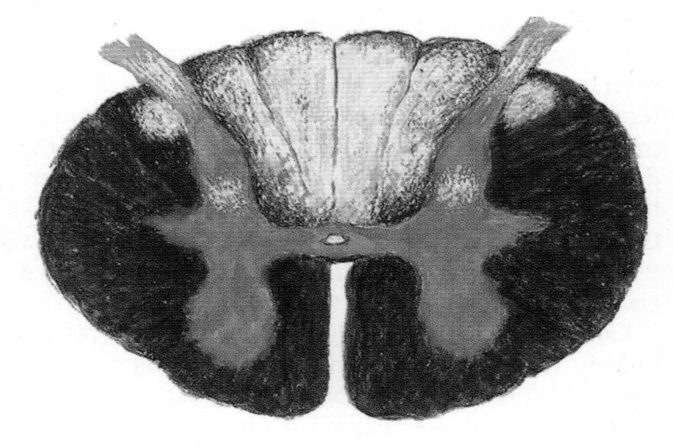

Degeneration in spinal cord

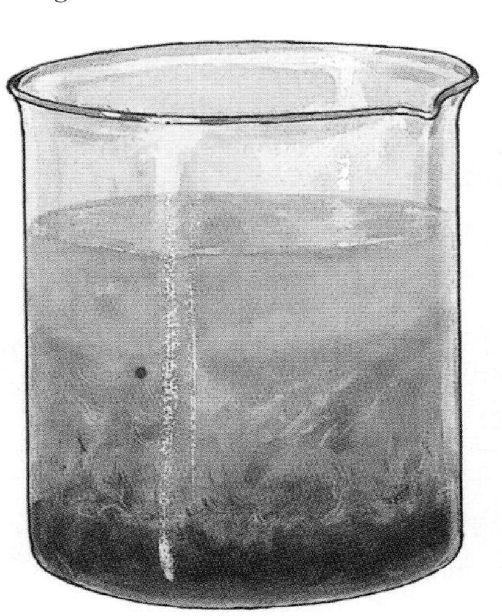

Aqueous stool in diarrhea of pellagra

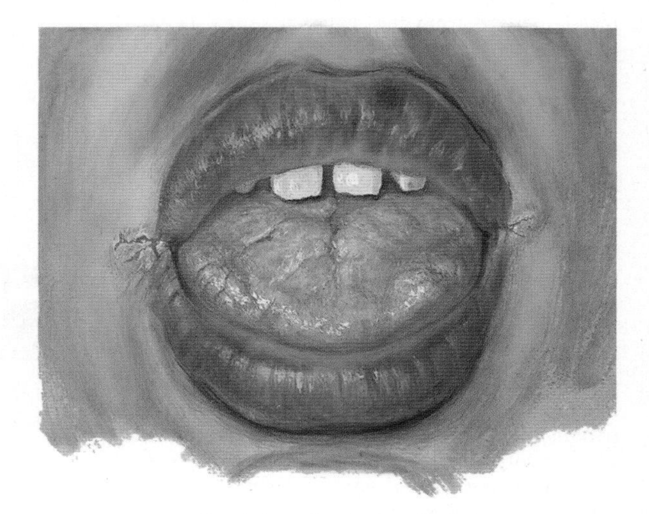

Glossitis and angular cheilitis are commonly seen in pellagra.

Pellagra (Continued)

Subtle neurologic findings precede full-blown encephalopathy in pellagra. These clinical findings include poor concentration, headaches, and apathy. Dementia eventually sets in as the disease causes a diffuse encephalopathy. The encephalopathy may mimic psychiatric disease, especially depression with suicidal tendency. Other well-defined symptoms include confusion, hallucination, delirium, insomnia, tremor, seizures, and extrapyramidal rigidity. The entire CNS is involved in severe pellagra. Cortical nerve cells show degeneration. The Betz cells show chromatolytic changes with displacement of the nucleus toward the cell wall. There is an increased amount of adipose in the nerve cells as well as an increase in the lipofuscin pigment within the cytoplasm of these cortical cells. The posterior columns may undergo demyelination, leading to tremor, gait disturbance, and movement difficulties. Chromatolysis has been shown to occur in the pontine nuclei, spinal cord nuclei, and multiple cranial nerve nuclei. As the encephalopathy progresses, disorientation and delirium take over, and the patient eventually slips into a coma. Death may shortly ensue unless the disease is diagnosed and treated appropriately. These unique clinical findings seen in pellagra can be simplified in the oft-quoted mnemonic, "4 D's": **d**ermatitis, **d**iarrhea, **d**ementia, and **d**eath.

The diagnosis is typically made on clinical grounds, and laboratory analysis is used for confirmation. Other vitamin deficiencies should also be considered when evaluating a patient with pellagra. The 24-hour urine secretion of *N*-methyl nicotinamide is normally in the range of 5 to 15 mg/day; in patients with pellagra, it is less than 1.5 mg/day. Measurement of this metabolite serves as an easy, noninvasive test to confirm the deficiency of niacin. Serum niacin levels can be measured directly, although they are not as accurate as the urinary excretion levels.

Pathogenesis: Niacin is an essential vitamin that is found in many food sources, including whole grain breads and meats. Patients whose diet is deficient in niacin are seen in regions of the world where corn is the main food source. Various levels of niacin deficiency occur. This disease can also be seen in persons with alcoholism who do not maintain a balanced diet and receive almost all of their caloric intake from alcoholic products. Patients who develop pellagra also have a diet deficient in tryptophan. Major sources of tryptophan include eggs and milk. Tryptophan is a precursor of niacin and can be converted to niacin. Niacin is required for the proper production of nicotinamide adenine dinucleotide and nicotinamide adenine dinucleotide phosphate, important coenzymes for many biochemical reactions. Both molecules are capable of acquiring two electrons and acting as reducing agents in various reduction-oxidation (redox) reactions. When a deficiency of niacin occurs, many biochemical reactions throughout the human body cannot be properly performed, and the clinical manifestations occur.

Carcinoid syndrome is a rare cause of pellagra. Carcinoid is a syndrome of excessive secretion of serotonin. Tryptophan is the precursor for serotonin as well as niacin, and in this syndrome all tryptophan is shunted to make serotonin at the expense of tryptophan. This results in decreased production of niacin and, potentially, the clinical symptoms of pellagra. Pellagra can also be caused by malabsorption syndromes, especially after bariatric surgery and from some medications such as isoniazid, 6-mercaptopurine, and phenobarbital.

Histology: The skin biopsy findings are nonspecific and show epidermal pallor with a mixed inflammatory infiltrate predominantly composed of lymphocytes in a perivascular location. Occasional areas of inflammatory vesiculation within the epidermis may be seen.

Treatment: Pellagra rapidly responds to supplementation with niacin. Niacin is given orally every 6 hours until the patient responds. If a patient does not respond, a coexisting vitamin deficiency should be sought. If possible, a nutritionist should be consulted to advise the patient on proper dietary intake. Persons with alcoholism, who can be deficient in many B vitamins, are often treated with multiple B vitamins. Patients with carcinoid syndrome need to take supplemental niacin to avoid pellagra symptoms, but the goal of therapy is to treat the underlying tumor.

PHENYLKETONURIA

Phenylalanine is an essential amino acid that serves as a substrate for many different biochemical pathways. Two end products that use phenylalanine as their precursors are melanin and epinephrine. Under normal physiologic and biochemical environments, any excess amount of phenylalanine is converted into tyrosine by the liver and used for a host of biochemical processes, including protein synthesis. In patients with phenylketonuria, the enzyme in the liver that converts phenylalanine into tyrosine is completely absent. This inborn error of metabolism is one of the most thoroughly researched disease states. With early detection and therapy, the severe sequelae of phenylketonuria can be avoided. Screening is performed soon after birth for all children in the United States and in most of the world. Children born in regions with poor medical infrastructure and no testing are at risk for the disease. Once the disease symptoms have appeared, therapy usually cannot reverse the damage that has been done. Phenylketonuria is inherited in an autosomal recessive manner and many genotypes have been described. The defect is located on the long arm of chromosome 12, where the *PAH* gene encodes the protein phenylalanine hydroxylase.

Clinical Findings: Phenylketonuria occurs in approximately 1 of every 10,000 births in the United States, with the White population being at highest risk. Worldwide, the Turkish population has the highest rate, 1 per 2500 newborns. Both sexes are affected equally. Infants appear normal at birth. The small load of phenylalanine that is derived from the maternal source in utero is typically not high enough to cause any symptoms or signs of phenylketonuria. Soon after birth, the first symptoms appear as the neonate, lacking the PAH enzyme, rapidly begins to accumulate phenylalanine in serum and tissues. Other biochemical pathways are enacted to try to rid the body of the excess phenylalanine, but these make matters worse. The degradation metabolites produced from various deamination and oxidation metabolic modification reactions can cause end-organ damage. Phenyl-lactic acid, phenylpyruvic acid, and phenylacetic acid are the main byproducts. Because of these byproducts, the urine takes on a characteristic "mousy" odor.

Affected neonates have blond hair and a generalized hypopigmentation. Children with darker-skinned parents often have a lighter skin tone and lighter hair and eye coloration than either parent. Most have blue eyes. Evidence of early-onset dermatitis that may appear as atopic dermatitis is often present. Other skin changes that have been described include sclerodermoid changes of the trunk and upper thighs.

The most dreaded sequela of phenylketonuria is the profound brain damage that can occur secondary to the elevated levels of phenylalanine. The neonatal brain is easily damaged by excessive levels of this amino acid. Global brain damage is caused by phenylalanine, and the damage is typically irreversible. This is the reason screening tests are performed on neonates. Mental delay, seizures, and tremors are common effects of phenylketonuria. Seizures can be of the grand mal or petit mal type and occur in infancy or childhood. The seizures are reversible once a low-phenylalanine diet is undertaken.

NORMAL AND ABNORMAL METABOLISM OF PHENYLALANINE

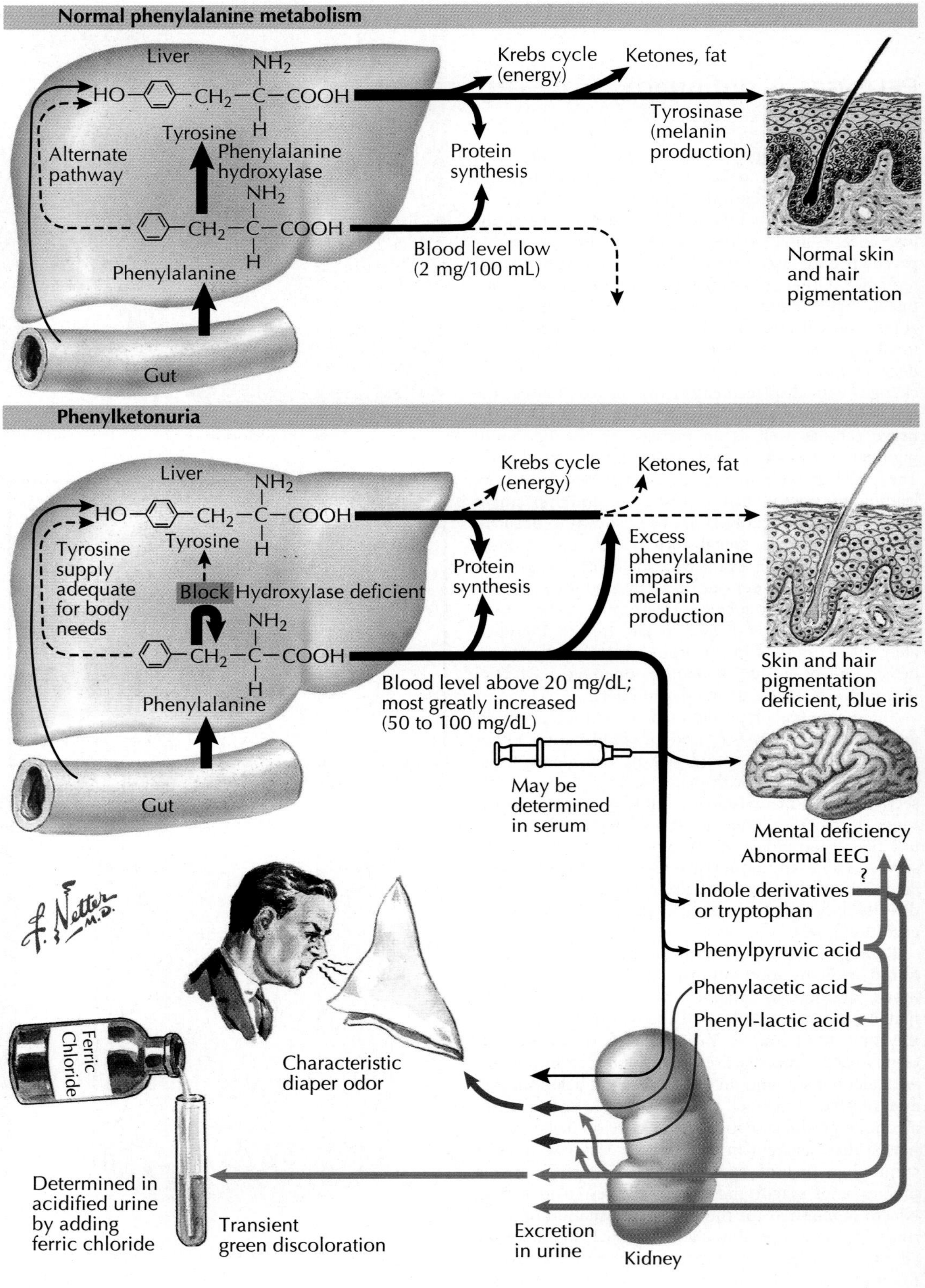

Normal phenylalanine metabolism

Phenylketonuria

The electroencephalogram of all infants and children with phenylketonuria shows abnormal results. As the child grows, the mental deficiencies begin to become more apparent. Physical growth and physical maturation are unaffected. Children tend to be hyperactive and are prone to develop self-mutilating rituals such as biting themselves or banging their heads violently against wall or floor. Tremors may be the only other neurologic finding observed.

Laboratory testing shows elevated levels of phenylalanine in the serum. Normal levels are between 1 and 2 mg/dL, and those with untreated phenylketonuria have levels greater than 20 mg/dL. Phenylpyruvic acid typically is not present in the urine in appreciable amounts in the normal physiologic state. In patients with phenylketonuria, urine levels are elevated. The addition of ferric chloride to the urine causes acidification of the urine, and a transient green discoloration is produced.

PHENYLKETONURIA (Continued)

All neonates should be tested for phenylketonuria within the first day or two of life as part of routine metabolic screening. This test can be followed up in 7 days if the initial test was performed within the first 24 hours of life or if the initial test was positive. In the past, testing was performed by the Guthrie inhibition assay or by the McCaman-Robins fluorometric test. These tests are highly accurate; levels greater than the normal value of 0.5 mg/dL are considered suspicious, and levels greater than 2 to 4 mg/dL are diagnostic. Tandem mass spectrometry is now the preferred method for diagnosis because of its speed and ability for simultaneous testing.

Pathogenesis: Phenylketonuria is an autosomal recessive disorder of the metabolism of phenylalanine. It is caused by a genetic defect in the long arm of chromosome 12 that results in a nonfunctional phenylalanine hydroxylase enzyme. Phenylalanine and its metabolites, via other metabolic pathways, lead to the clinical signs and symptoms. Excessive phenylalanine causes skin and hair hypopigmentation by direct inhibition of the tyrosinase enzyme, which decreases the amount of melanin and other molecules that are dependent on this enzyme pathway. Once the phenylalanine levels have dropped below the threshold of tyrosinase inhibition, enzyme function returns to normal and the pigmentary abnormalities resolve. Phenylalanine is directly toxic to brain cells, resulting in severe CNS abnormalities. Numerous mutations of *PAH* have been reported, making in utero diagnosis very difficult.

Histology: Findings on skin biopsy are nondiagnostic and are rarely helpful in this disease. Biopsy specimens of the hypopigmented skin appear normal. Those from areas of dermatitis show a nonspecific, spongiotic dermatitis with a lymphocytic infiltrate.

Treatment: The most important aspect of therapy is to maintain a low-phenylalanine diet. The goal should be to continue this diet lifelong because a subset of those who stop the diet early develop CNS disease. This is especially true for females of childbearing age. Deficiencies of phenylalanine hydroxylase in women who become pregnant can cause irreversible brain damage to their offspring if they do not control their phenylalanine level. These individuals should stay on a strict phenylalanine-free diet and be managed by a high-risk obstetrics team. Phenylalanine serum levels should be tested routinely to make sure the gravid parent keeps serum phenylalanine level below 5 to 10 mg/dL. Females who are considering getting pregnant should go on a low-phenylalanine diet before conception and should be under the care of an obstetrician. The diet is a prepared amino acid mixture. Strict elimination of foods high in phenylalanine is required, including meat, eggs, fish, milk, breads, and many other foodstuffs. The diet can be very difficult to follow for even the most dedicated of individuals. The artificial sweetener aspartame must also be avoided because it is made up of aspartate and phenylalanine.

Approximately 50% of cases of phenylketonuria respond to the medication tetrahydrobiopterin (BH4, sapropterin). BH4 has been found to help metabolize excess phenylalanine, and its starting dose and maintenance dose are based on patient weight and response to therapy. Some individuals with defects in BH4 have elevated levels of phenylalanine and normal phenylalanine hydroxylase function. Levels of phenylalanine must be measured over a few weeks to months to determine the effectiveness of the medication. Patients who are helped may potentially be able to increase the amount of protein in their diet. Phenylalanine ammonia lyase is an enzyme used to break down phenylalanine and is approved for use in adults with phenylketonuria.

During therapy, the skin disease, including discoloration of the hair and skin as well as dermatitis, disappears. The abnormal electroencephalogram pattern reverts to normal, and the patient's urine returns to normal. Mental performance may always lag, and permanent damage may be sustained early in the course of the disease. Only mild behavioral improvements have been reported. Children who were diagnosed before the onset of any abnormal symptoms and are maintained on a low-phenylalanine diet do not develop any of the sequelae of the disease.

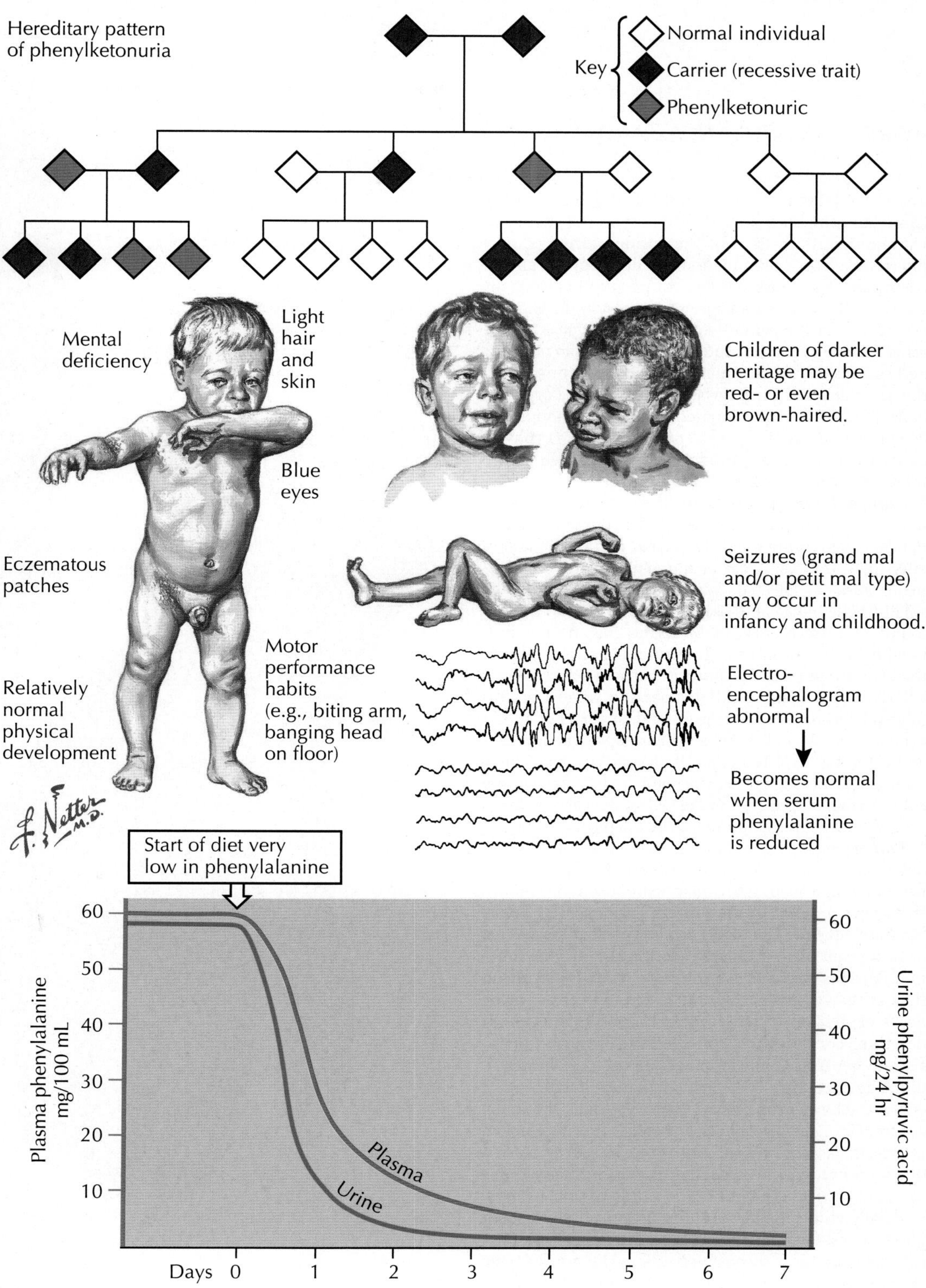

PORPHYRIA CUTANEA TARDA

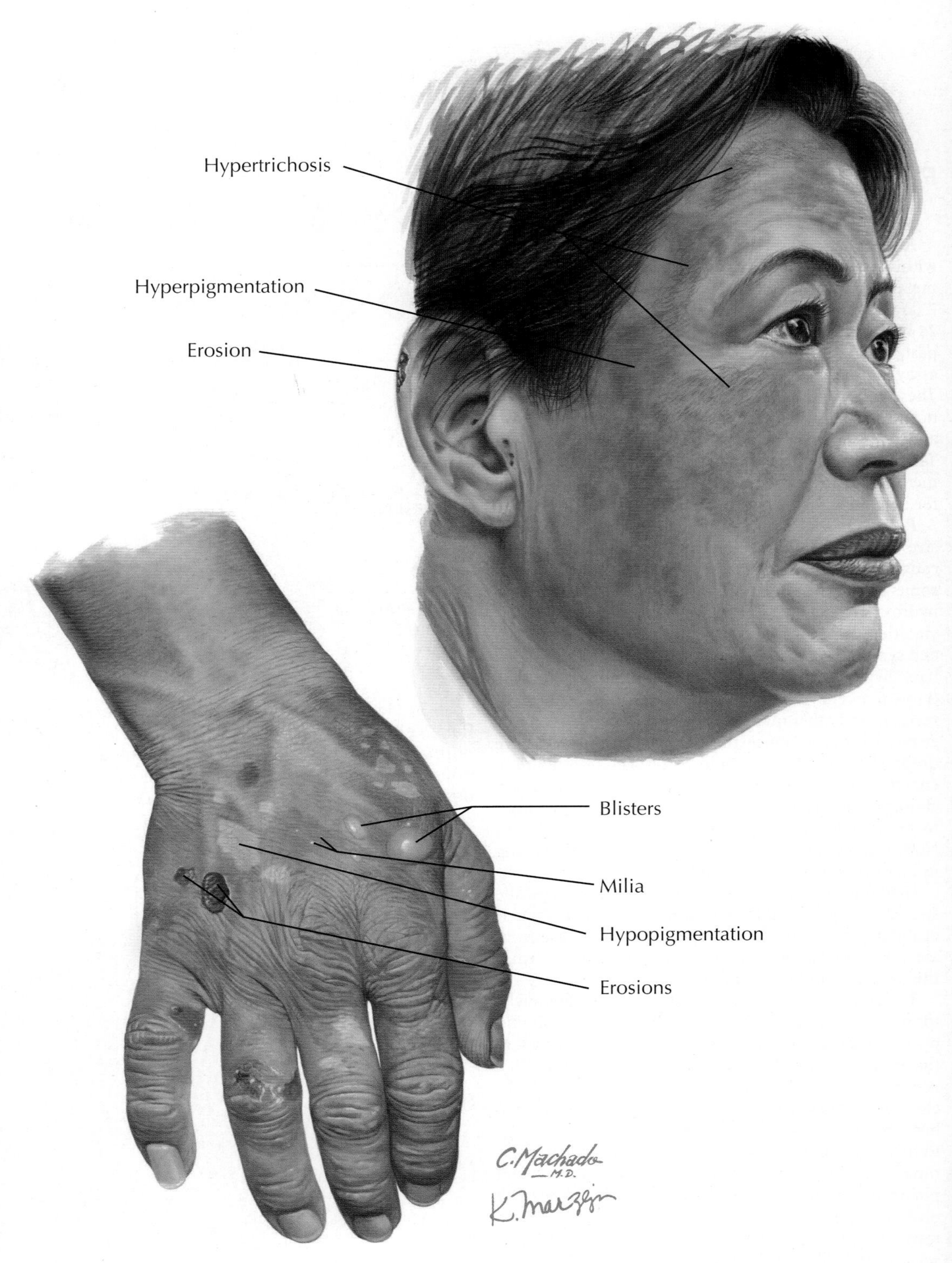

The porphyrias are a rare group of diseases resulting from abnormalities in the heme synthesis pathway. Unique defects in each of the various forms of porphyria result in accumulations of different porphyrin chemicals. The abnormal level of porphyrins leads directly to end-organ damage, which results in variable symptoms for the patient. Porphyrias can cause a wide range of symptoms, including acute neurologic signs and various cutaneous eruptions. The most common of the porphyrias is porphyria cutanea tarda. Porphyria cutanea tarda has an estimated incidence of about 1 in 20,000. There is no race or sex predilection in porphyria cutanea tarda. The acquired form is rarely seen before the fourth decade of life.

Clinical Findings: One of the first symptoms patients describe is an increased fragility to the skin of the dorsal hands. Patients note small erosions or peeling of the skin after slight trauma. Areas of sun exposure are the cutaneous surfaces affected. Small vesicles and eventually small fragile bulla can be seen. Milia formation is often found in former areas of blistering that have subsequently healed. Over time, hyperpigmentation and skin thickening with dermal fibrosis occur. Hypertrichosis will develop in long-standing cases and is most prominent on the temples, forehead, and upper cheeks. On exposure to a Wood's light, a urine sample will fluoresce and exhibit a coral-red color. If allowed to sit for a few hours, a urine sample will become a deep red-brown color. Urine, plasma, red blood cell, and fecal porphyrin testing may be needed to make the diagnosis.

Pathogenesis: During normal heme catabolism, various enzymes are required to properly break down the hemoglobin protein. Individuals with porphyria cutanea tarda have a defect in the uroporphyrinogen III decarboxylase enzyme. The defect can be genetically acquired or be a result of an acquired defect in the enzyme function. Various stressors that increase oxidative stress on the hepatocytes have been implicated in decreasing the liver's expression of the enzyme uroporphyrinogen III decarboxylase. Alcohol, iron overload, hemochromatosis, and hepatitis C infection have all been implicated in inducing acquired porphyria cutanea tarda. Once enzyme activity drops below 20% of normal, the initial accumulation of porphyrins begins. Porphyrinogen intermediates accumulate and are oxidized or broken down into photoactive porphyrins, which then are able to circulate in the bloodstream. On exposure to light, especially visible light at 410 nm, the porphyrins absorb photons and enter an excited state. The excited porphyrin molecule spontaneously reverts to the ground state after releasing energy. This released energy is believed to directly damage cutaneous structures, leading to the clinical signs of the disease.

Histology: The hallmark of porphyria cutanea tarda is a cell-poor subepidermal blister with festooning of the dermal papilla into the blister cavity. Caterpillar bodies will often be seen on the undersurface of the blister roof. These bodies are made of basement membrane zone proteins arranged in a linear fashion. Minimal to no inflammation is seen in the dermis.

Treatment: These is no cure for porphyria cutanea tarda, but it is not life-threatening. With treatment, individuals can have prolonged periods of remission. Exogenous factors such as estrogen, alcohol intake, and smoking should be discontinued. Screening for viral hepatitis, HIV, and hemochromatosis should occur. The mainstay of treatment is serial phlebotomy; 250 to 500 mL of whole blood is removed in order to remove iron as well as accumulated porphyrins. Monitoring of serum ferritin as well as hemoglobin levels should be performed to guide therapy. In individuals who cannot tolerate phlebotomy, low-dose hydroxychloroquine is an alternative therapy. Dosing is typically done once or twice a week. All individuals should be taught sun protection methods, and physical sun blockers should be used. Pseudoporphyria is a unique condition induced by various medications, most commonly nonsteroidal antiinflammatories. Individuals with pseudoporphyria have fragile skin, and vesicle and bulla formation occur in sun-exposed skin. Skin biopsy results can be nearly identical to those of porphyria cutanea tarda. These individuals will have no biochemical abnormalities, and the condition self-resolves after discontinuation of the medication.

SCURVY

Scurvy is a well-known nutritional disease that results from a lack of the water-soluble vitamin ascorbic acid (vitamin C). Scurvy has a well-documented history. It was first recognized in the 14th century in sailors who spent long amounts of time at sea. The symptoms were recognized as being related to a lack of fresh foods, especially citrus products. In 1753 James Lind, a British surgeon aboard the HMS *Salisbury,* performed the first documented clinical trial proving that scurvy was caused by a lack of citrus fruit in the diet of sailors. After Lind's discovery, citrus fruits were included in ships' provisions, and the incidence of scurvy in sailors plummeted. It was not until 1928 that ascorbic acid was isolated by the Hungarian chemist Albert von Szent-Györgyi, who was eventually awarded the Nobel Prize for this discovery. Scurvy is still present in some areas of the world because of inadequate dietary intake of vitamin C. Scurvy is uncommon in North America but can be seen in individuals with abnormal diets.

Clinical Findings: Scurvy is a disease that can affect a wide range of organ systems. The skin and mucous membranes are always involved and may display the initial symptoms of the disease. Recognition of these symptoms is critical in diagnosing the disease and preventing long-term illness. Scurvy is a rare disease in regions of the world with access to proper dietary intake of vitamin C. In North America and Europe, most cases are the result of abnormal dieting, psychiatric illness, or alcoholism. Prompt recognition of the cutaneous manifestations can lead to treatment and cure of the disease. Scurvy has an insidious onset with nonspecific constitutional symptoms such as generalized weakness, malaise, muscle and joint aches, and easy fatigability with shortness of breath. These symptoms may be related to the macrocytic anemia that is frequently seen in patients with scurvy and is believed to be caused by a coexisting folic acid deficiency.

The first clinical findings are often in the mucous membranes and the skin. There are a multitude of cutaneous manifestations. Early in the course of disease, the skin becomes dry and rough, in association with a dulling of the skin tone. Small, hyperkeratotic papules may be noticed and resemble those of keratosis pilaris. More specific and sensitive skin findings then develop, including perifollicular hemorrhage and "corkscrew hairs." The corkscrew hairs are most noticeable on the extremities. Swan-neck deformity of the extremity hair may also occur because of abnormal bending of the hair; this is less common than corkscrew hair. The nail bed shows splinter hemorrhages. All cutaneous findings appear to be more common on the lower extremities. This is believed to be a result of increased hydrostatic pressure in the lower extremities while upright, which leads to increased pressure on the small venules in the follicular locations, resulting in the perifollicular hemorrhages. These findings are also observed in areas of pressure directly on the skin, such as around the waistline. The Rumpel-Leede sign is positive: When a blood pressure cuff is inflated for 1 minute to a value that is greater than the diastolic pressure but less than the systolic pressure, numerous petechial hemorrhages occur distal to and underneath the blood pressure cuff.

DIETARY SOURCES OF VITAMIN C AND CLASSIC CUTANEOUS MANIFESTATIONS OF SCURVY

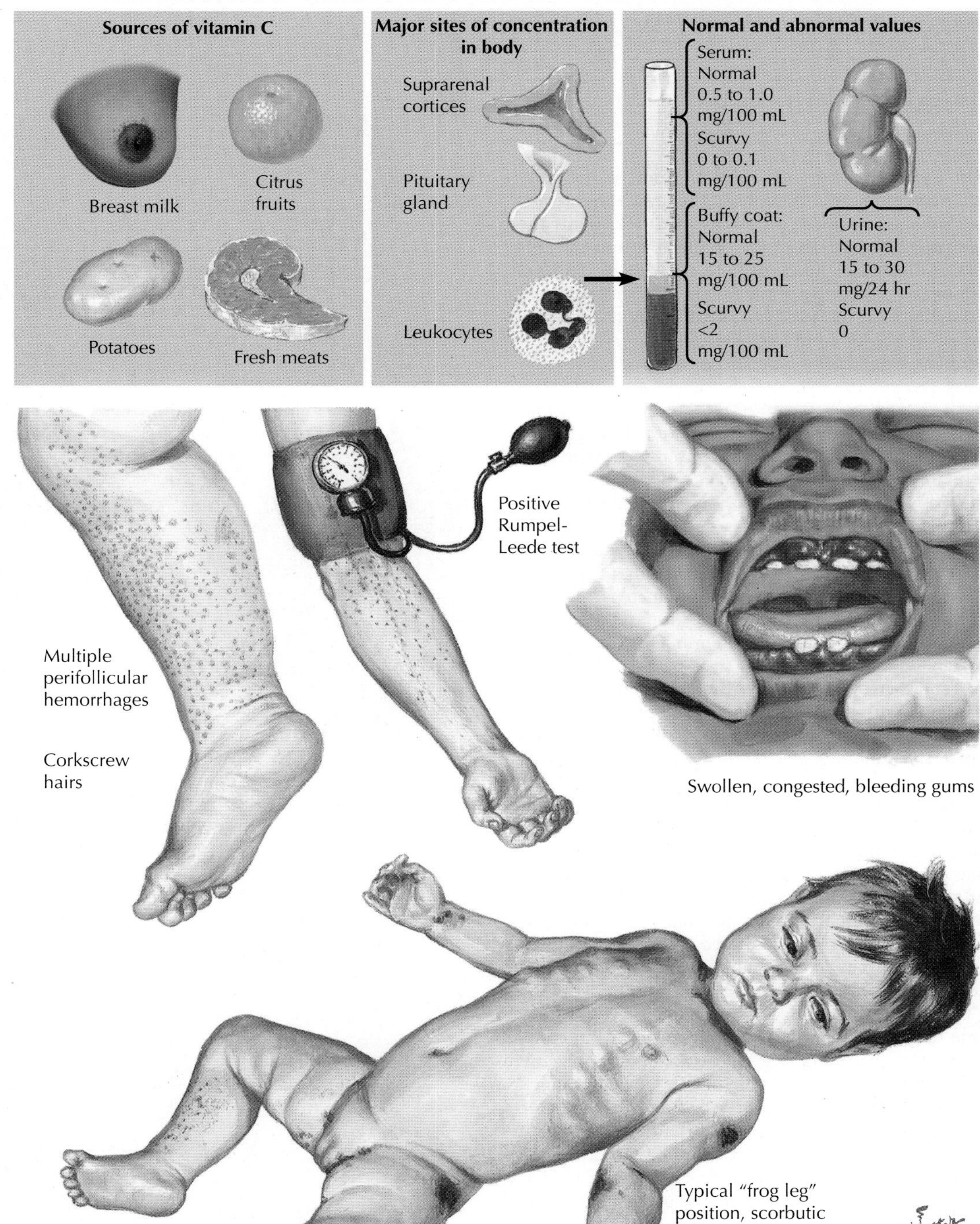

This test is a sign of capillary fragility induced by increased hydrostatic pressure.

The mucous membranes may show the first sign of the disease. The main finding is edematous, bleeding gums. As the disease progresses, the gums become friable and peel away from the teeth. The teeth may develop dental calculi at the base. This may result in loose teeth and pain. Teeth eventually become disrupted from their attachments and fall out.

Compared with scurvy in adults, congenital scurvy and scurvy during early childhood have unique manifestations related to bony development. Vitamin C is critically important for the development of collagen and cartilage, and abnormalities at a young age result in a variety of bony deformities. *Scorbutic rosary* is a term given to the prominence of the costochondral junctions. Infants with scurvy develop "frog legs" because of subperiosteal hemorrhage. This form of hemorrhage is painful, and the infant naturally relaxes the lower limbs in this pattern to relieve the pain. Healing of the subperiosteal hemorrhage often involves abnormal calcification of the region and the formation of a

SCURVY (Continued)

more club-shaped bone. This can lead to difficulty with movement. Radiographs of the long bones reveal the classic white line of Frankel, which represents the abnormal calcification of the cartilage within the epiphysial-diaphysial juncture. The periosteum appears ballooned out because of the presence of subperiosteal hemorrhage. Over time the hemorrhagic areas become partially or completed calcified.

Infants with scurvy may also develop severe ecchymosis around the eye and in the retrobulbar space, which, when severe, can result in proptosis. Child abuse may be considered in the differential diagnosis.

Breast milk contains adequate amounts of vitamin C, so infantile scurvy is more likely to occur in children who are not breastfed and are given a diet devoid of vitamin C.

Pathogenesis: Vitamin C is an essential vitamin that is acquired through dietary intake. Humans lack the enzyme L-gluconolactone oxidase, which is required for the synthesis of L-ascorbic acid from its precursor, glucose. Dietary sources of vitamin C include fruits, vegetables, and fresh meats. Citrus fruits are the main source of dietary vitamin C. All human tissues contain vitamin C, with the adrenal glands and pituitary glands having the highest concentrations. Leukocytes contain appreciable amounts of vitamin C, and the buffy coat level is helpful in diagnosis. The clinical manifestations of scurvy do not appear until the buffy coat concentration has fallen to less than 4 mg/100 mL or the serum level to less than 20 μmol/L. The normal buffy coat concentration is in the range of 15 to 25 mg/100 mL, and that of the serum is 40 to 120 μmol/L. The kidney has an extraordinary ability to adjust its vitamin C reabsorption and secretion based on serum levels. In scurvy, the kidney salvages all available vitamin C, and the urine concentration is 0 mg/24 hours.

Vitamin C is required as a cofactor for various enzyme functions. Vitamin C supplies electrons to enzymatic reactions. If these are absent, the enzymes are unable to properly produce their intended end product, and the manifestations of scurvy begin to develop. One of the most important functions of vitamin C is to serve as a cofactor, along with ferrous iron (Fe^{++}), for the enzymes prolyl hydroxylase and lysyl hydroxylase. These enzymes are responsible, respectively, for hydroxylation of the proline and lysine amino acid residues in collagen. If the proper ratio of proline and lysine hydroxylation is not present, the collagen molecule is unable to form a proper triple helix, and its function is compromised. Defective collagen production is the main deficiency responsible for the cutaneous signs of scurvy, as collagen is the major structural protein in blood vessel walls and in the dermis. Vitamin C is also responsible for electron donation in other enzymatic reactions, including those that synthesize tyrosine, dopamine, and carnitine.

Histology: Histology is not required for the diagnosis. Biopsy of a petechial lesion shows perifollicular red blood cell extravasation and a minimal lymphocytic inflammatory infiltrate. If the specimen includes the area around a hair follicle, close inspection will reveal a coiled or corkscrew appearance to the hair follicle. It should be remembered that patients with scurvy have impaired wound healing; after biopsy without proper therapy, the freshly incised skin may take weeks to months to heal, and large ecchymoses typically develop around the biopsy site.

Treatment: Therapy requires the replacement of vitamin C at a dosage of 300 to 500 mg daily until the symptoms resolve. Thereafter, the recommended daily allowance is required. Patients show rapid improvement. The root cause must be determined, and if the patient does not respond to therapy, serum levels should be rechecked. If they are still low, noncompliance with therapy should be considered. Often, patients with scurvy have an underlying alcoholism, eating disorder, or psychiatric illness that, if not properly addressed, will continue to occur. Patients should see a nutritionist, who can best educate them on the need for a balanced diet and which foods are high in vitamin C. Persons with alcoholism need to be referred to addiction experts who are adept at treating this common problem. Supplementation with the daily recommended amounts can be continued for life because any excess vitamin C is not stored in the body but excreted by the kidneys. Supplementation ensures the avoidance of further episodes of scurvy.

BONY AND SKIN ABNORMALITIES OF SCURVY

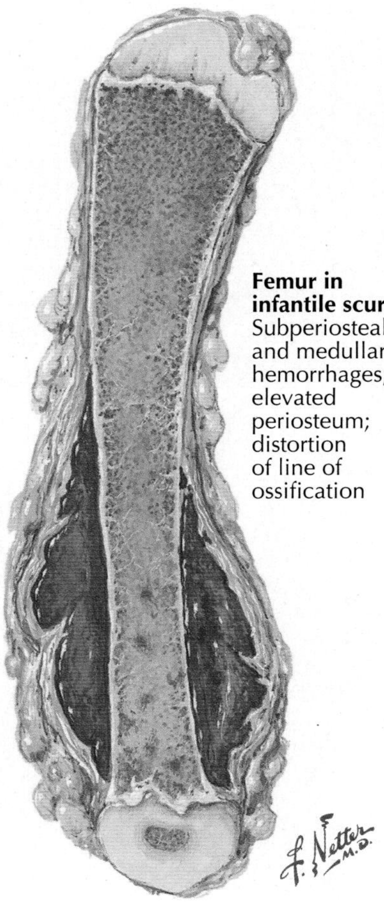

Femur in infantile scurvy. Subperiosteal and medullary hemorrhages; elevated periosteum; distortion of line of ossification

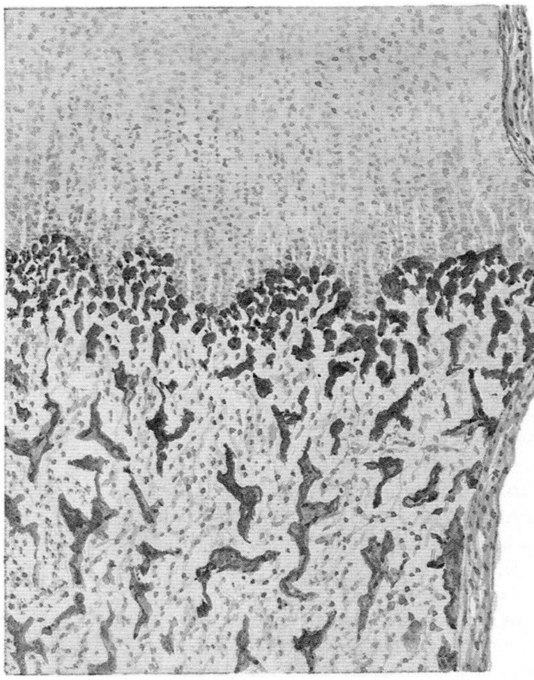

Scorbutic costochondral junction. Irregular masses of calcified matrix at junction; thin cortex; thin trabeculae imbedded in "framework marrow"

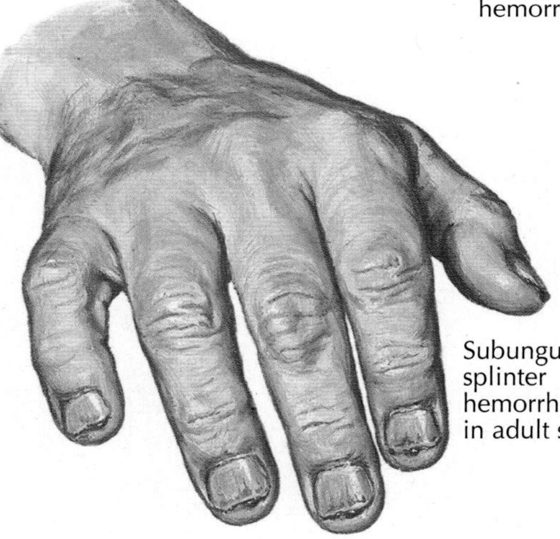

F. Netter M.D.

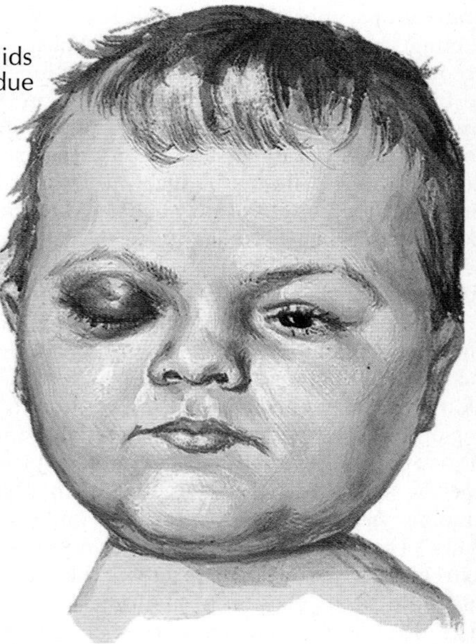

Ecchymosis of lids with proptosis due to retrobulbar hemorrhage

Subungual splinter hemorrhages in adult scurvy

VITAMIN A DEFICIENCY

Vitamin A deficiency, also known as *phrynoderma,* is a multisystem disorder caused by a deficiency of vitamin A, either from lack of intake or from a decrease in normal absorption. Vitamin A is a fat-soluble essential vitamin stored in the fatty tissue and liver. Humans require a nutritional source for this vitamin. Foods high in vitamin A include all yellow vegetables (including carrots), green leafy vegetables, liver, milk, eggs, tomatoes, and fish oils. Many other food staples contain vitamin A. Hippocrates may have been the first to describe vitamin A deficiency and a therapy for it. However, it was not until the early 20th century that scientists recognized the different forms of vitamin A and its carotene precursors.

Clinical Findings: Night blindness is one of the earliest findings in vitamin A deficiency. Vitamin A is crucially important for proper functioning of the retinal rods through the production of rhodopsin. Rhodopsin is the primary rod pigment that makes visual adaption in the dark possible. Xerophthalmia (dry eyes) often precedes the night blindness and is typically the first sign of vitamin A deficiency, although this sign is neither sensitive nor specific. As the deficiency progresses, the xerophthalmia may result in corneal dryness, abrasions, ulceration, and keratomalacia, which can lead to blindness. Bitot spots can be seen on the lateral conjunctiva of the eye. These are highly specific for vitamin A deficiency and appear as stuck-on foamy white papules and plaques that cannot be removed by swabbing. Bitot spots are caused by abnormal keratinization of the conjunctival epithelium. It is estimated that vitamin A deficiency is one of the leading causes of vision loss worldwide. Vitamin A deficiency can also cause growth impairment in children.

Phrynoderma is the name given to the skin findings in vitamin A deficiency. *Phrynoderma* means "toad-like" skin, and it is manifested by hyperkeratotic follicle-based papules. The skin is dry and rough. Patients with vitamin A deficiency may also have cheilitis and glossitis. These latter two conditions are nonspecific and can be seen in a variety of vitamin deficiencies.

Hypervitaminosis A can result from excessive vitamin A supplementation. It manifests as dry skin, hair loss, joint aches, bone pain, and headaches. Vitamin A can cause birth defects when taken in high doses during pregnancy.

Pathogenesis: Vitamin A deficiency in the United States is most frequently caused by strange dietary habits that avoid foods rich in vitamin A. Other conditions may predispose individuals to this deficiency, including cystic fibrosis, because of the difficulty in absorption of fat-soluble vitamins. Short gut syndrome that occurs after bariatric surgery may lead to vitamin A deficiency. Proper production of bile acids and pancreatic enzymes is required for absorption of vitamin A. Severe liver disease may result in functional vitamin A deficiency because the liver is required to convert carotene into vitamin A.

Vitamin A is found in foods predominantly as retinol or β-carotene. Vitamin A is critical for nuclear signaling through binding to its nuclear receptors, the retinoic acid receptors, and the retinoid X receptors. Once this binding occurs, the resulting complexes can affect the transcription of various gene products. The vitamin is responsible for maturation and proliferation of epithelial cells.

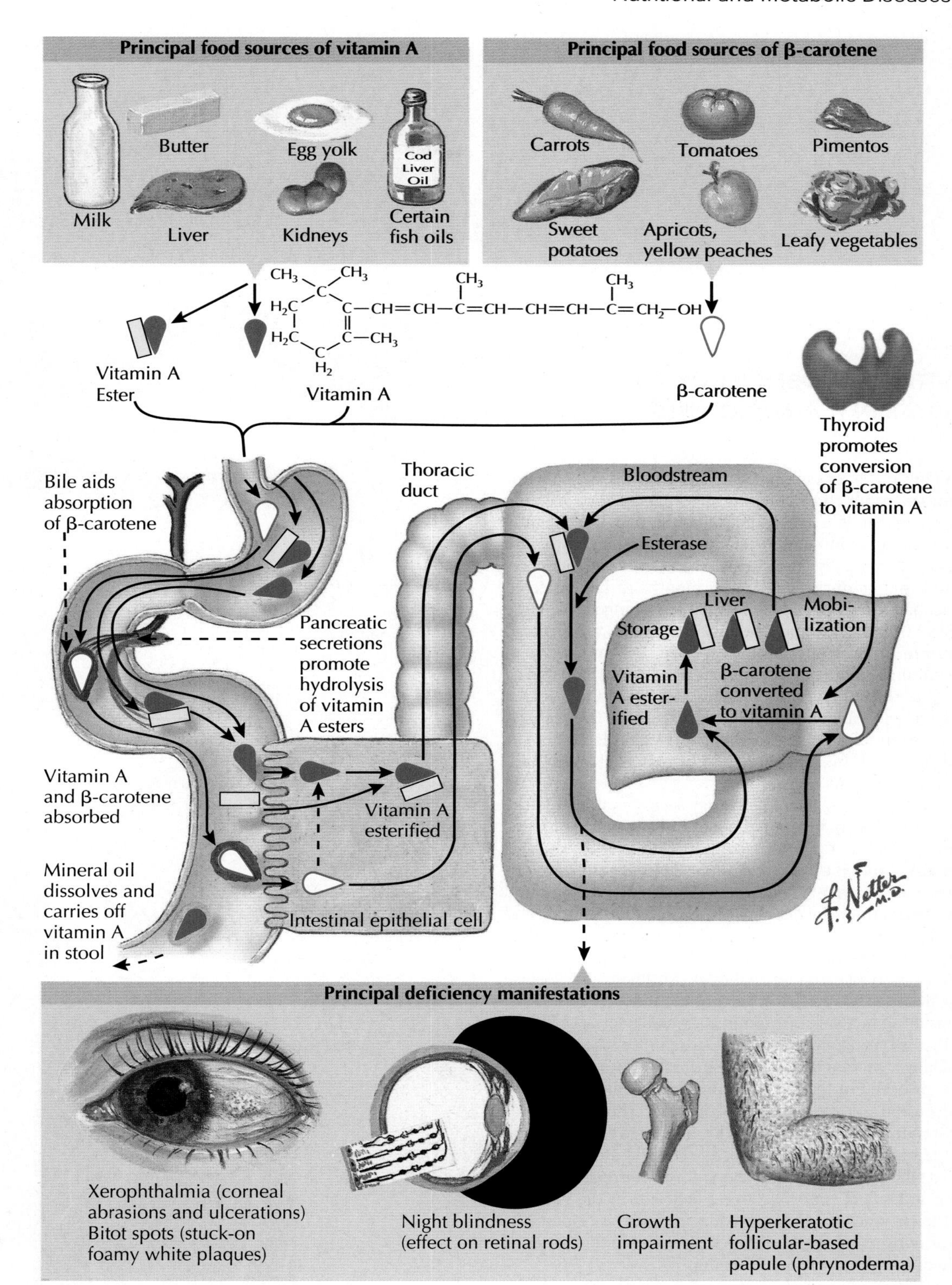

Histology: Cutaneous biopsies are nonspecific but may suggest a nutritional deficiency. There is pallor of the upper epidermis. Hyperkeratotic plugs are seen in follicles, with minimal to no inflammatory infiltrate.

Treatment: Treatment requires replacement of vitamin A and probably other essential vitamins in the patient's diet. The eye changes may be permanent, but the cutaneous findings respond well. Loss of only night vision has been shown to respond to therapy in some cases. Once blindness occurs, however, the only hope for vision is with corneal transplantation. Most cases in North America and Europe are caused by poor absorption due to an underlying cause, and the advice of a nutritionist who is an expert in malabsorption is indicated. These patients may require long-term replacement and monitoring of their vitamin A levels.

POTENTIAL CLINICAL CONSEQUENCES OF WARFARIN USE

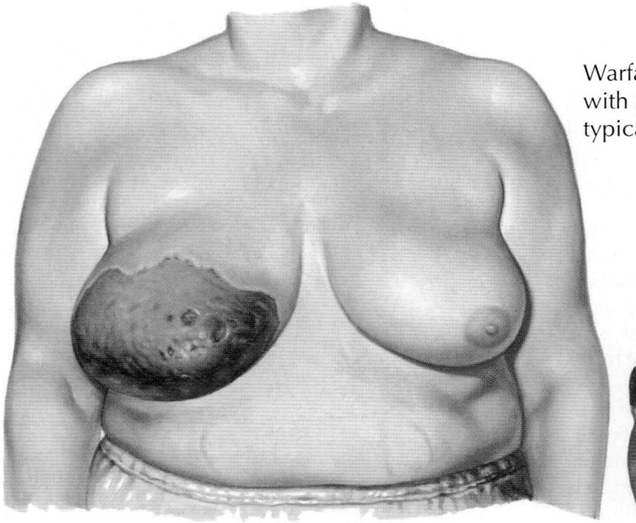

Warfarin-induced skin necrosis manifesting with purple hemorrhagic bullae and ulceration, typically over fatty tissue

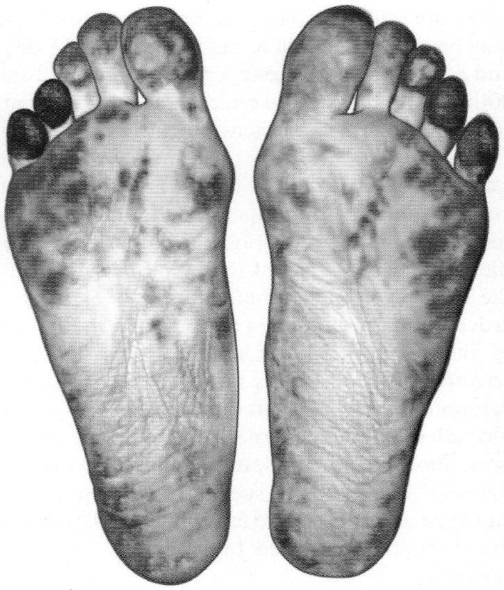

Vitamin K

Coumadin anticoagulants produce vitamin K deficiency.

Inactive K → Active K

Circulatory system

Purple toe syndrome associated with vitamin K antagonist therapy

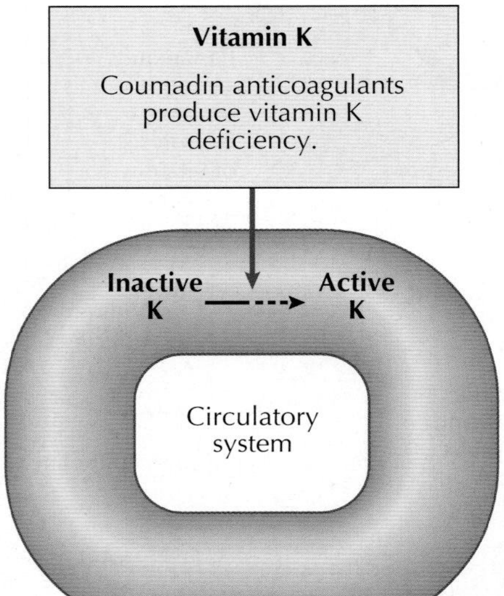

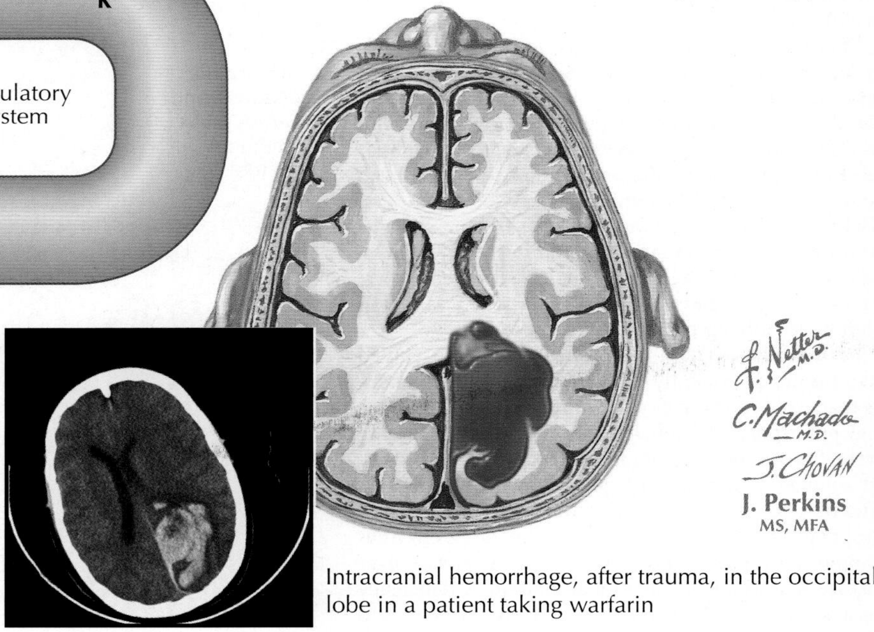

Intracranial hemorrhage, after trauma, in the occipital lobe in a patient taking warfarin

F. Netter M.D. C. Machado M.D. J. Chovan J. Perkins MS, MFA

VITAMIN K DEFICIENCY AND VITAMIN K ANTAGONISTS

Vitamin K is an essential nutrient required as a cofactor for the production of a handful of coagulation cascade proteins. It is a fat-soluble vitamin that is efficiently stored in the human body. Vitamin K deficiency is rare and is typically seen only transiently in neonates and infants during the first 6 months of life. Affected neonates may show abnormally prolonged bleeding after minor trauma. Patients may have an elevated prothrombin time and decreased serum levels of vitamin K and coagulation factors. Therapy consists of replacement of vitamin K to normal levels and a search for any possible underlying cause, such as liver or gastrointestinal disease. Neonatal and infantile vitamin K deficiency is most likely caused by maternal breast milk insufficiency of vitamin K.

Vitamin K deficiency is rarely seen in adults because most diets contain enough vitamin K for normal physiologic functioning. Adult patients with liver disease and malabsorption states are at highest risk for the development of vitamin K deficiency. Vitamin K may be found in two natural forms: vitamin K_1 (phylloquinone) and vitamin K_2 (menaquinone). K_1 is found in plants, and K_2 is produced by various bacteria that make up the normal flora of the gastrointestinal tract. Antibiotics may cause a decrease in the bacterial production of vitamin K_2, resulting in a lack of vitamin K available for absorption. This is typically not a clinical issue unless the patient is taking a vitamin K antagonist such as warfarin. Vitamin K is absorbed in the distal jejunum and ileum via passive diffusion across the cell membrane. The majority of vitamin K is stored normally in the liver. There, the vitamin is converted to its active state, hydroxyquinone. An efficient vitamin K salvage pathway normally prevents an individual from becoming deficient in the vitamin. The enzyme vitamin K epoxide reductase is responsible for converting the inactive epoxyquinone to the active hydroxyquinone form of vitamin K.

Warfarin is a synthetic analog of vitamin K and is the main vitamin K antagonist. It is indicated for use as an anticoagulant in the treatment of a number of conditions, including atrial fibrillation and deep venous thrombosis, and after heart valve replacement surgery. Warfarin acts by inhibiting the enzymes that are responsible for carboxylation of glutamate residues and epoxide reductase. This both decreases the available clotting factors and induces vitamin K deficiency, leading to added reduction of available clotting factors.

Clinical Findings: Vitamin K antagonists have been shown to cause a specific type of cutaneous eruption known as *warfarin necrosis,* which occurs in approximately 0.05% of patients taking the medication. Warfarin necrosis affects the areas of the body that have increased body fat, such as the breasts, the abdominal pannus, and the thighs. The feet are also particularly prone to development of warfarin necrosis. The skin initially develops small, red to violaceous petechiae and macules preceded by paresthesias. These regions become erythematous and purple (ecchymoses) with intense edematous skin. The lesions eventually ulcerate or form hemorrhagic bullae. The hemorrhagic bullae desquamate, leaving deep ulcers. Painful cutaneous ulcers may occur, with some extending into the subcutaneous tissue, including muscle. Most ulcers appear within 5 to 7 days after the initiation of warfarin therapy. Secondary infection may be a cause of significant morbidity. The affected areas continue to undergo necrosis unless the warfarin is withheld and the patient is treated with a different class of anticoagulant. The feet and lower extremities may have a reticulated, purplish discoloration called "purple toe syndrome." This cutaneous

VITAMIN K DEFICIENCY AND VITAMIN K ANTAGONISTS (Continued)

drug reaction can be eliminated or at least drastically decreased if the patient is pretreated with heparin or another equivalent anticoagulant before warfarin is initiated.

Pathogenesis: Vitamin K is needed for the modification of many coagulation cascade proteins, including protein C, protein S, factor II (prothrombin), factor VII, factor IX, and factor X. Factors II, VII, IX, and X are critical in forming a clot and are produced in the liver as inactive precursors. Preactivation of these clotting factors requires the action of vitamin K carboxylation on glutamate amino acid residues. Once preactivated, the clotting factors are available for full activation and clot formation when exposed to calcium and phospholipids on the surface of platelets.

Inhibition of these clotting factors by vitamin K antagonists leads to anticoagulation. Warfarin works by inhibiting the carboxylation of glutamate. On the other hand, protein C and protein S are responsible for turning off the clotting cascade and play a natural regulatory role in normal coagulation. When these proteins are inhibited, the clotting cascade may proceed unimpeded, allowing for excessive clotting. Protein C and protein S have shorter half-lives than factors II, VII, IX, and X. Therefore, when individuals are treated initially with warfarin, the levels of protein C and protein S are depleted before the other factors, leading to a prothrombic state. This initial prothrombic state is responsible for the clinical signs and symptoms of microvasculature blood clotting and skin necrosis. The clotting takes place in areas of increased adipose tissue because of the sluggish flow of blood through the fine vasculature in these regions. For this reason, most patients are given heparin or a similar anticoagulant until the full effect of warfarin on all clotting factors has occurred.

Histology: Skin biopsies from areas of warfarin necrosis show an ulcer with a mixed inflammatory infiltrate. Thrombosis is seen within the small vessels (venules and capillaries) of the cutaneous vasculature. Arterial involvement is absent. Minimal to no inflammatory infiltrate is present. Red blood cell extravasation is prominent. The main histopathologic finding is microthrombi. Findings of inflammation, a neutrophilic infiltrate, arterial involvement, a strong lymphocytic infiltrate, or the presence of bacteria in or around vessels mitigates against the diagnosis of warfarin necrosis. Bacteria will be present on the surface of the ulcer and are believed to be a secondary phenomenon.

Treatment: Treatment of warfarin necrosis requires discontinuation of warfarin and initiation of heparin anticoagulation and supportive care with fresh-frozen plasma to replace the lost protein C and protein S. Proper replacement of vitamin K is required. Menadione is a synthetic form of vitamin K that can be given therapeutically. Surgical debridement may be required, and one should be vigilant for any signs or symptoms of secondary infection.

Vitamin K deficiency in neonates and infants is diagnosed by an isolated elevation in the prothrombin time. The levels of the vitamin K–dependent clotting cofactors can each be measured, and vitamin K replacement should be administered to those who are deficient. Breast milk is not a strong source of vitamin K, and if the mother had previous children with vitamin K deficiency, the newborn should be given supplemental vitamin K. The best method for supplementation has yet to be determined, but it can be achieved with a one-time intramuscular injection or with oral replacement.

ANTICOAGULATION EFFECTS ON THE CLOTTING CASCADE

Cascade of clotting factors and sites of action of heparin and warfarin

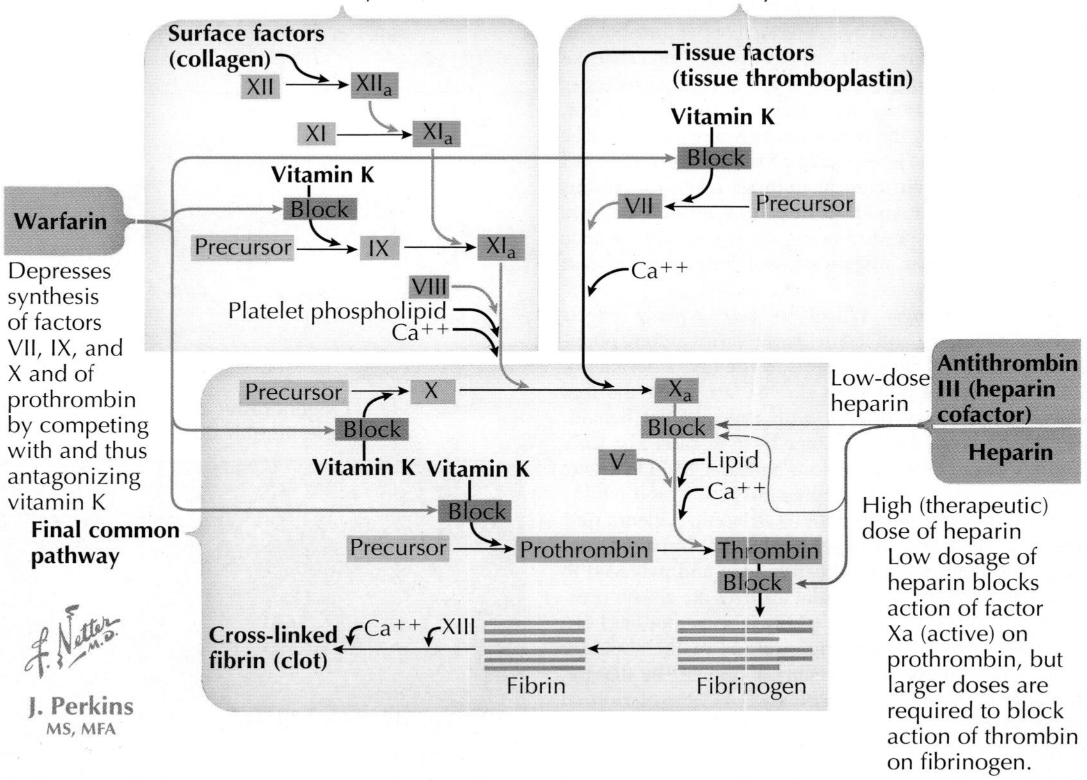

Intrinsic system **Extrinsic system**

Warfarin Depresses synthesis of factors VII, IX, and X and of prothrombin by competing with and thus antagonizing vitamin K

Low-dose heparin — **Antithrombin III (heparin cofactor)** — **Heparin**

High (therapeutic) dose of heparin

Low dosage of heparin blocks action of factor Xa (active) on prothrombin, but larger doses are required to block action of thrombin on fibrinogen.

J. Perkins MS, MFA

Element	Site of absorption	Mechanism
Ca^{++}	Duodenum and jejunum	Active
Fe^{++}	Duodenum and jejunum	Facilitated diffusion
Water-soluble vitamins		
Vitamin C	Ileum	Na^+-coupled/2° active
Thiamin (B_1)	Jejunum	Na^+-coupled/2° active
Riboflavin (B_2)	Jejunum	Na^+-coupled/2° active
Biotin	Jejunum	Na^+-coupled/2° active
Vitamin B_{12}	Ileum	Facilitated diffusion
Pyridoxine (B_6)	Jejunum and ileum	Passive diffusion
Fat-soluble vitamins		
Vitamin A	Jejunum and ileum	Passive diffusion
Vitamin D	Jejunum and ileum	Passive diffusion
Vitamin E	Jejunum and ileum	Passive diffusion
Vitamin K	Jejunum and ileum	Passive diffusion

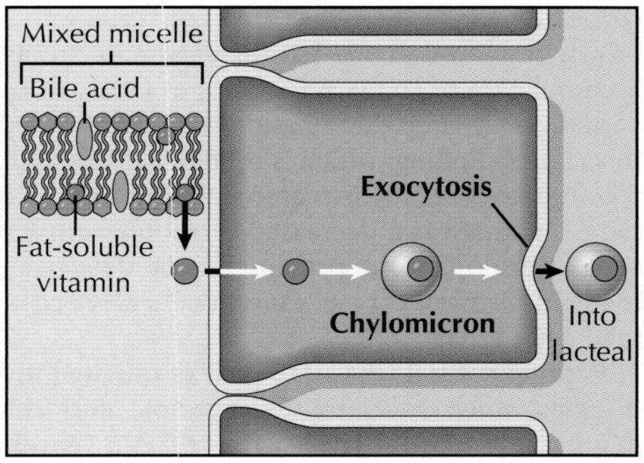

Wilson Disease

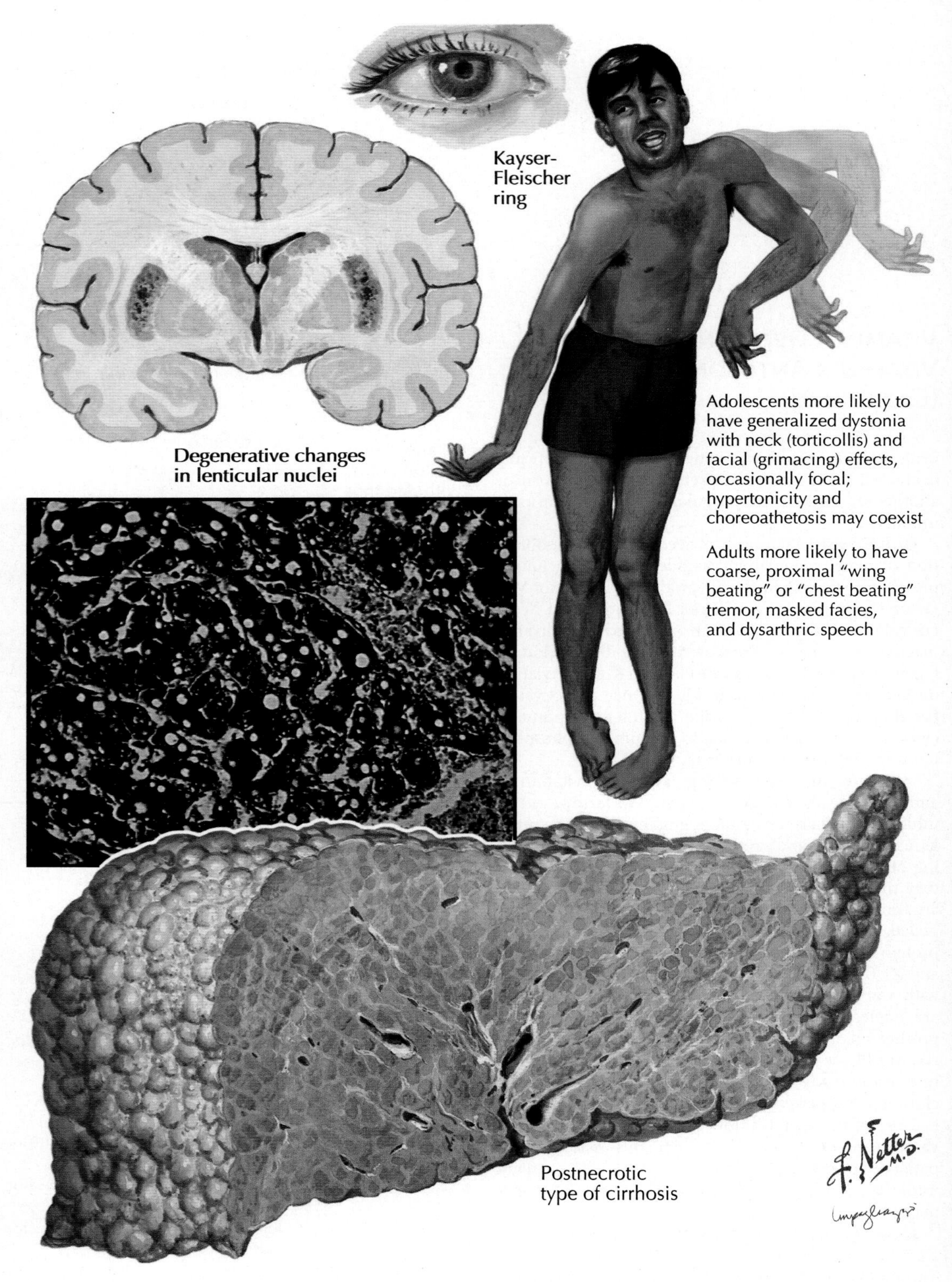

Wilson disease, also known as *hepatolenticular degeneration,* is a disorder caused by a defect in copper metabolism. The disease is rare, with a worldwide incidence of approximately 1 in 30,000. It is an autosomal recessive condition that is caused by a defect in the *ATP7B* gene, which is located on the long arm of chromosome 13. The product of this gene is responsible for the proper transport of copper. The main clinical findings relate to nervous system involvement and liver disease. Wilson disease has a variable phenotype depending on the specific genetic mutation. Cutaneous disease and ophthalmologic disease are frequently seen.

Clinical Findings: Wilson disease equally affects males and females, and its incidence varies among populations. The usual age at onset is in the first 2 decades of life. Liver disease and CNS disease are often the first signs. Patients may present with unexplained hepatomegaly, cirrhosis, and end-stage liver disease. The CNS findings can manifest in various patterns. Mild to severe psychiatric symptoms of depression and mood lability are common; the manifestations in some patients may approach the diagnosis of schizophrenia. Impaired cognition and memory are frequently seen and may lead to early dementia. Extrapyramidal features are always present and include tremor and rigidity. The tremor has been described as a "wing-beating" tremor of the shoulder girdle. Bradykinesia is invariably a part of the disease. Ataxia and chorea, along with dysfunction of normal motor coordination, are evident as time progresses.

The cutaneous findings, when present in conjunction with liver and CNS disease, can make the diagnosis. Patients have varying amounts of pretibial hyperpigmentation, the cause of which is poorly understood. Acanthosis nigricans is a common skin finding in these patients. Rarely, patients present with a blue discoloration to the lunula of the nail. The most pathognomonic sign is the presence of Kayser-Fleischer rings on the cornea. A Kayser-Fleischer ring is a yellow to orange-brown ring around the iris. It represents an abnormal accumulation of copper in Descemet's membrane of the cornea. A slit-lamp examination is required to appreciate this clinical finding, which is unique to Wilson disease.

Laboratory testing is required to confirm the diagnosis. A hallmark is a decreased ceruloplasmin level. The actual ceruloplasmin protein is not defective in any manner. Urinary copper excretion is elevated to more than 100 μg/day.

Pathogenesis: The *ATP7B* gene is mutated in Wilson disease, which leads to the systemic and cutaneous manifestations of the disease. *ATP7B* encodes the P-type adenosine triphosphatase (ATPase) that serves as a metal-binding and metal-carrying protein. This P-type ATPase is primarily responsible for the transport of copper. When it is defective, copper builds up to abnormal levels in the liver, the CNS, and to a lesser extent, the cornea. Many different mutations have been discovered in *ATP7B* and are responsible for the different phenotypes seen. Homozygous patients and compound heterozygotes have completely different phenotypes with some overlapping features. Certain mutations lead to liver and CNS disease or to a predominance of one over the other. The large number of mutations and the large size of the gene make it difficult to analyze. The prevalence of the different genetic mutations varies among populations.

Histology: Skin biopsies are not helpful in the diagnosis. Biopsies of the liver show varying degrees of portal inflammation and fibrosis with eventual cirrhosis. Hydropic degeneration of individual hepatocytes is seen to a varying degree depending on the timing of the biopsy. Special staining methods can highlight the elevated copper within the hepatocytes.

Treatment: The only cure for the disease is liver transplantation. This procedure is becoming more common and has led to excellent therapeutic responses. The transplanted normal liver produces adequate levels of the P-type ATPase to bring the copper levels to normal. CNS symptoms, if present at the time of transplantation, typically persist with minimal improvement over time. While awaiting liver transplantation, patients are usually treated with a combination of a low-copper diet, oral zinc supplementation, and D-penicillamine. Zinc competes with copper for absorption and decreases the amount of copper absorbed from the gastrointestinal tract. D-Penicillamine is a copper-chelating agent that helps to lower serum and tissue copper levels. Trientine is another copper-chelating agent that can be used if the patient is unable to tolerate D-penicillamine.

SECTION 9

GENODERMATOSES AND SYNDROMES

Addison Disease

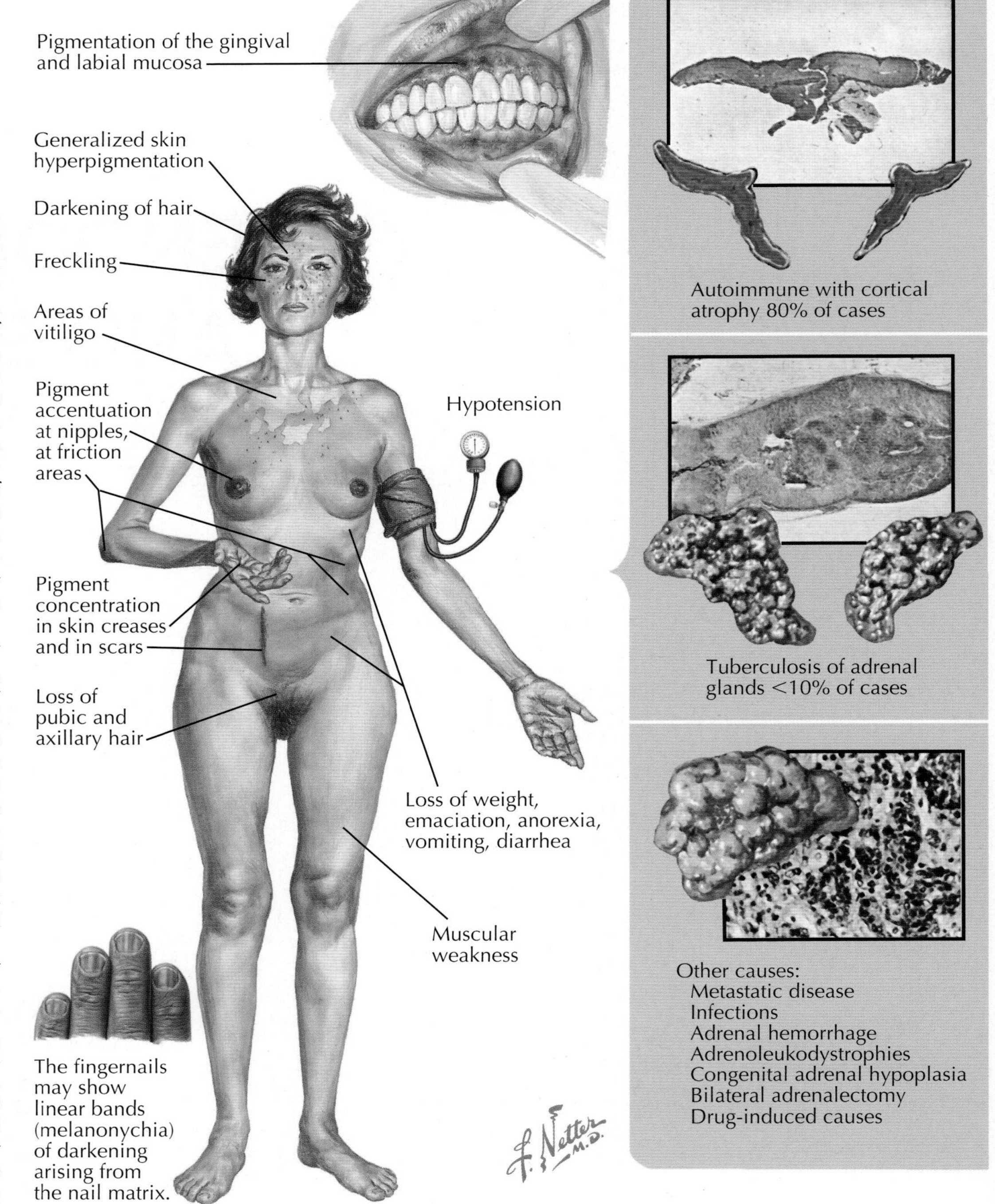

Addison disease (chronic primary adrenocortical insufficiency) occurs when the adrenal gland has lost most of its functional capacity. Addison disease can be caused by many different disease states that inhibit the functioning of the adrenal gland. The adrenal gland has a massive reserve capacity, and clinical manifestations of chronic adrenal insufficiency are not seen until the bilateral glands have lost at least 90% of their ability to produce adrenal hormones. Autoimmune destructive atrophy of the adrenal glands is the most common cause of Addison disease. Infectious processes can cause destruction of the adrenal gland, with tuberculosis one of the more common infectious causes of chronic adrenal gland insufficiency. Most cases of acute adrenal gland destruction are caused by other bacteria (i.e., meningococcal disease). Secondary adrenal insufficiency is similar clinically but is caused by pituitary dysfunction and lack of pituitary adrenocorticotropic hormone (ACTH) secretion.

Clinical Findings: Males and females are equally affected. It is estimated to affect 1 in 100,000 individuals, with those between the ages of 30 to 50 most commonly affected. The first symptoms are lethargy and generalized malaise. These symptoms may not be apparent until the affected patient undergoes a major stressful event, such as infection, which can lead to a prolonged disease course and a prolonged convalescence. Patients have excessive nervousness and may show emotional lability superimposed on periods of depression. Fatigue and weakness can be severe, to the point where even speaking causes fatigue. Weight loss and evidence of dehydration are present in most cases. Hypotension is frequently seen, and a small heart shadow is seen on chest radiography.

Cutaneous effects are always found in chronic primary adrenal insufficiency. Pigmentation is seen in many regions of the body and appears to occur in areas of friction, such as along the waistline, on elbows and knees, and over the knuckles. This is typically a generalized "bronze pigmentation," but it is accentuated in the groin, nipples, and scrotum. The hyperpigmentation in those with darker skin tones may be subtle. The palmar and plantar creases are accentuated. Hyperpigmentation may be prominent within previous scars. Vitiligo may be present in conjunction with autoimmune adrenal insufficiency. Increased pigmentation of hair is seen, but this may be subtle and may occur slowly. Pigmentary alterations of the gingival and labial mucosa may also be seen. Pigmentary anomalies are not seen in secondary adrenal insufficiency, which is caused by pituitary deficiency.

Body hair is dramatically decreased, with near total loss of axillary and pubic hair. The hair loss is more pronounced in females because males still produce androgens, primarily in the unaffected testes. Serum testing shows hyperkalemia and hyponatremia, with a low cortisol level. The diagnosis is confirmed by intravenously injecting a synthetic corticotropin and evaluating the adrenal gland's response by measuring cortisol levels after the injection. In patients with Addison disease, the serum cortisol level is not increased by stimulation testing.

Pathogenesis: The adrenal glands are responsible for making cortisol, aldosterone, and the 17-ketosteroiods. When the adrenal glands are no longer able to produce these molecules, Addison disease sets in. In the presence of low circulating levels of cortisol, the pituitary responds by increasing production of ACTH (corticotropin) and melanocyte-stimulating hormone (MSH). ACTH and MSH are derived from the same precursor protein, proopiomelanocortin (POMC). The pigmentary anomalies seen in Addison disease are directly related to increased release of MSH. The increase in MSH causes pigment production by melanocytes in skin, hair, and mucous membranes. Pubic and axillary hair loss is related to the lack of 17-ketosteroids, whereas hypotension is caused by the lack of aldosterone. The lack of aldosterone causes a decreased blood volume and decreased serum sodium. The lack of cortisol production is responsible for weakness, fatigue, weight loss, and decreased mentation.

Addison disease is seen frequently in association with other autoimmune endocrine disorders such as diabetes and autoimmune thyroiditis.

Histology: Skin biopsies are not helpful in making the diagnosis and are rarely performed. A normal number of melanocytes are present, with an increased amount of melanin pigment in the epidermis.

Treatment: Treatment requires the clearing of infection or addressing the underlying cause of adrenal gland dysfunction. Supplemental hydrocortisone and fludrocortisone are used as replacement therapy for those with inadequate adrenal function. Hydrocortisone is used primarily to replace the missing cortisol, and fludrocortisone is used to replace aldosterone. The skin hyperpigmentation improves with proper treatment.

Amyloidosis

The term *amyloidosis* refers to a heterogeneous group of diseases. Systemic and cutaneous forms of amyloidosis can occur and are caused by the deposition of one of many different amyloid proteins. The primary cutaneous forms are more frequently seen. They include nodular, lichen, and macular amyloidosis. The systemic form is a multisystem, life-threatening disorder that requires systemic therapy. Most systemic disease is caused by an abnormality in plasma cells; myeloma-associated amyloid is a distant second in incidence. In addition to amyloidosis of the skin, the central nervous system (CNS) may also be involved in cases of amyloidosis.

Clinical Findings: Systemic amyloidosis is caused by abnormal production of amyloid AL protein (immunoglobulin light chains) and its deposition in various organ systems. These effects can be seen in patients with plasma cell dyscrasia or myeloma. Mucocutaneous findings are often part of systemic amyloidosis, and on occasion they are the initial presentation of the disease. The hallmark cutaneous finding is translucent papules and plaques with varying degrees of hemorrhage. These papules are composed of the abnormal AL protein. Soft, rubbery papules may also occur within the oral mucous membranes. Pinch purpura of the skin is almost universal and results from weakening of the superficial cutaneous vessels by deposition of the AL protein. Periorbital ecchymoses may circumferentially surround the eye, which has led to the term "raccoon eyes." The ecchymoses may be induced by coughing or by superficial trauma. The palms and soles may have a waxy appearance. The tongue is often strikingly enlarged because of amyloid deposits.

Deposition of the AL protein in close approximation to the dermal elastic fibers produces a rare finding termed *amyloid elastosis*. Clinically, this may mimic cutis laxa; the skin is easily distensible and lacks elastic recoil.

Deposition of amyloid in the renal glomeruli, liver, or heart muscle can cause significant end-organ damage. Renal insufficiency leading to renal failure is a major cause of morbidity and mortality. Hepatomegaly, leading to fibrosis and liver failure, may occur. Amyloid protein that is deposited in the muscle of the heart may lead to arrhythmias and congestive heart failure.

The primary cutaneous diseases known as lichen amyloidosis and macular amyloidosis are localized to the leg and the back, respectively. Most cases are believed to be directly caused by keratinocyte-derived amyloid protein. There are no systemic symptoms. Patients present with pruritic hyperpigmented macules and papules that may coalesce into plaques. Nodular primary cutaneous amyloidosis is caused by the local production of AL protein by plasma cells in the skin. This condition is extremely rare and may progress to systemic amyloidosis.

Pathogenesis: Systemic AL amyloidosis results from plasma cell dyscrasia or from myeloma-associated disease. It is directly caused by a proliferation of abnormal plasma cells. The plasma cells produce excessive amounts of immunoglobulin light chains, predominantly λ chains. The excessive amounts of AL protein are deposited within the walls of the cutaneous vasculature; this leads to weakening of the vessel walls and is responsible for their easy rupture. The AL protein is deposited in many organ systems. Rarely, the plasma cells produce immunoglobulin heavy chains; this is termed AH protein.

Sites and Manifestations of Amyloid Deposition That May Occur in Various Combinations

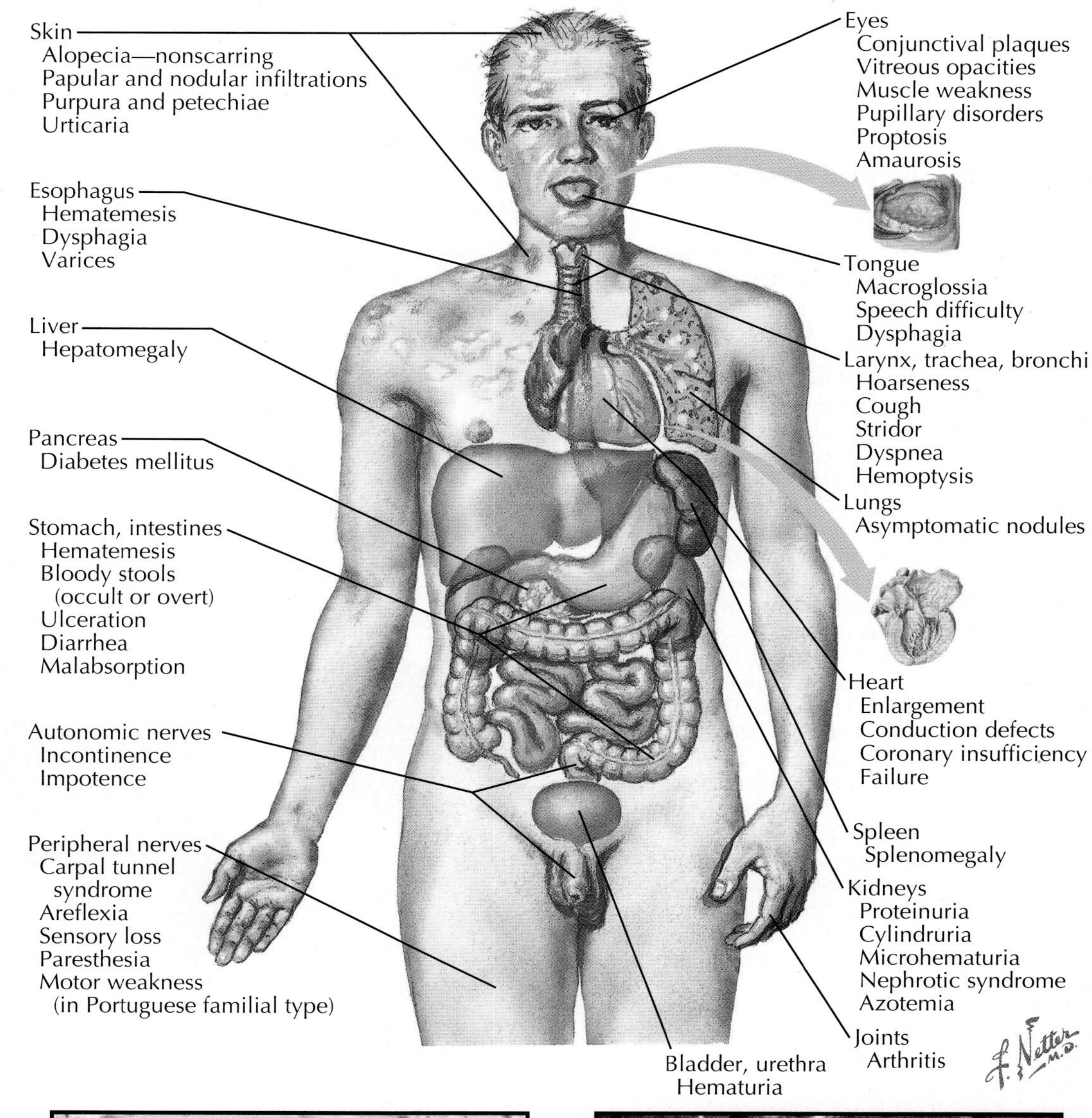

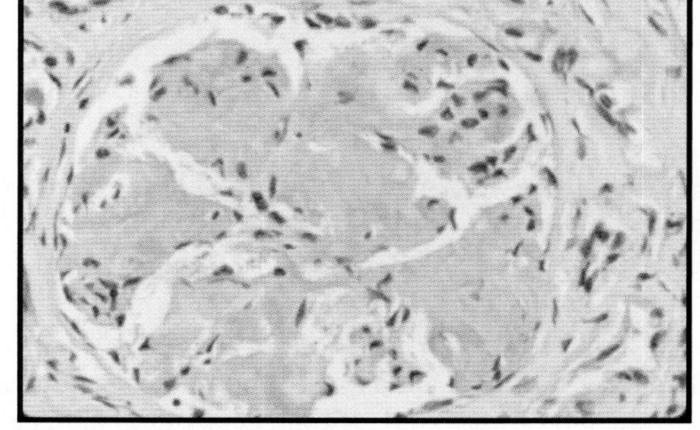

Extensive amyloid deposits in glomerulus of human kidney (Congo red and hematoxylin stain)

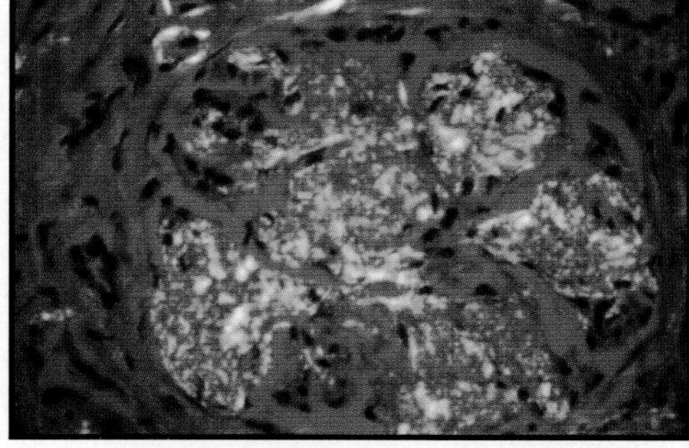

Same section, viewed under polarizing microscope, demonstrating green birefringence

Histology: Amyloidosis is a disease caused by the abnormal deposition of amorphous AL protein in the dermis and subcutaneous tissue. Biopsies of involved skin show eosinophilic deposits on routine staining. The amyloid protein is accentuated with special staining methods such as the Congo red stain, where it shows an apple-green birefringence under polarized light microscopy.

Treatment: Systemic amyloidosis is best treated with combination chemotherapy. Traditionally, prednisone and melphalan were the agents of choice. Proteosome inhibitors (bortezomib, ixazomib), immunomodulatory medications (thalidomide, lenalidomide), and anti-CD38 antibodies (daratumumab) are currently used. Bone marrow transplantation is performed in certain cases.

Therapy for primary cutaneous amyloidosis is directed at symptomatic control. Topical corticosteroids and oral antihistamines are used to control itching. Varying results have been reported with ultraviolet phototherapy. No randomized, prospective studies of the treatment of primary cutaneous amyloid have been published.

MANIFESTATIONS OF BASAL CELL NEVUS SYNDROME

Scoliosis. Ribs close together on concave side of curve, widely separated on convex side. Vertebrae rotated with spinous processes and pedicles toward concavity

Fibroma

Ovary

Medulloblastoma arising from vermis of cerebellum, filling 4th ventricle and protruding into cisterna magna

J

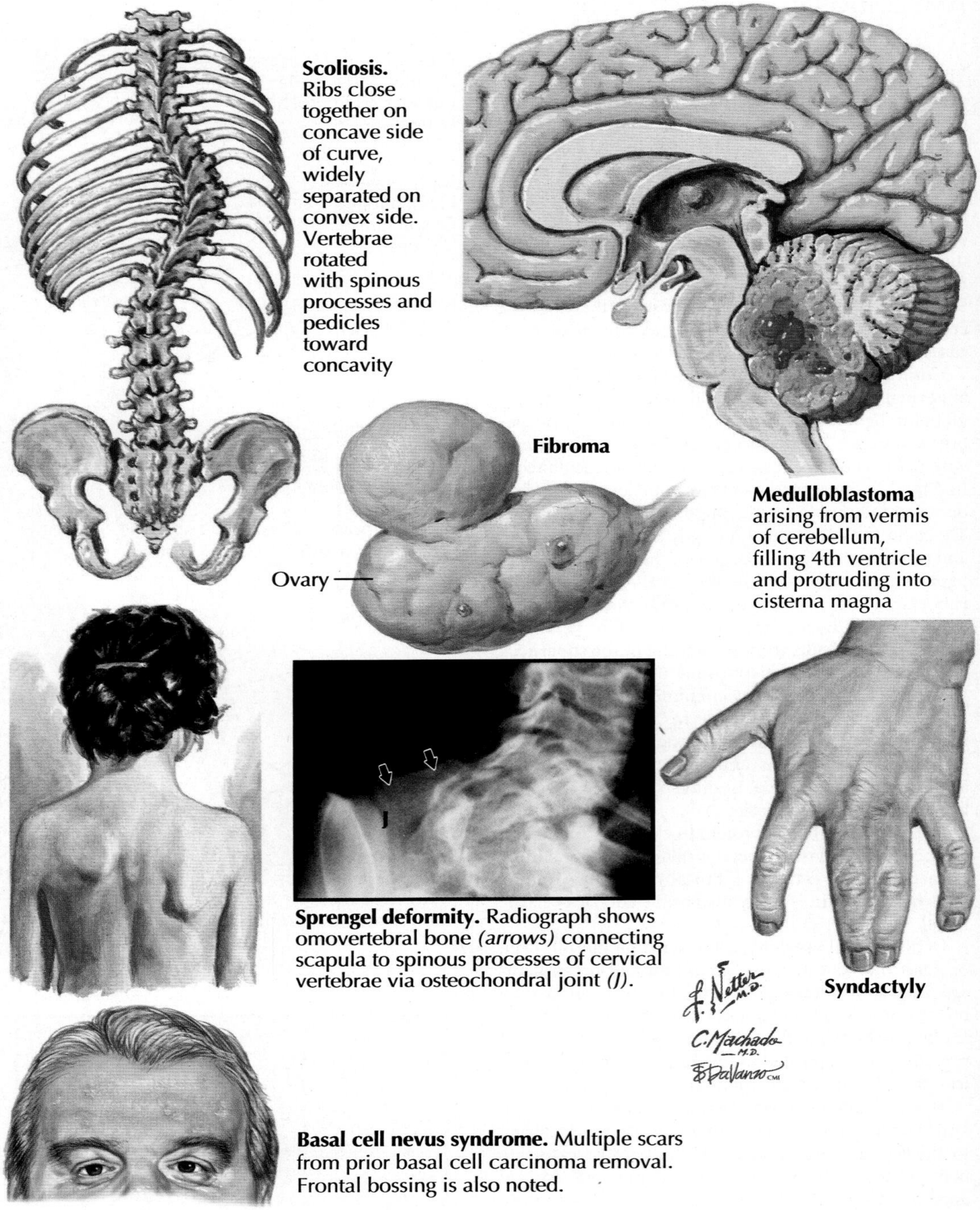

Sprengel deformity. Radiograph shows omovertebral bone *(arrows)* connecting scapula to spinous processes of cervical vertebrae via osteochondral joint *(J)*.

Syndactyly

F. Netter M.D.

C.Machado M.D.

DaVanzo CMI

Basal cell nevus syndrome. Multiple scars from prior basal cell carcinoma removal. Frontal bossing is also noted.

BASAL CELL NEVUS SYNDROME

Basal cell nevus syndrome (BCNS), also known as *nevoid basal cell carcinoma syndrome* or *Gorlin syndrome*, is an uncommon autosomal dominant genodermatosis caused by mutations in the *patched-1 (PTCH1)* gene on chromosome 9. Approximately 40% of cases represent new, spontaneous mutations. Affected individuals are predisposed to the development of multiple basal cell carcinomas (BCCs), often in the hundreds over their lifetime. The diagnosis of this syndrome is based on a number of established criteria. Mutations in the *PTCH2* and *SUFU* genes cause similar clinical outcomes. All three of these genetic mutations are grouped into one clinical diagnosis; separation of the genotypes into three distinct disease states may be possible as genetic research continues to develop.

Clinical Findings: The incidence of BCNS is estimated to be 1 in 100,000 persons, and there is no race or sex predilection. It is inherited in an autosomal dominant fashion. Often the first symptoms are painful keratogenic (odontogenic) jaw cysts. The early onset of BCCs often occurs before the age of 20 years.

Four of five patients with BCNS have odontogenic jaw cysts on dental examination or dental radiographs. In children, the BCCs have been shown to mimic skin tags. Because skin tags are highly unusual in children, any skin tags seen in a young child should be biopsied to evaluate for BCC. About 90% of affected individuals show evidence of palmar pitting, an abnormal keratinization of the palmar skin. The lesions manifest as small (1–2 mm), pink to red, shallow defects in the glabrous skin of the palms or soles.

Medulloblastoma is uncommonly seen in patients with BCNS, occurring in only 1% to 2% of patients. Interestingly, 1% to 2% of children diagnosed with medulloblastoma are also diagnosed with BCNS. The desmoplastic subtype of medulloblastoma appears to be more commonly seen in individuals with BCNS. Those individuals with a *SUFU* mutation appear to have a higher rate of medulloblastoma. This is likely the most serious sequela of the syndrome and carries significant morbidity and mortality.

Diagnosis of BCNS is based on fulfillment of well-developed criteria. Two major criteria or one major and two minor criteria must be met to make the diagnosis. The major criteria are (1) more than two BCCs; (2) palmar and plantar pitting; (3) odontogenic jaw cysts; (4) abnormalities of the ribs, including bifid or splayed ribs; (5) calcification of the falx cerebri; and (6) first-degree relative diagnosed with BCNS. The minor criteria are (1) congenital malformations (frontal bossing, hypertelorism, cleft palate, coloboma); (2) ovarian or cardiac fibromas; (3) macrocephaly; (4) skeletal abnormalities (scoliosis, syndactyly, Sprengel deformity of the scapula, pectus deformity); (5) medulloblastoma; (6) other radiologic abnormalities, including phalangeal lucencies in a flame shape, bridging of the sella turcica, and vertebral fusion; and (7) *PTCH* or *SUFU* mutation.

Pathogenesis: BCNS is caused by a defect in *PTCH1* on the long arm of chromosome 9, *PTCH2*, or *SUFU*. *PTCH1* is responsible for encoding the sonic hedgehog receptor protein that is found on many cell membranes. In normal physiologic states, the transmembrane protein encoded by *PTCH1* binds to the smoothened protein, turning off downstream cell signaling and ultimately decreasing cell proliferation. When the gene is mutated or when excessive sonic hedgehog protein is present, inhibition of the smoothened protein is removed, leading to uncontrolled cell signaling and a dramatically increased risk of cancer. Patients with BCNS are more sensitive to damage from ultraviolet light and radiation than normal controls.

Histology: BCC in the BCNS syndrome is histologically the same as any other BCC, and there are no distinguishing factors.

Treatment: BCCs tend to be multiple. Routine skin examinations and prompt removal of basal cell skin cancers help decrease the size of scarring and disfigurement resulting from surgery. All patients need to be educated at an early age on avoiding excessive sun exposure, tanning, and unnecessary radiation exposure from medical testing, because all of these increase the likelihood of BCC development. Jaw cysts are best removed surgically to relieve pain and discomfort.

Medulloblastoma is a serious, life-threatening tumor most commonly seen before the age of 4 years. Surgical and chemotherapeutic options exist. After prevention, surgical removal via Mohs surgery, standard excision, and electrodesiccation and curettage are the mainstays of therapy. Medical therapy includes topical agents such as 5-fluorouracil, imiquimod, and photodynamic therapy. The oral agents vismodegib and sonidegib are sonic hedgehog pathway inhibitors that have shown excellent efficacy in patients with BCNS.

Carney Complex

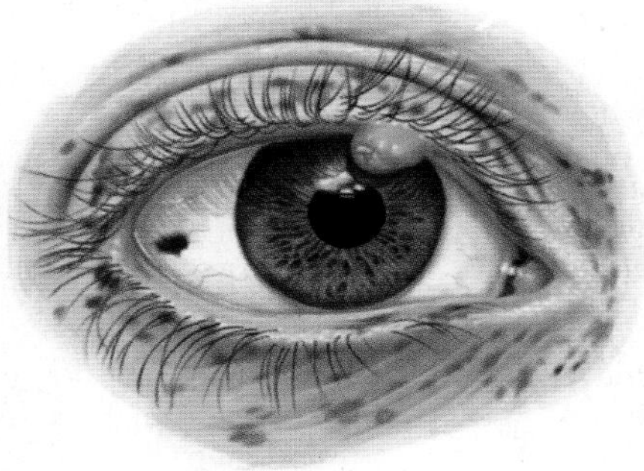

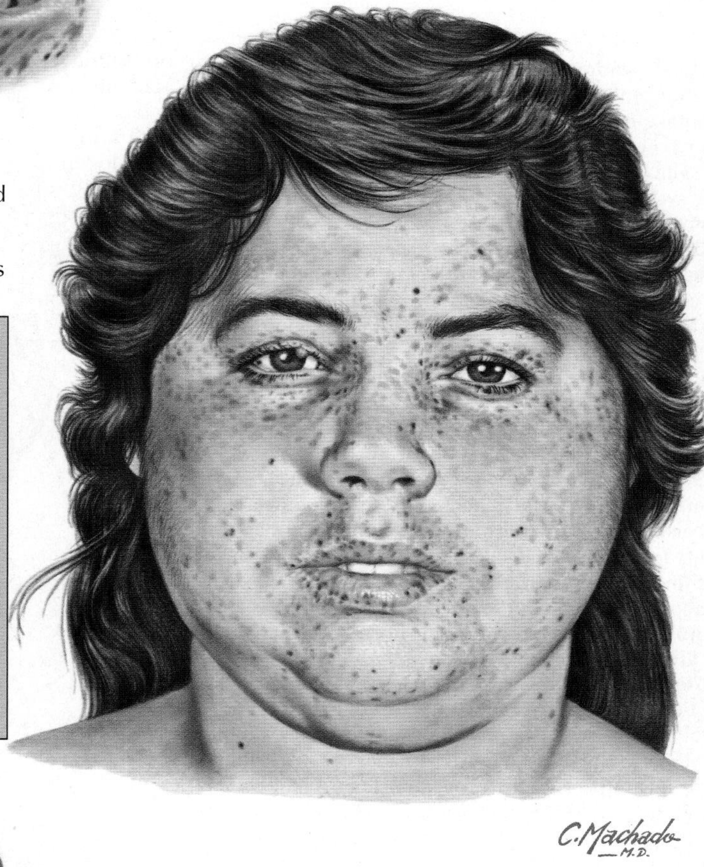

Carney complex, also known as *NAME syndrome* (**n**evi, **a**trial myxomas, **m**yxoid neurofibromas, **e**phelides) or *LAMB syndrome* (**l**entigines, **a**trial myxomas, **m**ucocutaneous myxomas, **b**lue nevi), is an autosomal dominant inherited disorder that affects the CNS and the integumentary, endocrine, and cardiovascular systems. This rare disorder is primarily (approximately 70% of cases) caused by a genetic mutation in the tumor suppressor gene *PRKAR1A* located at 17q24. Approximately 20% of patients have defects in an undescribed gene located at 2p16. Various genotypes and phenotypes exist, and the diagnosis is based on a complex list of major, supplemental, and minor criteria.

Clinical Findings: The phenotypic expression of the disease is variable, and research has shown the phenotype to be related to the underlying genotype of the disease. Cutaneous findings are often the first signs, and they are typically noticed in the first few months of life. Five prominent skin effects can be seen in isolation or, more commonly, in conjunction with one another. Multiple lentigines and common acquired nevi are the two most frequent skin findings. Multiple blue nevi are also seen. The blue nevi, lentigines, and nevi tend to group together on the head and neck region, lips, and sclerae. Mucocutaneous myxomas may be found at any location and appear as flesh-colored to slightly translucent, pedunculated papules that are soft and easily compressed. They vary widely in number from a few to hundreds. Subcutaneous myxomas are often found on the margin of the tarsal plate and can have a slightly pink-red to somewhat translucent appearance. They are not as soft to the touch as the mucocutaneous myxomas. Ephelides are also found in abundance, primarily in the head and neck region.

Cardiac myxomas are the leading cause of morbidity and mortality, and each patient diagnosed with Carney complex needs routine echocardiography and follow-up with cardiology. Male patients should be screened for testicular tumors and female patients for ovarian tumors with physical examinations and ultrasound evaluations. Pituitary adenomas may lead to a growth hormone–producing adenoma and subsequent evidence of acromegaly. Cushing syndrome may result from excessive cortisol production by the adrenal glands. This is a multisystem disorder with great variation in potential organ system involvement. Both benign and malignant thyroid tumors can be seen. Osteochondromyxomas are rare bone tumors seen in these patients. Carney complex is best treated and monitored with a multidisciplinary approach.

Pathogenesis: *PRKAR1A* encodes a regulatory subunit of a protein kinase A. Protein kinase A belongs to a family of regulatory proteins that are dependent on cyclic adenosine monophosphate for proper functioning. Many different mutations in *PRKAR1A* have been discovered, including missense, frameshift, and nonsense mutations, all leading to defects in the encoded protein. Because of the many unique mutations in this gene, researchers have been able to show that the type of genetic mutation correlates with the phenotype of the disease. As an example, mutations in the exon portions of the gene (compared with the intron portions) are much more likely to clinically express lentigines and cardiac myxomas.

Histology: Skin biopsies by themselves are not diagnostic, and the lentigines, myxomas, and blue nevi found in patients with this syndrome are not different histologically than those found outside the Carney complex. Testicular tumors usually show a Leydig cell or Sertoli cell tumor with various amounts of calcification. Histologic findings on biopsy of the adrenal gland characteristically show varying amounts of nodular pigmented regions; this has been termed *primary pigmented nodular adrenocortical disease* (PPNAD). Adrenal disease may lead to increased production of cortisol and ultimately to the signs and symptoms of Cushing syndrome. Psammomatous melanotic schwannomas are rare tumors that are almost entirely seen in individuals with Carney complex. These are not cutaneous tumors and are most likely to be found along the paraspinal sympathetic chain.

Treatment: Therapy for skin myxomas includes observation or excision of individual lesions. Lentigines and blue nevi can be removed for cosmetic purposes. Atrial myxomas are the leading cause of morbidity and mortality, and they require removal by cardiothoracic surgery. Patients must be monitored by cardiology and endocrinology specialists for their entire lifetime. Routine screening evaluations of the heart, pituitary, adrenal gland, thyroid, ovaries, and testicles must be performed.

Mucocutaneous manifestations of Carney complex characterized by pigmented lentigines, blue nevi, myxomas, common acquired nevi, and subcutaneous myxomas

Additional features of Carney complex can include:

- Myxomas: cardiac atrium, mucocutaneous myxoma
- Testicular large-cell calcifying Sertoli cell tumors
- Growth hormone–secreting pituitary adenomas
- Psammomatous melanotic schwannomas (found along the sympathetic nerve chain)

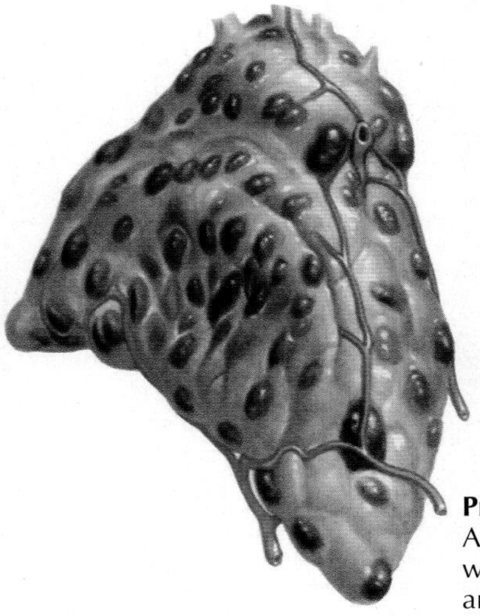

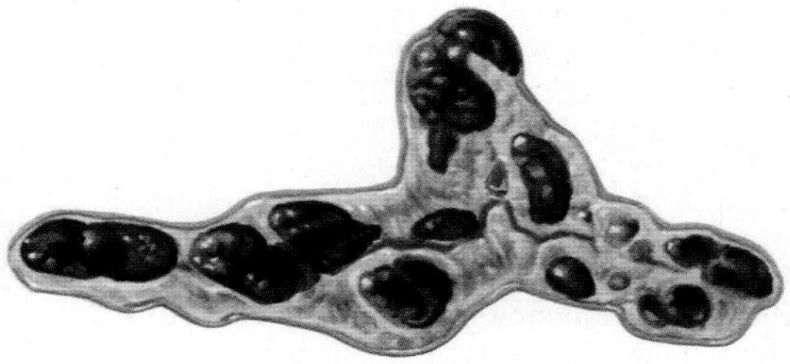

C. Machado M.D.

Primary pigmented nodular adrenocortical disease (PPNAD). Adrenal glands are usually of normal size and most are studded with black, brown, or red nodules. Most of the pigmented nodules are less than 4 mm in diameter and interspersed in the adjacent atrophic cortex.

CUSHING SYNDROME AND CUSHING DISEASE

Cushing syndrome is caused by excessive secretion of endogenous glucocorticoids or, more frequently, by intake of excessive exogenous glucocorticoids. The latter type is typically iatrogenic in nature. The excessive glucocorticoid levels lead to the many cutaneous and systemic signs and symptoms of Cushing syndrome and Cushing disease. Endogenous glucocorticoids are made and secreted by the adrenal glands, and benign adrenal adenomas are the most frequently implicated adrenal tumors causing Cushing syndrome. Cushing disease is caused by excessive secretion from the anterior pituitary of ACTH (corticotropin) as the result of a basophilic or chromophobe adenoma. The increased amount of ACTH causes the adrenal glands to hypertrophy and boost their production of cortisol, eventually leading to a state of hypercortisolism. Excessive release of corticotropin-releasing hormone (CRH) from the paraventricular nucleus of the hypothalamus can also cause the syndrome. Any tumor that has the ability to produce ACTH also has the potential to cause Cushing syndrome. The most frequently reported such tumor is the small cell tumor of the lung, which is able to produce many neuroendocrine hormones, including ACTH in large amounts.

Clinical Findings: Cushing disease is found more frequently in females than in males, and there is no race predilection. The most common age at onset of the disease is in the third to fourth decades of life. Cushing syndrome, especially the exogenous form, can be seen at any age, and ACTH-secreting tumors typically manifest in the sixth to eighth decades of life, particularly if caused by small cell lung cancer.

Cutaneous findings in Cushing syndrome and Cushing disease are almost identical. The skin findings, although frequently seen, are not universally present and can show varying degrees of severity. The excessive cortisol levels affect the skin, including the underlying subcutaneous adipose tissue. Patients have an insidious onset of fat redistribution. This leads to thinning of the arms and legs and deposition of adipose tissue in the abdomen and posterior cervical fat pad ("buffalo hump"). The fat redistribution also causes the face to have a full appearance ("moon facies"). Supraclavicular fat pads are frequently appreciated on physical examination. Large, thick, purple-red striae are seen along the areas of fat redistribution on the abdomen and buttocks, as well as on the breasts in female patients. Striae are caused by an increased production of fat and an increase in the catabolism of dermal elastic tissue. The catabolic effect of cortisol causes muscle wasting and the appearance of further thinning of the limbs. This also leads to weakness and easy fatigability. Cortisol directly causes thinning of the skin to the point that it appears translucent and almost paper-like. This thinning of the skin may impart a redness to the face (facial plethora) and other regions as the underlying vasculature becomes more noticeable. The skin is easily torn or bruised and shows poor wound-healing ability.

Cortisol decreases elastic tissue within the cutaneous vasculature, leading to easy and exaggerated bruisability and prominent ecchymoses. The excessive cortisol may also lead to increases in acne papules, pustules, and nodules; in some cases, this is quite severe, with cysts, nodules, and scarring. A rare cutaneous finding is excessive facial lanugo hair. In Cushing disease, the excessive production of ACTH is associated with an increase in the production of MSH and subsequent hyperpigmentation. This is not seen in untreated Cushing syndrome.

Cushing syndrome and Cushing disease also manifest systemically with myriad symptoms. Excessive cortisol may lead to mood changes, including depression, mania, and psychosis. Hypertension is common, and elevated blood sugar levels may occur and can be difficult to control. The skeletal system is always affected, and osteoporosis occurs early in the course of the disease; left untreated, this can lead to vertebral compression fractures and other bony fractures (e.g., femoral neck).

Treatment: Cushing syndrome of exogenous origin requires removal of the responsible agent. In most cases, this is difficult because these patients often require the life-saving exogenous corticosteroids (e.g., after transplantation). In such cases, the practitioner should decrease the dose to the minimum possible or try to change to a different immunosuppressant. Cushing syndrome caused by adrenal adenoma or bilateral adrenal hyperplasia requires surgical removal. After removal of both adrenal glands, the patient will need replacement therapy. If the syndrome is caused by abnormal secretion of ACTH from a malignant tumor such as a small cell carcinoma of the lung, the patient is best served by treating the underlying tumor. Cushing disease is best treated by neurosurgical removal of the tumor, with consideration of postoperative radiotherapy.

CLINICAL FINDINGS OF CUSHING SYNDROME

Facial plethora

Posterior cervical fat pads (buffalo hump)

Acne resistant to therapy

Moon face

Easy bruisability, ecchymoses

Supraclavicular fat pad

Thin skin (translucent, paper-like)

Wide marked purple-red striae

Hypertension

Thin arms and legs from fat redistribution and muscle wasting

Pendulous abdomen

Poor wound healing

Osteoporosis; compressed (codfish) vertebrae

Excess cortisol

Basophil adenoma

Overactive pituitary

Chromophobe adenoma

ACTH

ACTH

ACTH

Normal sella turcica

Enlarged sella turcica

Overactive adrenal cortex

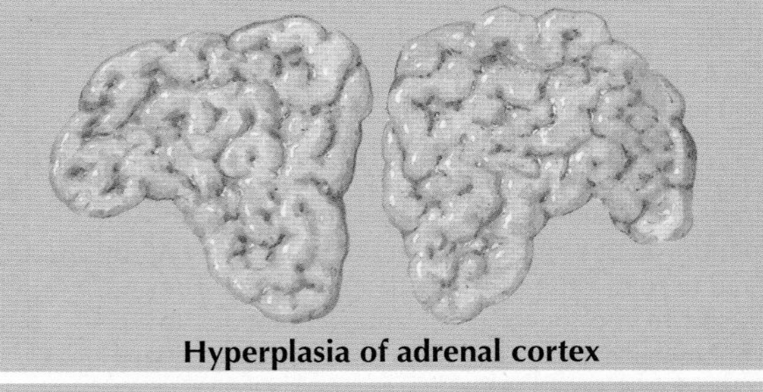

Hyperplasia of adrenal cortex

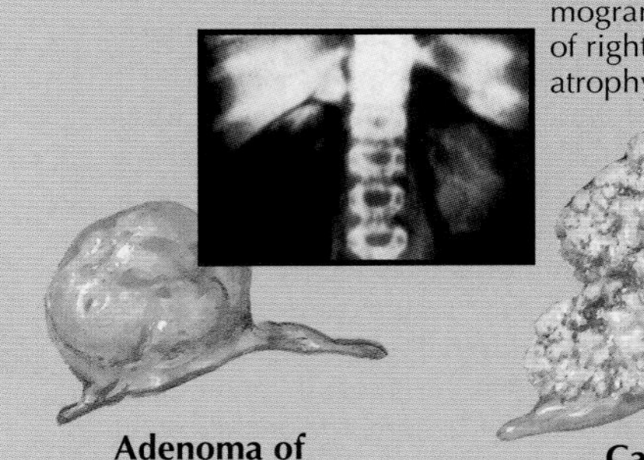

Retroperitoneal pneumogram (adenocarcinoma of right adrenal with atrophy of left adrenal)

Adenoma of adrenal cortex

Carcinoma of adrenal cortex

Cushing Syndrome: Pathophysiology

Cushing syndrome is directly caused by excessive amounts of glucocorticoids and their effects on numerous organ systems. Cortisol is strikingly elevated in all cases of Cushing syndrome. In some cases, levels of 17-ketosteroids and aldosterone are slightly elevated, and this plays a role in the clinical manifestations of the disease. Numerous disease states can cause hypercortisolemia, including excessive secretion of ACTH (corticotropin), adenoma and hyperplasia of the adrenal gland, carcinoma of the adrenal gland, PPNAD, and exogenous cortisol use. In all cases, marked elevation of cortisol ultimately is the cause of the disease.

Normally, ACTH is produced and regulated by the hypothalamic-pituitary-adrenal (HPA) axis. CRH is the main hypothalamic regulator of pituitary ACTH production. CRH acts on the corticotroph cells of the anterior pituitary, causing them to secrete POMC, which is posttranslationally modified into ACTH. ACTH then acts on the adrenal glands to increase production of cortisol. Normally, cortisol and ACTH both act in a negative feedback loop to inhibit excessive secretion of CRH.

Excessive ACTH may be produced in several ways. Most often it is produced from a basophilic adenoma of the anterior stalk of the pituitary gland. The term *Cushing disease* should be used in cases of anterior pituitary ACTH-secreting tumors. All other forms of the condition should be referred to as *Cushing syndrome*. In basophilic adenomas of the pituitary, the size of the sella turcica can range from normal to dramatically enlarged. ACTH production is elevated and is not suppressed by the increase in the cortisol level. Bilateral adrenal hyperplasia is seen because ACTH acts to increase the production of cortisol by the adrenal glands.

ACTH is produced in the pituitary by posttranslational modification of the protein POMC. POMC is modified by various enzymes to produce ACTH, β-lipotropin, and MSH. ACTH is further broken down to produce MSH. β-Lipotropin is broken down to produce β-endorphin. Cushing disease is associated with a generalized skin hyperpigmentation caused by increased melanin production that is directly related to the effects of MSH on the cutaneous melanocytes. Hyperpigmentation of the skin is seen only in patients with an abnormally elevated ACTH secretion.

Excessive ACTH may also be produced from ectopic ACTH-producing tumors, most frequently bronchogenic small cell tumors. Most patients present with signs and symptoms of Cushing syndrome before the underlying tumor is diagnosed. This form of Cushing syndrome can be very difficult to differentiate from Cushing disease in the early stages of each, and the clinician needs to be aware of the various pathophysiologic mechanisms involved in excessive ACTH production. When faced with a patient with excessive ACTH production, the clinician must perform a thorough evaluation, including history, physical examination, and laboratory and radiologic testing, to determine the etiology.

Cortisol excess may also be seen in primary adrenal disease caused by benign bilateral adrenal hyperplasia, a cortisol-secreting adenoma, or, less likely, a carcinoma. In these cases, plasma ACTH levels are reduced to near zero because of the effect of the negative feedback loop on the HPA axis. The uninvolved adrenal gland is typically atrophic. Exogenous steroid use can also lead to Cushing syndrome. In those cases, the ACTH level is decreased and the adrenal glands are atrophic.

Regardless of the etiology of Cushing disease or endogenous Cushing syndrome, the clinical manifestations are caused entirely by excessive cortisol production in the zona fasciculata of the adrenal gland. Cortisol is a catabolic steroid and causes profound muscle weakness if allowed to persist. Adipose tissue redistribution is prominent. Central obesity is easily observed, with a thinning of the extremities. Supraclavicular and posterior cervical ("buffalo hump") fat pads are frequently encountered. Cortisol has negative effects on the connective tissue of the skin, leading to a decrease in collagen. This, in turn, leads to an increase in capillary fragility, easy bruising, ecchymoses, and a thin or translucent appearance to the skin. Prominent purple to red striae are seen as a result of the loss of normal connective tissue function within the skin. The striae are most prominent in areas of obesity and are made more noticeable by the central fat redistribution. Facial plethora is regularly seen and is likely caused by thinning of the skin and an underlying polycythemia. Excessive cortisol leads to increased blood glucose levels; this in turn can lead to poor wound healing and an increase in skin infections. Hyperglycemia can lead to polyuria and polydipsia.

Most patients with elevated cortisol levels exhibit some degree of CNS involvement. Fatigue, lethargy, emotional disturbance, depression, and occasionally psychosis can be diagnosed in these patients. Excess cortisol can cause an increase in gastric acidity, leading to severe peptic ulcer disease. Patients with Cushing syndrome are more likely to have severe recalcitrant peptic ulcer disease than the average peptic ulcer patient.

In some patients, levels of 17-ketosteroids and aldosterone are moderately elevated. This leads to acne, which is often nodulocystic and recalcitrant to therapy. Hirsutism and premature or accelerated androgenetic alopecia may be seen. In rare cases, clitoral enlargement and breast atrophy are seen. A decrease in libido is extremely common. Excessive aldosterone may lead to hypertension, hyponatremia, and a metabolic hypokalemic alkalosis. The elevation of 17-ketosteroids and aldosterone is most frequently associated with adrenal carcinoma.

Plate 9.6 continued on next page

CUSHING SYNDROME: PATHOPHYSIOLOGY (Continued)

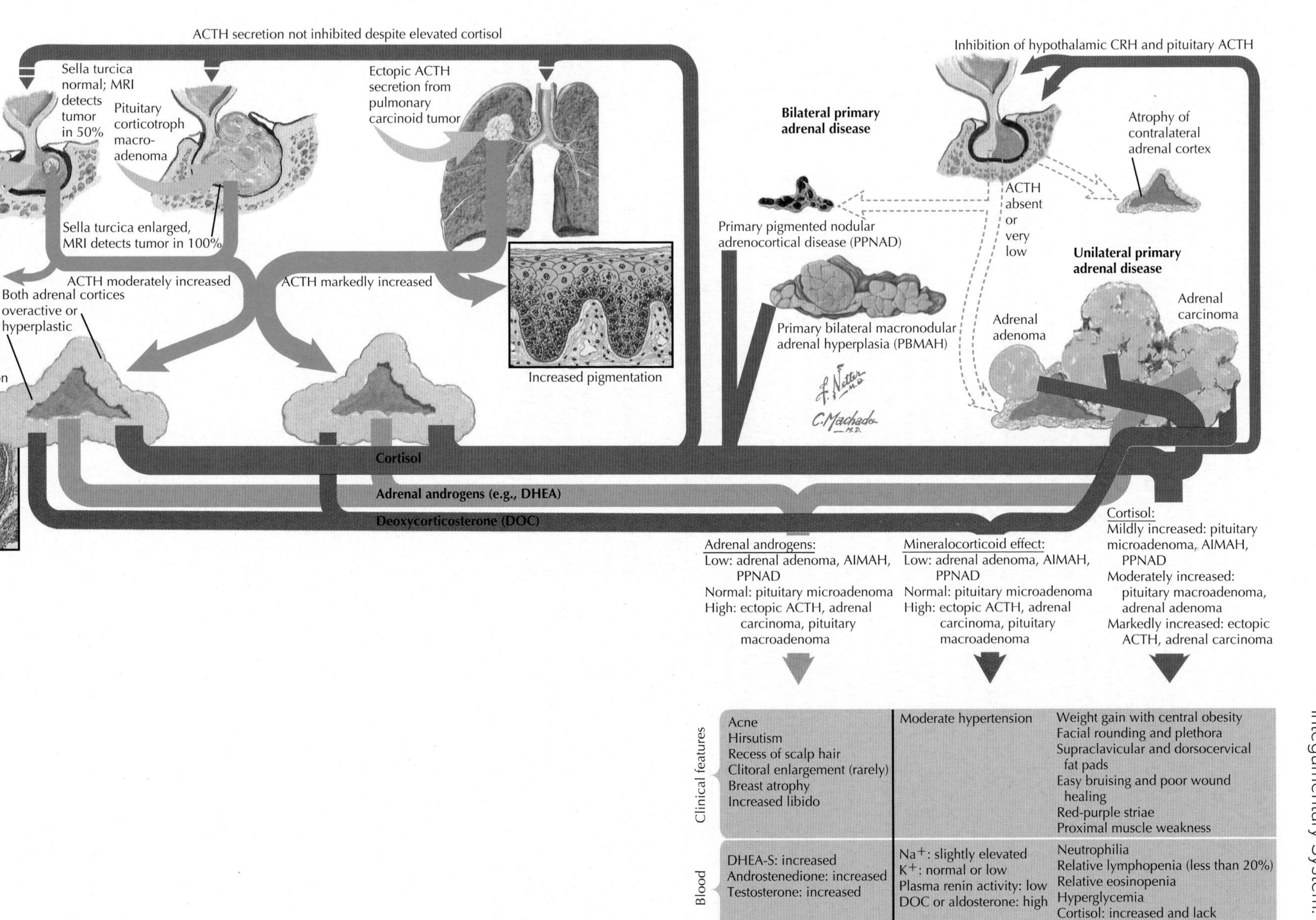

Down Syndrome

Down syndrome is a genetic disorder caused by trisomy of chromosome 21. Trisomy 21 occurs in approximately 1 of every 500 to 1000 births. Chromosome 21 is an acrocentric chromosome, and trisomy 21 is the most common form of chromosomal trisomy. Trisomy 21 most often occurs as the result of nondisjunction of meiosis, which leads to an extra copy of chromosome 21. Some patients with Down syndrome have a Robertsonian translocation to chromosome 14 or chromosome 22, which are two other acrocentric chromosomes. In these cases, the number of total chromosomes is normal at 46, but the extra chromosome 21 material is translocated to another chromosome. This, in effect, causes an extra chromosome 21. All or part of chromosome 21 may be translocated, leading to variations in phenotype. Mosaicism is a rare cause of trisomy 21 in partial cell lines, and the clinical phenotype depends on how early the genetic defect occurred during embryogenesis.

Clinical Findings: There is no race predilection in Down syndrome and only a slightly increased incidence in males. Down syndrome has been shown to increase in incidence with increasing maternal age. The estimated incidence increases to 1 in every 25 to 50 births for mothers who are 45 years of age. The clinical manifestations of Down syndrome are wide reaching and affect every organ system. Patients with Down syndrome have a decreased life span, although modern medicine continues to improve these patients' quality and quantity of life. Congenital heart disease is one of the most frequent problems and leads to a plethora of complications and increased morbidity and mortality. Endocardial cushion defects are the most frequently seen heart abnormality in Down syndrome. CNS involvement leads to mental and physical delay. The incidence of childhood leukemia is increased in these patients, the most frequent type being acute megakaryoblastic leukemia, followed by acute lymphoblastic leukemia.

The cutaneous findings in Down syndrome are vast. All patients with Down syndrome have cutaneous disease, but because of the variation in phenotype, not all have the same findings. Patients with Down syndrome are more likely to develop atopic dermatitis, which may be mild or severe. Generalized xerosis is universally found in Down syndrome. Patients may have an increase from the normal number of nuchal skin folds in infancy as well as a characteristic facies. Epicanthic folds and a flat-appearing face with small ears and a flattened nose are common. Ophthalmologic findings include Brushfield spots and strabismus.

Syringomas are frequently seen in Down syndrome and affect the eyelids and upper cheeks. Elastosis perforans serpiginosa (EPS) is a rare disease caused by the transepidermal elimination of fragmented elastic tissue. EPS is seen with a higher incidence in Down syndrome. The appearance is often that of a thin patch with a peripheral elevated rim and a polycyclic border or serpentine course. Acanthosis nigricans was shown to be present in approximately 50% of individuals with Down syndrome. It can be located in any flexural area, and the etiology is unknown. The external ear canal has been shown to be narrowed in most patients with Down syndrome; this predisposes them to an increased number of external and middle ear infections. Macroglossia with a geographic and/or fissured tongue is frequently encountered.

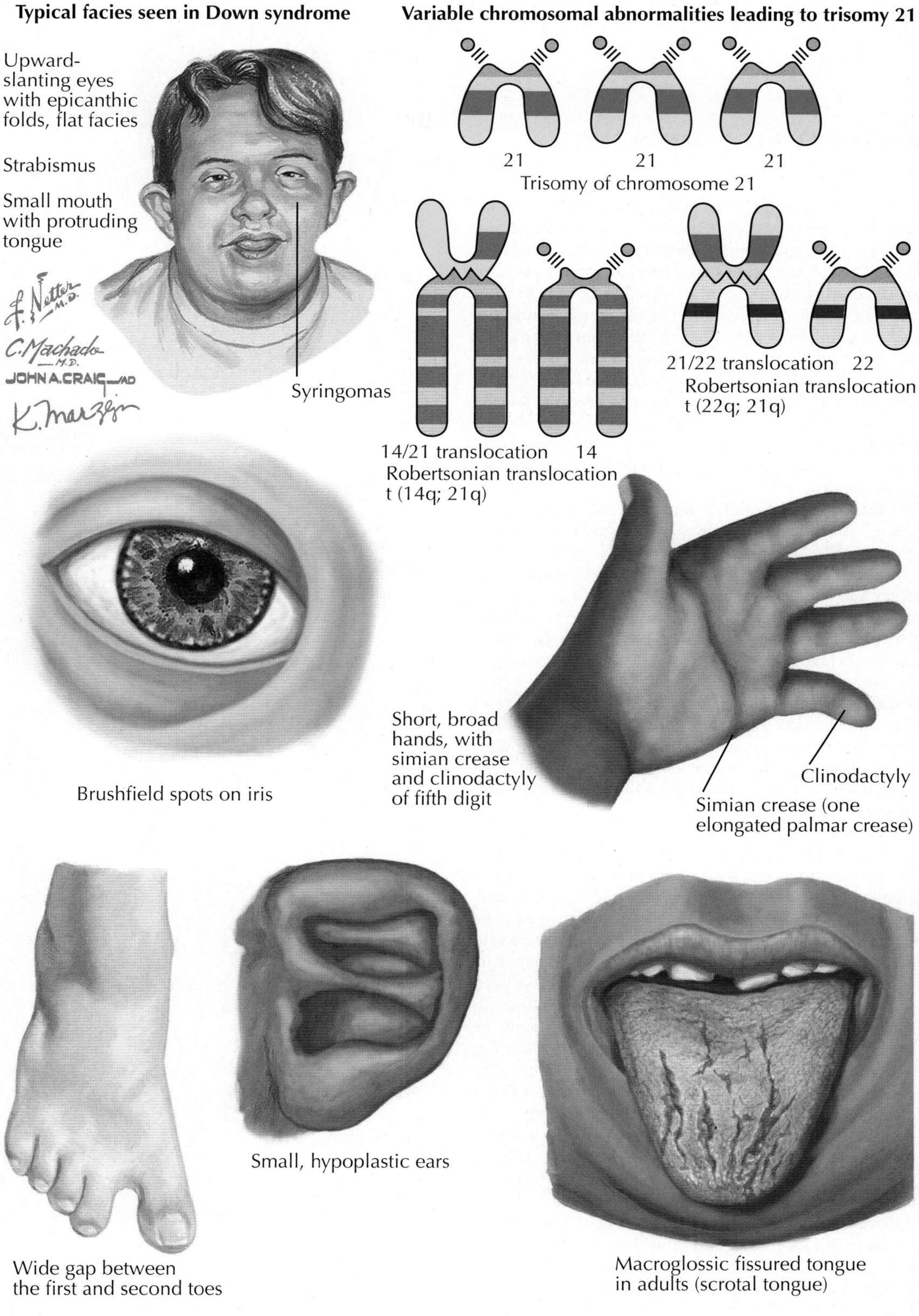

Typical facies seen in Down syndrome

Upward-slanting eyes with epicanthic folds, flat facies

Strabismus

Small mouth with protruding tongue

Syringomas

Variable chromosomal abnormalities leading to trisomy 21

21 21 21

Trisomy of chromosome 21

14/21 translocation 14

Robertsonian translocation t (14q; 21q)

21/22 translocation 22

Robertsonian translocation t (22q; 21q)

Brushfield spots on iris

Short, broad hands, with simian crease and clinodactyly of fifth digit

Simian crease (one elongated palmar crease)

Clinodactyly

Wide gap between the first and second toes

Small, hypoplastic ears

Macroglossic fissured tongue in adults (scrotal tongue)

A single transverse palmar crease (simian crease) is unique to patients with Down syndrome. Shortened metacarpal bones lead to smaller-than-normal hands, and an extra-wide gap between the first and second toes is usually prominent. Alopecia areata and seborrheic dermatitis are both found with increased incidence in Down syndrome.

Treatment: Patients with Down syndrome require a multidisciplinary approach. Cardiac defects tend to cause the most morbidity and mortality, and surgical intervention to correct underlying heart defects is often required. Patients must be monitored regularly by a pediatrician and then an internist or family physician who is well aware of the complications and care of patients with Down syndrome. The dermatologic manifestations are treated as in any other individual, and no special considerations are needed. Xerosis should be managed with excellent daily skin care. It is important for clinicians to recognize the common cutaneous findings in Down syndrome so that they can educate parents and patients alike.

EHLERS-DANLOS SYNDROME

Ehlers-Danlos syndrome (EDS) is a heterogeneous disease of defective connective tissue production. There are many subtypes, most caused by defects in collagen formation or in the posttranslational modification of collagen. This grouping of diseases has been confusing because of the variable nature of the subtypes and the lack of a universally adopted classification system. The most recent international classification system was adopted in 2017 and includes 13 separate types of EDS. The new classification system has not been universally adopted, which contributes to the confusion. As the genetic defects behind each subtype are determined, researchers and clinicians will gain a better understanding of the syndrome.

Clinical Findings: EDS is a grouping of connective tissue diseases. Each subtype is distinct and has a unique underlying genetic defect. Taken as a whole, the syndrome is estimated to occur in approximately 1 of every 400,000 persons. Because of the variation in phenotypic expression, the syndrome is likely underreported. Most cases are termed classic EDS (formerly designated types I and II). The onset of signs and symptoms occurs in early childhood and can even be manifested at birth. Each subtype has a different mode of inheritance. Most are inherited in an autosomal dominant manner, with autosomal recessive inheritance the next most prolific mode of transmission. X-linked inheritance has been described. EDS affects males and females equally.

Cutaneous findings are seen in most subtypes of the syndrome. The skin, when stretched, is hyperextensible, but it recoils to its resting position promptly and entirely after being released. Easy bruisability and excessive scarring are noticed soon after the child begins to crawl. The scarring has a characteristic "fish mouth" appearance, in that the normally thin linear scars stretch abnormally and leave a profoundly wider scar than would have been predicted. The scar tissue is extremely thinned and can appear translucent. The underlying vasculature can be seen prominently through the atrophic skin, further worsening the appearance of the scar tissue. Piezogenic pedal papules are seen and are caused by fat herniation on the lateral or medial aspects of the heel. Molluscoid pseudotumors and calcified subcutaneous nodules (spheroids) occur along regions of repetitive trauma. Epicanthic folds and elastosis perforans serpiginosa are two cutaneous findings that can be seen in cases of EDS. Rare occurrences of blue sclerae have been reported.

The major morbidity and mortality in EDS is seen in the vascular subtype (type IV). Vascular-type EDS is subdivided into three similar variants and is caused by a defect in the *COL3A1* gene. The skin in this subtype is not hyperextensible but is rather translucent. Joint laxity is absent or minimally present. Individuals with this subtype are more prone than others with EDS to arterial aneurysms and rupture leading to death. Both large and medium-sized vessels are involved. The wall of the colon is easily ruptured, and abdominal pain in these patients can be an impending sign of colonic rupture.

Pathogenesis: Most forms of EDS are caused directly by a genetic defect in collagen synthesis or indirectly by a defect in posttranslational modification of collagen. These defects lead to an abnormal amount as well as abnormal functioning of the underlying collagen and the properties it imparts to the connective tissue. The vascular subtype is caused by a defect in *COL3A1* that leads to minimal or no functional type III collagen. Because type III collagen is a critical component of the walls of the vasculature and colon, these structures are weakened and are prone to distention and breakage. Classic EDS is caused by defects in *COL5A1* and *COL5A2* that lead to defective type V collagen. Defects in the enzymes lysyl hydroxylase and procollagen peptidase, which are responsible for posttranslational modifications of collagen, are present, respectively, in the kyphoscoliosis and dermatosparaxis subtypes of EDS.

Treatment: Patients with EDS need to be under the supervision of a pediatrician who understands the disease. Referral to tertiary care centers is an appropriate course of action. Patients need to avoid unnecessary trauma. They should refrain from contact sports. The orthopedic complications can be treated by an experienced orthopedic surgeon. Patients with vascular-type EDS need to be monitored routinely by a cardiologist and a cardiothoracic surgeon. This subtype is the most difficult to manage because of its unpredictable nature.

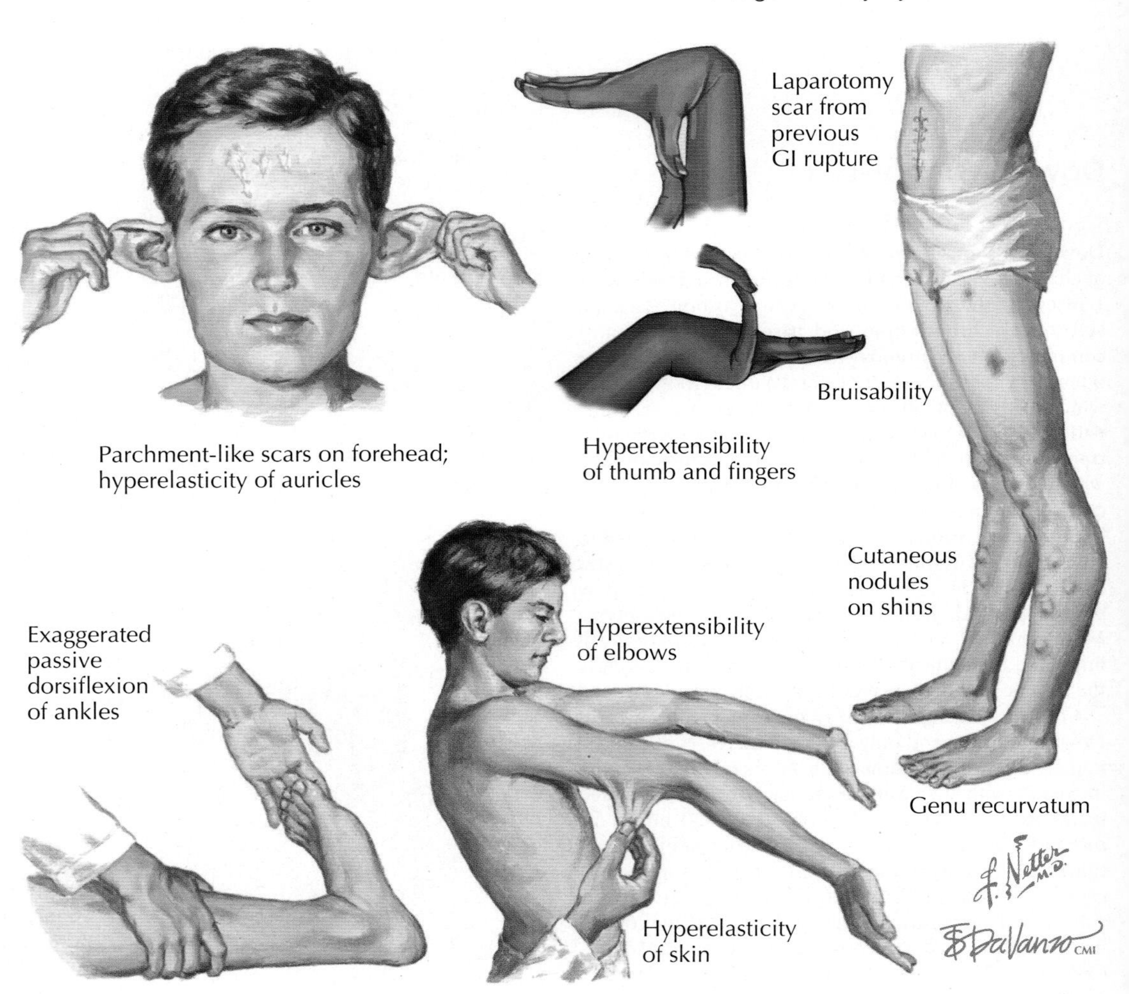

Type	Inheritance	Gene defect (protein)
Classic	AD, AR	*COL5A1, COL5A2* (collagen V)
Hypermobility	AD	Unknown, *TNXB* (tenascin XB) in a small subset
Vascular	AD, AR	*COL3A1* (collagen III)
Kyphoscoliosis	AR	*PLOD1* (lysyl hydroxylase)
Arthrochalasis	AD	*COL1A1, COL1A2* (collagen I)
Dermatosparaxis	AR	*ADAMTS2* (procollagen N-proteinase)
Other	AR, AD, X	*FN1* (fibronectin), and some unknown

AD, autosomal dominant; AR, autosomal recessive; X, X-linked

Marfan Syndrome

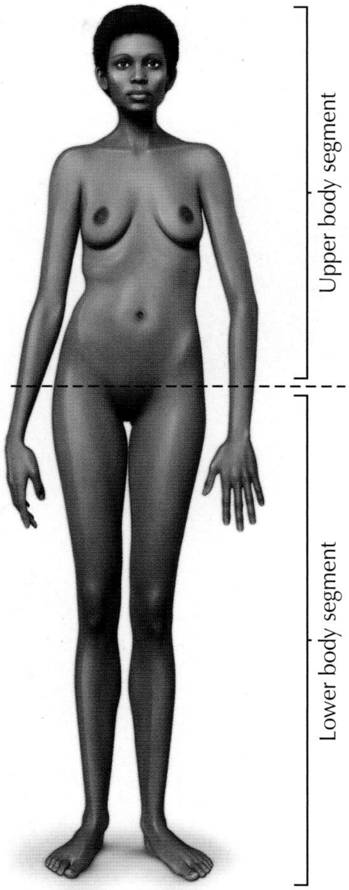

Marfan syndrome is an autosomal dominant inherited disorder of connective tissue that is caused by a genetic defect in the *FBN1* gene located on chromosome 15. The disorder leads to a defect in the fibrillin-1 protein, which is a component of the extracellular matrix of connective tissue. The defect leads to many clinical findings in the cardiovascular, ocular, skeletal, integumentary, and respiratory systems. The diagnosis is made based on multiple criteria that include major and minor features of the syndrome. Cardiovascular disease is a major cause of morbidity and mortality in this syndrome.

Clinical Findings: Marfan syndrome has an estimated incidence of approximately 1 per 5000 people. It affects all populations and has no sex differential. Many of the manifestations of the syndrome are present at the time of birth. As the child grows, the findings become more evident and the severity may worsen. The diagnosis of Marfan syndrome does not imply any specific prognosis because the syndrome has a range of clinical manifestations. There are numerous genotypes of Marfan that lead the wide variability in phenotype. On one end of the spectrum is the patient with life-threatening disease, and at the other end is the patient who has only the musculoskeletal clinical features of the syndrome.

Many skeletal anomalies can be seen, including arachnodactyly, pectus excavatum, scoliosis, pes planus, hindfoot valgus, acetabular protrusion, high palate, and an increased lower to–upper body ratio. The most striking features are tall stature, thin body habitus, long arms, and disproportionate lower-to–upper body ratio.

Cutaneous findings of Marfan syndrome may be subtle. The presence of striae distensae is almost universal. Adipose tissue is decreased, and patients often appear extremely thin. Elastosis perforans serpiginosa is seen with a high incidence in Marfan syndrome and is caused by the extrusion of abnormal elastic tissue through the epidermis.

Ocular involvement often leads to an upward displacement of the lens (ectopia lentis). Myopia is often seen, as well as a decreased ability to constrict the pupil.

The respiratory and cardiovascular systems are commonly affected. Pulmonary blebs can be seen in an apical location. The blebs may spontaneously rupture, causing a pneumothorax. Severity of involvement of the cardiovascular system is the best prognostic indicator in Marfan syndrome. Prolapse of the mitral valve, aortic root dilation, and early-onset calcification of the mitral valve anulus are a few of the cardiovascular findings. The leading cause of mortality is rupture of an aortic aneurysm or aortic dissection.

Pathogenesis: Fibrillin-1 is a glycoprotein found in a wide range of connective tissues. Fibrillin-1 is required for proper elasticity and strength properties of the extracellular matrix. Many hundreds of mutations have been reported in the gene that encodes fibrillin-1. There is a wide phenotypic variability in Marfan syndrome, due in some part to the different mutations of the gene but also to other, as yet undescribed factors. This leads to a large variation in phenotype among individuals with even the same genotypic mutation.

Defects in the fibrillin-1 protein lead to a decreased ability to bind to calcium. This ultimately manifests as abnormalities of the microfibrils throughout the connective tissue. These abnormal microfibrils are more susceptible to degradation by matrix metalloproteinases, and when they occur within the connective tissue lining of the vascular walls, the lining's elastic and strength properties are compromised. This may lead to dilation, increased stiffness, aneurysm, and eventual dissection of arterial walls, with the aorta being the most commonly affected vessel.

Treatment: All patients with Marfan syndrome should be monitored directly by a cardiologist and a cardiothoracic surgeon as needed. Routine echocardiograms and evaluations for aortic aneurysms are required. β-Blockade has been shown to be helpful to decrease mean arterial pressure. This reduces the pressure on the weakened vessel walls and subsequently decreases the likelihood of arterial dilation, dissection, and aneurysms. Angiotensin-converting enzyme inhibitors or angiotensin II receptor blockers are second-line agents. Calcium channel blockers have fallen out of favor because some studies have shown worse cardiovascular outcomes in these patients. Patients with Marfan syndrome who are closely followed and treated promptly may live a normal life span. They must be educated to avoid strenuous physical activity and contact sports. Surgery to repair aortic dilation and aneurysm should be considered if the caliber of the aorta reaches 4.2 cm or if the rate of enlargement is greater than 0.5 cm/year. Ocular disease should be evaluated and treated promptly by an ophthalmologist.

Upper body segment

Lower body segment

Tall, thin person with skeletal disproportion. Upper body segment (top of head to pubis) shorter than lower body segment (pubis to soles of feet). Fingertips reach almost to knees (arm span–to-height ratio greater than 1.05). Long, thin fingers (arachnodactyly). Scoliosis, chest deformity, inguinal hernia, flatfoot.

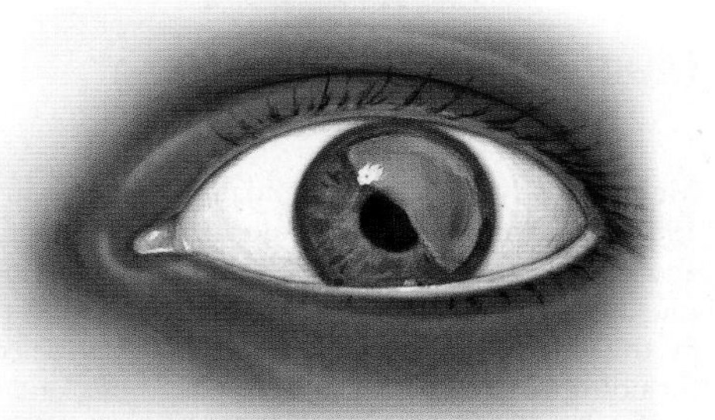

Ectopia lentis (upward and temporal displacement of eye lens). Retinal detachment, myopia, and other ocular complications may occur.

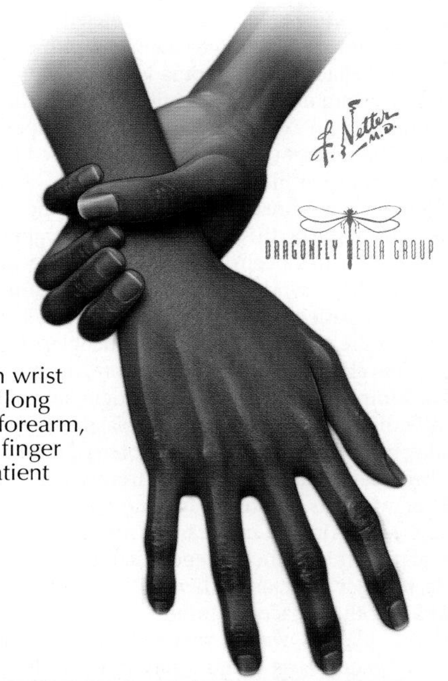

Walker-Murdoch wrist sign. Because of long fingers and thin forearm, thumb and little finger overlap when patient grasps wrist.

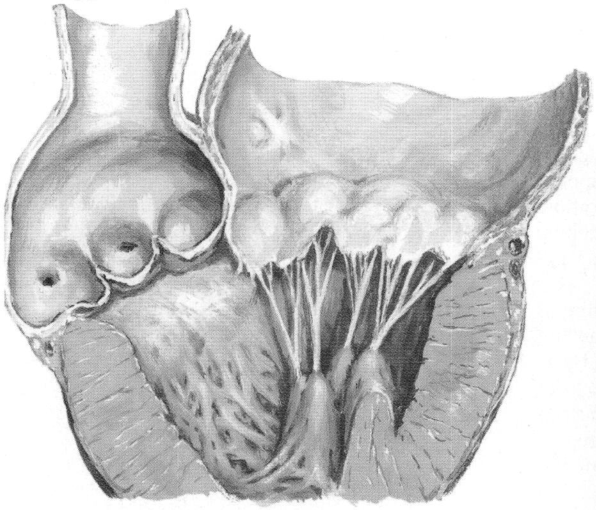

F. Netter M.D.

DRAGONFLY MEDIA GROUP

Dilation of aortic ring and aneurysm of ascending aorta due to cystic medial necrosis cause aortic insufficiency. Mitral valve prolapse causes regurgitation. Heart failure is common.

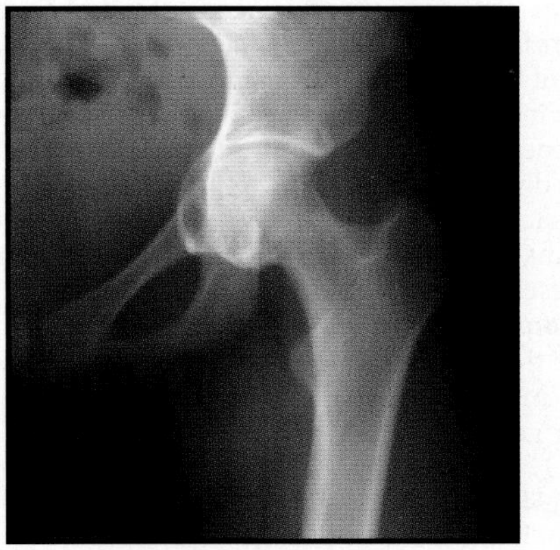

Radiograph shows acetabular protrusion (unilateral or bilateral).

MUIR-TORRE SYNDROME

Muir-Torre syndrome was initially described in the late 1960s. It is inherited in an autosomal dominant manner and has been determined to be caused by various DNA mutations in mismatch repair genes. Individuals afflicted by this condition develop various sebaceous neoplasms, including sebaceous carcinomas, adenomas, and epitheliomas as well as keratoacanthomas. Muir-Torre syndrome is believed to be a phenotypic variant of Lynch syndrome. Individuals with Muir-Torre are at a higher risk for developing colorectal cancer. Lynch syndrome is also known as *hereditary nonpolyposis colorectal cancer*.

Clinical Findings: Individuals inflicted with Muir-Torre syndrome will typically manifest with sebaceous neoplasms. Sebaceous carcinoma is the most frequently encountered tumor with sebaceous differentiation in this patient population and is regularly seen in the periocular location. The sebaceous adenoma is considered the most specific tumor seen in Muir-Torre syndrome. A diagnosis of any sebaceous neoplasm should alert the clinician to the possibility of this syndrome. A straightforward scoring system has been developed and is termed the Mayo Muir-Torre syndrome risk score algorithm, which considers the patient's age, personal and family history of cancer, and the number of sebaceous neoplasms the patient has developed. The higher the score, the more likely one has Muir-Torre syndrome. If a patient has been diagnosed with multiple sebaceous neoplasms, they almost certainly have Muir-Torre. Various internal malignancies have been reported with this syndrome, the most frequent of which is colorectal carcinoma. These tend to develop earlier in life and can be multiple in nature. Visceral tumors seen include endometrial, kidney, breast, gastric, lung, ovarian, and others.

Clinically the sebaceous tumors will present early as papules to plaques with a yellowish hue. If neglected, these can become large plaques and nodules with varying degrees of tissue infiltration and ulceration. Sebaceous tumors tend to occur more frequently in the sun-exposed areas of the head and neck but can occur at any location. These individuals are also at a higher risk for developing keratoacanthomas and basal cell carcinomas with sebaceous differentiation.

Sebaceous hyperplasia is a near universal finding as humans age. It is not part of Muir-Torre syndrome and its presence is not an indication of any underlying issue.

Pathogenesis: Microsatellite instability is the root cause that leads to the genetic mutations in various DNA mismatch repair genes. A number of mismatch repair genes have been implicated and include *MLH1*, *MLH3*, *MSH2*, *MSH3*, *MSH6*, *PMS1*, and *PMS2*. The *EBCAM* and *MUTYH* genes have also been implicated, although they are not DNA mismatch repair genes. There are numerous DNA repair mechanisms. One such method to repair DNA damage that accumulates in a cell is DNA mismatch repair. During normal DNA replication, errors can be made because of both exogenous and endogenous factors. Cells repair these mismatched DNA bases via various proteins that replace the mismatched DNA pair with the correct DNA base. This allows for protection of the genome. If they were not to be corrected, various mutations in both somatic and germline cells could occur and lead to myriad deleterious effects, including cancer.

Individuals with Muir-Torre syndrome have varying phenotypes, which for the most part can be explained by the underlying genetic defect. Germline genetic testing is available.

Solitary keratoacanthoma. Typical keratoacanthomas manifest as crateriform nodules with hyperkeratosis on sun-exposed skin.

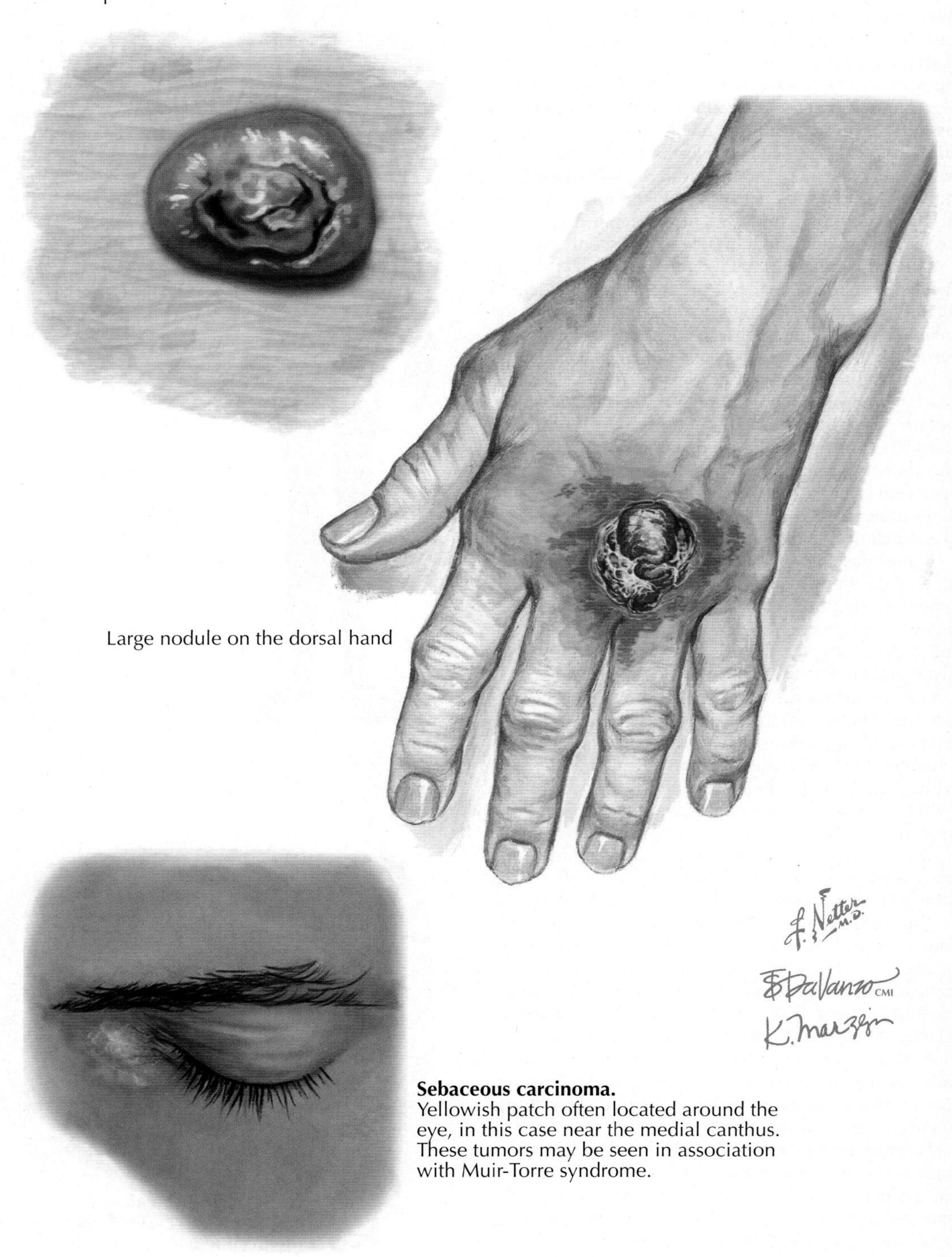

Large nodule on the dorsal hand

Sebaceous carcinoma. Yellowish patch often located around the eye, in this case near the medial canthus. These tumors may be seen in association with Muir-Torre syndrome.

Histology: Sebaceous adenomas will have two distinct cell populations within a well-circumscribed tumor. There are peripherally located basaloid cells with more mature centrally located sebaceous cells. Sebaceous carcinomas seen in Muir-Torre syndrome can show deep infiltrative growth patterns. Histologically they are essentially identical to solitary sebaceous carcinomas that are not associated with Muir-Torre syndrome. Immunohistochemical testing can be performed on pathology specimens if requested. These techniques use antibodies against the various mismatch repair proteins. Their absence indicates an abnormality.

Treatment: Skin cancers should be promptly treated surgically. Mohs surgery or standard excisions are used to treat sebaceous carcinomas and keratoacanthomas. Sebaceous adenomas and epitheliomas typically will not recur after excision. All patients will need lifelong dermatology screening to diagnose skin cancers early. Referral to a gastrointestinal disease specialist is necessary. Routine colonoscopy screening is done frequently. The patient's primary care physician should be aware and perform age-appropriate cancer screening and an annual urinalysis with cytologic exam. Female patients should be screened for endometrial and ovarian cancer.

NEUROFIBROMATOSIS

There are various distinct clinical forms of neurofibromatosis. The two most studied and clinically important forms are type I and type II. Neurofibromatosis type I (von Recklinghausen disease) and neurofibromatosis type II are autosomal dominant disorders involving the skin, the CNS, and various other organ systems. Type II has many overlapping features that are also seen in patients with type I disease. The genetic bases for type I and type II neurofibromatosis have been determined, and the specific gene for each type has been isolated. The skin findings can be instrumental in the diagnosis of neurofibromatosis type I.

Clinical Findings: Type I neurofibromatosis is usually diagnosed in early childhood. It has an estimated incidence of 1 per 3000 births and occurs worldwide. There is no sex or race predilection, and type I accounts for 85% to 90% of all cases of neurofibromatosis. There is wide clinical variability in neurofibromatosis. Diagnostic criteria have been established by the US National Institutes of Health. Two or more of the following seven criteria are needed for diagnosis: (1) six or more café-au-lait macules ($\geq$5 mm in size in prepuberty patients; $>$1.5 cm in postpuberty patients); (2) one plexiform neurofibroma or two or more neurofibromas; (3) axillary or inguinal freckling; (4) optic glioma; (5) two or more Lisch nodules of the iris; (6) sphenoid dysplasia or other distinctive bone abnormality, such as pseudarthrosis of a long bone; or (7) a first-degree relative with neurofibromatosis.

The cutaneous findings, and in particular the café-au-lait macules, are often the presenting sign of the disease. Solitary café-au-lait macules are seen in a large percentage of the normal population, and the diagnostic criteria for neurofibromatosis require the presence of at least six such lesions. Spinal dysraphism may be present if the skin overlying the spine is involved with a café-au-lait macule. The onset of axillary and inguinal freckling is often during puberty. Axillary freckling is also known as the Crowe sign. Cutaneous neurofibromas are the most common benign tumor found in patients with neurofibromatosis. The tumors tend to be plentiful and to increase in number and size with time. They are soft and often exhibit the "buttonhole" sign when compressed. These tumors may have an overlying pink to light violet coloration. Plexiform neurofibromas are large dermal and subcutaneous tumors specific to type I neurofibromatosis. They can cause compression of underlying structures and wrap themselves around nerves. Compared with the typical neurofibroma, they are firm and larger and have an ill-defined border. Both forms of neurofibromas can produce varying amounts of pruritus. Patients with plexiform neurofibromas have hypertrichosis with and without hyperpigmentation. The presence of multiple neurofibromas can cause psychological disease. Individuals with neurofibromas that develop juvenile xanthogranulomas should be screened for acute myeloid leukemia.

Lisch nodules are hamartomas of the iris. They are observed under slit-lamp examination and can be seen by approximately 6 years of age. Optic gliomas are seen in about one of every eight patients with neurofibromatosis. Optic gliomas may be asymptomatic, or they may cause compression of the pituitary gland, resulting in precocious puberty. Gliomas can also cause visual disturbance and proptosis. The best method to detect an optic glioma is with brain magnetic resonance imaging. Other ophthalmologic findings that may be present include hypertelorism and congenital glaucoma. Breast cancer risk is increased, and early screening is recommended. Malignant peripheral nerve sheath tumors can be seen and are best evaluated with functional MRI or positron emission tomography scans. These can be aggressive sarcomas.

Type II neurofibromatosis has a very different phenotype than type I disease, with some overlap. Onset of disease is often not until the second or third decade of life. The main aspect of type II neurofibromatosis is the formation of bilateral acoustic neuromas (vestibular schwannomas). These tumors can lead to headaches, vertigo, and various degrees of hearing loss. Schwannomas may occur in any cranial nerve. The criteria used to establish the diagnosis are (1) the presence of bilateral schwannomas, (2) the combination of a first-degree relative with type II neurofibromatosis and a unilateral vestibular schwannoma, or (3) a first-degree relative with type II neurofibromatosis and any two of the following tumors: neurofibroma, glioma,

CUTANEOUS MANIFESTATIONS OF NEUROFIBROMATOSIS

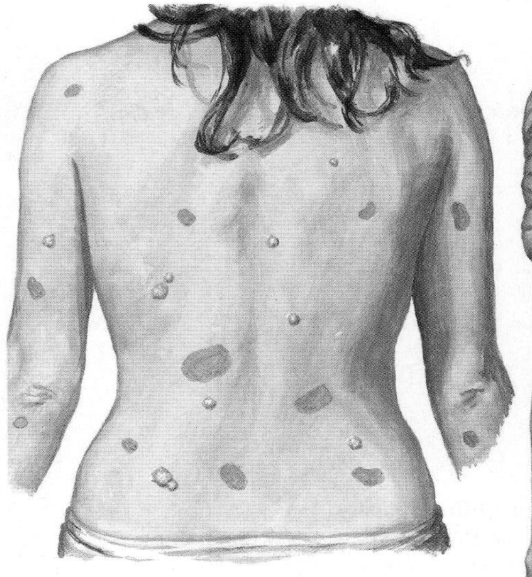

Multiple café-au-lait spots and nodules (fibroma molluscum) are the most common manifestations.

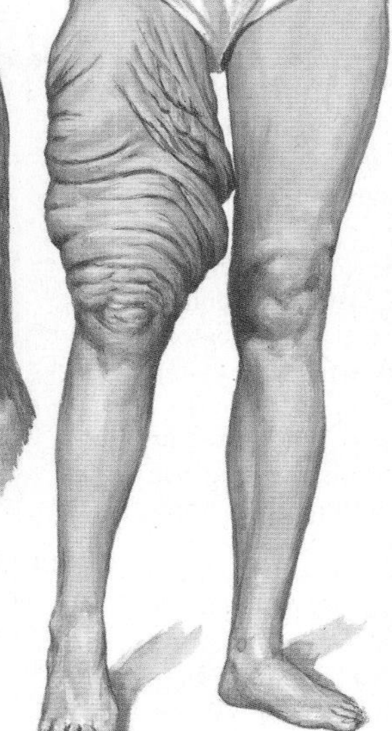

Localized elephantiasis of thigh with redundant skinfolds overlying a plexiform neurofibroma.

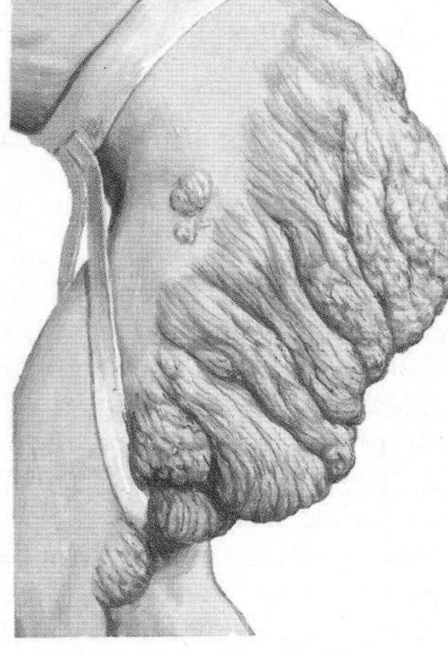

Verrucous hyperplasia. Maceration of velvety-soft skin may cause weeping and infection in crevices overlying a plexiform neurofibroma.

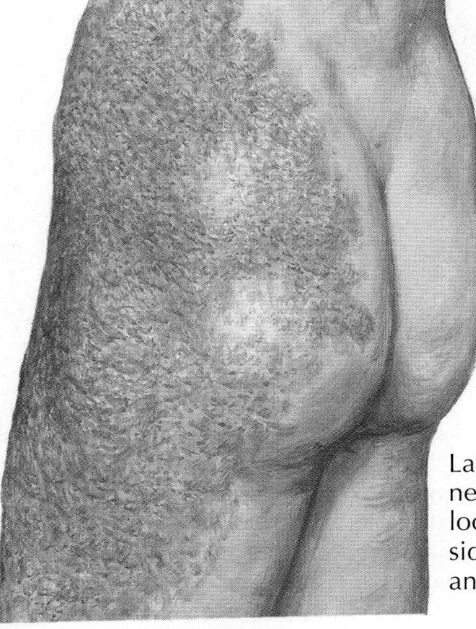

Large plexiform neurofibroma localized to one side of trunk and thigh

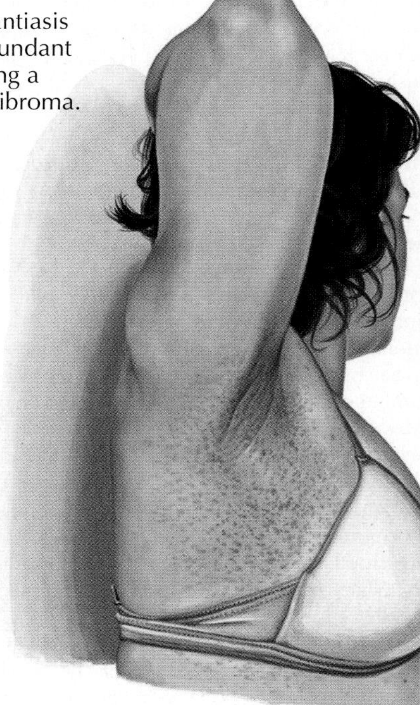

Dense axillary and inguinal freckling is rarely found in the absence of NF1.

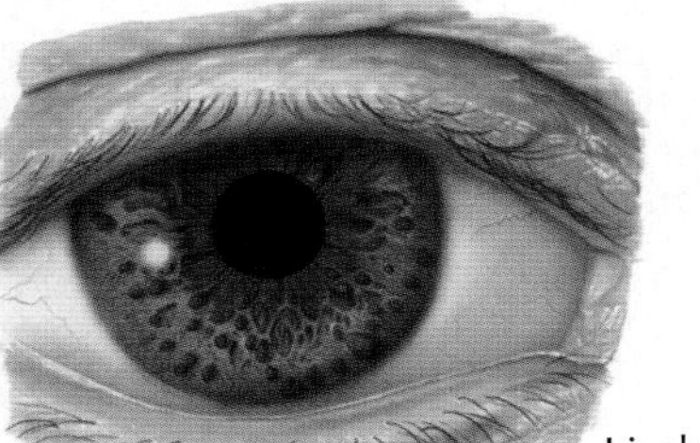

F. Netter M.D.
C. Machado M.D.

Lisch nodules are hamartomas of the iris. They are raised and frequently pigmented.

NEUROFIBROMATOSIS (Continued)

schwannoma, meningioma, or juvenile posterior subcapsular lenticular opacity.

Cutaneous findings in type II neurofibromatosis include neurofibromas and café-au-lait macules. Although both findings are less numerous than in type I neurofibromatosis, most patients have only one or two café-au-lait macules. Cutaneous schwannomas are common in type II disease but are not seen in type I disease. A unique form of cataracts can be seen in neurofibromatosis type II; these are termed *juvenile posterior subcapsular lenticular cataracts.*

Pathogenesis: Type I neurofibromatosis is caused by a mutation in *NF1*. This gene is located on the long arm of chromosome 17 and encodes the protein neurofibromin. Defects in *NF1* are responsible for most cases of neurofibromatosis, making type I the most common type of neurofibromatosis. Because of the large size of *NF1,* many spontaneous mutations occur and result in cases of neurofibromatosis. The neurofibromin protein has been determined to be a tumor suppressor protein. It regulates the *ras* family of protooncogenes. When neurofibromin is defective, the *ras* protooncogene loses its negative regulatory protein and is able to signal continuously.

Type II neurofibromatosis is caused by a genetic defect in the *SCH (NF2)* gene on the long arm of chromosome 22. *NF2* is approximately one-third the size of *NF1*. It encodes the schwannomin (merlin) protein, a tumor suppressor protein that helps act as a go-between in the interactions between the cell cytoskeleton/membrane and the extracellular matrix. Loss of function of the protein results in abnormal cell signaling and unabated cell growth in various tissues.

Histology: Skin biopsies of café-au-lait macules show epidermal hyperpigmentation. There is no increase in the number of melanocytes, and no nevus cells are present. Macromelanosomes can be seen. Neurofibromas can be located within the dermis or subcutaneous tissue. Histologic evaluation shows a well-circumscribed tumor composed of uniform-appearing spindle cells of nerve origin. Special immune histochemical stains can be performed to confirm the nerve derivation of the tumors. Many mast cells are seen intermingled within the spindle cell tumor.

Treatment: Once the diagnosis has been established, patients need lifelong monitoring for the development of various complications related to their disease. Family members should be screened for the disease, and genetic counseling should be offered to affected patients. Adolescents and young adults may benefit from annual physical examinations, and routine ophthalmologic examinations should be recommended. Screening in childhood for the development of scoliosis should be recommended. Patients should be screened for hypertension at each visit because of the increased incidence of pheochromocytoma. Patients with neurofibromatosis are at increased risk for development of malignant transformation of their neurofibromas into neurofibrosarcomas. These rare sarcomas can be located anywhere, and any major change, pain, or growth of a preexisting neurofibroma should make the clinician consider performing a biopsy to rule out malignant degeneration. Optic gliomas are best surgically excised if indicated, though removal of the optic glioma typically results in blindness.

Patients with type II disease should have screening MRI studies of the brain and the rest of the central nervous system to look for schwannomas. Type II disease, because of the presence of bilateral schwannomas, is a much more serious and life-altering disease than type I. The follow-up management of type II neurofibromatosis requires a multidisciplinary approach. Ophthalmology, otolaryngology, neurosurgery, and internal medicine physicians need to coordinate care for these patients. Neurosurgery and localized radiotherapy have been used to treat the brain tumors. Surgical treatment has been the mainstay of therapy for symptomatic plexiform neurofibromas as well as other benign and malignant tumors in neurofibromatosis. Selumetinib, an MEK inhibitor, was the first medicine approved by the US Food and Drug Administration for the treatment of plexiform neurofibromas. It has been shown to decrease the size and pain of symptomatic plexiform neurofibromas. Sirolimus and a plethora of tyrosine kinase inhibitors and other medications are being studied.

Cutaneous and Skeletal Manifestations of Neurofibromatosis

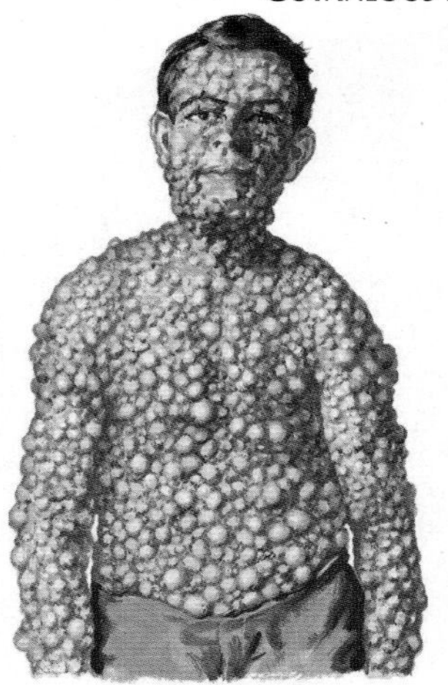

Neurofibromatosis. One of von Recklinghausen's original patients, who had extensive subcutaneous nodules but no neurologic symptoms. Such widespread skin involvement is uncommon.

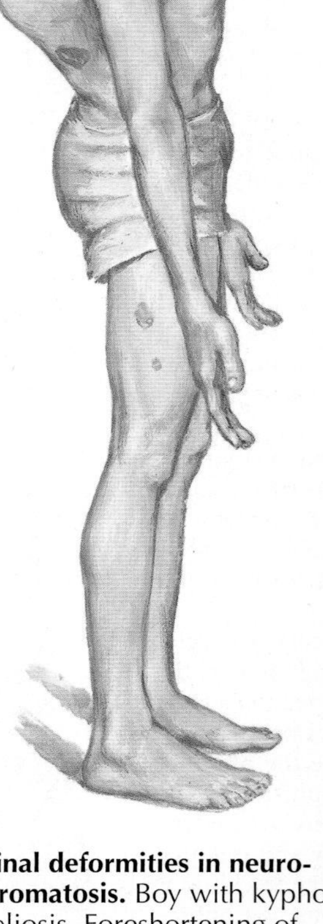

Spinal deformities in neurofibromatosis. Boy with kyphoscoliosis. Foreshortening of trunk secondary to kyphosis gives appearance of longer upper limbs.

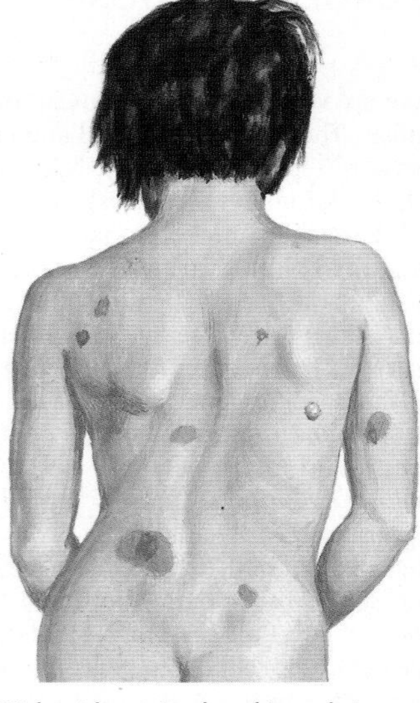

Girl with typical café-au-lait spots but only a few skin nodules. Relatively mild neurofibromatous scoliosis is present.

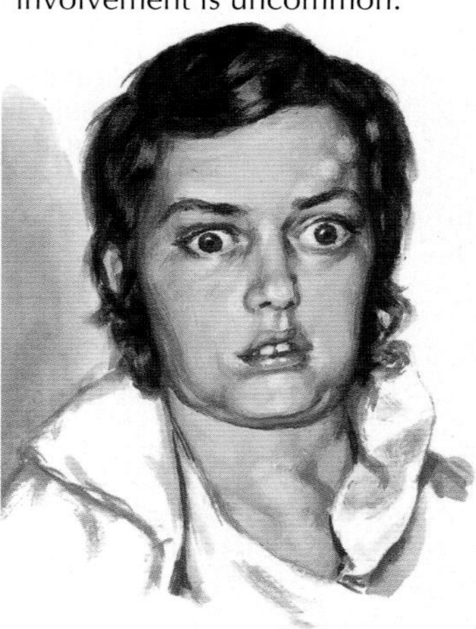

Young woman with bilateral facial palsy. Note drooping of cheeks due to compression of both facial (VII) nerves by acoustic neuromas, which also caused hearing loss. Proptosis resulted from bilateral optic (II) nerve tumors. Subcutaneous nodules developed on her forehead, and masses in her neck compressed the trachea. Disease was fatal in this patient.

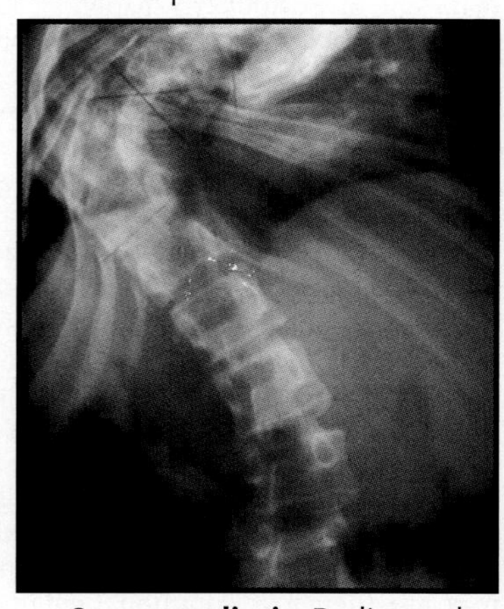

Severe scoliosis. Radiograph shows typical sharp angulation unresponsive to corrective measures, often seen in neurofibromatosis.

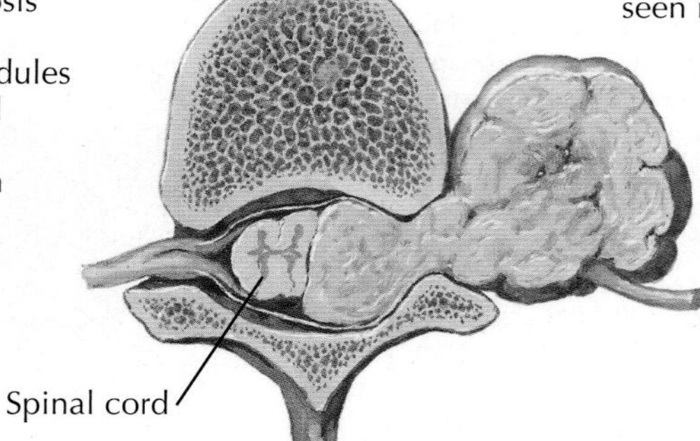

Dumbbell tumor of spinal nerve root

TUBEROUS SCLEROSIS

Tuberous sclerosis (Bourneville syndrome) is a multisystem disease that often manifests with cutaneous findings. It is inherited in an autosomal dominant manner and is directly caused by a defect in one of two genes, *TSC1* or *TSC2*, usually because of a spontaneous mutation. *TSC1* has been shown to encode the hamartin protein, whereas *TSC2* encodes the tuberin protein. The skin, CNS, cardiovascular, respiratory, visual, and musculoskeletal systems are affected. This genodermatosis has an extremely variable phenotype. At one extreme is the severely disabled and intellectually delayed individual with severe seizure disorders; at the other end of the spectrum is the individual with mild skin disease and unappreciable CNS disease.

Clinical Findings: The incidence of tuberous sclerosis is approximately 1 in 10,000, and the disease affects all races and both sexes equally. Infants and young children may present with primary CNS disease with the onset of seizures. All children with new-onset seizures should be evaluated for the cutaneous findings of tuberous sclerosis; if these are located, the child should be further evaluated for the possibility of this diagnosis. Mental delay may be noticeable because the child may not meet normal developmental milestones. Other brain anomalies have been reported to occur in tuberous sclerosis, including astrocytomas, hydrocephalus, cortical tubers, and subependymal tumors. Cardiac rhabdomyomas may manifest with a murmur and are best evaluated with the use of an echocardiogram. In adulthood, the lungs are rarely involved with lymphangiomyomatosis.

Cutaneous findings are often the earliest findings of the disease, even before the onset of CNS disease. The "ash leaf" macule is the first cutaneous finding; it is represented by a hypopigmented to depigmented macule in the shape of an ash leaf. Other hypopigmented macules are prominent components of tuberous sclerosis and include "confetti" macules and polygonal hypopigmented macules. The isolated finding of a hypopigmented macule in infants should trigger an evaluation for the diagnosis of tuberous sclerosis. Approximately 0.25% of normal newborns have a hypopigmented macule with no other evidence of tuberous sclerosis. The pigment alteration is best appreciated with the use of a Wood's light.

Connective tissue nevi are frequently seen in this disease and can manifest as small plaques or dermal nodules. These nevi have been termed "shagreen patches." Skin biopsies are required to diagnose a connective tissue nevus. Koenen tumors, a type of periungual fibroma, are a feature of the disease and can be seen on a solitary digit or on multiple digits of the hands and feet. Café-au-lait macules are occasionally seen. At puberty or slightly before, the presence of facial angiofibromas may become noticeable. These facial tumors tend to increase in size and number over time. They cause significant morbidity and psychological harm to the affected individual. These angiofibromas have been given the name *adenoma sebaceum,* and in some cases they are the initial sign of the disease. They are frequently misdiagnosed as early acne, and only after lack of response to therapy or referral to a dermatologist are they accurately identified. These facial growths cause significant disfigurement, and many individuals seek therapy to lessen the appearance of these tumors.

Pathogenesis: When defective, hamartin and tuberin have been shown to cause tuberous sclerosis. They are both tumor suppressor proteins that function by interacting with a G protein. This interaction inhibits the so-called mammalian target of rapamycin (mTOR) signaling pathway. When these proteins are mutated, the inhibition is removed, and the mTOR pathway is allowed to signal uncontrolled. This leads to unregulated cell division and the production of various tumors.

Treatment: Therapy needs to be individualized for each patient. Those with seizure disorders and CNS tumors require the expertise of a neurologist, neurosurgeon, or both. Antiseizure medications are frequently required for prolonged periods. Routine ophthalmologic examinations should be recommended to evaluate for the possibility of retinal astrocytic hamartomas (phakomas). Facial angiofibromas can be surgically removed by many means. Laser vaporization and more traditional surgical methods have been used to remove or lessen the appearance of these tumors. Topical application of sirolimus, an mTOR inhibitor, has been shown to decrease the size of the facial angiofibromas and the subungual fibromas. No therapy is required for the hypopigmented macules or the connective tissue nevi. All children should have routine physical examinations by their pediatrician and be monitored routinely to ensure they achieve their developmental milestones.

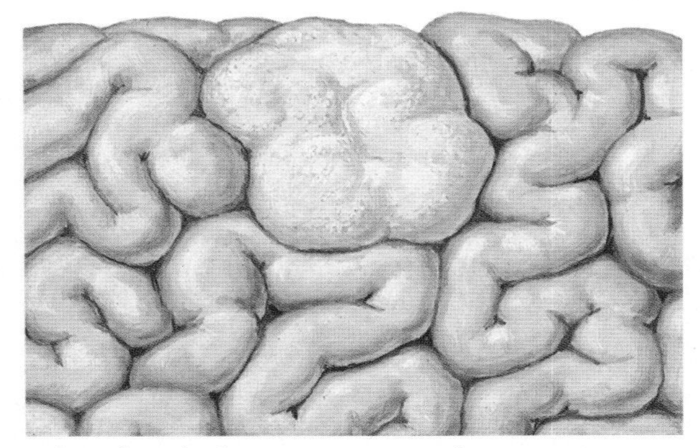

Tuber of cerebral cortex consisting of many astrocytes, scanty nerve cells, and some abnormal sites

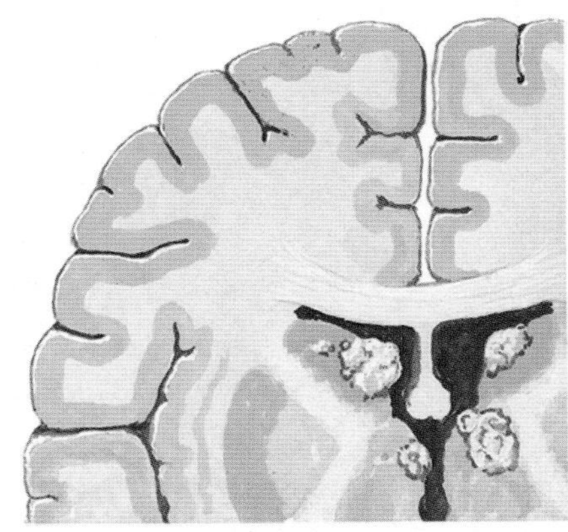

Multiple small tumors. Caudate nucleus and thalamus project into ventricles.

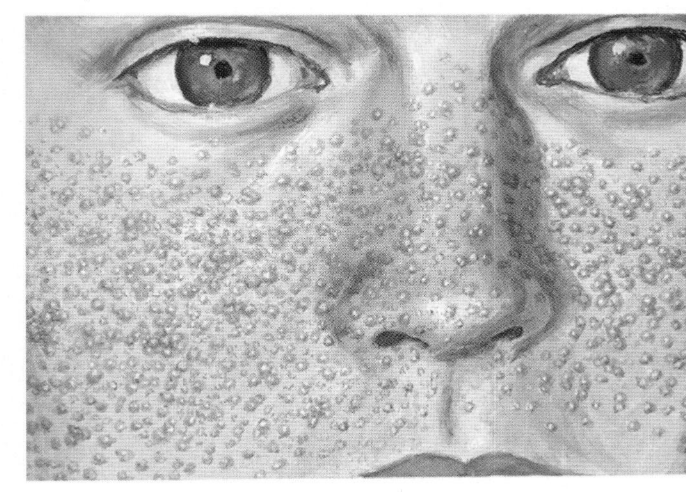

Adenoma sebaceum over both cheeks and bridge of nose

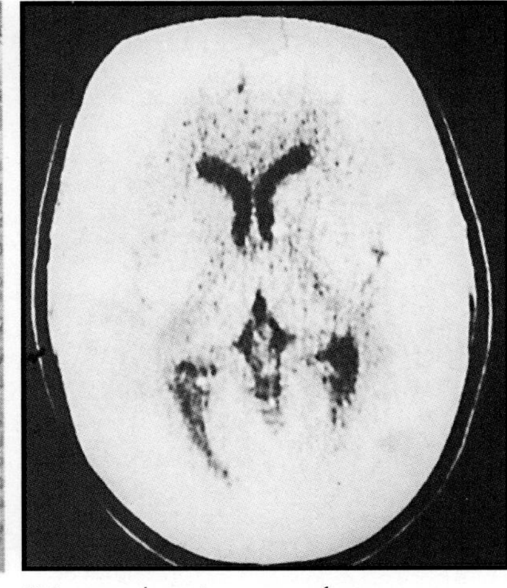

CT scan showing one of many calcified lesions in periventricular area

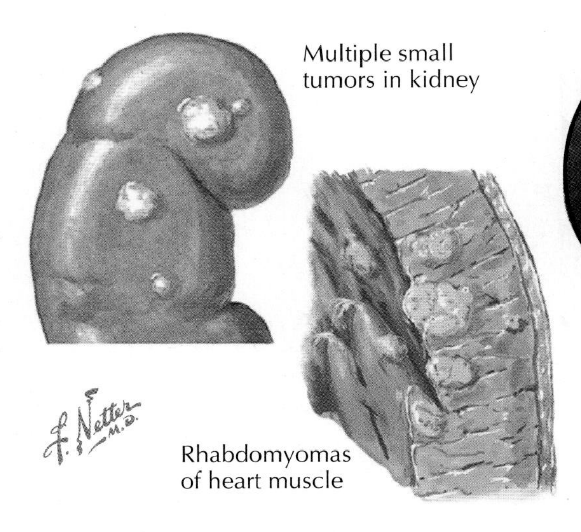

Multiple small tumors in kidney

Rhabdomyomas of heart muscle

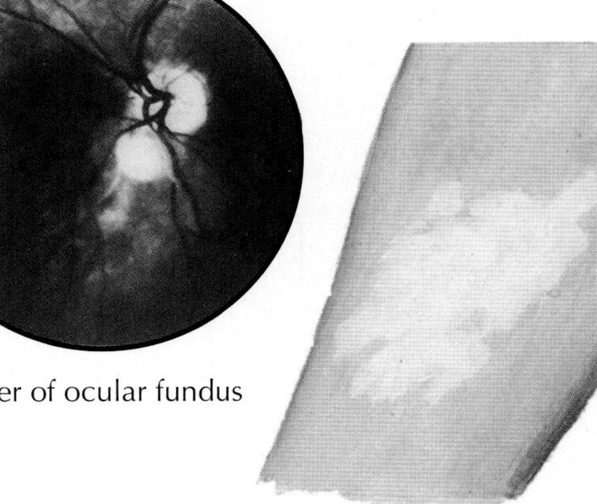

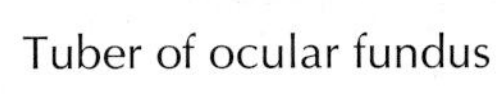

Tuber of ocular fundus

Depigmented skin area

SELECTED REFERENCES

Section 1: Anatomy, Embryology, and Physiology

Anjum F, Manzoor H, et al. Molecular characterization and antibiogram studies of bacterial flora of human facial skin. *Nat Volatiles & Essent Oils*. 2021;8(5):9735-9741.

Bolognia J, Jorizzo JL, Rapini RP. *Dermatology*. 2nd ed. St. Louis: Mosby; 2008.

Elias PM, Hatano Y, Williams ML. Basis for the barrier abnormality in atopic dermatitis: outside-inside-outside pathogenic mechanisms. *J Allergy Clin Immunol*. 2008;121:1337-1343.

James WD, Berger TG, Elston DM. *Andrews' Diseases of the Skin: Clinical Dermatology*. 10th ed. Philadelphia: Saunders; 2006.

Kabashima K, Honda T, Ginhoux F, Egawa G. The immunological anatomy of the skin. *Nat Rev Immunol*. 2019;21:19-30.

Khavkin J, Elis DAF. Aging skin: histology, physiology, and pathology. *Facial Plast Surg Clin North Am*. 2011;19:229-234.

Navarro-Triviño FJ, Arias-Santiago S, Gilaberte-Calzada Y. Vitamin D and the skin: a review for dermatologists. *Actas Dermo-Sifiliográficas*. 2019;110(4):262-272.

Sandilands A, Sutherland C, Irvine AD, McLean WHI. Filaggrin in the frontline: role in skin barrier function and disease. *J Cell Sci*. 2009;122(9):1285-1294.

Saponaro F, Saba A, Zucchi R. An update on vitamin D metabolism. *Int J Mol Sci*. 2020;21:6573.

Som PM, Laitman JT, Mak K. Embryology and anatomy of the skin, its appendages, and physiologic changes in the head and neck. *Neurographics*. 2017;7(5):390-415.

Sorg H, Tilkorn DJ, Hager S, Hauser J, Mirastschijski U. Skin wound healing: an update on the current knowledge and concepts. *Eur Surg Res*. 2017;58:81-94.

Section 2: Benign Growths

Agero AL, Lahmer JJ, Holzborn RM, et al. Naevus of Ota presenting in two generations: a mother and daughter. *J Eur Acad Dermatol Venereol*. 2009;23:102-104.

Arneja JS, Gosain AK. Giant congenital melanocytic nevi. *Plast Reconstr Surg*. 2007;120:26e-40e.

Boon LM, Mulliken JB, Enjolres O, et al. Glomuvenous malformation (glomangioma) and venous malformation: distinct clinicopathologic and genetic entities. *Arch Dermatol*. 2004;140:971-976.

Brodsky J. Management of benign skin lesions commonly affecting the face: actinic keratosis, seborrheic keratosis, and rosacea. *Curr Opin Otolaryngol Head Neck Surg*. 2009;17:315-320.

Ferrari A, Soyer HP, et al. Central white scarlike patch: a dermatoscopic clue for the diagnosis of dermatofibroma. *J Am Acad Dermatol*. 2000; 43(6):1123-1125.

Fink AM, Filz D, Krajnik G, et al. Seborrhoeic keratoses in patients with internal malignancies: a case-control study with prospective accrual of patients. *J Eur Acad Dermatol Venereol*. 2009;23:1316-1319.

Golod O, Soriano T, Craft N. Palisaded encapsulated neuroma—a classic presentation of a commonly misdiagnosed neural tumor. *J Drugs Dermatol*. 2005;4:92-94.

Hafner C, Stoehr R, van Oers JM, et al. The absence of BRAF, FGFR3, PIK3CA mutations differentiates lentigo simplex from melanocytic nevus and solar lentigo. *J Invest Dermatol*. 2009;129:2730-2735.

Hagen R, Kolodney JA, Patterson J, et al. Genetic relationship between pilar cysts, pilar tumors and pilar carcinomas. *J Clin Oncol*. 2019; 37:(15 Suppl):e21063-e21063.

Herranz P, Pizarro A, De Lucas R, et al. High incidence of porokeratosis in renal transplant recipients. *Br J Dermatol*. 1997;136:176-179.

Juckett G, Hartman-Adams H. Management of keloids and hypertrophic scars. *Am Fam Physician*. 2009;80:253-260.

Kapoor S, Gogia S, Paul R, et al. Albright's hereditary osteodystrophy. *Indian J Pediatr*. 2006;73:153-156.

Kim HJ, Lee JY, Kim SH, et al. Stromelysin-3 expression in the differential diagnosis of dermatofibroma and dermatofibrosarcoma protuberans: comparison with factor XIIIa and CD34. *Br J Dermatol*. 2007;157: 319-324.

Liu K, DeAngelo P, Mahmet K, et al. Cytogenetics of neurofibromas: two case reports and literature review. *Cancer Genet Cytogenet*. 2010;196:93-95.

Losee JE, Serletti JM, Pennino RP. Epidermal nevus syndrome: a review and case report. *Ann Plast Surg*. 1999;43:211-214.

Manonukul J, Omeapinyan P, Vongjirad A. Mucoepidermoid (adenosquamous) carcinoma, trichoblastoma, trichilemmoma, sebaceous adenoma, tumor of the follicular infundibulum and syringocystadenoma papilliferum arising within 2 persistent lesions of nevus sebaceous: report of a case. *Am J Dermatopathol*. 2009;31:658-663.

Menascu S, Donner EJ. Linear sebaceous syndrome: case reports and review of the literature. *Pediatr Neurol*. 2008;38:207-210.

Miettinen M, Fetsch JF. Reticulohistiocytoma (solitary epitheloid histiocytoma): a clinicopathologic and immunohistochemical study of 44 cases. *Am J Surg Pathol*. 2006;30:521-528.

Misago N, Kimura T, Narisawa Y. Fibrofolliculoma/trichodiscoma and fibrous papule (perifollicular fibroma/angiofibroma): a reevaluation of the histopathological and immunohistochemical features. *J Cutan Pathol*. 2009;36:943-951.

Mones JM, Ackerman AB. "Atypical" Spitz's nevus, "malignant" Spitz's nevus and "metastasizing" Spitz's nevus: a critique in historical perspective of three concepts flawed fatally. *Am J Dermatopathol*. 2004;26:310-333.

Myers RS, Lo AK, Pawel BR. The glomangioma in the differential diagnosis of vascular malformations. *Ann Plast Surg*. 2006;57:443-446.

Newman MD, Milgraum S. Palisaded encapsulated neuroma (PEN): an often misdiagnosed neural tumor. *Dermatol Online J*. 2008;14:12.

Pandya KA, Radke F. Benign skin lesions: lipomas, epidermal inclusion cysts, muscle and nerve biopsies. *Surg Clin North Am*. 2009;89:677-687.

Person JP, Longcope C. Becker's nevus: an androgen-mediated hyperplasia with increased androgen receptors. *J Am Acad Dermatol*. 1984;10:235-238.

Płachta I, Kleibert M, Czarnecka AM, et al. Current diagnosis and treatment options for cutaneous adnexal neoplasms with apocrine and eccrine differentiation. *Int J Mol Sci*. 2021;22:5077.

Requena C, Requena L, Kutzner H, et al. Spitz nevus: a clinicopathological study of 349 cases. *Am J Dermatopathol*. 2009;31: 107-116.

Saravana GH. Oral pyogenic granuloma: a review of 137 cases. *Br J Oral Maxillofac Surg*. 2009;47:318-319.

Sowa J, Kobayashi H, Ishii M, et al. Histopathologic findings in Unna's nevus suggest it is a tardive congenital nevus. *Am J Dermatopathol*. 2008;30:561-566.

Sperling LC, Sakas EL. Eccrine hidrocystomas. *J Am Acad Dermatol*. 1982;7:763-770.

Spitz JL. *Genodermatosis: A Clinical Guide to Genetic Skin Disorders*. 2nd ed. Philadelphia: Lippincott Williams & Wilkins; 2005.

Stewart L, Glenn GM, Stratton P, et al. Association of germline mutations in the fumarate hydratase gene and uterine fibroids in women with hereditary leiomyomatosis and renal cell cancer. *Arch Dermatol*. 2008;144:1584-1592.

Suzuki H, Anderson RR. Treatment of melanocytic nevi. *Dermatol Ther*. 2005;18:217-226.

Tang S, Hoshida H, Kamisago M, et al. Phenotype-genotype correlation in a patient with co-occurrence of Marfan and LEOPARD syndromes. *Am J Med Genet A*. 2009;149A:2216-2219.

Walsh JJ, Eady JL. Vascular tumors. *Hand Clin*. 2004;20:261-268.

Wang W, Qu M, Xu L, et al. Sorafenib exerts an anti-keloid activity by antagonizing TGF-β/Smad and MAPK/ERK signaling pathways. *J Mol Med (Berl)*. 2016;94(10):1181-1194.

Zaballos P, Blazquez S, Puig S, et al. Dermoscopic pattern of intermediate stage in seborrhoeic keratosis regressing to lichenoid keratosis: report of 24 cases. *Br J Dermatol*. 2007;157:266-272.

Zalaudek I, Hofmann-Wellenhof R, Kittler H, et al. A dual concept of nevogenesis: theoretical considerations based on dermoscopic features of melanocytic nevi. *J Dtsch Dermatol Ges*. 2007;5:985-992.

Zhong Y, Yang B, Huang L, Elias PM, Man MQ. Lasers for Becker's nevus. *Lasers Med Sci*. 2019;34(6):1071-1079

Section 3: Malignant Growths

Abrams TA, Schuetze SM. Targeted therapy for dermatofibrosarcoma protuberans. *Curr Oncol Rep*. 2006;8:291-296.

Aydin F, Senturk N, Sabanciler MT, et al. A case of Ferguson-Smith type multiple keratoacanthomas associated with keratoacanthoma centrifugum marginatum: response to oral acitretin. *Clin Exp Dermatol*. 2007;32:683-686.

Budd GT. Management of angiosarcoma. *Curr Oncol Rep*. 2002;4: 515-519.

Buitrago W, Joseph AK. Sebaceous carcinoma: the great masquerader: emerging concepts in diagnosis and treatment. *Dermatol Ther*. 2008;21:459-466.

Conry RM, Westbrook B, McKee S, et al. Talimogene laherparepvec: first in class oncolytic virotherapy. *Hum Vaccin Immunother*. 2018;14(4):839-846.

Cox NH, Eedy DJ, Morton CA. Guidelines for management of Bowen's disease: 2006 update. *Br J Dermatol*. 2007;156:11-21.

Criscione VD, Weinstock MA, Naylor MF, et al. Actinic keratosis: natural history and risk of malignant transformation in the Veterans Affairs Topical Tretinoin Chemoprevention Trial. *Cancer*. 2009; 115:2523-2530.

De Giorgi V, Salvati L, Barchielli A, et al. The burden of cutaneous adnexal carcinomas and the risk of associated squamous cell carcinoma: a population-based study. *Br J Dermatol*. 2019;180(3): 565-573.

DiLorenzo G. Update on classic Kaposi sarcoma therapy: new look at an old disease. *Crit Rev Oncol Hematol*. 2008;68:242-249.

Dimitropoulos VA. Dermatofibrosarcoma protuberans. *Dermatol Ther*. 2008;21:447-451.

Dubina M, Goldenberg G. Viral-associated nonmelanoma skin cancers: a review. *Am J Dermatopathol*. 2009;31:561-573.

Eisen DB, Michael DJ. Sebaceous lesions and their associated syndromes: part I. *J Am Acad Dermatol*. 2009;61:549-560.

Elder DE, Gimotty PA, Guerry D. Cutaneous melanoma: estimating survival and recurrence risk based on histopathologic features. *Dermatol Ther*. 2005;18:369-385.

Epstein EH. Basal cell carcinomas: attack of the hedgehog. *Nat Rev Cancer*. 2008;8:743-754.

Eroglu Z, Ribnas A. Combination therapy with BRAF and MEK inhibitors for melanoma: latest evidence and place in therapy. *Ther Adv Med Oncol*. 2016;8(1):48-56.

Farley CR, Perez MC, Soelling SJ, et al. Merkel cell carcinoma outcomes: does AJCC8 underestimate survival? *Ann Surg Oncol* 2020;27:1978-1985.

Farzaliyev F, Hamacher R, Steinau HU, et al. Secondary angiosarcoma: a fatal complication of chronic lymphedema. *J Surg Oncol*. 2020;121:85-90.

Gaertner WB, Hagerman GF, Goldberg SM, et al. Perianal Paget's disease treated with wide excision and gluteal skin flap reconstruction: report of a case and review of the literature. *Dis Colon Rectum*. 2008;51:1842-1845.

Goerdt LV, Schneider SW, Booken N. Cutaneous angiosarcomas: molecular pathogenesis guides novel therapeutic approaches. *J German Soc Derm*. 2022;20:1-15.

Gremel G, Rafferty M, Lau TY, et al. Identification and functional validation of therapeutic targets for malignant melanoma. *Crit Rev Oncol Hematol*. 2009;72:194-214.

Hanrahan AJ, Solit DB. BRAF mutations: the discovery of allele- and lineage-specific differences. *Cancer Res*. 2022;82(1):12-14.

Houben R, Schrama D, Becker JC. Molecular pathogenesis of Merkel cell carcinoma. *Exp Dermatol*. 2009;18:193-198.

Kanitakis J. Mammary and extramammary Paget's disease. *J Eur Acad Dermatol Venereol*. 2007;21:581-590.

Kirkwood JM, Jukic DM, Averbook BJ, et al. Melanoma in pediatric, adolescent and young adults. *Semin Oncol*. 2009;36:419-431.

Lansigan F, Foss FM. Current and emerging treatment strategies for cutaneous T-cell lymphoma. *Drugs*. 2010;70:273-286.

Larkin J, Chiarion-Sileni V, Gonzalez R, et al. Combined nivolumab and ipilimumab or monotherapy in untreated melanoma. *N Engl J Med*. 2015;373:23-34.

Liao PB. Merkel cell carcinoma. *Dermatol Ther*. 2008;21:447-451.

Llombart B, Serra C, Requena C, et al. Guidelines for diagnosis and treatment of cutaneous sarcomas: dermatofibrosarcoma protuberans. *Actas Dermo-Sifiliográficas*. 2018;109(10):868-877.

Lookingbill DP, Spangler N, Helm KF. Cutaneous metastases in patients with metastatic carcinoma: a retrospective study of 4020 patients. *J Am Acad Dermatol*. 1993;29:228-236.

Mendenhall WM, Mendenhall CM, Werning JW, et al. Cutaneous angiosarcoma. *Am J Clin Oncol*. 2006;29:524-528.

Migden M, Farberg AS, Dummer R, et al. A review of hedgehog inhibitors sonidegib and vismodegib for treatment of advanced basal cell carcinoma. *J Drugs Dermatol*. 2021;20(2):156-165.

Ntomouchtsis A, Vahtsesevanos K, Patrikidou A, et al. Adnexal skin carcinomas of the face. *J Craniofac Surg*. 2009;20:134-137.

O'Connell KA, Okhovat JP, Zeitouni NC. Photodynamic therapy for Bowen's disease (squamous cell carcinoma in situ) current review and update. *Photodiag Photodyn Ther*. 2018;24:109-114.

Owen JL, Kibbi N, Worley B, et al. Sebaceous carcinoma: evidence-based clinical practice guidelines. *Lancet Oncol*. 2019;20(12): e699-e714.

Paradisi A, Abeni D, Rusciani A, et al. Dermatofibrosarcoma protuberans: wide local excision vs. Mohs micrographic surgery. *Cancer Treat Rev*. 2008;34:728-736.

Robert C, Schachter J, Long GV, et al. Pembrolizumab versus ipilimumab in advanced melanoma. *N Engl J Med*. 2015;372:2521-2532.

Serrone L, Zeuli M, Sega FM, et al. Dacarbazine-based chemotherapy for metastatic melanoma: thirty-year experience overview. *J Exp Clin Cancer Res*. 2000;19(1):21-34.

Shalin SC, Lyle S, Calonje E, et al. Sebaceous neoplasia and the Muir-Torre syndrome: important connections with clinical implications. *Histopathology*. 2010;56:133-147.

Simonds RM, Segal RJ, Sharma A. Extramammary Paget's disease: a review of the literature. *Int J Dermatol*. 2019;58(8):871-879.

Telfer NR, Clover GB, Morton CA. Guidelines for the management of basal cell carcinoma. *Br J Dermatol*. 2008;159:35-48.

Valantin MA, Royston L, Hentzien M, et al. Therapeutic perspectives in the systemic treatment of Kaposi's sarcoma. *Cancers*. 2022;14(3):484.

Vergilis-Kalner IJ, Kriseman Y, Goldberg LH. Keratoacanthomas: overview and comparison between Houston and Minneapolis experiences. *J Drugs Dermatol*. 2010;9:117-121.

Weinberg AS, Ogle CA, Shim EK. Metastatic cutaneous squamous cell carcinoma: an update. *Dermatol Surg*. 2007;33:885-899.

Yu F, Finn DT, Rogers GS. Microcystic adnexal carcinoma: a rare locally aggressive cutaneous tumor. *Am J Clin Oncol*. 2010;33: 196-197.

Zinzani PL, Ferreri AJM, Cerroni L. Mycosis fungoides. *Crit Rev Oncol Hematol*. 2008;65:172-182.

Section 4: Rashes

Abla O, Egeler RM, Weitzman S. Langerhans cell histiocytosis: current concepts and treatments. *Cancer Treat Rev*. 2010;36:354-359.

Adelborg K, Larsen JB, Hvas AM. Disseminated intravascular coagulation: epidemiology, biomarkers, and management. *Br J Haematol*. 2021;192(5):803-818.

Ahdout J, Haley JC, Chiu MW. Erythema multiforme during anti-tumor necrosis factor treatment for plaque psoriasis. *J Am Acad Dermatol*. 2010;62:874-879.

Ahmadi S, Powell FC. Pruritic urticarial papules and plaques of pregnancy: current status. *Australas J Dermatol*. 2005;46:53-58.

Akin C, Valent P, Escribano L. Urticaria pigmentosa and mastocytosis: the role of immunophenotyping in diagnosis and determining response to treatment. *Curr Allergy Asthma Rep*. 2006;6:282-288.

Ale IS, Maibacht HA. Diagnostic approach in allergic and irritant contact dermatitis. *Expert Rev Clin Immunol*. 2010;6:291-310.

Al Hammadi A, Asai Y, Patt ML, et al. Erythema annulare centrifugum secondary to treatment with finasteride. *J Drugs Dermatol*. 2007;6:460-463.

Alikhan A, Kurek L, Feldman SR. The role of tetracyclines in rosacea. *Am J Clin Dermatol*. 2010;11:79-87.

Al-Mahfoudh R, Clark S, Buxton N. Alkaptonuria presenting with ochronotic spondyloarthropathy. *Br J Neurosurg*. 2008;22:805-807.

Antia C, Baquerizo K, Korman A, et al. Urticaria: a comprehensive review: treatment of chronic urticaria, special populations, and disease outcomes. *J Am Acad Dermatol*. 2018;79(4):617-633.

Antonelli A, Ferrari SM, Ragusa F, et al. Graves' disease: epidemiology, genetic and environmental risk factors and viruses. *Best Pract Res Clin Endocrinol Metab*. 2020;34(1):101387.

Antoniu SA. Targeting the TNF-alpha pathway in sarcoidosis. *Expert Opin Ther Targets*. 2010;14:21-29.

Aractingi S, Chosidow O. Cutaneous graft-versus-host disease. *Arch Dermatol*. 1998;134:602-612.

Arias-Santiago S, Aneiros-Fernandez J, Girón-Prieto MS, et al. Palpable purpura. *Cleve Clin J Med*. 2010;77:205-206.

Armstrong AW, Read C. Pathophysiology, clinical presentation, and treatment of psoriasis: a review. *JAMA*. 2020;323(19):1945-1960.

Avena-Woods C. Overview of atopic dermatitis. *Am J Manag Care*. 2017;23(8 Suppl)l:S115-S123.

Badea I, Taylor M, Rosenberg A, et al. Pathogenesis and therapeutic approaches for improved topical treatment in localized scleroderma and systemic sclerosis. *Rheumatology*. 2009;48:213-221.

Bandino JP, Wohltmann WE, Bray DW, et al. Naproxen-induced generalized bullous fixed drug eruption. *Dermatol Online J*. 2009;15:4.

Bechara FG, Podda M, Prens EP, et al. Efficacy and safety of adalimumab in conjunction with surgery in moderate to severe hidradenitis suppurativa: the SHARPS randomized clinical trial. *JAMA Surg*. 2021;156(11):1001-1009.

Ben-Amitai D, Metzker A, Cohen HA. Pediatric cutaneous mastocytosis: a review of 180 patients. *Isr Med Assoc J*. 2005;7:320-322.

Bergqvist C, Ezzedine K. Vitiligo: A focus on pathogenesis and its therapeutic implications. *J Dermatol*. 2021;48:252-270.

Beyens A, Boel A, Symoens S, et al. Cutis laxa: a comprehensive overview of clinical characteristics and pathophysiology. *Clinical Genetics*. 2020;99(1):53-66.

Bieber T, Novak N. Pathogenesis of atopic dermatitis: new developments. *Curr Allergy Asthma Rep*. 2009;9:291-294.

Blair JE. State-of-the-art treatment of coccidioidomycosis: skin and soft-tissue infections. *Ann N Y Acad Sci*. 2007;1111:411-421.

Boch K, Langan EA, Khalaf K. Lichen planus. *Front Med*. 2021:8.

Boguniewicz M, Leung DY. Recent insights into atopic dermatitis and implications for management of infectious complications. *J Allergy Clin Immunol*. 2010;125:4-13.

Boissan M, Feger F, Guillosson J, et al. c-Kit and c-kit mutations in mastocytosis and other hematological diseases. *J Leukoc Biol*. 2000;67:135-148.

Borda LJ, Wikramanayake TC. Seborrheic dermatitis and dandruff: a comprehensive review. *J Clin Investig Dermatol*. 2015;3(2):10.

Brahimi N, Routier E, Raison-Peyron N, et al. A three-year-analysis of fixed drug eruptions in hospital settings in France. *Eur J Dermatol*. 2010;20:461-464.

Brickman WJ, Huang J, Silverman BL, et al. Acanthosis nigricans identifies youth at high risk for metabolic abnormalities. *J Pediatr*. 2010;156:87-92.

Buck T, González LM, Lambert WC, et al. Sweet's syndrome with hematologic disorders: a review and reappraisal. *Int J Dermatol*. 2008;47:775-782.

Buyon JP, Clancy RM, Friedman DM. Cardiac manifestations of neonatal lupus erythematosus: guidelines to management, integrating clues from the bench and bedside. *Nat Clin Pract Rheumatol*. 2009;5:139-148.

Camelo-Piragua S, Zambrano E, Pantanowitz L. Langerhans cell histiocytosis. *Ear Nose Throat J*. 2010;89:112-113.

Carlson JA. The histological assessment of cutaneous vasculitis. *Histopathology*. 2010;56:3-23.

Chang KL, Snyder DS. Langerhans cell histiocytosis. *Cancer Treat Res*. 2008;142:383-398.

Chassaing N, Martin L, Calvas P, et al. Pseudoxanthoma elasticum: a clinical, pathophysiological and genetic update including 11 novel ABCC6 mutations. *J Med Genet*. 2005;42:881-892.

Chasset F, Francès C. Current concepts and future approaches in the treatment of cutaneous lupus erythematosus: a comprehensive review. *Drugs*. 2019;79:1199-1215.

Chen YJ, Wu CY, Huang YL, et al. Cancer risks of dermatomyositis and polymyositis: a nationwide cohort study in Taiwan. *Arthritis Res Ther*. 2010;12:R70.

Chu C, Marks JG Jr, Flamm A. Occupational contact dermatitis: common occupational allergens. *Dermatol Clin*. 2020;38(3):339-349.

Clark SC, Zirwas MJ. Management of occupational dermatitis. *Dermatol Clin*. 2009;27:365-383.

Cohen PR. Neutrophilic dermatoses: a review of current treatment options. *Am J Clin Dermatol*. 2009;10:301-312.

Cohen PR. Sweet's syndrome-a comprehensive review of an acute febrile neutrophilic dermatosis. *Orphanet J Rare Dis*. 2007;26:34.

Cox V, Lesesky EB, Garcia BD, et al. Treatment of juvenile pityriasis rubra pilaris with etanercept. *J Am Acad Dermatol*. 2008;59(Suppl 5):S113-S114.

Crispín JC, Liossis SN, Kis-Toth K, et al. Pathogenesis of human systemic lupus erythematosus: recent advances. *Trends Mol Med*. 2010;16:47-57.

Crowson AN, Mihm MC Jr, Magro CM. Cutaneous vasculitis: a review. *J Cutan Pathol*. 2003;30:161-173.

Dahl M. Granuloma annulare: long-term follow up. *Arch Dermatol*. 2007;143:946-947.

Das A, Datta D, Kassir M, et al. Acanthosis nigricans: a review. *J Cosmet Dermatol*. 2020;19(8):1857-1865.

Das AM, Naim HY. Biochemical basis of Fabry disease with emphasis on mitochondrial function and protein trafficking. *Adv Clin Chem*. 2009;49:57-71.

da Silva Santos PS, Fontes A, Andrade F, et al. Gingival leukemic infiltration as the first manifestation of acute myeloid leukemia. *Otolaryngol Head Neck Surg*. 2010;143:465-466.

Deeg HJ, Antin JH. The clinical spectrum of acute graft-versus-host disease. *Semin Hematol*. 2006;43:24-31.

DeWane ME, Waldman R, Lu J. Dermatomyositis: clinical features and pathogenesis. *J Am Acad Dermatol*. 2020;82(2):267-281.

Díaz-Pérez JL, De Lagrán ZM, Díaz-Ramón JL, et al. Cutaneous polyarteritis nodosa. *Semin Cutan Med Surg*. 2007;26:77-86.

Domm JM, Wootton SK, Medin JA, et al. Gene therapy for Fabry disease: progress, challenges, and outlooks on gene-editing. *Mol Genet Metab*. 2021;134(1-2):117-131.

Drago F, Rebora A. Treatments for pityriasis rosea. *Skin Therapy Lett*. 2009;14:6-7.

Drent M, Crouser ED, Grunewald J. Challenges of sarcoidosis and its management. *N Engl J Med*. 2021;385:1018-1032.

Dubrey SW, Falk RH. Diagnosis and management of cardiac sarcoidosis. *Prog Cardiovasc Dis*. 2010;52:336-346.

Egeler RM, van Halteren AG, Hogendoorn PC, et al. Langerhans cell histiocytosis: fascinating dynamics of the dendritic cell-macrophage lineage. *Immunol Rev*. 2010;234:213-232.

Eisendle K, Zelger B. The expanding spectrum of cutaneous borreliosis. *G Ital Dermatol Venereol*. 2009;144:157-171.

Eisman S, Sinclair R. Pityriasis rosea. *Br Med J*. 2015;351.

Elewski BE. Safe and effective treatment of seborrheic dermatitis. *Cutis*. 2009;83:333-338.

Elston DM. Tick bites and skin rashes. *Curr Opin Infect Dis*. 2010;23:132-138.

Elston DM. What's eating you? Chiggers. *Cutis*. 2006;77:350-352.

Esler-Brauer L, Rothman I. Tender nodules on the palms and soles: palmoplantar eccrine hidradenitis. *Arch Dermatol*. 2007;143:1201-1206.

Espírito Santo J, Gomes MF, Gomes MJ, et al. Intravenous immunoglobulin in lupus panniculitis. *Clin Rev Allergy Immunol*. 2010;38:307-318.

Farasat S, Aksentijevich I, Toro J. Autoinflammatory diseases: clinical and genetic advances. *Arch Dermatol*. 2008;144:392-402.

Ferreira M, Sanches M, Lobo I, et al. Alkaptonuric ochronosis. *Eur J Dermatol*. 2007;17:336-337.

Finger RP, Charbel Issa P, Ladewig MS, et al. Pseudoxanthoma elasticum: genetics, clinical manifestations and therapeutic approaches. *Surv Ophthalmol*. 2009;54:272-285.

Florez-Pollack S, Kunzler E, Jacobe HT. Morphea: current concepts. *Clin Dermatol*. 2018;36(4):475-486.

Fraticelli P, Benfaremo D, Gabrielli A. Diagnosis and management of leukocytoclastic vasculitis. *Intern Emerg Med*. 2021;16:831-841.

Frazier W, Bhardwaj N. Atopic dermatitis: diagnosis and treatment. *Am Fam Physician*. 2020;101(10):590-598.

Fred HL, Accad M. Images in clinical medicine. Lipemia retinalis. *N Engl J Med*. 1999;340:1969.

French LE (ed). Adverse cutaneous drug eruptions. *Chem Immunol Allergy*. 2012;97:106-121.

Frisoli, ML, Essien K, Harris JE. Vitiligo: mechanisms of pathogenesis and treatment. *Annu Rev Immunol*. 2020;38:621-648.

Funabiki M, Tanioka M, Miyachi Y, et al. Sudden onset of calciphylaxis: painful violaceous livedo in a patient with peritoneal dialysis. *Clin Exp Dermatol*. 2009;34:622-624.

Gendernalik SB, Galeckas KJ. Fixed drug eruptions: a case report and review of the literature. *Cutis*. 2009;84:215-219.

Grönhagen CM, Nyberg F. Cutaneous lupus erythematosus: an update. *Indian Dermatol Online J*. 2014;5(1):7-13.

Gupta N, Phadke SR. Cutis laxa type II and wrinkly skin syndrome: distinct phenotypes. *Pediatr Dermatol*. 2006;23:225-230.

Habeshian KA, Cohen BA. Current issues in the treatment of acne vulgaris. *Pediatrics*. 2020;145(Suppl 2):S225-S230.

Hacihamdioglu B, Ozcan A, Kalman S. Subcutaneous granuloma annulare in a child: a case report. *Clin Pediatr*. 2008;47:306-308.

Hamilton BK. Updates in chronic graft-versus-host disease. *Hematology*. 2021;(1):648-654.

Häusermann P, Walter RB, Halter J, et al. Cutaneous graft-versus-host disease: a guide for the dermatologist. *Dermatology*. 2008;216:287-304.

Hazel K, O'Connor A. Emerging treatments for inflammatory bowel disease. *Ther Adv Chronic Dis*. 2020;11:1-12.

Heath MS, Ortega-Loayza AG. Insights into the pathogenesis of Sweet's syndrome. *Front Immunol*. 2019;12(10):414.

Heffernan MP. Combining traditional systemic and biological therapies for psoriasis. *Semin Cutan Med Surg*. 2010;29:67-69.

Hengstman GJ, van den Hoogen FH, van Engelen BG. Treatment of the inflammatory myopathies: update and practical recommendations. *Expert Opin Pharmacother*. 2009;10:1183-1190.

Herbert CR, Russo GG. Polyarteritis nodosa and cutaneous polyarteritis nodosa. *Skinmed*. 2003;2:277-285.

Higgins SP, Freemark M, Prose NS. Acanthosis nigricans: a practical approach to evaluation and management. *Dermatol Online J*. 2008;14:2.

Hoesly FJ, Huerter CJ, Shehan JM. Purpura annularis telangiectodes of Majocchi: case report and review of the literature. *Int J Dermatol*. 2009;48:1129-1133.

Hoffmann B. Fabry disease: recent advances in pathology, diagnosis, treatment and monitoring. *Orphanet J Rare Dis*. 2009;4:21.

Hoffman HM. Therapy of autoinflammatory syndromes. *J Allergy Clin Immunol*. 2009;124:1129-1138.

Hosaka H, Ohtoshi S, Nakada T, et al. Erythema multiforme, Stevens-Johnson syndrome and toxic epidermal necrolysis: frozen-section diagnosis. *J Dermatol*. 2010;37:407-412.

Hossani-Madani AR, Halder RM. Topical treatment and combination approaches for vitiligo: new insights, new developments. *G Ital Dermatol Venereol*. 2010;145:57-78.

Hymes SR, Turner ML, Champlin RE, et al. Cutaneous manifestations of chronic graft-versus-host disease. *Biol Blood Marrow Transplant*. 2006;12:1101-1113.

Hymes SR, Strom EA, Fife C. Radiation dermatitis: clinical presentation, pathophysiology, and treatment. *J Am Acad Dermatol*. 2006;54:28-46.

Ishiguro N, Kawashima M. Cutaneous polyarteritis nodosa: a report of 16 cases with clinical and histopathological analysis and a review of the published work. *J Dermatol*. 2010;37:85-93.

Janmohamed SR, Madern GC, de Laat PCJ, et al. Educational paper: pathogenesis of infantile hemangioma, an update 2014 (part I). *Eur J Pediatr*. 2014;174:97-103.

Joshi TP, Duvic M. Granuloma annulare: an updated review of epidemiology, pathogenesis, and treatment options. *Am J Clin Dermatol*. 2020;23:37-50.

Kanazawa N, Furukawa F. Autoinflammatory syndromes with a dermatological perspective. *J Dermatol*. 2007;34:601-618.

Karadag O, Jayne DJ. Polyarteritis nodosa revisited: a review of historical approaches, subphenotypes and a research agenda. *Clin Exp Rheumatol*. 2018;36:S135-S142.

Katoh N. Future perspectives in the treatment of atopic dermatitis. *J Dermatol*. 2009;36:367-376.

Kazandjieva J, Tsankov N. Drug-induced acne. *Clin Dermatol*. 2017;35(2):156-162.

Kennedy Carney C, Cantrell W, Elewski BE. Rosacea: a review of current topical, systemic and light-based therapies. G Ital Dermatol Venereol. 2009;144:673-688.

Khan IJ, Azam NA, Sullivan SC, et al. Necrobiotic xanthogranuloma successfully treated with a combination of dexamethasone and oral cyclophosphamide. *Can J Ophthalmol*. 2009;44:335-336.

Khanna S, Reed AM. Immunopathogenesis of juvenile dermatomyositis. *Muscle Nerve*. 2010;41:581-592.

King CS, Kelly W. Treatment of sarcoidosis. *Dis Mon*. 2009;55:704-718.

Kiss JE. Thrombotic thrombocytopenic purpura: recognition and management. *Int J Hematol*. 2010;91:36-45.

Klein A, Landthaler M, Karrer S. Pityriasis rubra pilaris: a review of diagnosis and treatment. *Am J Clin Dermatol*. 2010;11:157-170.

Knowles S, Shear NH. Clinical risk management of Stevens-Johnson syndrome/toxic epidermal necrolysis spectrum. *Dermatol Ther*. 2009;22:441-451.

Kok K, Zwiers KC, Boot RG, Overkleeft HS, Aerts JMFG, Artola M. Fabry disease: molecular basis, pathophysiology, diagnostics and potential therapeutic directions. *Biomolecules*. 2021;11(2):271.

Krawczyk M, Mykala-Ciesla J, Kolodziej-Jaskula A. Acanthosis nigricans as a paraneoplastic syndrome. Case reports and review of literature. *Pol Arch Med Wewn*. 2009;119:180-183.

Krowchuk DP, Frieden IJ, Mancini AJ, et al. Infantile hemangiomas. *Pediatrics*. 2019;143(1):e20183475.

Kumar R, Das A, Das S. Management of Stevens-Johnson syndrome—toxic epidermal necrolysis: looking beyond guidelines! *Indian J Dermatol*. 2018;63(2):117-124.

Kung AC, Stephens MB, Darling T. Phytophotodermatitis: bulla formation and hyperpigmentation during spring break. *Mil Med*. 2009;174:657-661.

Kwaku MP, Burman KD. Myxedema coma. *J Intensive Care Med*. 2007;22:224-231.

Langley RGB, Krueger GG, Griffiths CEM. Psoriatic arthritis and psoriasis: classifications, clinical features, pathophysiology, immunology, genetics. *Ann Rheum Dis*. 2005;64:18-23.

Larsen S, Bendtzen K, Nielsen OH. Extraintestinal manifestations of inflammatory bowel disease: epidemiology, diagnosis, and management. *Ann Med*. 2010;42:97-114.

Laube S, Moss C. Pseudoxanthoma elasticum. *Arch Dis Child*. 2005; 90:754-756.

Laufer F. The treatment of progressive pigmented purpura with ascorbic acid and a bioflavonoid rutoside. *J Drugs Dermatol*. 2006;5:290-293.

Lause M, Kamboj A, Fernandez-Faith E. Dermatologic manifestations of endocrine disorders. *Transl Pediatr*. 2017;6(4):300-312.

Lavogiez C, Delaporte E, Darras-Vercambre S, et al. Clinicopathological study of 13 cases of squamous cell carcinoma complicating hidradenitis suppurativa. *Dermatology*. 2010;220:147-153.

Leask A. Signaling in fibrosis: targeting the TGF beta, endothelin-1 and CCN2 axis in scleroderma. *Front Biosci*. 2009;1:115-122.

Lee DY, Lee JH. Epidermal grafting for vitiligo: a comparison of cultured and noncultured grafts. *Clin Exp Dermatol*. 2010;35:325-326.

Lee LA. The clinical spectrum of neonatal lupus. *Arch Dermatol Res*. 2009;301:107-110.

Lee WJ, Kim CH, Chang SE, et al. Generalized idiopathic neutrophilic eccrine hidradenitis in childhood. *Int J Dermatol*. 2010;49:75-78.

Lepe K, Riley CA, Salazar FJ. Necrobiosis lipoidica. [Updated 2021 Aug 26]. In: StatPearls. Treasure Island (FL): StatPearls Publishing; 2022.

Levi M. Disseminated intravascular coagulation in cancer patients. *Best Pract Res Clin Haematol*. 2009;22:129-136.

Levy Bencheton A, Pagès F, Berenger JM, et al. Bedbug dermatitis (*Cimex lectularius*). *Ann Dermatol Venereol*. 2010;137:53-55.

Li Q, Jiang Q, Pfendner E, et al. Pseudoxanthoma elasticum: clinical phenotypes, molecular genetics and putative pathomechanisms. *Exp Dermatol*. 2009;18:1-11.

Lim SH, Kim SM, Oh BH, et al. Low-dose ultraviolet A1 phototherapy for treating pityriasis rosea. *Ann Dermatol*. 2009;21:230-236.

Lipozencić J, Wolf R. The diagnostic value of atopy patch testing and prick testing in atopic dermatitis: facts and controversies. *Clin Dermatol*. 2010;28:38-44.

Lo YH, Cheng GS, Huang CC, et al. Efficacy and safety of topical tacrolimus for the treatment of face and neck vitiligo. *J Dermatol*. 2010;37:125-129.

Lolis MS, Bowe WP, Shalita AR. Acne and systemic disease. *Med Clin North Am*. 2009;93:1161-1181.

Lowes MA, Bowcock AM, Krueger JG. Pathogenesis and therapy of psoriasis. *Nature*. 2007;445:866-873.

Luch A. Mechanistic insights on spider neurotoxins. *EXS*. 2010;100: 293-315.

Madan V, Chinoy H, Griffiths CE, et al. Defining cancer risk in dermatomyositis. Part I. *Clin Exp Dermatol*. 2009;34:451-455.

Madrigal-Martínez-Pereda C, Guerrero-Rodríguez V, Guisado-Moya B, et al. Langerhans cell histiocytosis: literature review and descriptive analysis of oral manifestations. *Med Oral Patol Oral Cir Bucal*. 2009;14:E222-E228.

Mammen AL. Dermatomyositis and polymyositis: clinical presentation, autoantibodies, and pathogenesis. *Ann N Y Acad Sci*. 2010;1184: 134-153.

Mana J, Marcoval J. Erythema nodosum. *Clin Dermatol*. 2007;25: 288-294.

Marqueling AL, Gilliam AE, Prendiville J, et al. Keratosis pilaris rubra. A common but underrecognized condition. *Arch Dermatol*. 2006;142:1611-1616.

Martinez-Cibrian N, Zeiser R, Perez-Simon JA. Graft-versus-host disease prophylaxis: pathophysiology-based review on current approaches and future directions. *Blood Reviews*. 2021;48:100792.

Marzano AV, Vezzoli P, Crosti C. Drug-induced lupus: an update on its dermatologic aspects. *Lupus*. 2009;18:935-940.

Mataix J, Betlloch I. Langerhans cell histiocytosis: an update. *G Ital Dermatol Venereol*. 2009;144:119-134.

Matusiak Ł, Bieniek A, Szepietowski JC. Hidradenitis suppurativa markedly decreases quality of life and professional activity. *J Am Acad Dermatol*. 2010;62:706-708.

Matz H, Orion E, Wolf R. Pruritic urticarial papules and plaques of pregnancy: polymorphic eruption of pregnancy (PUPPP). *Clin Dermatol*. 2006;24:105-108.

Mazereeuw-Hautier J, Bezio S, Mahe E, et al. Segmental and nonsegmental childhood vitiligo has distinct clinical characteristics: a prospective observational study. *J Am Acad Dermatol*. 2010;62:945-949.

McDaniel B, Cook C. Erythema annulare centrifugum. [Updated 2021 Aug 27]. In: StatPearls. https://www.ncbi.nlm.nih.gov/books/NBK482494/

McIntosh BC, Lahinjani S, Narayan D. Necrobiosis lipoidica resulting in squamous cell carcinoma. *Conn Med*. 2005;69:401-403.

Mill J, Wallis B, Cuttle L, et al. Phytophotodermatitis: case reports of children presenting with blistering after preparing lime juice. *Burns*. 2008;34:731-733.

Mok CC. Update on emerging drug therapies for systemic lupus erythematosus. *Expert Opin Emerg Drugs*. 2010;15:53-70.

Mold JW, Thompson DM. Management of brown recluse spider bites in primary care. *J Am Board Fam Pract*. 2004;17:347-352.

Morava E, Guillard M, Lefeber DJ, et al. Autosomal recessive cutis laxa syndrome revisited. *Eur J Hum Genet*. 2009;17:1099-1110.

Mosher DB, Parrish JA, Fitzpatrick TB. Monobenzylether of hydroquinone: a retrospective study of treatment of 18 vitiligo patients and a review of the literature. *Br J Dermatol*. 1977;97:669-679.

Musso CG, Enz PA, Guelman R, et al. Non-ulcerating calcific uremic arteriolopathy skin lesion treated successfully with intravenous ibandronate. *Perit Dial Int*. 2006;26:717-718.

Nassau S, Fonacier L. Allergic contact dermatitis. *Med Clin North Am*. 2020;104(1):61-76.

Neogi T. Clinical practice. Gout. *N Engl J Med*. 2011;364:443-452.

Neoh CY, Tan AW, Mohamed K, et al. Characterization of the inflammatory cell infiltrate in herald patches and fully developed eruptions of pityriasis rosea. *Clin Exp Dermatol*. 2010;35:300-304.

Newkirk RE, Fomin DA, Braden MM. Erythema multiforme versus Stevens-Johnson syndrome/toxic epidermal necrolysis: subtle difference in presentation, major difference in management. *Mil Med*. 2020;185(9-10):e1847-e1850.

Ng ES, Aw DC, Tan KB, et al. Neutrophilic eccrine hidradenitis associated with decitabine. *Leuk Res*. 2010;34:e130-e132.

Nigliazzo A, Khoo S, Saxe A. Calciphylaxis. *Am Surg*. 2009;75: 516-518.

Nigwekar SU, Thadhani R, Brandenburg VM. Calciphylaxis. *N Engl J Med*. 2018;378:1704-1714.

Nosbaum A, Vocanson M, Rozieres A, et al. Allergic and irritant contact dermatitis. *Eur J Dermatol*. 2009;19:325-332.

Obradović R, Kesić L, Mihailović D, et al. Malignant transformation of oral lichen planus. A case report. *West Indian Med J*. 2009;58:490-492.

O'Connell S. Lyme borreliosis: current issues in diagnosis and management. *Curr Opin Infect Dis*. 2010;23:231-235.

Ogunbiyi A. Acne keloidalis nuchae: prevalence, impact, and management challenges. *Clin Cosmet Investig Dermatol*. 2016;14(9):483-489.

Oh BH, Lee YW, Choe YB, et al. Epidemiologic study of *Malassezia* yeasts in seborrheic dermatitis patients by the analysis of 26S rDNA PCR-RFLP. *Ann Dermatol*. 2010;22:149-155.

Ong VH, Denton CP. Innovative therapies for systemic sclerosis. *Curr Opin Rheumatol*. 2010;22:264-272.

O'Regan GM, Sandilands A, McLean WHI, Irvine AD. Filaggrin in atopic dermatitis. *J Allergy Clin Immunol*. 2008;122(4):689-693.

Osterne RL, Matos Brito RG, Pacheco IA, et al. Management of erythema multiforme associated with recurrent herpes infection: a case report. *J Can Dent Assoc*. 2009;75:597-601.

Owlia MB, Eley AR. Is the role of Chlamydia trachomatis underestimated in patients with suspected reactive arthritis? *Int J Rheum Dis*. 2010;13:27-38.

Panasiti V, Devirgiliis V, Curzio M, et al. Erythema annulare centrifugum as the presenting sign of breast carcinoma. *J Eur Acad Dermatol Venereol*. 2009;23:318-320.

Panopoulos S, Chatzidionysiou K, Tektonidou, MG, et al. Treatment modalities and drug survival in a systemic sclerosis real-life patient cohort. *Arthritis Res Ther*. 2020;22:56.

Pardanani A, Tefferi A. Systemic mastocytosis in adults: a review on prognosis and treatment based on 342 Mayo Clinic patients and current literature. *Curr Opin Hematol*. 2010;17:125-132.

Parrillo SJ. Stevens-Johnson syndrome and toxic epidermal necrolysis. *Curr Allergy Asthma Rep*. 2007;7:243-247.

Patel K, Nixon R. Irritant contact dermatitis—a review. *Curr Dermatol Rep*. 2022;11(2):41-51.

Pauli I, Puka J, Gubert IC, et al. The efficacy of antivenom in loxoscelism treatment. *Toxicon*. 2006;48(2):123-137.

Pérez-Garza DM, Chavez-Alvarez S, Ocampo-Candiani J, et al. Erythema nodosum: a practical approach and diagnostic algorithm. *Am J Clin Dermatol*. 2021;22(3):367-378.

Pierce J, Patel T, Scott C. Eruptive xanthomas. *Mayo Clin Proc*. 2021; 96(12):3097-3098.

Pitt JJ. Newborn screening. *Clin Biochem Rev*. 2010;31:57-68.

Polańska A, Bowszyc-Dmochowska M, Żaba RW, et al. Elastosis perforans serpiginosa: a review of the literature and our own experience. *Postepy Dermatol Alergol*. 2016;33(5):392-395.

Postlethwaite AE, Harris LJ, Raza SH, et al. Pharmacotherapy of systemic sclerosis. *Expert Opin Pharmacother*. 2010;11:789-806.

Raju S, Hollis K, Neglen P. Use of compression stockings in chronic venous disease: patient compliance and efficacy. *Ann Vasc Surg*. 2007;21:790-795.

Ranque B, Mouthon L. Geoepidemiology of systemic sclerosis. *Autoimmun Rev*. 2010;9:A311-A318.

Raymond CB, Wazny LD, Sood AR. Sodium thiosulfate, bisphosphonates, and cinacalcet for calciphylaxis. *CANNT J*. 2009;19:25-29.

Renner R, Sticherling M. The different faces of cutaneous lupus erythematosus. *G Ital Dermatol Venereol*. 2009;144:135-147.

Rigopoulos D, Larios G, Katsambas AD. The role of isotretinoin in acne therapy: why not as first-line therapy? Facts and controversies. *Clin Dermatol*. 2010;28:24-30.

Rijal A, Agrawal S. Outcome of Stevens Johnson syndrome and toxic epidermal necrolysis treated with corticosteroids. *Indian J Dermatol Venereol Leprol*. 2009;75:613-614.

Rodrigue-Gervais IG, Saleh M. Generics of inflammasome-associated disorders: a lesson in the guiding principles of inflammasome function. *Eur J Immunol*. 2010;40:643-648.

Rodriguez Bandera AI, Sebaratnam DF, Wargon O, et al. Infantile hemangioma. Part 1: epidemiology, pathogenesis, clinical presentation, and assessment. *J Am Acad Dermatol*. 2021;85(6):1379-1392.

Rodriguez-Galindo C, Allen CE. Langerhans cell histiocytosis. *Blood*. 2020;135(16):1319-1331.

Roenneberg S, Biedermann T. Pityriasis rubra pilaris: algorithms for diagnosis and treatment. *JEADV*. 2018;32:889-898.

Ryan C, Menter A, Warren RB. The latest advances in pharmacogenetics and pharmacogenomics in the treatment of psoriasis. *Mol Diagn Ther*. 2010;14:81-93.

Saeki H, Tomita M, Kai H, et al. Necrobiotic xanthogranuloma with paraproteinemia successfully treated with melphalan, prednisolone and skin graft. *J Dermatol*. 2007;34:795-797.

Sălăvăstru C, Tiplica GS. Therapeutic hotline: ulcerative lichen planus—treatment challenges. *Dermatol Ther*. 2010;23:203-205.

Sasseville D. Clinical patterns of phytodermatitis. *Dermatol Clin*. 2009;27:299-308.

Satter EK, High WA. Langerhans cell histiocytosis: a review of the current recommendations of the Histiocyte Society. *Pediatr Dermatol*. 2008; 25:291-295.

Sawamura A, Hayakawa M, Gando S, et al. Disseminated intravascular coagulation with a fibrinolytic phenotype at an early phase of trauma predicts mortality. *Thromb Res*. 2009;124:608-613.

Scheinfeld N. Pruritic urticarial papules and plaques of pregnancy wholly abated with one week twice daily application of fluticasone propionate lotion: a case report and review of the literature. *Dermatol Online J*. 2008;15:14-4.

Scheinfeld N, Berk T. A review of the diagnosis and treatment of rosacea. *Postgrad Med*. 2010;122:139-143.

Schlieper G, Brandenburg V, Ketteler M, et al. Sodium thiosulfate in the treatment of calcific uremic arteriolopathy. *Nat Rev Nephrol*. 2009;5:539-543.

Schmitt SK. Reactive arthritis. *Infect Dis Clin North Am*. 2017;31:265-277.

Schmutz, JL. Neutrophilic eccrine hidradenitis. In: Wallach, D., Vignon-Pennamen, MD., Valerio Marzano, A. (eds) *Neutrophilic Dermatoses*. Springer; 2018.

Scott AT, Metzig AM, Hames RK, et al. Acanthosis nigricans and oral glucose tolerance in obese children. *Clin Pediatr*. 2010;49:69-71.

Sebaratnam DF, Rodriguez Bandera AI, Wong LF, et al. Infantile hemangioma. Part 2: management. *J Am Acad Dermatol*. 2021;85(6): 1395-1404.

Shaw MG, Burkhart CN, Morrell DS. Systemic therapies for pediatric atopic dermatitis: a review for the primary care physician. *Pediatr Ann*. 2009;38:380-387.

Shen Z, Hao F, Wei P. HAIR-AN syndrome in a male adolescent with concomitant vitiligo. *Arch Dermatol*. 2009;145:492-494.

Shimizu S, Yasui C, Shiroshita K, et al. Calciphylaxis with unusual skin manifestations. *Eur J Dermatol*. 2010;20:241-242.

Shinkai K, McCalmont TH, Leslie KS. Cryopyrin-associated periodic syndromes and autoinflammation. *Clin Exp Dermatol*. 2008;33:1-9.

Shiohara T. Fixed drug eruption: pathogenesis and diagnostic tests. *Curr Opin Allergy Clin Immunol*. 2009;9:316-321.

Sierra-Sepúlveda A, Esquinca-González A, Benavides-Suárez SA. Systemic sclerosis pathogenesis and emerging therapies, beyond the fibroblast. *Biomed Res Int*. 2019;2019:1-15.

Silapunt S, Chon SY. Generalized necrobiotic xanthogranuloma successfully treated with lenalidomide. *J Drugs Dermatol*. 2010;9:273-276.

Silver RM, Major H. Maternal coagulation disorders and postpartum hemorrhage. *Clin Obstet Gynecol*. 2010;53:252-264.

Simpson EL. Atopic dermatitis: a review of topical treatment options. *Curr Med Res Opin*. 2010;26:633-640.

Singh JA, Gaffo A. Gout epidemiology and comorbidities. *Semin Arthritis Rheum*. 2020;50(3):S11-S16.

Soter NA. Mastocytosis and the skin. *Hematol Oncol Clin North Am*. 2000;14:537-555.

Sotozono C, Ueta M, Kinoshita S. Systemic and local management at the onset of Stevens-Johnson syndrome and toxic epidermal necrolysis with ocular complications. *Am J Ophthalmol*. 2010; 149:354.

Spałek M. Chronic radiation-induced dermatitis: challenges and solutions. *Clin Cosmet Investig Dermatol*. 2016;9(9):473-482.

Sperling LC, Nguyen JV. Commentary: treatment of lichen planopilaris: some progress, but a long way to go. *J Am Acad Dermatol*. 2010;62: 398-401.

Spicknall KE, Mehregan DA. Necrobiotic xanthogranuloma. *Int J Dermatol*. 2009;48:1-10.

Spigariolo CB, Giacalone S, Nazzaro G. Pigmented purpuric dermatoses: a complete narrative review. *J Clin Med*. 2021;10:2283.

Stefanaki I, Katsambas A. Therapeutic update on seborrheic dermatitis. *Skin Therapy Lett*. 2010;15:1-4.

Steinhelfer L, Kühnel T, Jägle H, et al. Systemic therapy of necrobiotic xanthogranuloma: a systematic review. *Orphanet J Rare Dis*. 2022;17:132.

Szudy-Szczyrek A, Bachanek-Mitura O, Gromek T, et al. Real-world efficacy of midostaurin in aggressive systemic mastocytosis. *J Clin Med*. 2021;10(5):1109.

Takai T, Matsunaga A. A case of neutrophilic eccrine hidradenitis associated with streptococcal infectious endocarditis. *Dermatology*. 2006;212:203-205.

Tchernev G, Patterson JW, Nenoff P, et al. Sarcoidosis of the skin—a dermatological puzzle: important differential diagnostic aspects and guidelines for clinical and histopathological recognition. *J Eur Acad Dermatol Venereol*. 2010;24:125-137.

ThibOutot DM, Fleischer AB, Del Rosso JQ Jr, et al. Azelaic acid 15% gel once daily versus twice daily in papulopustular rosacea. *J Drugs Dermatol.* 2008;7:541-546.
Thiboutot DM, Gollnick H, Bettoli V, et al. New insights into the management of acne: an update from the Global Alliance to Improve Outcomes in Acne Group. *J Am Acad Dermatol.* 2009;60:S1-S50.
Thyssen JP, Johansen JD, Linneberg A, et al. The epidemiology of hand eczema in the general population—prevalence and main findings. *Contact Dermatitis.* 2010;62:75-87.
Tlougan BE, Podjasek JO, Dickman PS, et al. Painful plantar papules and nodules in a child. Palmoplantar eccrine hidradenitis (PEH). *Pediatr Ann.* 2008;37:83-84.
Toh CH, Hoots WK. SSC on disseminated intravascular coagulation of the ISTH. The scoring system of the Scientific and Standardisation Committee on Disseminated Intravascular Coagulation of the International Society on Thrombosis and Haemostasis: a 5-year overview. *J Thromb Haemost.* 2007;5:604-606.
Tsai H. Pathophysiology of thrombotic thrombocytopenic purpura. *Int J Hematol.* 2010;91:1-9.
Uzzan B, Konate L, Diop A, et al. Efficacy of four insect repellents against mosquito bites: a double-blind randomized placebo-controlled field study in Senegal. *Fundam Clin Pharmacol.* 2009;23:589-594.
Valent P, Akin C, Metcalfe DD. Mastocytosis: 2016 updated WHO classification and novel emerging treatment concepts. *Blood.* 2017;129(11):1420-1427.
van Zuuren EJ. Rosacea. *N Engl J Med.* 2017;377:1754-1764.
Ventura F, Vilarinho C, da Luz Duarte M, et al. Two cases of annular elastolytic granuloma: different response to the treatment. *Dermatol Online J.* 2010;16:11.
Vergilis-Kalner IJ, Mann DJ, Wasserman J, et al. Pityriasis rubra pilaris sensitive to narrow band-ultraviolet B light therapy. *J Drugs Dermatol.* 2008;8:270-273.
Villalón G, Martin JM, Monteagudo C, et al. Eruptive xanthomas after onset of diabetes mellitus. *Actas Dermosifiliogr.* 2008;99:426-427.
Vineetha M, Palakkal S, Skaria L, et al. Autoinflammatory syndromes: a review. *J Skin Sex Transm Dis.* 2020;2(1):5-12.
Wada H, Asakura H, Okamoto K, et al. Expert consensus for the treatment of disseminated intravascular coagulation in Japan. Japanese Society of Thrombosis Hemostasis/DIC subcommittee. *Thromb Res.* 2010;125:6-11.
Waldman R, DeWane ME, Lu J. Dermatomyositis: diagnosis and treatment. *J Am Acad Dermatol.* 2020;82(2):283-296.
Walling HW, Sontheimer RD. Cutaneous lupus erythematosus: issues in diagnosis and treatment. *Am J Clin Dermatol.* 2009;10:365-381.
Walling HW, Swick BL. Pityriasis rubra pilaris responding rapidly to adalimumab. *Arch Dermatol.* 2009;145:99-101.
Walton KE, Bowers EV, Drolet BA, et al. Childhood lichen planus: demographics of a U.S. population. *Pediatr Dermatol.* 2010;27:34-38.
Warren RB, Griffiths CE. The future of biological therapies. *Semin Cutan Med Surg.* 2010;29:63-66.
Wedderburn LR, Rider LG. Juvenile dermatomyositis: new developments in pathogenesis, assessment and treatment. *Best Pract Res Clin Rheumatol.* 2009;23:665-678.
Wenzel D, Haddadi NS, Afshari K, et al. Upcoming treatments for morphea. *Immun Inflamm Dis.* 2021;9(4):1101-1145.
Wetter DA, Camilleri MJ. Clinical, etiologic, and histopathologic features of Stevens-Johnson syndrome during an 8-year period at Mayo Clinic. *Mayo Clin Proc.* 2010;85:131-138.
Windebank K, Nanduri V. Langerhans cell histiocytosis. *Arch Dis Child.* 2009;94:904-908.
Wolinsky CD, Waldorf H. Chronic venous disease. *Med Clin North Am.* 2009;93:1333-1346.
Wood AJ, Wagner MV, Abbott JJ, et al. Necrobiotic xanthogranuloma: a review of 17 cases with emphasis on clinical and pathologic correlation. *Arch Dermatol.* 2009;145:279-284.
Yang CC, Shih IH, Lin WL, et al. Juvenile pityriasis rubra pilaris: report of 28 cases in Taiwan. *J Am Acad Dermatol.* 2008;59:943-948.
Yang Y, Xu J, Li F, et al. Combination therapy of intravenous immunoglobulin and corticosteroid in the treatment of toxic epidermal necrolysis and Stevens-Johnson syndrome: a retrospective comparative study in China. *Int J Dermatol.* 2009;48:1122-1128.
Youn SW. The role of facial sebum secretion in acne pathogenesis: facts and controversies. *Clin Dermatol.* 2010;28:8-11.
Zancanaro PC, Isaac AR, Garcia LT, et al. Localized scleroderma in children: clinical, diagnostic and therapeutic aspects. *An Bras Dermatol.* 2009;84:161-172.
Zatkova A, Ranganath L, Kadasi L. Alkaptonuria: current perspectives. *Appl Clin Genet.* 2020;13:37-47.
Ziemer M, Eisendle K, Zelger B. New concepts on erythema annulare centrifugum: a clinical reaction pattern that does not represent a specific clinicopathological entity. *Br J Dermatol.* 2009;160:119-126.

Section 5: Autoimmune Blistering Diseases

Al-Amoudi A, Frangakis AS. Structural studies on desmosomes. *Biochem Soc Trans.* 2008;36(Pt 2):181-187.
Alonso-Llamazares J, Gibson LE, Rogers RS 3rd. Clinical, pathologic, and immunopathologic features of dermatitis herpetiformis: review of the Mayo Clinic experience. *Int J Dermatol.* 2007;46:910-919.
Aryanian Z, Balighi K, Daneshpazhooh M, et al. Rituximab exhibits a better safety profile when used as a first line of treatment for pemphigus vulgaris: a retrospective study. *Int Immunopharmacol.* 2021;96:107755.
Barnadas M, Roe E, Brunet S, et al. Therapy of paraneoplastic pemphigus with rituximab: a case report and review of literature. *J Eur Acad Dermatol Venereol.* 2006;20:69-74.
Baroni A, Lanza A, Cirillo N, et al. Vesicular and bullous disorders: pemphigus. *Dermatol Clin.* 2007;25:597-603.
Bruch-Gerharz D, Hertl M, Ruzicka T. Mucous membrane pemphigoid: clinical aspects, immunopathological features and therapy. *Eur J Dermatol.* 2007;17:191-200.
Caproni M, Antiga E, Melani L, et al. Guidelines for the diagnosis and treatment of dermatitis herpetiformis. *J Eur Acad Dermatol Venereol.* 2009;23:633-638.
Chang JH, McCluskey PJ. Ocular cicatricial pemphigoid: manifestations and management. *Curr Allergy Asthma Rep.* 2005;5:333-338.
Culton DA, Qian Y, Li N, et al. Advances in pemphigus and its endemic pemphigus foliaceus (fogo selvagem) phenotype: a paradigm of human autoimmunity. *J Autoimmun.* 2008;31:311-324.
Daniel E, Thorne JE. Recent advances in mucous membrane pemphigoid. *Curr Opin Ophthalmol.* 2008;19:292-297.
Dart J. Cicatricial pemphigoid and dry eye. *Semin Ophthalmol.* 2005; 20:95-100.
Dasher D, Rubenstein D, Diaz LA. Pemphigus foliaceus. *Curr Dir Autoimmun.* 2008;10:182-194.
Díaz MS, Morita L, Ferrari B, et al. Linear IgA bullous dermatosis: a series of 17 cases. *Actas Dermo-Sifiliográficas.* 2019;110(8): 673-680.
Edgin WA, Pratt TC, Grimwood RE. Pemphigus vulgaris and paraneoplastic pemphigus. *Oral Maxillofac Surg Clin North Am.* 2008;20: 577-584.
Flores G, Qian Y, Díaz LA. The enigmatic autoimmune response in endemic pemphigus foliaceus. *Actas Dermosifiliogr.* 2009;100 (Suppl 2):40-48.
Georgoudis P, Sabatino F, Szentmary N, et al. Ocular mucous membrane pemphigoid: current state of pathophysiology, diagnostics and treatment. *Ophthalmol Ther.* 2019;8:5-17.
Giovanni G, Di Zenzo G, Emanuele C. New insights into the pathogenesis of bullous pemphigoid: 2019 update. *Front Immunol.* 2019;10:1506.
Handler NS, Handler MZ, Stephany MP, et al. Porphyria cutanea tarda: an intriguing genetic disease and marker. *Int J Dermatol.* 2017;56(6):e106-117.
Hernandez L, Green PH. Extraintestinal manifestations of celiac disease. *Curr Gastroenterol Rep.* 2006;8:383-389.
Hingorani M, Lightman S. Ocular cicatricial pemphigoid. *Curr Opin Allergy Clin Immunol.* 2006;6:373-378.
Kasperkiewicz M, Schmidt E. Current treatment of autoimmune blistering diseases. *Curr Drug Discov Technol.* 2009;6:270-280.
Kasperkiewicz M, Zillikens D. The pathophysiology of bullous pemphigoid. *Clin Rev Allergy Immunol.* 2007;33:67-77.
Kharfi M, Khaled A, Karaa A, et al. Linear IgA bullous dermatosis: the more frequent bullous dermatosis of children. *Dermatol Online J.* 2010;16:2.
Kitajima Y. Cross-talk between hemidesmosomes and focal contacts: understanding subepidermal blistering diseases. *J Invest Dermatol.* 2010;130:1493-1496.
Kridin K, Kneiber D, Kowalski EH, et al. Epidermolysis bullosa acquisita: a comprehensive review. *Autoimmunity Rev.* 2019;18(8):786-795.
Lessey E, Li N, Dias L, et al. Complement and cutaneous autoimmune blistering diseases. *Immunol Res.* 2008;41:223-232.
McDonald HC, York NR, Pandya AG. Drug-induced linear IgA bullous dermatosis demonstrating the isomorphic phenomenon. *J Am Acad Dermatol.* 2010;62:897-898.
Melchionda V, Harman KE. Pemphigus vulgaris and pemphigus foliaceus: an overview of the clinical presentation, investigations and management. *Clin Exp Dermatol.* 2019;44:740-746.
Onodera H, Mihm MC Jr, Yoshida A, et al. Drug-induced linear IgA bullous dermatosis. *J Dermatol.* 2005;32:759-764.
Reunala T, Hervonen K, Salmi T. Dermatitis herpetiformis: an update on diagnosis and management. *Am J Clin Dermatol.* 2021;22:329-338.
Salameh H, Sarairah H, Rizwan M et al. Relapse of porphyria cutanea tarda after treatment with phlebotomy or 4-aminoquinoline antimalarials: a meta-analysis. *Brit J Dermatol.* 2018;179(6):1351-1357.
Sehgal VN, Srivastava G. Paraneoplastic pemphigus/paraneoplastic autoimmune multiorgan syndrome. *Int J Dermatol.* 2009;48: 162-169.
Shah A, Bhatt H. Cutanea tarda porphyria. *StatPearls.* 2022.
Shinkuma S, Nishie W, Shibaki A, et al. Cutaneous pemphigus vulgaris with skin features similar to the classic mucocutaneous type: a case report and review of the literature. *Clin Exp Dermatol.* 2008;33: 724-728.
Singal, AK. Porphyria cutanea tarda: recent update. *Mol Genet Metab.* 2109;128(3):271-281.
Stirling L, Kirsner RS. Evidence-based pemphigus treatment? *J Invest Dermatol.* 2010;130:1963.
Stozel U, Doss MO, Schuppan D. Clinical guide and update on porphyrias. *Gastroenterology.* 2019;157(2):365-384.
Svoboda SA, Huang S, Liu X, et al. Paraneoplastic pemphigus: revised diagnostic criteria based on literature analysis. *J Cutan Pathol.* 2021;48:1133-1138.
Templet JT, Welsh JP, Cusack CA. Childhood dermatitis herpetiformis: a case report and review of the literature. *Cutis.* 2007;80:473-476.
Woodley DT, Remington J, Chen M. Autoimmunity to type VII collagen: epidermolysis bullosa acquisita. *Clin Rev Allergy Immunol.* 2007;33: 78-84.
Zhu X, Zhang B. Paraneoplastic pemphigus. *J Dermatol.* 2007;34:503-511.

Section 6: Infectious Diseases

Adams BB. New strategies for the diagnosis, treatment, and prevention of herpes simplex in contact sports. *Curr Sports Med Rep.* 2004;3: 277-283.
Adams EN, Parnapy S, Bautista P. Herpes zoster and vaccination: a clinical review. *Am J Health Syst Pharm.* 2010;67:724-727.
Alfa M. The laboratory diagnosis of *Haemophilus ducreyi*. *Can J Infect Dis Med Microbiol.* 2005;16:31-34.
Anderson AL, Chaney E. Pubic lice *(Pthirus pubis)*: history, biology and treatment vs. knowledge and beliefs of US college students. *Int J Environ Res Public Health.* 2009;6:592-600.
Andina D, Belloni-Fortina A, Bodemer C, et al. Skin manifestations of COVID-19 in children: Part 1. *Clin Exp Dermatol.* 2021;46:444-450.
Andina D, Belloni-Fortina A, Bodemer C, et al. Skin manifestations of COVID-19 in children: Part 2. *Clin Exp Dermatol.* 2021;46:451-460.
Andina D, Belloni-Fortina A, Bodemer C, et al. Skin manifestations of COVID-19 in children: Part 3. *Clin Exp Dermatol.* 2021;46:462-472.
Andrews MD, Burns M. Common tinea infections in children. *Am Fam Physician.* 2008;77:1415-1420.
Ayyadurai S, Sebbane F, Raoult D, et al. Body lice, *Yersinia pestis orientalis*, and Black Death. *Emerg Infect Dis.* 2010;16:892-893.
Azar MM, Loyd JL, Relich RF. Current concepts in the epidemiology, diagnosis, and management of histoplasmosis syndromes. *Semin Respir Crit Care Med.* 2020;41:13-30.
Bachmeyer C, Buot G, Binet O, et al. Fixed cutaneous sporotrichosis: an unusual diagnosis in West Europe. *Clin Exp Dermatol.* 2006;31:479-481.
Baringer JR. Herpes simplex infections of the nervous system. *Neurol Clin.* 2008;26:657-674.
Bauer ME, Janowicz DM. Chancroid. In: Singh S, editor. *Diagnostics to Pathogenomics of Sexually Transmitted Infections.* Wiley; 2018.
Baughn RE, Musher DM. Secondary syphilitic lesions. *Clin Microbiol Rev.* 2005;18:205-216.
Bechah Y, Capo C, Mege JL, et al. Epidemic typhus. *Lancet Infect Dis.* 2008;8:417-426.
Biolcati G, Alabiso A. Creeping eruption of larva migrans—a case report in a beach volley athlete. *Int J Sports Med.* 1997;18:612-613.
Blackwell V, Vega-Lopez F. Cutaneous larva migrans: clinical features and management of 44 cases presenting in the returning traveller. *Br J Dermatol.* 2001;145:43-437.
Bonilla DL, Kabeya H, Henn J, et al. Bartonella quintana in body lice and head lice from homeless persons in San Francisco, California, USA. *Emerg Infect Dis.* 2009;15:912-915.
Bosis S, Mayer A, Esposito S. Meningococcal disease in childhood: epidemiology, clinical features and prevention. *J Prev Med Hyg.* 2015;56(3):E121-E124.
Bowman DD, Montgomery SP, Zajac AM, et al. Hookworms of dogs and cats as agents of cutaneous larva migrans. *Trends Parasitol.* 2010;26:162-167.
Bradsher RW, Chapman SW, Pappas PG. Blastomycosis. *Infect Dis Clin North Am.* 2003;17:21-40.
Bratton RL, Whiteside JW, Hovan MJ, et al. Diagnosis and treatment of Lyme disease. *Mayo Clin Proc.* 2008;83:566-571.
Brown M, Paulson C, Henry SL. Treatment for anogenital molluscum contagiosum. *Am Fam Physician.* 2009;80:864.
Burgess IF. Current treatments for pediculosis capitis. *Curr Opin Infect Dis.* 2009;22:131-136.
Carpenter JB, Feldman JS, Leyva WH, et al. Clinical and pathologic characteristics of disseminated cutaneous coccidioidomycosis. *J Am Acad Dermatol.* 2010;62:831-837.
Chen X, Anstey AV, Bugert JJ. Molluscum contagiosum virus infection. *Lancet Infect Dis.* 2013;13(10):877-888.
Clarridge JE 3rd, Zhang Q. Genotypic diversity of clinical *Actinomyces* species: phenotype, source, and disease correlation among genospecies. *J Clin Microbiol.* 2002;40:3442-3448.
Currie BJ, McCarthy JS. Permethrin and ivermectin for scabies. *N Eng J Med.* 2010;362:717-725.
Davies HD, Sakuls P, Keystone JS. Creeping eruption. A review of clinical presentation and management of 60 cases presenting to a tropical disease unit. *Arch Dermatol.* 1993;129:588-591.
Dean D, Bruno WJ, Wan R, et al. Predicting phenotype and emerging strains among *Chlamydia trachomatis* infections. *Emerg Infect Dis.* 2009;15:1385-1394.
Deps P, Lockwood DN. Leprosy presenting as immune reconstitution inflammatory syndrome: proposed definitions and classification. *Lepr Rev.* 2010;81:59-68.
Domantay-Apostol GP, Handog EB, Gabriel MT. Syphilis: the international challenge of the great imitator. *Dermatol Clin.* 2008;26:191-202.
Frankowski BL, Bocchini JA Jr. Head lice. *Pediatrics.* 2010;126: 392-403.
Gallo ES, Peboushek JF, Crowson AN. An exophytic nasal nodule. Coccidioidomycosis. *Arch Dermatol.* 2010;146:789-794.

Genovese G, Moltrasio C, Bertio E, et al. Skin manifestations associated with COVID-19: current knowledge and future perspectives. *Dermatology.* 2021;237:1-12.
Geria AN, Schwartz RA. Impetigo update: new challenges in the era of methicillin resistance. *Cutis.* 2010;85:65-70.
Ghaninejad H, Hasibi M, Moslehi H, et al. Primary cutaneous actinomycosis of the elbow with an exceptionally long incubation period. *Int J Dermatol.* 2008;47:304-305.
Gisondi P, Di Leo S, Bellinato F, et al. Time of onset of selected skin lesions associated with COVID-19: a systematic review. *Dermatol Ther.* 2021;11:695-705.
Gnat S, Lagowski D, Nowakiewicz A. Major challenges and perspectives in the diagnostics and treatment of dermatophyte infections. *J Appl Microbiol.* 2020;129:212-232.
Goulart LR, Goulart IM. Leprosy pathogenic background: a review and lessons from other mycobacterial diseases. *Arch Dermatol Res.* 2009;301:123-127.
Guo F, Cofie LE, Berenson AB. Cervical cancer incidence in young U.S. females after human papillomavirus vaccine introduction. *Am J Prevent Med.* 2018;55(2):197-204.
Gupta AK, Cooper EA. Update in antifungal therapy of dermatophytosis. *Mycopathologia.* 2008;166:353-367.
Hardman S, Stephenson I, Jenkins DR, et al. Disseminated *Sporothix schenckii* in a patient with AIDS. *J Infect.* 2005;51:e73-e77.
Harrison LH. Epidemiological profile of meningococcal disease in the United States. *Clin Infect Dis.* 2010;50(Suppl 2):S37-S44.
Hay RJ. Scabies and pyodermas—diagnosis and treatment. *Dermatol Ther.* 2009;22:466-474.
Hernández-Castro R, Pinto-Almazán R, Arenas R, et al. Epidemiology of clinical sporotrichosis in the Americas in the last ten years. *J Fungi.* 2022;8(6):588.
Heukelbach J, Wilcke T, Feldmeier H. Cutaneous larva migrans (creeping eruption) in an urban slum in Brazil. *Int J Dermatol.* 2004;43:511-515.
Hicks MI, Elston DM. Scabies. *Dermatol Ther.* 2009;22:279-292.
Hindy JR, Haddad SF, Kanj SS. New drugs for methicillin-resistant *Staphylococcus aureus* skin and soft tissue infections, *Curr Opin Infect Dis.* 2022;35(2):112-119.
Hochedez P, Caumes E. Hookworm-related cutaneous larva migrans. *J Travel Med.* 2007;14:326-333.
Hope-Rapp E, Anyfantakis V, Fouéré S, et al. Etiology of genital ulcer disease. A prospective study of 278 cases seen in an STD clinic in Paris. *Sex Transm Dis.* 2010;37:153-158.
Howell ER, Phillips CM. Cutaneous manifestations of *Staphylococcus aureus* disease. *Skinmed.* 2007;6:274-279.
Janowicz DM, Li W, Bauer ME. Host-pathogen interplay of *Haemophilus ducreyi. Curr Opin Infect Dis.* 2010;23:64-69.
Jones S, Kress D. Treatment of molluscum contagiosum and herpes simplex virus cutaneous infections. *Cutis.* 2007;79(Suppl 4):S11-S17.
Jouan Y, Grammatico-Guillon L, Espitalier F, et al. Long-term outcome of severe herpes simplex encephalitis: a population-based observational study. *Critical Care.* 2015;19(1):345.
Kakourou T, Uksal U. Guidelines for the management of tinea capitis in children. *Pediatr Dermatol.* 2010;27:226-228.
Kil EH, Heymann WR, Weinberg JM. Methicillin-resistant *Staphylococcus aureus*: an update for the dermatologist, part 1: epidemiology. *Cutis.* 2008;81:227-233.
Kil EH, Heymann WR, Weinberg JM. Methicillin-resistant *Staphylococcus aureus*: an update for the dermatologist, part 2: pathogenesis and cutaneous manifestations. *Cutis.* 2008;81:247-254.
Kim KS. Acute bacterial meningitis in infants and children. *Lancet Infect Dis.* 2010;10:32-42.
Könönen E, Wade WG. Actinomyces and related organisms in human infections. *Clin Microbiol Rev.* 2015;28(2):419-442.
Lamers MM, Haagmans BL. SARS-COV-2 pathogenesis. *Nat Rev Microbiol.* 2022;20:270-284.
Lautenschlager S. Cutaneous manifestations of syphilis: recognition and management. *Am J Clin Dermatol.* 2006;7:291-304.
Lee SJ, Kim H, Hong KJ, et al. Immune responses to varicella zoster virus and effective vaccines. *Korean Soc Microbiol.* 2021;51(3):103-111.
Lefèvre B, Poinsignon Y, Piau C. Chronic meningococcemia: a report of 26 cases and literature review. *Infection.* 2019;47:285-288.
Lübbe J. Secondary infections in patients with atopic dermatitis. *Am J Clin Dermatol.* 2003;4:641-654.
Martinez R. New trends in paracoccidioidomycosis. Epidemiology. *J Fungi.* 2017;3(1):1.
Marzano AV, Genovese G, Moltrasio C, et al. The clinical spectrum of COVID-19-associated cutaneous manifestations: an Italian multicenter study of 200 adult patients. *J Am Acad Dermatol.* 2021;84:1356-1363.
Mazi PB, Rauseo AM, Spec A. Blastomycosis. *Infect Dis Clin.* 2021;35(2):515.
McElhaney JE. Herpes zoster: a common disease that can have a devastating impact on patients' quality of life. *Expert Rev Vaccines.* 2010;9(Suppl 3):S27-S30.
McKinnell JA, Pappas PG. Blastomycosis: new insights into diagnosis, prevention, and treatment. *Clin Chest Med.* 2009;30:227-239.
Mele JA 3rd, Linder S, Capozzi A. Treatment of thromboembolic complications of fulminant meningococcal septic shock. *Ann Plast Surg.* 1997;38:283-290.
Mick G. Vaccination: a new option to reduce the burden of herpes zoster. *Expert Rev Vaccines.* 2010;9(Suppl 3):S31-S35.
Morar N, Ramdial PK, Naidoo DK, et al. Lues maligna. *Br J Dermatol.* 1999;140:1175-1177.
Mourad A, Perfect JR. Present and future therapy of cryptococcus infections. *J Fungi.* 2018;4(3):79.
Müllegger RR, Glatz M. Skin manifestations of Lyme borreliosis: diagnosis and management. *Am J Clin Dermatol.* 2008;9:355-368.
Murray TS, Shapiro ED. Lyme disease. *Clin Lab Med.* 2010;30:311-328.
Naka W, Masuda M, Konohana A, et al. Primary cutaneous cryptococcosis and *Cryptococcus neoformans* serotype D. *Clin Exp Dermatol.* 1995;20:221-225.
Newton HR, Lambiase MC. Disseminated cutaneous coccidioidomycosis masquerading as lupus pernio. *Cutis.* 2010;86:25-28.
Nordlund JJ. Cutaneous ectoparasites. *Dermatol Ther.* 2009;22:503-517.
Odell CA. Community-associated methicillin-resistant *Staphylococcus aureus* (CA-MRSA) skin infections. *Curr Opin Pediatr.* 2010;22:273-277.
Ohno S, Tanabe H, Kawasaki M, et al. Tinea corporis with acute inflammation caused by Trichophyton tonsurans. *J Dermatol.* 2008;35:590-593.
Panackal AA, Halpern EF, Watson AJ. Cutaneous fungal infections in the United States: analysis of the National Ambulatory Medical Care Survey (NAMCS) and National Hospital Ambulatory Medical Care Survey (NHAMCS), 1995–2004. *Int J Dermatol.* 2009;48:704-712.
Patel AR, Romanelli P, Roberts B, et al. Treatment of herpes simplex virus infection: rationale for occlusion. *Adv Skin Wound Care.* 2007;20:408-412.
Patel GA, Wiederkehr M, Schwartz RA. Tinea cruris in children. *Cutis.* 2009;84:133-137.
Patil D, Siddaramappa B, Manjunathswamy BS, et al. Primary cutaneous actinomycosis. *Int J Dermatol.* 2008;47:1271-1273.
Paul AY, Aldrich S, Scott RS, et al. Disseminated histoplasmosis in a patient with AIDS: case report and review of the literature. *Cutis.* 2007;80:309-312.
Peel TN, Bhatti D, De Boer JC, et al. Chronic cutaneous ulcers secondary to Haemophilus ducreyi infection. *Med J Aust.* 2010;192:348-350.
Perna A, Passiatore M, Massaro, et al. Skin manifestations in COVID-19 patients, state of the art. a systemic review. *Int J Dermatol.* 2021;60:547-553.
Pietras TA, Baum CL, Swick BL. Coexistent Kaposi sarcoma, cryptococcosis, and Mycobacterium avium intracellulare in a solitary cutaneous nodule in a patient with AIDS: report of a case and literature review. *J Am Acad Dermatol.* 2010;62:676-680.
Ramos-E-Silva M, Saraiva Ldo E. Paracoccidioidomycosis. *Dermatol Clin.* 2008;26:257-269.
Ramos-E-Silva M, Vasconcelos C, Carneiro S, et al. Sporotrichosis. *Dermatol Clin.* 2007;25:181-187.
Romano C, Castelli A, Laurini L, et al. Case report. Primary cutaneous histoplasmosis in an immunosuppressed patient. *Mycoses.* 2000;43:151-154.
Rosen T, Brown TJ. Cutaneous manifestations of sexually transmitted diseases. *Med Clin North Am.* 1998;82:1081-1104.
Rosen T, Hwong H. Pedal interdigital condylomata lata: a rare sign of secondary syphilis. *Sex Transm Dis.* 2001;28:184-186.
Rutman H. Ivermectin versus malathion for head lice. *N Engl J Med.* 2010;362:2426-2427.
Saberi A, Syed SA. Meningeal signs: Kernig's sign and Brudzinski's sign. *Hosp Physician.* 1999;24:23-24.
Saccente M, Woods GL. Clinical and laboratory update on blastomycosis. *Clin Microbiol Rev.* 2010;23:367-381.
Sanchezruiz WL, Nuzum DS, Kouzi SA. Oral ivermectin for the treatment of head lice infestation. *Am J Health-Sys Pharm.* 2018;75(13):937-943.
Scheurich D, Woeltje K. Skin and soft tissue infections due to CA-MRSA. *Mo Med.* 2009;106:274-276.
Schmid DS, Jumaan AO. Impact of varicella vaccine on varicella-zoster virus dynamics. *Clin Microbiol Rev.* 2010;23:202-217.
Schubach A, Barros MB, Wanke B. Epidemic sporotrichosis. *Curr Opin Infect Dis.* 2008;21:129-133.
Sehgal VN, Srivastava G. Chancroid: contemporary appraisal. *Int J Dermatol.* 2003;42:182-190.
Silverberg NB. Human papillomavirus infections in children. *Curr Opin Pediatr.* 2004;16:402-409.
Snoeck R. Papillomavirus and treatment. *Antiviral Res.* 2006;71:181-191.
Stanek G, Strle F. Lyme borreliosis-from tick bite to diagnosis and treatment. *FEMS Microbiol Rev.* 2018;42(3):233-258.
Sunderkötter C, Wohlrab J, Hamm H. Scabies: epidemiology, diagnosis, and treatment. *Deutsches Arzteblatt Int.* 2021;118(41):695-704.
Tan LK, Carlone GM, Borrow R. Advances in the development of vaccines against *Neisseria meningitidis. N Engl J Med.* 2010;362:1511-1520.
Thompson GR, Lewis JS, Nix DE, et al. Current concepts and future directions in the pharmacology and treatment of coccidioidomycosis. *Med Mycol.* 2019;57:S76-S84.
Thurnheer MC, Weber R, Toutous-Trellu L, et al. Occurrence, risk factors, diagnosis and treatment of syphilis in the prospective observational Swiss HIV Cohort Study. *AIDS.* 2010;24:1907-1916.
Tucker JD, Shah S, Jarell AD, et al. Lues maligna in early HIV infection: case report and review of the literature. *Sex Transm Dis.* 2009;36:512-514.
Tuddenham S, Hamill MM, Ghanem KG. Diagnosis and treatment of sexually transmitted infections: a review. *JAMA.* 2022;327(2):161-172.
Ulusoy S, Ozkan G, Bektaş D, et al. Ramsay Hunt syndrome in renal transplantation recipient: a case report. *Transplant Proc.* 2010;42:1986-1988.
Walsh DS, Portaels F, Meyers WM. Recent advances in leprosy and Buruli ulcer (Mycobacterium ulcerans infection). *Curr Opin Infect Dis.* 2010;23:445-455.
Watkins P. Identifying and treating plantar warts. *Nurs Stand.* 2006;20:50-54.
Williamson DA, Chen MY. Emerging and reemerging sexually transmitted infections. *N Engl J Med.* 2020;382:2023-2032.
Wolf R, Davidovici B. Treatment of scabies and pediculosis: facts and controversies. *Clin Dermatol.* 2010;28:511-518.
World Health Organization *Guidelines for the Diagnosis, Treatment and Prevention of Leprosy.* World Health Organization; 2018.
Worobec SM. Treatment of leprosy/Hansen's disease in the early 21st century. *Dermatol Ther.* 2009;22:518-537.

Section 7: Hair and Nail Diseases

Avram M, Rogers N. Contemporary hair transplantation. *Dermatol Surg.* 2009;35:1705-1719.
Basmanav FBU, Cau L, Tafazzoli A, et al. Mutations in three genes encoding proteins involved in hair shaft formation cause uncombable hair syndrome. *Am J Human Genetics.* 2016;99(6):1292-1304.
Baswan S, Kasting, GB, Li SK, et al. Understanding the formidable nail barrier: a review of the nail microstructure, composition and diseases. *Mycoses.* 2018;60(5):284-295.
Burk C, Hu S, Lee C, et al. Netherton syndrome and trichorrhexis invaginata—a novel diagnostic approach. *Pediatr Dermatol.* 2008;25:287-288.
Calderon P, Otberg N, Shapiro J. Uncombable hair syndrome. *J Am Acad Dermatol.* 2009;61:512-515.
Camacho FM, Randall VA, Proce VH, eds. *Hair and Its Disorders: Biology, Pathology, and Management.* London: Martin Dunitz Ltd.; 2000.
Cashman MW, Sloan SB. Nutrition and nail disease. *Clin Dermatol.* 2010;28:420-425.
Chamberlain SR, Odlaug BL, Boulougouris V, et al. Trichotillomania: neurobiology and treatment. *Neurosci Biobehav Rev.* 2009;33:831-842.
Cohen PR, Scher RK. Geriatric nail disorders: diagnosis and treatment. *J Am Acad Dermatol.* 1992;26:521-531.
Darwin E, Hirt PA, Fertig R, et al. Alopecia areata: review of epidemiology, clinical features, pathogenesis, and new treatment options. *Int J Trichology.* 2018;10(2):51-60.
DeBerker D. Childhood nail diseases. *Dermatol Clin.* 2006;24:355-363.
Duarte AF, Correia O, Barros AM, et al. Nail matrix melanoma in situ: conservative surgical management. *Dermatology.* 2010;220:173-175.
Duke DC, Keeley ML, Geffken GR, et al. Trichotillomania: a current review. *Clin Psychol Rev.* 2010;30:181-193.
Fabbrocini G, Cantelli M, Masarà A, et al. Female pattern hair loss: a clinical, pathophysiologic, and therapeutic review. *Int J Women's Dermatol.* 2018;4(4):203-211.
Harrison S, Bergfeld WF. Diseases of the hair and nails. *Med Clin North Am.* 2009;93:1195-1209.
Harrison S, Sinclair R. Telogen effluvium. *Clin Exp Dermatol.* 2002;27:389-395.
Heidelbaugh JJ, Lee H. Management of the ingrown toenail. *Am Fam Physician.* 2009;79:303-308.
Jadhav VM, Mahajan PM, Mhaske CB. Nail pitting and onycholysis. *Indian J Dermatol Venereol Leprol.* 2009;75:631-633.
Jaks V, Kasper M, Toftgård R. The hair follicle—a stem cell zoo. *Exp Cell Res.* 2010;316:1422-1428.
Kos L, Conlon J. An update on alopecia areata. *Curr Opin Pediatr.* 2009;21:475-480.
Lee JY. Severe 20-nail psoriasis successfully treated with low dose methotrexate. *Dermatol Online J.* 2009;15:8.
Mancini C, Van Ameringen M, Patterson B, et al. Trichotillomania in youth: a retrospective case series. *Depress Anxiety.* 2009;26:661-665.
Mirmirani P, Samimi SS, Mostow E. Pili torti: clinical findings, associated disorders, and new insights into mechanisms of hair twisting. *Cutis.* 2009;84:143-147.
Myung P, Andl T, Ito M. Defining the hair follicle stem cell (part I). *J Cutan Pathol.* 2009;36:1031-1034.
Myung P, Andl T, Ito M. Defining the hair follicle stem cell (part II). *J Cutan Pathol.* 2009;36:1134-1137.
Rathnayake D, Sinclair R. Male androgenetic alopecia. *Exp Opin Pharmacother.* 2010;11:1295-1304.
Rigopoulos D, Larios G, Gregoriou S, et al. Acute and chronic paronychia. *Am Fam Physician.* 2008;77:339-346.
Schweizer J. More than one gene involved in monilethrix: intracellular but also extracellular players. *J Invest Dermatol.* 2006;126:1216-1219.
Seavolt MB, Sarro RA, Levin K, et al. Mees' lines in a patient following acute arsenic intoxication. *Int J Dermatol.* 2002;41:399-401.
Stefanato CM. Histopathology of alopecia: a clinicopathological approach to diagnosis. *Histopathology.* 2010;56:24-38.
Trüeb RM. Chemotherapy-induced alopecia. *Semin Cutan Med Surg.* 2009;28:11-14.

Welsh O, Vera-Cabrera L, Welsh E. Onychomycosis. *Clin Dermatol.* 2010;28:151-159.

Wosicka H, Cal K. Targeting to the hair follicles: current status and potential. *J Dermatol Sci.* 2010;57:83-89.

Section 8: Nutritional and Metabolic Diseases

Adams PC, Barton JC. How I treat hemochromatosis. *Blood.* 2010; 116:317-325.

Akikusa JD, Garrick D, Nash MC. Scurvy: forgotten but not gone. *J Paediatr Child Health.* 2003;39:75-77.

Balotti RF Jr, Malone RJ, Schanzer RJ. Warfarin necrosis. *Am J Phys Med Rehabil.* 2009;88:263.

Betrosian AP, Thireos E, Toutouzas K, et al. Occidental beriberi and sudden death. *Am J Med Sci.* 2004;327:250-252.

Beyzaei Z, Geramizadeh B. Molecular diagnosis of glycogen storage disease type I: a review. *EXCLI J.* 2019;30(18):30-46.

Cancado RD, Alvarenga AM, Santos P. HFE hemochromatosis: an overview about therapeutic recommendations, *Hematol Trans Cell Ther.* 2022;44(1):95-99.

Cederbaum S. Phenylketonuria: an update. *Curr Opin Pediatr.* 2002; 14:702-706.

Chalmers EA. Neonatal coagulation problems. *Arch Dis Child Fetal Neonatal Ed.* 2004;89:F475-F478.

Chaudhry SI, Newell EL, Lewis RR, et al. Scurvy: a forgotten disease. *Clin Exp Dermatol.* 2005;30:735-736.

Cope-Yokoyama S, Finegold MJ, Sturniolo GC, et al. Wilson disease: histopathological correlations with treatment on follow-up liver biopsies. *World J Gastroenterol.* 2010;16:1487-1494.

Delgado-Sanchez L, Godkar D, Niranjan S. Pellagra: rekindling of an old flame. *Am J Ther.* 2008;15:173-175.

Dolberg OJ, Elis A, Lishner M. Scurvy in the 21st century. *Isr Med Assoc J.* 2010;12:183-184.

Englander L, Friedman A. Iron overload and cutaneous disease: an emphasis on clinicopathological correlations. *J Drugs Dermatol.* 2010;9:719-722.

Feillet F, van Spronsen FJ, MacDonald A, et al. Challenges and pitfalls in the management of phenylketonuria. *Pediatrics.* 2010;126:333-341.

Inayatullah S, Phadke G, Vilenski L, et al. Warfarin-induced skin necrosis. *South Med J.* 2010;103:74-75.

Lau H, Massasso D, Joshua F. Skin, muscle and joint disease from the 17th century: scurvy. *Int J Rheum Dis.* 2009;12:361-365.

Levy PA. An overview of newborn screening. *J Dev Behav Pediatr.* 2010;31:622-631.

Lichter-Konecki U, Vockley J. Phenylketonuria: current treatments and future developments. *Drugs.* 2019;79:495-500.

Lind, J. *A Treatise of the Scurvy. In Three Parts.* Edinburgh: Sands Murray and Cochran; 1753.

Mulligan C, Bronstein JM. Wilson disease an overview and approach to management. *Neurol Clin.* 2020;38:417-432.

Nazarian RM, Van Cott EM, Zembowicz A, et al. Warfarin-induced skin necrosis. *J Am Acad Dermatol.* 2009;61:325-332.

Nguyen RT, Cowley DM, Muir JB. Scurvy: a cutaneous clinical diagnosis. *Australas J Dermatol.* 2003;44:48-51.

Patterson MC, Garver WS, Giugliani R, et al. Long-term survival outcomes of patients with Niemann-Pick disease type C receiving miglustat treatment: a large retrospective observational study. *J Inherit Metab Dis.* 2020;43(5):1060-1069.

Popovich D, McAlhany A, Adewumi AO, et al. Scurvy: forgotten but definitely not gone. *J Pediatr Health Care.* 2009;23:405-415.

Prabhu D, Dawe RS, Mponda, K. Pellagra a review exploring causes and mechanisms, including isoniazid-induced pellagra. *Photodermatol Photoimmunol Photomed.* 2021;37:99-104.

Tanumihardjo SA. Assessing vitamin A status: past, present and future. *J Nutr.* 2004;134:290s-293s.

Towbin A, Inge TH, Garcia VF, et al. Beriberi after gastric bypass surgery in adolescence. *J Pediatr.* 2004;145:263-267.

Underwood BA. Vitamin A deficiency disorders: international efforts to control a preventable "pox." *J Nutr.* 2004;134:231s-236s.

Vanier MT, Millat G. Niemann-Pick disease type C. *Clin Genet.* 2003;64:269-281.

Vanier MT. Prenatal diagnosis of Niemann-Pick diseases types A, B, and C. *Prenat Diagn.* 2002;22:630-632.

van Spronsen FJ. Phenylketonuria: a 21st century perspective. *Nat Rev Endocrinol.* 2010;6:509-514.

Walshe JM. Monitoring copper in Wilson's disease. *Adv Clin Chem.* 2010;50:151-163.

Zacharski LR. Hemochromatosis, iron toxicity and disease. *J Intern Med.* 2010;268:246-248.

Section 9: Genodermatoses and Syndromes

Antal Z, Zhou P. Addison disease. *Pediatr Rev.* 2009;30:491-493.

Barbagallo JS, Kolodzieh MS, Silverberg NB, et al. Neurocutaneous disorders. *Dermatol Clin.* 2002;20:547-560.

Barbot M, Zilio M, Scaroni C, et al. Cushing's syndrome: overview of clinical presentation, diagnostic tools and complications. *Best Pract Res Clin Endocrinol Metab.* 2020;34(2):1-23.

Bleicken B, Hahner S, Ventz M, et al. Delayed diagnosis of adrenal insufficiency is common: a cross-sectional study in 216 patients. *Am J Med Sci.* 2010;339:525-531.

Bouys, L, Bertherat J. Carney complex: clinical and genetic update 20 years after the identification of the CNC1 (PRKAR1A) gene. *Eur J Endocrinol.* 2021;184(3):R99-R109.

Callewaert B, Malfait F, Loeys B, et al. Ehlers-Danlos syndromes and Marfan syndrome. *Best Pract Res Clin Rheumatol.* 2008;22:165-189.

Casaletto JJ. Is salt, vitamin, or endocrinopathy causing this encephalopathy? A review of endocrine and metabolic causes of altered level of consciousness. *Emerg Med Clin North Am.* 2010;28:633-662.

Chakera AJ, Vaidya B. Addison disease in adults: diagnosis and management. *Am J Med.* 2010;123:409-413.

Choi J, An S, Lim SY, et al. Current concepts of neurofibromatosis type 1: pathophysiology and treatment. *Arch Craniofac Surg.* 2022;23(1):6-16.

Feldman DS, Jordan C, Fonseca L. Orthopaedic manifestations of neurofibromatosis type 1. *J Am Acad Orthop Surg.* 2010;18:346-357.

Ferner RE. The neurofibromatoses. *Pract Neurol.* 2010;10:82-93.

Figueroa A, Correnti M, Avila M, et al. Keratocystic odontogenic tumor associated with nevoid basal cell carcinoma syndrome: similar behavior to sporadic type? *Otolaryngol Head Neck Surg.* 2010;142:179-183.

Fotiou D, Dimopoulos MA, Kastritis E. Systemic AL amyloidosis: current approaches to diagnosis and management. *Hemasphere.* 2020;4(4):e454.

García de Marcos JA, Dean-Ferrer A, Arroyo Rodríguez S, et al. Basal cell nevus syndrome: clinical and genetic diagnosis. *Oral Maxillofac Surg.* 2009;13:225-230.

Gawthrop F, Mould R, Sperritt A, et al. Ehlers-Danlos syndrome. *Br Med J.* 2007;335:448-450.

Goldberg LH, Firoz BF, Weiss GJ, et al. Basal cell nevus syndrome: a brave new world. *Arch Dermatol.* 2010;146:17-19.

Horvath A, Bertherat J, Groussin L, et al. Mutations and polymorphisms in the gene encoding regulatory subunit type 1-alpha of protein kinase A (PRKAR1A): an update. *Hum Mutat.* 2010;31:369-379.

Isaacs H. Perinatal (fetal and neonatal) tuberous sclerosis: a review. *Am J Perinatol.* 2009;26:755-760.

Jett K, Friedman JM. Clinical and genetic aspects of neurofibromatosis 1. *Genet Med.* 2010;12:1-11.

Keane MG, Pyeritz RE. Medical management of Marfan syndrome. *Circulation.* 2008;117:2802-2813.

Luo C, Ye W-R, Shi W, et al. Perfect match: mTOR inhibitors and tuberous sclerosis complex. *Orphanet J Rare Dis.* 2022;17:106.

Malfait F, Francomano C, Byers P, et al. The 2017 international classification of the Ehlers-Danlos syndromes. *AM J Med Genet (Semin Medi Genet).* 2017;175C:8-26.

Mann JA, Siegel DH. Common genodermatoses: what the pediatrician needs to know. *Pediatr Ann.* 2009;38:91-98.

Oldfeld EH. Cushing disease. *J Neurosurg.* 2003;98:948-951.

Orlova KA, Crino PB. The tuberous sclerosis complex. *Ann N Y Acad Sci.* 2010;1184:87-105.

Pitak-Arnnop P, Chaine A, Oprean N, et al. Management of odontogenic keratocysts of the jaws: a ten-year experience with 120 consecutive lesions. *J Craniomaxillofac Surg.* 2010;38:358-364.

Pursnani AK, Levy NK, Benito M, et al. Carney's complex. *J Am Coll Cardiol.* 2010;55:1395.

Rabin KR, Whitlock JA. Malignancy in children with trisomy 21. *Oncologist.* 2009;14:164-173.

Santos-Briz A, Cañueto J, Antúnez P, et al. Primary cutaneous localized amyloid elastosis. *Am J Dermatopathol.* 2010;32:86-90.

Staser K, Yang FC, Clapp DW. Mast cells and the neurofibroma microenvironment. *Blood.* 2010;116:157-164.

Storr HL, Chan LF, Grossman AB, et al. Paediatric Cushing's syndrome: epidemiology, investigation and therapeutic advances. *Trends Endocrinol Metab.* 2007;18:167-174.

Valin N, De Castro N, Garrait V, et al. Iatrogenic Cushing's syndrome in HIV-infected patients receiving ritonavir and inhaled fluticasone: description of 4 new cases and review of the literature. *J Int Assoc Physicians AIDS Care.* 2009;8:113-121.

Vandersteen A, Turnbull J, Jan W, et al. Cutaneous signs are important in the diagnosis of the rare neoplasia syndrome Carney complex. *Eur J Pediatr.* 2009;168:1401-1404.

Williams A, Davies S, Stuart AG, et al. Medical management of Marfan syndrome: a time for change. *Heart.* 2008;94:414-421.

Wiseman FK, Alford KA, Tybulewicz VL, et al. Down syndrome—recent progress and future prospects. *Hum Mol Genet.* 2009;18:R75-R83.

Zhang L, Smyrk TC, Young WF, et al. Gastric stromal tumors in Carney triad are different clinically, pathologically, and behaviorally from sporadic gastric gastrointestinal stromal tumors: findings in 104 cases. *Am J Surg Pathol.* 2010;34:53-64.

INDEX

E

F

G

H

T

U

V

W

X

Y

Z